American Red Cross

Nurse Assistant Training

This textbook was developed and produced through the combined efforts of American Red Cross Chapter staff, subject matter experts in the field, American Red Cross national headquarters and StayWell. Without the commitment to excellence of both employees and volunteers, this textbook could not have been created.

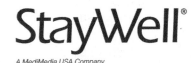

StayWell®

A MediMedia USA Company

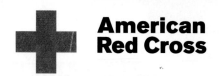

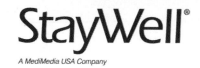

A MediMedia USA Company

Content reflects the *American Red Cross 2005 Guidelines for Emergency Care and Education* and the *2005 Guidelines for First Aid.*

This participant's textbook is an integral part of the American Red Cross Nurse Assistant Training Program. By itself, this book does not constitute comprehensive American Red Cross certified training for nurse assistants. Please contact your Red Cross unit for further information on this program.

These materials contain training and information on infection control practices for use in those settings and situations most commonly encountered by nurse assistants. Because regulations influencing the infection control procedures outlined in this book change frequently due to periodic revisions of standards and guidelines of the Centers for Disease Control (CDC) and Occupational Safety and Health Administration (OSHA) in the United States *and* because laws and procedures may be periodically redefined, it is the reader's responsibility to stay current with information such as infection control by attending inservice courses offered by employers or through other sources.

Printed in the United States of America
Printed by Banta Book Group

StayWell
780 Township Line Rd.
Yardley, PA 19067

Library of Congress Cataloging-in-Publication Data
Nurse assistant training / American Red Cross. — [2nd ed.]
    p. ; cm.
  Includes bibliographical references and index.
  ISBN 978-1-58480-414-7
 1. Nurses aides—Programmed instruction.   I. American Red Cross.
  [DNLM: 1. Nursing Care—methods—Problems and Exercises. 2. Nurses'
Aides—education—Problems and Exercises. 3. Professional
Competence—Problems and Exercises. WY 18.2 N97362 2008]

RT84.N867 2008
610.7306'98—dc22

                                        2008029260

ISBN-13: 978-1-58480-414-7

        11 / 9 8 7 6

How far you go in life depends on your being tender with the young,

compassionate with the aged, sympathetic with the striving, and

tolerant of the weak and strong—because someday in life you will

have been all of these.

– George Washington Carver

Acknowledgments

This manual is dedicated to all the individuals who care deeply about the quality of care they and their loved ones will receive within the long-term care system. And the thousands of employees and volunteers of the American Red Cross who contribute their time and talent to supporting and teaching life-saving skills worldwide.

We have endeavored to improve and polish this manual and course, which reflects the *American Red Cross 2005 Guidelines for Emergency Care and Education and the 2005 Guidelines for First Aid.* Many individuals shared in the development and revision process in various supportive, technical and creative ways. Both editions could not have been developed without the dedication and support of employees and volunteers.

The American National Red Cross Team for this text and the previous edition included:

Pat Bonifer
Director
Research and Product Development

Emilie Sparks Parker
Project Manager
Research and Product Development

John Beales
Manager
Business Planning

Jennifer Deibert
Project Manager
Research and Product Development

Jean Erdtmann, RN
Director
Program Management and Field Support

Kelly Fischbein
Associate, Evaluation
Research and Product Development

Don Lauritzen
Senior Associate
Operations

Nancy McKelvey, RN
Chief Nurse/Healthcare Partnerships Lead

Adreania McMillian
Senior Associate, Technical Development
Research and Product Development

Greta Petrilla
Manager
Communication and Marketing

John Thompson
Senior Associate
Program Administration and Support

Betty J. Williams Butler
Administrative Assistant
Research and Product Development

Rhadamés Avila
Administration Associate
Research and Product Development

Guidance and support was provided by the following individuals:

Scott Connor
Vice President
Preparedness and Health and Safety Services

Don Vardell
National Chair
Preparedness and Health and Safety Services

Deborah Carman, RN, MNSc
Executive Advisor
Preparedness and Health and Safety Services

The StayWell team for this edition included:

Nancy Monahan
Senior Vice President

Paula Batt
Executive Director
Sales and Business Development

Reed Klanderud
Executive Director, Marketing

Ellen Beal
Director, Editorial

Mary Ellen Curry
Director, Publication Production

Shannon Bates
Managing Editor

Stephanie Weidel
Senior Production Editor

Carolyn Lemanski
Business Development National Sales

Pam Billings
Marketing Manager

The following members of the American Red Cross Advisory Council on First Aid, Aquatics, Safety and Preparedness (ACFASP) also provided guidance and review:

David Markenson, MD, FAAP, EMT-P
Chair, American Red Cross Advisory Council on
First Aid, Aquatics, Safety and Preparedness
Chief, Pediatric Emergency Medicine
Maria Fareri Children's Hospital
Westchester Medical Center
Valhalla, NY

Richard Ellis, BSOE, NREMT-P
Chief Master Sergeant
United States Air Force
Warner Robins, GA

Jeffrey H. Fox, PhD
Psychologist, Private Practice
Schenectady, NY

Janice Taylor MNS, GNP, RN
Clinical Instructor
UAMS College of Nursing
Bigelow, AR

The American Red Cross thanks the following individuals for their reviews of this text and the previous edition:

Anika Bailey, RN, MSN
Health Care Training Program Manager
American Red Cross of Southeastern Michigan
Detroit, MI

Margaret Bercaw, RN, BS
American Red Cross of Greater Los Angeles
Los Angeles, CA

Susan Chase
Director, Health and Safety Services
Tampa Bay Chapter
Tampa Bay, FL

Leslie Chmielewski, RN, BSN
Home Care Supervisor
Henry Ford Health Systems
Detroit, MI

Renay Clark, RN, BSN
Manager, Employment Training
Greater Cleveland Chapter
Cleveland, OH

Karen Cook, LPN
Tampa Bay Chapter
Tampa Bay, FL

Marnie Dodson, BSN, RN
Senior Associate, Nursing Development
American Red Cross National Headquarters
Washington, DC

Gail Esterson, RN, BSN
Clinical Instructor
Central Maryland Chapter
Baltimore, MD

Pearlie Faulkner, RN
Home Care Nurse
Henry Ford Health Systems
Detroit, MI

Fay Flowers, RN, BS, MEd
Southeastern Michigan Chapter
Detroit, MI

Genevieve Gipson, RN, MEd, RNC
National Network of Career Nursing Assistants
Career Nurse Assistants Programs, Inc.
Norton, OH

Peggy Ann Graf, RN, BSN
Home Care Nurse
Henry Ford Health Systems
Detroit, MI

Constance Grimaldi-Schwartzman, RN, BSN, MPH
Instructor Trainer
American Red Cross of Greater Los Angeles
Los Angeles, CA

Demetria Gross, RN
Southeastern Michigan Chapter
Detroit, MI

Martha Gross, RN, BSN, MA
Supervisor, Nursing Programs
Central Maryland Chapter
Baltimore, MD

Charles James
American Red Cross of Greater Los Angeles
Los Angeles, CA

Peggy Kirk, RN
Nurse Assistant Training Program Administrator
Tampa Bay Chapter
Tampa Bay, FL

Judith Kurtz, RN
Instructor
Central Maryland Chapter
Baltimore, MD

Patricia LaBrie, RN, CMH, CAI
Director of Nurses
American Red Cross of Greater Los Angeles
Los Angeles, CA

Rhonda Lee, LPN
Home Care Nurse
Henry Ford Health Systems
Detroit, MI

Shirley Lewis, RN, BSN
Nurse Assistant Training Instructor
Greater Cleveland Chapter
Cleveland, OH

Lydia Marien, MS, ARNP, BC, FNP
Gopper/Trinity Family Care
Kansas City, KS

Marianne Mastrangelo, BSN, RN
Director Health Care Training
American Red Cross of Massachusetts Bay
Cambridge, MA

Virginia Mateo, RNC, EMT
Instructor Trainer
American Red Cross of Greater Los Angeles
Los Angeles, CA

Edith J. McCall, RN, BSN, MBA
Senior Manager
Southeastern Pennsylvania Chapter
Philadelphia, PA

Norma Olsen, RN, CSA
Health Care and Public Safety Programs Manager
American Red Cross of the Twin Cities Area
Minneapolis, MN

John Pacheco, MA
American Red Cross of Greater Los Angeles
Los Angeles, CA

Joyce Russell, RN, BSN
Southeastern Michigan Chapter
Detroit, MI

Linda Schulman, RNC
Nursing Supervisor, Program Coordinator
Greater Cleveland Chapter
Cleveland, OH

Carole Staley Collins, PhD, RN
Nursing Instructor
Annapolis, MD

Lisa Straight, RN
American Red Cross of the Twin Cities Area
Minneapolis, MN

Angie Turner, RN, BSN
San Gabriel Valley Chapter
Pasadena, CA

Althea Zanecosky, MS, RD, LDN
Past Spokesperson, American Diatetic Association
Philadelphia, PA

The American Red Cross gives special thanks to the following:

Patrice Acosta and Glenda Nelson, Beverly Healthcare Corporation, Fort Smith, AK; Deborah Gale, Consultant, San Mateo, CA; Debra Kania, RN, California Association of Health Facilities, Sacramento, CA; Allison Ascher Webber, ESL Instructor, Arriba Juntos; Donna Schwan, BS, MEd; Larissa Barclay, RN, MSN and Lindsay Miller, MPA, Southeastern Michigan Chapter of the American Red Cross, Detroit, MI; Dana T. Bass, RN, DSD, Consultant, Sacramento, CA; East San Gabriel Valley Regional Occupational Program and Technical Center, West Covina, CA; Ginger Fallesen, RN, and Marcia Easterling, Job Developer, Los Angeles County Office of Education, Regional Occupational Program, Downey, CA; Edward Hector, Mathematics Professor, Los Angeles Southwest College; Mary P. Cadogan, RN, PhD, CGNP Associate Adjunct Professor, UCLA School of Nursing; and Linda Wendling, MA, MFA.

The American Red Cross thanks the following organizations for their helpful staff's time and the use of their facilities.

Gladys Spellman Specialty Hospital & Nursing Center
Cheverly, MD

Beverly Health and Rehabilitation Services Inc.
Costa Mesa, CA

Ramona Care Center
El Monte, CA

The American Red Cross and StayWell thank Rick Brady for his contributions to this project.

Table of Contents

List of Nurse Assistant Skills

Introduction

Welcome to the *American Red Cross Nurse Assistant Training Textbook.* Whether you are training to become a certified nurse assistant or a caregiver for a friend or family member at home, this book will be an invaluable resource for you. The authors of this book and accompanying materials believe that caregiving is an art, applied creatively and compassionately, using carefully established principles of care.

THE NURSE ASSISTANT TRAINING PROGRAM

Nurse Assistant Training continues the focus on providing concerned, individualized care begun in the American Red Cross Nurse Assistant Training program (NATP) of 1989. The Nurse Assistant Training program consists of this textbook and the materials that supplement it. The program meets the federal requirements of the Omnibus Reconciliation Act (OBRA) of 1987 for training nurse assistants and updates the *Foundations for Caregiving Textbook*, endorsed by the National League for Nursing. It adds special information for life skills training, conflict resolution skills and effective interview techniques, more coverage of medical terminology, as well as supplemental math for nurse assistants, to be used as needed. Both the textbook and instructor's manual also include a stand-alone module for providing care as a nurse assistant in the home. The 2007 revision includes 160 new photos. The skill sheets have been enhanced with color and photographic icons for preparations, precautions and completion steps.

If you use this book as part of an American Red Cross course preparing you to become a certified nurse assistant, you gain these added benefits: being taught by an American Red Cross–trained instructor; viewing the skills, demonstrations on DVD or Video; using the skill sheets in the textbook, which describe step by step how to perform all essential skills; and being awarded an American Red Cross Nurse Assistant pin and certificate on successful completion of the course.

SIX PRINCIPLES OF CARE

Focusing on concerned, individualized caregiving, this program continues to adhere to the six principles of care unique to the American Red Cross Nurse Assistant Training program: safety, privacy, dignity, communication, independence and infection control.

PATTERNS OF THE BOOK

The *Nurse Assistant Training Textbook* is fun and easy to use. Each chapter begins with a list of goals, a relevant scenario and a Key Terms box and ends with Information Review questions and Questions to Ask Yourself. In between, the chapters include photos, illustrations, boxes, skill sheets and tables—all of which make learning more interesting.

GOALS

The goals listed at the beginning of each chapter provide a road map for the chapter; they tell you which ideas are most important to learn. As you complete each chapter, reread the goals to see whether you grasped the key information.

SCENARIOS

Following the list of goals in each chapter is a scenario depicting an event that involves a person who is receiving care or a person who is providing care. The characters that appear in the scenarios are purely fictional and represent no persons who are alive or who have lived; however, they *do* represent the human aspects of providing and receiving care: health problems, moods, behavior quirks and opinions. They also demonstrate the importance of providing care in a way that makes the person feel important, special and respected. Characters and scenarios also appear within the chapters and challenge you to be a compassionate caregiver.

INCLUSION

The people served by nurse assistants are, of course, both men and women. Rather than say "he or she" every time, this book switches back and forth when discussing care tactics, sometimes using "he" and sometimes "she."

KEY TERMS

As you read the *Nurse Assistant Training Textbook*, you will learn many new words; key words are **boldfaced** in the text. As a learning and reference aid, each boldfaced term in the text also appears in a Key Terms box at the beginning of each chapter along with its pronunciation, if necessary, and its meaning.

Look at the way words in the Key Terms box are divided into syllables. When saying a word out loud, place the greatest stress on the capitalized part of the word. Note how small, familiar words often are used in the pronunciations and how each word is spelled to represent the correct way it should sound. Every vowel has several sounds, as demonstrated in the chart of vowel sounds in this Introduction. For quick reference, a Word Element Usage guide also appears at the end of this book. Refer to this chart often as you learn to pronounce new words.

FIGURES

Figures may be either illustrations, depicting the characters in the scenarios, or photographs. Each figure is positioned on a page near its reference in the text. A description of the figure provides additional information to support the text.

SKILL SHEETS

Included at the end of appropriate chapters are the skill sheets enhanced with color and icons that will guide you step by step to perform skills you must learn to be a nurse assistant. Most skills are presented in the same brief, easy-to-follow format.

Every skill begins with **Precautions**. This section provides you with a list of things you should think about before you start the skill. Pre-cautions are often based on the principle of safety. The icon for precautions is handwashing because handwashing is a safeguard against disease.

In most skills, a section called **Preparation** follows the precautions. Preparation standards are set up in a shortened form, which will be described later in this section. They are concerned mainly with practicing infection control, providing privacy, promoting dignity and independence and communicating. The icon for preparations is putting on disposable gloves because gathering supplies such as disposable gloves and putting them on is an important preparation step for many nursing skills.

The **Procedure** section describes the steps you take that are specific to a particular skill. You will notice two small boxes inside each of the buttons and beside each step of the procedure. These are called check-off boxes and will be used by your instructor. When you believe you can perform the skill without coaching, you will demonstrate the skill for your instructor. The instructor will then place a check in the first box as you do each step. Should you have difficulty and need to demonstrate the skill another time; the instructor will check the second box.

The last section of each skill contains **Completion** standards, which are concerned mainly with leaving the person safe and comfortable. You will notice that the layout of the preparation and completion sections is similar. The icon for completion steps is a call signal because leaving the call signal in an easy-to-reach location is often the last completion step.

In some cases, an Additional Information section provides you with a list of things you need to think about as you perform a skill.

INFORMATION REVIEW

The Information Review questions, when answered correctly, provide a summary of the chapter; and an answer key at the back of the book provides the list of correct answers for each chapter.

QUESTIONS TO ASK YOURSELF

The Questions to Ask Yourself sections pose real-life situations that encourage you to apply your knowledge in decision making. These questions may have several correct answers. They are issues to think about and to discuss with your classmates and your instructor.

APPENDICES

Appendix A, "Medical Terminology and Supplemental Activities," provides additional activities that will help you to develop skills needed to learn the special language used by caregivers.

Appendix B, "Body Basics," provides brief descriptions and illustrations about organs and systems in the human body.

Appendix C, "Home Health Care," offers guidelines for quality caregiving in a private home setting.

Appendix D, "Math Applications," provides supplemental math skills frequently needed and used by nurse assistants; these will be used as needed.

Appendix E, "Taking a Temperature with a Glass Thermometer," provides additional optional information which is needed by several States for their Nurse Assistant Training certifications.

VOWEL SOUNDS CHART

For the sound of …	As in …	We use …	As in …
short a	apple	ah	**adaptation** (ah-dap-TAY-shun)
short a	attend	uh	**assertive** (uh-SER-tiv)
long a	stable	ay	**patient** (PAY-shent)
short e	enter	e	**gender** (JEN-der)
short e	estate	uh	**eliminate** (uh-LIM-uh-nate)
long e	east	ee	**dyspnea** (disp-NEE-uh)
short i	liver	i	**clinic** (KLIN-ik)
short i	chemical	uh	**cuticles** (KYU-tuh-kuhls)
long i	ivy	eye	**IV** (eye-VEE)
long i	ivy	i	**dehydrated** (dee-HI-dray-ted)
long i	ivy	y	**miter** (MY-ter)
short o	obvious	o	**obstetric** (ob-STET-rik)
short o	oven	uh	**suffocate** (SUF-uh-kate)
long o	only	oe	**mobility** (moe-BIL-uh-tee)
long o	only	oh	**obesity** (oh-BEE-suh-tee)
short u	under	u	**custom** (KUS-tum)
long u	dune	ew	**nutrient** (NEW-tre-ent)
long u	human	you	**regulation** (reg-you-LAY-shun)

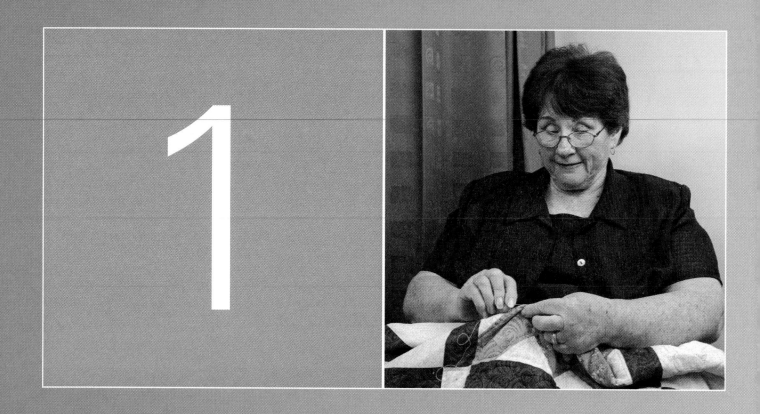

1

The Art of Caregiving

GOALS

After reading this chapter, you will have the information needed to:

Discuss why caregiving is an art.

Identify three health care settings where you may work.

Describe two types of specialized hospitals.

Describe three things that a nurse assistant may do in a hospital setting.

Describe the type of resident that may be in a nursing home.

Describe three things that a home health aide may do when providing care.

Describe ways in which nurse assistants are similar in all the health care settings.

You walk into Mrs. Agnes Ryan's room to take her for one of her three daily walks. Mrs. Ryan says she isn't ready to go because she is working on her quilt and wants to finish one more section. You remind her that her walk is important to keep her strong, and then you ask her how long it will take to finish the section of quilting. She says it will take about 10 minutes, so you mentally adjust your schedule and decide to change the bed of Mrs. Ryan's roommate, Mrs. Louise Wang, who is at physical therapy.

As you change the bed, you marvel at how beautifully Mrs. Ryan sews. You ask her how long she has been quilting, and she begins to tell you how her grandmother made quilts. "When my older sister made our dresses," Mrs. Ryan remembers, "she would cut

KEY TERMS

acute illness: An illness that begins suddenly.

AIDS: an abbreviation for acquired immunodeficiency syndrome. AIDS is caused by the human immunodeficiency virus (HIV), which results in a breakdown of the body's defense systems.

art: a skill attained by study, practice or observation.

chronic illness: (KRAHN-ik) a long-lasting condition or illness that may not subside or that may occur again.

client: (KLY-ent) a person who receives health care at home.

general hospital: a facility that provides care for people of all ages and with almost any type of illness or injury.

Health Insurance Portability and Accountability Act (HIPAA): The Health Insurance Portability and Accountability Act (HIPAA) includes rules covering administrative simplification, including making health care delivery more efficient. It also provided standardization of electronic transmittal of billing and claims information. A key part of the act also increased and standardized confidentiality and security of health data. HIPAA privacy regulations require that access to patient info be limited to only those authorized, and that only the information necessary for a task be available. And finally that personal health information must be protected and kept confidential.

home health aide: a nurse assistant with additional training who works in home health care.

home health care: health care provided in private homes to people who do not need to stay in hospitals or nursing homes.

home health care agency: A health organization that employs home health aides and others who provide health care and other services to people in their homes.

hospice: (HOS-pis) a program of medical and emotional care and support for people who are dying, as well as for their families.

hospital clinic: a hospital department that provides care to patients who do not need to stay overnight.

inpatient: a patient who must stay overnight in a hospital.

Medicaid: a state-administered federal program that provides health coverage for persons with very low incomes.

Medicare: a federal health insurance program for persons over age 65 or persons of any age who are disabled or have permanent kidney failure.

monitor: (MON-e-ter) to check regularly for the quality of a person's physical or emotional condition.

nausea: discomfort in throat or chest that often precedes vomiting.

orthopedic: (or-tho-PEE-dik) a type of medicine or care provided for people who have problems with their bones or joints.

outpatient: a patient who receives care in a hospital but does not need to stay overnight.

patient: a person who receives health care in a hospital or an outpatient facility.

personal care assistant: assists elderly or disabled adults with daily living activities at the person's home or in a daytime non-residential facility.

referral process: (re-FER-uhl) a set of procedures that allows one member of the health care system to recommend to other members that a person needs their kind of specialized care.

rehabilitation: (re-huh-bil-e-TAY-shun) the process of regaining physical and emotional health.

resident: (REZ-e-dent) a person who receives health care in a nursing home or long-term facility.

specialized hospital: a facility that provides care for people with only certain types of diseases or illnesses.

subacute care: care provided to residents who are stable and not acutely ill. Usually requires special services such as rehabilitation, ventilator care, wound treatments; usually requires a higher skill-level staff than in a traditional nursing facility.

terminal illness: (TER-muh-nul) a serious illness or condition that a person is not expected to survive.

therapeutic: healing, beneficial.

walk-in clinic: a hospital department that provides care for patients without requiring appointments.

out the pattern and then give the left-over pieces of fabric to my grand-mother, who was so happy to receive these scraps of cloth. Bags of gold would not have made her happier. She loved making quilts.

"Grandmother taught me to cut the fabric into different shapes, sort them by color and shape, and stack them neatly on the table. Then we began to sew them together, one stitch at a time. The tiny pieces took on new shapes, sizes and arrangements of color until we had sewn all the little pieces into one piece large enough to cover a bed. Then Grandmother put thick cotton between the pieced top layer and a bottom sheet, and we stitched the layers together to provide softness and warmth for the lucky person who would sleep beneath this masterpiece. It took lots of practice for me to get it just right. The hardest parts were having enough strength to push the needle through the many layers of fabric and the patience to finish all the tasks. My mother always said that Grandmother sewed the quilts together not with thread, but with love."

CAREGIVING IS AN ART

Caregiving in a health care setting is like *quilt making*. As a caregiver, you make decisions, fit many pieces of work into a day, pay attention to the details of each person's life and use personal strength to handle the many complex parts of your job. You work with patience and devotion while helping ill or disabled people feel comfortable, important and respected. All of us are caregivers at one time or another when we provide important and necessary care to a friend or family member who needs help because of an illness or disability. Being employed as a trained caregiver, however, requires us not only to provide the best care that we can but also to take on additional kinds of responsibili-

ties, such as providing social and emotional support.

It takes a special person to provide quality health care in a caring way. As a nurse assistant, you are a valuable and special caregiver who can make a difference in the lives of people receiving care. You blend your knowledge of people and the accurate performance of skills with your caring spirit. Many people learn the skills of caregiving, but not everyone can deliver those skills with kindness and compassion. Skillful care provided in a thoughtful way is an **art.**

This chapter explores the art of caregiving and also introduces you to the information that you must know to be a skilled caregiver and to make each person feel that he or she has received a gift—the best care possible. As you prepare for your job—whether you are called a *nurse assistant, nursing assistant, nurse aide, home health aide* or *geriatric aide*—you will learn the difference between just getting

your job done and providing the quality of care expected from a good nurse assistant. The art of caregiving, the art of treating each person as an individual, makes the difference. Getting to know each person as an individual is the key (Figure 1-1). Each person receiving care is different, as is each situation. This book provides guidelines to help you make the best decisions to provide the best care to each person.

WORKING IN THE HEALTH CARE SYSTEM

Nurse assistants work with a variety of health professionals, such as nurses, physical therapists and dietitians. These health care professionals provide many kinds of health care, depending on the needs of the person receiving care. For example, health care professionals in a hospital clinic provide regular medical checkups to help healthy people stay well and avoid health problems.

FIGURE 1-1 The art of caregiving focuses on providing care for each person as an individual. This nurse assistant takes time to listen to a resident's utmost concern—the outcome of last night's televised football game.

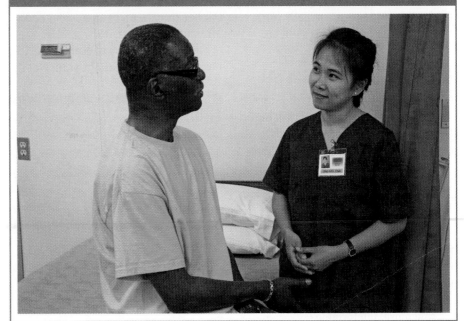

Health care professionals in a hospital find and treat problems, such as high blood pressure, before they become serious. Health care professionals cannot cure some health problems, such as diabetes, but they can help people learn to live with them and keep them under control. When people have health problems from which they cannot recover, health care workers strive to make them as comfortable as possible.

People choose health care services depending on where they live, the kind of care they need, and how they will pay for their care. In the United States, people pay for health care in a variety of ways. Some people receive health insurance through government programs like **Medicare** and **Medicaid.** Others have insurance coverage through their employment or organizations. Some people may choose to pay for their own personal insurance coverage. There are some individuals that do not have any health insurance because they cannot afford to pay for it.

The health care system has many parts, each with a special function. In some instances, a person may use three parts of the system—the hospital, a nursing home and home health care—to meet his or her health care needs. Nurse assistants usually work in one of these health care settings.

WORKING IN A HOSPITAL

When a 72-year-old resident at Morningside Nursing Home woke up in her hospital room after hip surgery, she looked up and saw some strange-looking equipment beside her bed. She felt afraid. She was in pain and wondered how long it would take to get better. She didn't like being in this unfamiliar place. What were those sounds she heard? She just wanted to be back home. Then someone gently took her hand and said, "Hello, Mrs. Garcia. I'm your nurse assistant. How can I help you feel more comfortable?"

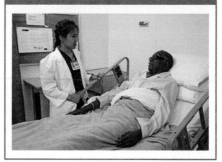

FIGURE 1-2 You will have many opportunities to comfort and reassure the people in your care.

What is Hospital Care?

When Mrs. Garcia needed surgery to repair her broken hip, her doctor admitted her to a hospital. A hospital provides care for people who have major illnesses, become sick or injured suddenly, require surgery or need tests to find out whether they have an illness or disease. To keep serious illnesses from occurring, hospital clinics promote wellness through health maintenance and health education. When Mrs. Garcia receives care in the hospital, she is called a **patient.** Part of your job as a nurse assistant is to help patients feel comfortable, as well as to assist nurses and other members of the health care team in providing care for patients. (Figure 1-2)

People who stay overnight in a hospital receive **inpatient** care. Not all hospital patients stay overnight, however. Some people have regular doctor appointments at a **hospital clinic.** For example, at a **walk-in clinic,** people can come in without an appointment. They may also go to a clinic to see another health professional, such as a physical therapist, speech therapist or dietitian. A hospital may also have a surgery clinic, where people go for same-day surgical procedures that do not require them to stay overnight. Individuals visiting hospital clinics receive **outpatient** care.

Two major types of hospitals are **specialized hospitals** and general hospitals. A specialized hospital provides services for only one type of health care need. A children's or pediatric hospital is an example of a specialized hospital. Look at Table 1-1, which lists several types of specialized hospitals and the care each provides.

A **general hospital** usually provides care for patients of all ages and with almost any type of illness or injury. It also provides outpatient care, surgical services, emergency care services, health education classes and testing procedures to identify illnesses.

Most general hospitals provide this wide variety of care through individual departments, which help their staffs to focus primarily on one type of patient or illness. This focus allows staff members to become experts in providing specialized care. In fact, even with one

TABLE 1-1 EXAMPLES OF SPECIALIZED HOSPITALS

Type of Hospital	Service and Care Provided for ...
Obstetric	Pregnant women and those with newborn babies; women with diseases of the reproductive system
Orthopedic	People with broken bones; people with diseases of bones or joints
Pediatric	Children with illnesses or injuries
Psychiatric	People with mental or emotional problems

single need, a patient may encounter several types of caretakers. For example, when Mrs. Garcia broke her hip, she was admitted in the emergency room. The staff then moved her to the operating room, where the surgeon fixed her hip. Finally she woke up in the **orthopedic** unit.

What is it Like to Work in a Hospital?

Working in a hospital can be exciting, since it is an intense place, full of vigorous activity. Because most patients do not stay a long time, the people in your care may change fairly often. Patients may have fairly serious illnesses or injuries. Being cared for in a hospital is very expensive, so patients usually are discharged to their own homes or to nursing homes as soon as they no longer require the kind of care a hospital provides.

A hospital can be a difficult place in which to create comfortable, familiar surroundings. Often there is not much space for personal items, and patients are encouraged to leave anything of value at home. Sometimes, for health reasons, even flowers are not permitted. For example, a person with **nausea** may not be able to tolerate strong smells.

Most hospitals have some single rooms, but patients usually share a room with one or more people. Team members can pull curtains around a space so that others cannot see the patient, but it is hard to keep conversations private. Hospitals permit all but the most seriously ill people to have visitors. The number of visitors and visiting hours may be limited so that patients can receive the care and rest they need. The hospitals may also have rules regarding the ages of visitors who come to the hospital.

For all these reasons, a nurse assistant working in a hospital must have a special ability to form effective relationships quickly with people who are under stress. You become an

important person for patients who may be afraid of having surgery or tests or who may be in pain. Family or friends may not be around when the patient needs comfort and support. Things happen quickly in a hospital, and patients ask many questions that they may not have had a chance to ask other members of the health care team. Perhaps something was explained to them, but they do not remember what they heard or do not understand. Family members and friends may have similar concerns, and other members of the health care team may not be available to talk with them during visiting hours. It is important for you to tell your supervising nurse about any questions and con-

cerns the patient or the patient's family may discuss with you. Information concerning a patient's condition is limited to only those authorized to know.

As a nurse assistant in a hospital, you are a vital member of the health care team. You may provide basic nursing care under the supervision of a licensed nurse, or you may assist the nursing staff in a certain department by transporting patients to and from the department or helping with examinations. Some of these departments you work in might include obstetrics, pediatrics, orthopedics and surgical (Table 1-2).

Remember that whatever department you are assigned to, each patient is unique and should be treated as a

TABLE 1-2 EXAMPLES OF DEPARTMENTS IN A GENERAL HOSPITAL	
Department	Service and Care Provided for ...
Medical	Patients who need medical care
Surgical	Patients who need surgery
Cardiology	Patients with heart diseases
Clinic	Patients who need medical care but who do not need to stay overnight at the hospital
Emergency	People with emergency medical needs
Intensive care unit	Patients with life-threatening illnesses or conditions
Nursery	Newborn babies
Obstetric	Pregnant women and newborn babies
Oncology	Patients with cancer
Operating room	Patients who undergo surgery
Orthopedic	Patients with bone and joint problems
Pediatric	Children up to 18 years of age
Psychiatric/ mental health	Patients with mental or emotional problems

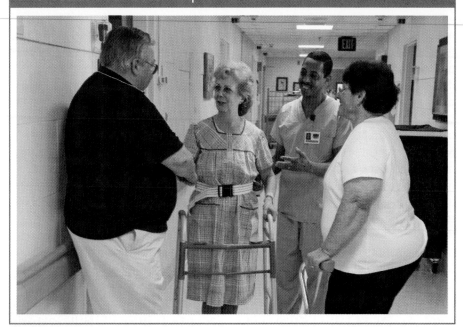

person, not as an illness. The compassionate care you provide can make a difference in how a patient feels about his or her time in the hospital.

WORKING IN LONG-TERM CARE

On a sunny day in March, you help Mrs. Garcia pack the small suitcase her children have brought to the hospital. She is feeling much better, and her hip is getting stronger since she has started the exercises recommended by the physical therapist. Still, she needs more care before she can return home, so she is going to continue her recovery at a nursing home. As she prepares to go to Morningside Nursing Home, Mrs. Garcia has many questions: "Who else lives in the home? Will I make friends? (Figure 1-3) What will I do with my time? Will the nurses be nice to me? Will I get the kind of treatment I need? Will they treat me with respect?" Her children also have questions: "Will we be able to visit? Will they take good care of Mother?"

What is a Nursing Home?

A nursing home or nursing facility, which are the most frequently used terms, is a place where long-term care is provided for people who need regular or continuous skilled care. People may also receive long-term care in assisted-living communities, group homes and residential care facilities (Box 1-1). A person who receives care in a nursing facility is called a **resident**. The average stay for a person in a nursing home is 7 months to 2 years.

Some people may stay in a nursing home for a few days or for a few weeks to regain their physical and emotional health through **rehabilitation.** Residents in nursing facilities can be categorized by how long they stay in the facility. Short-term residents are those who leave the facility in 3 to 6 months. They tend to be younger, and may be admitted from a hospital. The increase in **subacute care** units in nursing facilities has also added to the increase in short-term residents. Long-term residents stay in the facility for 6 months or more. As a nurse assistant, you work with the health care team to provide daily care and help residents live as fully and independently as possible.

What is it Like to Work in a Nursing Home?

Working in a nursing home can be both challenging and rewarding. You have the same responsibility that all nurse assistants have: to provide basic nursing care. In addition, you do certain things that are specific to working in a nursing home. For example, one of the most important needs of residents is talking with other people. Often nursing home residents do not have

---

BOX 1-1

OTHER TERMS FOR NURSING HOME

Assisted-living community
Care center
Convalescent center
Geriatric center
Group home
Health center
Health care center
Long-term care center

Nursing center
Nursing facility
Nursing and rehabilitative treatment center
Rehabilitation center
Residential care facility
Skilled care center

family members nearby who can come to visit regularly. You can fill some of their needs by talking with them and encouraging them to talk with one another and to get involved in activities. Most people like to be asked about their lives, accomplishments and families. Try and remember these events in their lives so that at a later date the information can be used in a **therapeutic** manner as you work with the nursing home resident.

In many instances, the nursing home setting may be your first introduction to caregiving. You may have challenges because you may have to work long hours. But you will find that the work you do is highly valued by the resident, the family and nursing staff.

WORKING IN HOME HEALTH CARE

The Move to Home Health Care

After Mrs. Garcia receives physical therapy and other rehabilitative care at the nursing home, her doctor decides that her walking has improved and that she can go home. However, he also decides that she will still need some assistance, so he refers her to a home health care agency. The **referral process** allows one member of the health care system to let other members know that a person requires their kind of specialized care.

Although the doctor or nurse typically makes a home health care referral, anyone in the community can call a home health care agency and ask for services. The home health care agency evaluates each case to see whether they can provide services.

Clients pay for home health care in a number of different ways: through Medicare, Medicaid, private insurance and private pay. Rules and regulations govern how each of these methods of payment covers the cost. Because these rules differ from agency to agency, a client should check with a local home health care agency for the rules that apply in his or her state.

Mrs. Garcia is happy to be back at home. She likes sleeping in her own bed and enjoys being alone. She gets in and out of bed by herself, fixes her own simple meals and even manages to get dressed by herself. But Mrs. Garcia needs help with bathing, changing the bed linens and shopping for groceries. She also needs help with doing the exercises recommended by the physical therapist (Figure 1-4). The **home health aide** visits with Mrs. Garcia twice each week to help her with these tasks.

What is Home Health Care?

A **home health care agency** provides health care services to people in their homes so that they safely get the care they need, while feeling secure within their own homes and with their families. When Mrs. Garcia receives home health care, she is called a **client**. Typically, clients receive home health care from a registered nurse, who **monitors** their health and plans their care, and from a home health aide, who helps them with their daily care.

For many years people were afraid to go to the hospital. They thought that they would get better care at home. As time went on, it became more common for people who were very sick to get health care in a hospital. Today, **home health care** is again popular because it encourages people to receive individualized care in their own homes, and it does not cost as much as hospital care.

Two purposes of home health care are to help people get better and to promote independence of clients in the comfort of their homes. A client with a **chronic illness** may choose to be cared for at home. A client with a **terminal illness** is not expected to recover and may also use home health care. Many elderly people require some assistance because they are frail and not able to do certain things for themselves.

Home health aides receive training similar to that of nurse assistants

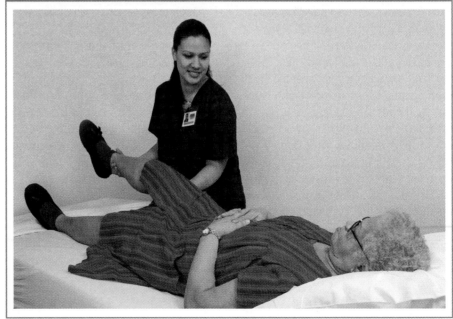

FIGURE 1-4 By helping Mrs. Garcia with her hip exercises, the home health aide is helping her reach her goal of living independently

and provide the same basic nursing care. Sometimes home health care workers teach family members or friends to provide care for their loved ones at home.

Clients receiving home health care can be young or old, male or female, and of any race, religion or ethnic background. They all have special medical problems that require different kinds of care in their homes to maintain or recover their health. People who require home health care want to know that they will receive good care. To guarantee that people receive a certain level of care, federal and state governments established standards for staffing and operation that all home health agencies must meet. In 1987, these new home health requirements, which state that home health agencies are responsible for providing good care to their clients, became effective. When working in home health care, you hear people talking about these "OBRA" requirements. You will learn more about OBRA requirements in the next chapter.

What is it Like to Work as a Home Health Aide?

To be a good home health aide, you must be professional and mature. Home health aides often work alone, but their duties and responsibilities are clearly outlined in the job description. Because home health aides fill a very important need they also have special training needs that include home management and home safety, as well as food planning and preparation. The law requires that they be tested by their employer to make sure they are qualified. Depending on your client's needs, your responsibilities will include providing personal care, such as bathing and grooming, and making sure your client is safe. Some clients

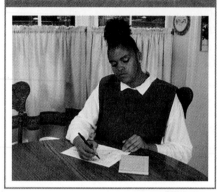

FIGURE 1-5 Because a home health aide often works alone providing care to the client, she must carefully document her activities and observations.

may need help cooking a meal. Other clients may have to be reminded to take their medications. Finally, you will carefully document all your activities and observations (Figure 1-5).

All nurse assistants deal with families, but in the home health care setting you talk with household members in their own environments. Sometimes you may find working in their homes to be a warm and rewarding experience. At other times you may not like how some people behave. You may be exposed to values that are different from your own.

If your client's home is a caring and safe place, it will probably be a pleasant setting for caregiving. However, some people may not keep their homes as clean as you keep your own. You may also observe or suspect alcohol abuse, drug abuse, physical abuse or illegal activity while you are providing care in the home. You should report any concerns you have about your client's well-being to your supervising nurse, who will help you decide what to do.

THE ROLE OF A PERSONAL CARE ASSISTANT

A caregiver is sometimes referred to as a **personal care assistant** or informal caregiver. This person assists elderly or disabled adults with daily living activities at the person's home or in a daytime non-residential facility. Duties performed at a place of residence may include:

- keeping house (making beds, doing laundry, washing dishes) and preparing meals.
- providing meals and supervised activities at non-residential care facilities.
- advising families, the elderly and disabled on such things as nutrition, cleanliness and household utilities.

USING COMMUNITY RESOURCES

Many services are available in the community to help people get well, help them learn to adapt to their illnesses or offer emotional support. Some organizations provide information about particular illnesses or conditions, such as cancer, diabetes or cystic fibrosis. Others offer community lectures and support groups for people with specific needs. Some community services offer rides to and from doctors' appointments, deliver meals to people's homes and provide child care. Check with your supervising nurse or the social worker if you think someone in your care would benefit from one of these community services. In addition, **AIDS** service organizations and **hospice** offer special care and sometimes offer special training programs for nurse assistants and home health aides.

Circle the correct answers and fill in the blanks.

1. Three parts of the health care system in which nurse assistants may work are _hospital_, _nursing home_, and _home setting_.

2. A person receiving care in a hospital is called a _patient_.

3. Signing a person into a health care facility is called:
   a. certifying.
   b. referring.
   (c.) admitting.
   d. discharging.

4. A nurse assistant who provides care in people's homes is often called a:
   a. maintenance employee.
   (b.) home health aide.
   c. nurse practitioner.
   d. social worker.

5. A person receiving health care at home is called a _client_.

6. One thing a caregiver working in home health care is permitted to do is:
   a. give medication.
   b. prepare medication.
   (c.) remind the person to take medication.
   d. none of the above.

7. Some people stay in nursing facilities for a short period of time to regain their physical and emotional health. We call this situation:
   a. activity of daily living.
   b. cognitive impairment.
   (c.) rehabilitation.
   d. chronic illness.

8. A person receiving care in a nursing facility is called a _resident_.

1. *What are your reasons for wanting to become a nurse assistant in a hospital, nursing facility or home setting?*

2. *What do you think your duties will be in this job?*

3. *What do you think will be the rewards of this work?*

4. *What do you think will be the challenges of this work?*

5. *Think of someone you know who received care in one of the three major parts of the health care system. What did the person think of the care he or she received?*

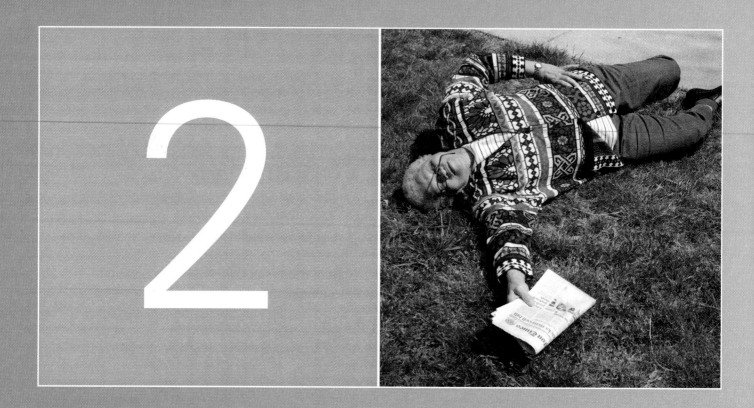

2

Working in Long-Term Care

GOALS

After reading this chapter, you will have the information needed to:

Discuss regulations in OBRA '87 that affect nurse assistants.

Describe the people who live in a long-term care facility.

List three qualities of a good nurse assistant.

Name four parts of your role as a nurse assistant.

List five members of the health care team and explain their roles.

Describe the six principles of care and explain why you should practice them.

Discuss how to put the individual first in caregiving.

Discuss upward mobility for nurse assistants.

It was raining when 72-year-old Alma Garcia went outside to get her morning newspaper. As she walked back toward the front door, she slipped and fell. She lay unnoticed until a neighbor walked by and saw her lying on the ground. The neighbor phoned for an ambulance, which took her to the hospital. There, a doctor examined her and gave her the bad news: she had broken her hip.

After she began to recover from surgery, Mrs. Garcia worked with a physical therapist, who helped exercise her hip so that she could later learn to use a walker. Nurse assistants helped her bathe and get out of bed and worked with the supervising nurse to provide the best possible care. Over time, she got stronger and no longer needed hospital care, but she wasn't well enough to go home. A hospital staff member referred her to a nursing home.

At Morningside Nursing Home, Mrs. Garcia received nursing care and physical therapy to help strengthen her hip and help her learn to walk with a walker. Nurse assistants helped with bathing, dressing and walking and also assisted her with special exercises that she learned from the physical therapist. As time passed, she became stronger and more independent and walked longer distances with her walker.

After several months, Mrs. Garcia was able to walk without help and she was discharged from the nursing facility and returned home.

WHAT IS OBRA '87?

People like Mrs. Garcia, who live in a nursing home, want to know that they will receive good care. To guarantee that people receive a certain level of care, federal and state governments have established standards for staffing and operation that all nursing homes must meet. In 1987, the United States Congress passed a law to improve the quality of health care in this country. This law is known as **OBRA '87** because it was part of the 1987 Omnibus Budget Reconciliation Act. Later, in 1990, new federal nursing home requirements also became effective.

These OBRA **regulations** are a way to improve the quality of care that is given in a nursing facility.

They set the standards that nurse assistants must meet in order to work in **Medicare-** and **Medicaid-** reimbursed facilities. This federal law requires that nurse assistants complete a minimum 75-hour state-approved nurse assistant training program or pass a state **competency evaluation program** to obtain state **certification** (Box 2-1). Nurse assistants must then renew their certification periodically. Each state offers specific guidelines for both certification and renewal.

OBRA regulations also emphasize respect for the rights of residents in nursing facilities; for example, people in nursing homes and those receiving home health care have the right to be treated with dignity and the right to make choices. You will read more about these rights in Chapter 3, "Protecting People's Rights." OBRA also emphasizes the responsibility of nursing facilities and home health agencies to provide residents with the most comfortable and fulfilling lifestyle and to promote their physical, mental, emotional and spiritual well-being to the highest degree possible.

KEY TERMS

activities of daily living (ADLs): daily self-care activities that help keep a person independent and healthy.

certification: (ser-te-fuh-KAY-shun) having skills that have been tested and approved.

cognitive impairment: (KOG-nuh-tiv/ im-PARE-ment) a condition that decreases a person's ability to think clearly.

compassion: (kum-PASH-un) a feeling of sorrow for another person's hardship that leads to help.

competency evaluation program: state-operated program to certify skills of persons wanting to work as nurse assistants.

health care team: a group headed by the person receiving care. Includes doctors, nurses, nurse assistants, therapists, secretaries and other people involved in the caregiving process.

Medicaid: a state-administered federal program that provides health coverage for persons with very low incomes.

Medicare: a federal health insurance program for persons over age 65 or persons of any age who are disabled or have permanent kidney failure.

nurture: (NUR-tyur) to promote and encourage good care.

OBRA '87: (OH-brah) an abbreviation for the 1987 Omnibus Budget Reconciliation Act, which provides certain standards for nursing homes and home health care.

patient-focused care: treating each patient as an individual when providing care.

principles of care: (PRIN-suh-puls) basic rules of caregiving that guide caregivers in making decisions about providing individualized care for each person.

regulation: (reg-you-LAY-shun) a rule that must be followed.

BOX 2-1

SUMMARY OF OBRA REGULATIONS FOR NURSE ASSISTANTS*

As a nurse assistant you must:

1. Pass a competency evaluation program and/or
2. Complete an approved nurse assistant training program, content to include:
   - Basic nursing skills
   - Basic restorative services
   - Resident rights
   - Safety and emergency care
3. Understand mental health and social needs of residents
4. Know how to provide care for people with cognitive impairment
5. Practice infection control
6. Work at least 8 hours in a 12-month period (for pay)
7. Complete ~~X~~ hours of inservice per year 24hrs. Renew

*These are minimum requirements; each state may increase the requirements. Be sure to discuss with your instructor about your particular state requirements that may be needed for certification in your state.

WHO ARE THE PEOPLE IN NURSING FACILITIES?

The average age of nursing home residents is 85 years. Two-thirds of these are women (Figure 2-1). How would you feel about living in a place with twice as many women as men?

Why do you think these very old people, mostly women, live in nursing facilities? Almost all people in nursing facilities go there because of one of the following conditions: cognitive or emotional disorder (including Alzheimer's disease), circulatory disease (including heart disease and stroke), diabetes, cancer, hip or other fracture or musculoskeletal system disorder (including arthritis). More than for any other reason, residents go to nursing homes to receive care because they are mentally unable to take care of themselves. Over 50% of all nursing facility residents have some type of **cognitive impairment**. The

FIGURE 2-1 Residents in a nursing facility may be similar in age and medical condition but have a wide variety of experiences and accomplishments.

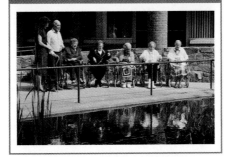

most common cause of cognitive impairment is Alzheimer's disease. Many people also go to nursing homes because they cannot function alone as a result of circulatory disease.

Most residents have more than one medical condition. For example, a

resident may have heart disease and a cognitive or emotional disorder. The heart disease may be the reason for admission, but the resident also needs care because of the cognitive impairment.

The effects of these medical conditions on some people, rather than the conditions themselves, often lead to the need for nursing home care. For example, someone who has arthritis may no longer be able to get in and out of bed, go to the toilet, or dress without help. Someone with Alzheimer's disease may be physically able to function but may need constant reminders to eat, get dressed, and stay out of danger because she cannot remember to do these things.

You may be surprised to learn that some children and younger people live in nursing homes. A child or a younger person may live there because of an injury to the head, neck or back (called a *spinal cord injury*); a mental disability; or a serious, disabling handicap. No matter how old or young they are, all residents in nursing homes have one thing in common: they cannot take care of themselves completely and have special health care needs that cannot be met at home. Nurse assistants are the key staff in providing for the needs of nursing home residents.

THE HEALTH CARE TEAM

No matter where people go, they want to receive skilled, compassionate and individualized care. In every place where care is provided, many staff members work together to meet people's needs. Each staff member has special training and skills that contribute to the kind of health care being provided. Along with the person receiving care, these staff members form a **health care team** that plans and provides the necessary services (Figure 2-2). People often think that the team includes only doctors and nurses. Although doctors and nurses

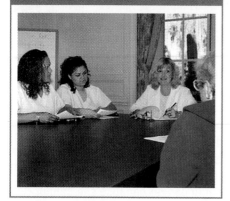

have important positions on the team, every member has an important role on the team. Some have a higher level of skill. You, as a nurse assistant, are also part of the health care team. The person *receiving the care* is considered the "captain" of the team. Whenever Mrs. Garcia received care, she was in charge of the team and the care she received, even though she was disabled. The other people on the team worked for Mrs. Garcia. If she had not been able to make decisions or be in charge, the team would have worked for her family.

Wherever you work, you will be part of a health care team.

Look at Table 2-1 to learn about the part or role each team member plays in different health care settings.

The specific members of your team will vary, depending on where you work. In Figure 2-3 on page 17, the person receiving care is surrounded by members of the health care team who have the most direct contact with her. Team members in the base of the figure may not have much contact with the person, but they support the health care team, and the work they do is important to the caregiving process.

TABLE 2-1 WHAT HEALTH CARE TEAM MEMBERS DO

Team Member*	Role	Setting
Person receiving care (patient, resident, client)	Is the "captain" of the health care team; is in charge of the care she receives; works with the team, which helps her make decisions about needed care	Hospital Nursing facility Home health care
Family members and friends	Should be encouraged to help with care if the captain wants them to help; often are important sources of emotional support; may decide about the kinds of care the person receives if the person turns this responsibility over to them	Hospital Nursing facility Home health care
Registered nurse (RN)	Supervises the nursing care team members as they plan and provide care	Hospital Nursing facility Home health care
Licensed practical nurse (LPN) or licensed vocational nurse (LVN)	Helps plan and supervise some types of care under the direction of a registered nurse	Hospital Nursing facility Home health care
Certified nurse assistant (CNA) or home health aide (HHA)	Helps plan care and assists with care under the supervision of a registered or licensed nurse	Hospital Nursing facility Home health care
Doctor	Determines the person's illness or condition and supervises medical care; writes medical orders and prescribes medication when needed	Hospital Nursing facility Home health care

*This list of team members represents only some of the many people on the health care team. The team varies from one facility to another and from one setting to another and includes many different specialists and assistants.

TABLE 2-1 WHAT HEALTH CARE TEAM MEMBERS DO (continued)

Team Member*	Role	Setting
Discharge planner (Continuing Care Nurse, Case Manager or Utilization Manager)	Meets with members of the health care team to develop a plan that will meet the patient's medical needs after discharge; often works with the social services department to make appropriate referrals	Hospital
Nurse practitioner	A nurse with a graduate degree in advance practice nursing. Activities can include: taking the patient's history, performing a physical exam, and ordering appropriate laboratory tests and procedures, diagnosing, treating and managing acute and chronic diseases, providing prescription and coordinating referrals and promoting healthy activities in collaboration with the patient.	Hospital Nursing facility Home health care
Activities director (or recreational therapist)	Plans and coordinates activities that provide opportunities for socializing, spiritual support, creativity, entertainment, exercise and citizen activities, such as voting	Hospital Nursing facility
Dentist	Provides dental care	Nursing facility
Housekeeper	Makes sure rooms and other parts of the facility are cleaned each day	Hospital Nursing facility
Laundry employee	Washes and mends linens, bedding and clothing	Hospital Nursing facility
Maintenance employee	Makes repairs in the facility and takes care of the grounds around the facility	Hospital Nursing facility
Dietitian	Talks with the person/family about food and nutrition; serves as a resource for staff members	Hospital Nursing facility Home health care
Social worker	Helps admit people to and discharge them from a hospital, a nursing home, or home health care; works with people and their families to make sure their needs are met	Hospital Nursing facility Home health care
Medical director (physician)	Serves as the head of the medical staff	Hospital Nursing facility Home health care
Psychologist	Provides mental health assessment services	Hospital Home health care Nursing facility

Continued

TABLE 2-1 WHAT HEALTH CARE TEAM MEMBERS DO (continued)

Team Member*	Role	Setting
Pharmacist	Provides medications ordered by the doctor and keeps a record of all medications	Hospital Nursing facility
Religious leader (priest, minister, rabbi)	Provides spiritual support, as needed and requested, for the person receiving care, her family and staff members	Hospital Nursing facility Home health care
Administrator	Directs the overall operation of the facility or agency	Hospital Nursing facility Home health care
Bookkeeper	Takes care of paperwork for paying all bills and salaries	Hospital Nursing facility Home health care
Secretary or administrative assistant	Helps staff members in different departments to communicate with one another; often interacts with the public and family members over the phone; often keeps people's charts in order	Hospital Nursing facility Home health care
Speech therapist	Helps people improve their speech and language; helps people who have trouble swallowing	Hospital Nursing facility Home health care
Physical therapist	Helps people improve their ability to move their bodies	Hospital Nursing facility Home health care
Occupational therapist	Helps people regain their independence in daily living tasks	Hospital Nursing facility Home health care

WHO CAN BE A GOOD NURSE ASSISTANT?

It takes a special person to be a good nurse assistant. Box 2-2 lists these basic qualities.

No matter where you work, your primary role is to assist the people in your care to do the things they cannot do for themselves. It is also important for you as a nurse assistant to understand your own fears and feelings about aging and the very old. Feelings that you have, particularly negative feelings that you may have about the elderly, can affect the people in your care. Being able to recognize what is a fact and what is a myth about aging will help you to be a better nurse assistant. The greatest strengths for this job, though, are your special qualities of caring, compassion, respect and kindness.

YOUR ROLE AS A NURSE ASSISTANT

Your role of caregiving is the same in all parts of the system, but the people you help may be more or less ill, more or less independent, and more or less able to recover fully. Your tasks vary, depending on the needs of the people in your care and your employer's requirements. Your role as a nurse assistant includes four important parts: providing direct

FIGURE 2-3 The health care team.

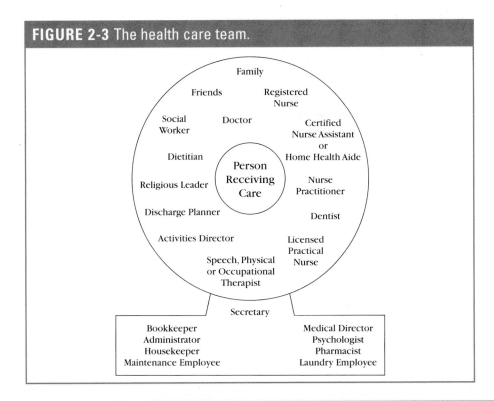

care, providing emotional support, participating as a team member, and promoting the six principles of care.

Providing Direct Care

Most people in nursing homes require your help with **activities of daily living** (Box 2-3), such as walking, eating, bathing and dressing (Figure 2-4). You also provide a safe, comfortable environment for the person in your care. You will learn the skills to help with these activities later in this book.

Providing Emotional Support

You can show thoughtfulness and compassion for people by listening and paying attention to them. The people in your care have health problems, but they also have all the other day-to-day worries and concerns we all have. Often they just need to talk to someone who

BOX 2-2

BASIC QUALITIES OF A GOOD NURSE ASSISTANT

Health/Hygiene
A good nurse assistant:
- Eats a well-balanced diet
- Gets plenty of rest
- Has good posture
- Never takes alcoholic beverages or illegal drugs before or during work
- Cares about his or her appearance and dresses in a professional manner.
- Bathes frequently enough so that he or she has no body odors
- Shampoos hair often, uses deodorant and wears clean clothing
- Exercises
- Wears comfortable shoes that provide support

Social
A good nurse assistant:
- Is able to get along with other people
- Is a good listener
- Is able to talk with families and other staff members
- Is able to tell someone when he or she has a problem or needs something

Character
A good nurse assistant:
- Keeps private information to himself or herself; does not gossip about a person with staff or other people
- Is truthful
- Is polite to everyone

- Treats others with respect
- Respects and protects people's personal belongings
- Is dependable; does what he or she is supposed to do
- Is reliable; reports to work as scheduled and on time
- Behaves in a professional manner; uses good judgment when asked to give advice to the person receiving care
- Never accepts money or a gift as a bribe for special treatment
- Is energetic—has lots of energy to put into his or her job and to give to the people with whom he or she works

BOX 2-3

ACTIVITIES OF DAILY LIVING

- Eating
- Bathing
- Dressing
- Grooming
- Using the toilet
- Walking/moving
- Communicating

FIGURE 2-5 By giving this resident her full attention, the nurse assistant lets him know that she is interested in what he is saying.

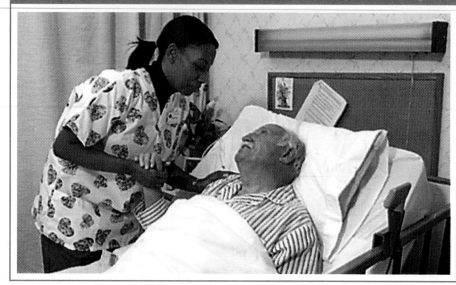

FIGURE 2-4 Sometimes all you have to do is steady a person's hand so that she can feed herself.

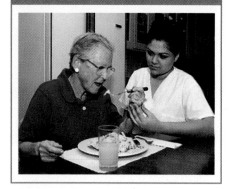

listens to them. Listening may seem simple, but it is one of the most important parts of good caregiving (Figure 2-5).

Participating as a Team Member

Regardless of where you work in health care, you are part of a team providing health care for ill, hurt or disabled people. The nurse assistant is often the eyes and ears for the rest of the health care team. Because of the amount of time you spend with a person, you may see and hear things the rest of the team does not. For example, if someone is afraid of having a test or procedure done, you can relay her fear to your supervising nurse, and

together you can help comfort the person. You may also notice that someone does not eat. Your supervising nurse may not be aware of this situation. It is your responsibility to tell your supervising nurse your concerns. When you help the person in your care, you also are assisting your supervising nurse, who helps and supports you by giving you your assignments, receiving your reports and answering your questions. Your supervising nurse may be called the *charge nurse, head nurse, primary nurse, supervisor* or *team leader.* Regardless of where you work, your employer provides you with a list of basic tasks and procedures called a *job description.* Look at the sample job description for nurse assistants in Box 2-4. Job descriptions vary from employer to employer, so you must always read each new job description carefully to make sure you know your responsibilities. Perform only the tasks listed in your job description.

Promoting and Practicing the Six Principles of Care

The ill, injured or disabled people in your care need more than your assistance. They need your assistance delivered with **compassion** and thoughtfulness, according to the six principles of care. These principles will provide you with a good framework for caregiving.

For instance, as you help Mrs. Ryan get ready for an important day, let the six **principles of care**—*safety, privacy, dignity, communication, independence* and *infection control*—guide every decision you make and every action that you take (Box 2-5).

These principles of care help you remember to put the person first. When making decisions about the person in your care, always ask yourself the following: Is the person *safe*? Am I protecting her *privacy*? Am I promoting her *dignity*? Does she want to talk? Do I need to say something to her? How can I *communicate* to her? How can I encourage her to be as *independent* as possible? Would a particular action prevent the spread of germs and promote *infection control*? These principles also help you consider the whole person. Although the care you provide for Mrs. Ryan may seem ordinary, there will be many opportunities to practice these principles of care.

BOX 2-4

SAMPLE JOB DESCRIPTION

As a nurse assistant, you:

1. Assist with the activities of daily living for the person in your care. This includes providing assistance with complete and partial baths, mouth care, skin and nail care, dressing, using the toilet and exercise.
2. Use safe and correct techniques to assist the person with moving, walking and positioning in bed.
3. Provide nutritional care, which includes delivering food trays and other nourishment, helping people eat, observing and recording a person's ability to take nourishment and reporting anything unusual to your supervising nurse.
4. Practice Standard Precautions and Isolation Precautions.
5. Take and record the person's blood pressure, temperature, pulse rate and respirations. Measure intake, output, height and weight.
6. Assist with the collection of urine, stool and sputum specimens for lab tests.
7. Help a person with admitting, transferring and discharging.
8. Observe the person's general physical and emotional condition and report significant observations, reactions or changes in the person to your supervising nurse.
9. Respond to call signals to determine the person's needs. Communicate these needs to appropriate health care team members.
10. Provide your supervising nurse with written and/or oral reports of the person's status, nursing care and services provided. Record information on appropriate nursing forms, bedside charts, flow sheets and progress/nursing notes.
11. Cooperate with all members of the health care team to provide quality care.
12. Participate in staff and care conferences.
13. Participate in nursing education programs designed for nurse assistants.
14. Respect the person's rights, provide privacy and maintain confidentiality.
15. Respond properly to emergencies and know how to perform all safety procedures.
16. Follow your employer's policies when using and caring for equipment.
17. Follow all of your employer's policies.

When you apply these principles of care to caregiving, it is like Mrs. Ryan's grandmother sewing cotton into her quilt to provide substance and warmth. By applying the principles of care, you provide substance and warmth to the everyday skills of caregiving (Figure 2-6).

PUTTING THE PERSON IN YOUR CARE FIRST

A generation ago, providing health care was different than it is today. Back then, caregivers believed that the fewer things people in their care had to do for themselves, the better. Caregivers made people stay in bed, fed them and bathed them. They gave everyone the same care, focusing on treating everyone the same instead of as individuals with special needs and differences. Over time, health care professionals came to understand that people got better and stronger much more quickly if they were encouraged to do more things for themselves (Figure 2-7). They recovered faster if they were encouraged to do things when and how they liked to do them. People also responded better to treatment if their conditions were explained and if they participated in planning their care.

This discovery has changed the way health care professionals provide care. Although you still **nurture** the people in your care, you no longer do everything for them. You still may have to help them with many things, such as bathing, eating and using the toilet, but you also encourage them to do as much as possible for themselves.

BOX 2-5

PRACTICING THE SIX PRINCIPLES OF CARE

To learn more about these principles, read the chapters indicated in parentheses.

Safety: Keep a person free from harm by preventing injuries (Chapter 8, "Keeping People Safe").

Privacy: Keep a person's private business private, and do not allow private things to be seen or overheard by other people (Chapter 3, "Protecting People's Rights").

Dignity: Treat each person with respect at all times (Chapter 3, "Protecting People's Rights"). Report information about the person to your supervising nurse.

Communication: Be available to talk, listen and respond to a person's thoughts and feelings. Tell the person about the care you plan to provide. Report information about the person to your supervising nurse (Chapter 5, "Communicating with People").

Independence: Encourage each person to do as much as possible (Chapter 3, "Protecting People's Rights"; Chapter 5, "Communicating with People").

Infection Control: Help control the spread of germs (Chapter 7, "Controlling the Spread of Germs").

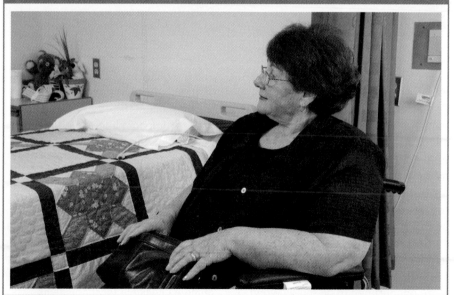

FIGURE 2-6 Respect for Mrs. Ryan's needs as she prepares for a special day enables her now to feel proud as she waits for the arrival of her birthday visitors.

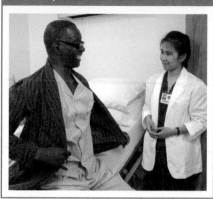

FIGURE 2-7 Completing even the smallest task gives a person a sense of accomplishment.

In caregiving, focusing on the person and his or her individual needs is important. Daily care must be individualized to meet the needs of each person; this is called **patient-focused care**. Care should not become routine or automatic. Anything can easily become automatic. For example, have you ever ridden home from your job, walked up to the front door of your home, and suddenly realized that you did not even remember your trip home?

What did you miss seeing along the way? The flowers? Budding trees? A beautiful sunset in the sky? Had your trip home from work become so automatic that you forgot to think about it and to enjoy how special that ride was?

As a nurse assistant, you must see each person as an individual with special needs. That person is more than a body or a disease that you fit into your schedule. Your schedule may make you feel comfortable, but that is not as important as what makes the person feel comfortable. You need to remember that each person is a human being who also has favorite routines. For instance, Mrs. Ryan needs to bathe when she wants to bathe, not when you have written her into your schedule. She needs to use the toilet when she needs to, not when you have time to help her. You must readjust your schedule, sometimes putting your own needs aside to take care of her needs.

While you are on the job you must always put your personal thoughts, feelings and troubles second to those of the person in your care, even though it may upset you. You *have* your own feelings, but you cannot *act* on them or let your mind rest on your own concerns while you provide care for someone. When you are distracted by your personal thoughts, you cannot give good care to an individual. If your thoughts and feelings get in the way of your work, talk to a co-worker, your supervising nurse, or someone else who may be able to help. You may need to continue to work for a while before you

get a chance to talk, but often, making the decision to talk with someone helps you clear your mind so that you can focus on the person in your care.

UPWARD MOBILITY FOR NURSE ASSISTANTS

Your job as a nurse assistant may be your first entry into the health care field. As competition for nurse assistants continues to grow, nursing facilities are looking at ways to hire more nurse assistants and to keep their nurse assistants. One way of doing this is by creating a career ladder within the facility, providing a means

for a nurse assistant to move up on the job. Some career ladders help nurse assistants to move into professional positions such as practical or vocational nurse or registered nurse positions. Other career ladder programs focus on improving the status of nurse assistants by offering opportunities for growth and development within the current employment setting and designing special recognition events for nurse assistants. The work of the nurse assistant is demanding. Facilities that offer programs that will improve nurse assistant morale will be more successful in recruiting and retaining quality nurse assistants.

INFORMATION REVIEW

Circle the correct answers and fill in the blanks.

1. The "captain" of the health care team is the:
   a. doctor.
   b. registered nurse.
   c. administrator.
   (d.) person receiving care.
2. A health care worker who helps people learn about what they eat is a:
   a. nurse practitioner.
   (b.) dietitian.
   c. pharmacist.
   d. physical therapist.

3. In addition to helping the person in your care, you assist your <u>supervising nurse</u>, who gives you your assignments, receives your reports and answers your questions.
4. The law passed by Congress that ensures that residents receive the best care possible is known as OBRA '87.
5. The condition that affects most residents living in nursing facilities is cognitive impairment.

QUESTIONS TO ASK YOURSELF

1. *What are some of the most important qualities a nurse assistant should have?*
2. *What special qualities would you bring to your work as a nurse assistant?*
3. *Think of someone you know who is in a nursing facility. What does the person (or a family member) think of the care he or she receives?*
4. *At Morningside Nursing Facility, Mr. Flanagan spends a lot of time holding a picture of his wife. Sometimes he talks to the picture. Every*

day he tells you that he wants to go home. How would you respond?
5. *Mrs. Landers clearly loves the fresh flowers her daughter brought her and wants to keep them on her bedside table, but her roommate is allergic to flowers. What would you do?*
6. *In the activity lounge, two residents are arguing over which television show to watch. What would you say when they ask you, "Who is right?"*

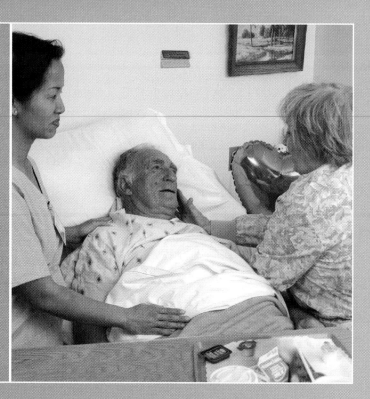

3

Protecting People's Rights

GOALS

After reading this chapter, you will have the information needed to:

Explain what legal rights are and how they came into being.

Give five examples of the rights of people receiving health care.

Discuss your role in resolving residents' complaints.

Explain the difference between legal and ethical responsibilities.

Discuss your role as a caregiver in protecting rights and behaving in an ethical manner.

Describe what you should do if you suspect that a person in your care is being neglected or abused.

At 11 A.M., you knock on Mr. Rivera's door. You listen carefully for his response because he has difficulty speaking as a result of paralysis from a stroke.

"Come in," says Mr. Rivera. When you walk in, you are surprised to see Mrs. Rivera sitting on the edge of the bed. Mrs. Rivera normally visits her husband every day around 2 P.M.

Not only is Mrs. Rivera there, but she has already served up two plates of food on the overbed table and she brought a balloon. This is not what you were expecting. You had already scheduled Mr. Rivera's bath for 11:15, just as you do every day.

"It's the 60th anniversary of the day we met," explains Mrs. Rivera. "Victor and I met at my cousin's 15th birthday party. When I saw him, I knew he was the right man for me." Mrs. Rivera smiles at her husband, who is sitting up in bed against some pillows. She touches his face gently and then starts to cut his food.

You ask Mr. Rivera if he would still like to take his bath at 11:15. Mr. Rivera shakes his head from side to side as he chews his food. "Not today," he finally replies, after swallowing. Then he pats Mrs. Rivera on the hand.

Mr. O'Reilly, Mr. Rivera's roommate, has physical therapy from 11:00 to 12:00, so you usually make his bed before assisting Mr. Rivera with his bath at 11:15. As you start to make Mr. O'Reilly's bed, however, Mr. Rivera clears his throat a couple of times. "Mrs. Rivera and I would like some time alone to celebrate our special day," he says with difficulty.

At first you feel a little annoyed. "Why didn't Mr. Rivera tell me about this change so that I could schedule

KEY TERMS

abuse: (ah-BYOOS) the willful infliction of injury, unreasonable confinement, intimidation or punishment with resulting physical harm, pain or mental anguish.

advance medical directive: document that allows a person to express written wishes regarding health care decisions to be used when and if the person is unable to speak for himself or herself.

advocate: (noun) a person who speaks on behalf of someone else; (verb) to speak on behalf of someone else.

client rights: a document listing the rights and expectations provided to a resident who receives care in her or his home; must be signed by the client.

durable power of attorney: type of advance directive that gives someone power to make health care decisions for another person.

emotional abuse: (e-MO-shun-uhl/ah-BYOOS) harm that occurs when one person's words or actions lead to another person feeling sad or feeling afraid.

endangerment: placement of an individual in a life-threatening situation that the person cannot respond to.

ethical: (ETH-e-kuhl) that which is morally and professionally correct.

ethical dilemma: (ETH-uh-kuhl/de-LEM-uh) a problem or situation in which a nurse assistant must decide what is the correct, moral and professional thing to do.

exploitation: (eks-ploy-TAY-shun) the act of taking advantage of someone.

grievance process: procedure in which a person may make a complaint about services or care received.

health care proxy: (PROK-see) a legal document that names a person to make health care decisions if the person receiving care is unable to.

incapacitated: (in-kuh-PAH-se-tay-ted) being unable to act for oneself.

informed consent: permission given after full disclosure of the facts.

legal right: (LEE-gul) a privilege that is protected by law.

living will: a legal document, prepared by a person receiving care, that directs which measures to take or not take to prolong life when death seems likely.

maltreatment: providing poor or improper treatment or using inappropriate responses (e.g., employee isolation, confinement or restraint of a patient as a disciplinary action).

neglect: (nuh-GLEKT) failure to provide goods and services necessary to avoid physical harm, mental anguish or mental illness.

ombudsman: (OM-buds-man) a person who acts as a mediator between a resident and the nursing facility. The ombudsman listens to the resident's concerns and complaints and resolves conflicts with the health care provider.

patient rights: a document listing the rights and expectations provided to a resident who receives care in a hospital; must be signed by the patient.

physical abuse: (FIZ-e-kull/ah-BYOOS) harm that occurs when a person's body is purposely hurt.

resident council: a group made up of nursing facility residents and residents' family members, who work together to solve problems or disagreements.

resident rights: a document listing the rights and expectations provided to a resident in a nursing facility; must be signed by the resident or family.

sexual abuse: (SEK-shue-al/ah-BYOOS) harm that occurs when a person's body is mistreated for sexual reasons or when they are forced or coerced into unwanted or improper sexual activity.

my day differently?" you wonder. Your routine normally works so well. Then you try to put yourself in Mr. Rivera's place. This room is his home, after all, and today is a very important day. You also know that Mr. Rivera has a right to his privacy.

"Congratulations," you say as you close the door on your way out. "I'll be down the hall if you need me."

Do you know what the word *right* means? You probably have heard people using the word all your life. If you look in a dictionary, you will find many different meanings for the word *right*. In your work as a nurse assistant, three meanings will be important to you:

- *Right* means "correct and true," based on some standard of quality or correctness. For example, if you have to take Mr. Rivera's temperature, you want to be sure you take it the right way. Only then will you get a correct reading.
- *Right* also means "a privilege" that belongs to a person and is protected by law. For example, does Mr. Rivera have the right not to take his bath? Or to refuse the medication ordered by his doctor? He has the legal right to refuse his bath and the medication, even though he needs the bath to stay clean and the medication to stay healthy. Legal rights vary from state to state, and you must check with your supervising nurse to make sure you understand how **legal rights** are defined in the state where you work.
- *Right* also means "good and virtuous," based on the concepts of justice and morality. For example, what if another nurse assistant tells you that she is wearing one of Mrs. Wang's necklaces today? The nurse assistant tells you that Mrs. Wang has so many necklaces that she won't miss this one for just one day. The right thing for

you to do is to take steps to make sure the necklace is returned to its rightful owner as soon as possible.

Throughout this book you will read about the right way to do different nursing procedures so that you can provide care that meets the standard for quality. In this chapter, you will read about the legal rights of the people in your care and how you can help protect those rights. You also will read about your **ethical** responsibility to do what is morally right when providing care for people.

THE RIGHTS OF PEOPLE RECEIVING HEALTH CARE

Individuals living in the United States have certain individual rights. These rights are guaranteed by law, and no one can take them away. The Constitution and the Bill of Rights guarantee U.S. citizens the right to speak their thoughts freely, worship in any way they want (Figure 3-1), gather together in groups and decide freely what to print.

During our nation's history, many people have fought for legal rights by

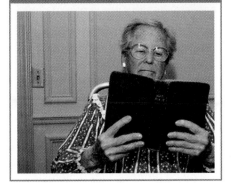

FIGURE 3-1 Resident rights guarantee a person's right to practice her or his own religion. As a nurse assistant, you are responsible for helping to protect this right for the people in your care.

writing letters, carrying signs and protesting in front of government buildings and marching down city streets. Because people are free to demonstrate for something they believe in, situations can be changed. Some changes today that were brought about by demonstration include the following: women have the right to vote; African Americans have rights to equal education, jobs and housing; children have the right to be protected from **abuse;** and minorities and the elderly have the right to be protected against discrimination.

A person's rights are protected by law because rights are crucial to a person's freedom. People who receive health care have these same rights and privileges. They are dependent on others for care; therefore, they have additional rights that are protected by special laws. These laws guarantee that people receiving health care have the right to competent, considerate care that is delivered with respect. They have the right to know the kind of care they will receive and the cost of that care, as well as the right to help decide about the care and who will provide it. In addition, people receiving health care now have the right to confidentiality and privacy and the right to be free from restraints and abuse. These rights about health care exist as law because many people, including families, friends and health care professionals, fought for and won them.

Today, when a person is admitted into a hospital, nursing home or home health care agency, signing a list of rights is part of that process. In the nursing facility, the rights are called **resident rights.** The rights of persons admitted to hospitals are called **patient rights,** and people receiving care at home have **client rights.** Discussing these rights helps consumers and their families know more about what they can expect.

Over the last several decades, as more people in our society grew older, the need increased for places to provide care for older people who could not take care of themselves because of mental and physical disabilities. Nursing homes evolved to fill this need. Initially, these facilities were not regulated, and families began to report that their loved ones were being tied in chairs, developing bedsores and experiencing other difficulties. It became clear that residents needed to know that they had specific rights under the law. These rights guaranteed that residents could be more involved in their care and make decisions about the care that they received. Ideas such as **informed consent** took on more meaning.

In 1991, the federal government passed the Patient Self-Determination Act. This law gives the person the right to make decisions about his or her care. It also requires hospitals, nursing homes and other health care facilities receiving Medicare and Medicaid funds to give residents written information that explains their rights. These rights include the right to accept or refuse care and to develop **advance medical directives.** An advance directive is a legal document stating how a person wants health decisions made if he or she is unable to make decisions alone in the future.

Let's suppose that Josie Miller, a resident in your care, wants to create a document that describes how she wants the medical staff to proceed if she is too ill to decide for herself. She tells you she does not want any life support. One document that can protect her rights is a **living will,** which gives specific directions about what steps to take or not take to prolong the person's life when death seems near (Figure 3-2). Some prefer that no steps be taken to prolong life at that point. If someone is unclear about his or her rights, you can arrange for the patient and family members to meet with the social worker or supervising nurse,

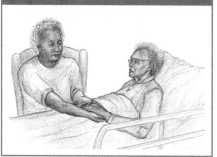

FIGURE 3-2 Josie Miller tells her sister Arlene about her living will, which states her decision not to be put on life support systems. Josie made this difficult decision so Arlene wouldn't have to decide for her.

who can provide a copy of these rights and explain them. Examples of a person's legal rights, along with specific things you can do to protect them, are listed in Table 3-1.

People who receive health care also have the right to name someone to make health care decisions for them if they become **incapacitated.** This is a specific type of advance directive called **durable power of attorney.** You and other members of the health care team are responsible for telling each patient, resident or client about this right. Anyone can use a legal document called a **health care proxy** to name a friend or family member to fill this role.

Protecting the rights of people receiving health care is one of your most important responsibilities as a nurse assistant, and you can help ensure that the person in your care does not give up any of these rights. It is important to remember that resident rights must never be violated. Even when all their rights are protected, residents may still have complaints. The resident has the right to a **grievance process,** whereby resi-

dents and families can challenge the care that is given and you as the nurse assistant must respond to these complaints. You may respond formally or informally, and you can help residents to voice and resolve their complaints (Table 3-2). Let's look at an example of an informal response.

Suppose that Mrs. Wang's granddaughter and her three children visit every Wednesday afternoon. The lively chatter annoys Mrs. Wang's roommate, Mrs. Ryan, who likes to nap after lunch. Mrs. Ryan complains to you about the noise. As a nurse assistant, you can help resolve this problem by negotiating informally with the two roommates. However, sometimes a more formal response is needed. We'll look at how to help in a more formal way in the next section.

ADVOCATING PATIENT RIGHTS

The person receiving care, the family and all members of the health care team need to know what the patient's rights are, how to protect them, how to promote them and how to report situations in which they have been violated. If a resident in a nursing home thinks that his or her rights are being violated, he or she can talk to the **resident council.** The resident council is a group made up of residents and residents' families who work together to solve problems, complaints and disagreements in the nursing home. Another group that can be used to **advocate** for the resident is the Long-Term Care Ombudsman Program. The federal government requires each state to have an ombudsman program that serves nursing homes. These **ombudsmen** are volunteers who act on behalf of nursing home residents and their loved ones to obtain a good quality of life in nursing homes. The most frequent complaints investigated by

TABLE 3-1 RESPECTING AND PROTECTING RIGHTS

A Person Has the Right to ...	You Can ...
Know his or her rights.	Remind the person to meet with your supervising nurse or the social worker to get a copy of the rights and discuss them.
Be treated with dignity and respect without discrimination because of race, color, sex, culture, sexual orientation, disability or diagnosis.	Call the person by name.
Receive considerate care.	Explain the care that you are going to provide. Get permission to provide care. Involve the person in his or her own care.
Have his or her needs met.	Do everything possible to take care of the person's needs.
Be told about his or her condition and what the doctor recommends for treatment (informed consent).	Communicate the person's needs to the other team members. Encourage the person to ask questions of the appropriate person.
Know the cost of care.	Refer the person to the social worker or the accounting department. Encourage the person and family members to ask about fees. Provide any literature about cost.
Refuse care or treatment and be given information about what may happen because he or she has refused treatment. Refuse to be part of experimental treatments.	Encourage the person to ask questions. Suggest getting a second opinion, if the person has the resources to pay for one. Offer to come back at a better time. Talk to your supervising nurse about changing the care plan. Work with him or her to rearrange scheduling to meet needs. Ask your supervisor to meet with the person to talk about what may happen if treatment is refused.
Keep records private and confidential and be able to see his or her own clinical record.	Keep information about the person to yourself when talking with people in or out of the hospital who are not involved in the person's care. Show the clinical record only to those who are authorized to see it.
Know, and have in writing, the services and items that are covered or not covered by Medicaid or Medicare.	Encourage the person to talk with the social worker and ask questions.
Be treated by the doctor and caregivers of choice.	Make sure your supervising nurse knows which caregivers the person prefers.
Know about own medical condition and be given current and complete information about the diagnosis, treatment, alternatives, risks, and prognosis.	Encourage the person to talk with your supervising nurse or the doctor and ask specific questions.
Know about all services and the frequency of visits, as well as help plan for care and treatment.	Involve the person and family members in writing the care plan. (Remember that the person is the head of the team.)

Continued

TABLE 3-1 RESPECTING AND PROTECTING RIGHTS continued

A Person Has the Right to ...	You Can ...
Make a complaint or suggest changes in health care services or staff without being threatened or discriminated against.	Communicate a complaint to your supervising nurse, and modify care to meet the person's needs.
Be free from abuse.	Treat everyone with dignity and respect. Report incidents of abuse.
Be free from restraints.	Never use restraints without a doctor's order.
Be told in writing if care is going to be denied, changed, or ended. Appeal when this situation occurs (in a nursing home or home health care setting).	Remind the person of the right to appeal and that someone who is not involved with the original decision will review the case.
Privacy.	Get permission to provide care. Keep the person covered, and pull the curtain when providing care. Ask permission to open bedside drawers and closets. Talk about the person's medical condition or personal affairs only with others who are authorized to know about it.
Manage his or her own money matters.	Never take money or gifts from the person in your care. Never discuss the person's finances. Refer the person to the social worker if he or she has concerns about finances.
Send and receive mail that has not been opened.	Deliver unopened mail to the person. Offer to help open or read mail.
Practice his or her religion.	Help the person get to religious services. Call the clergy of choice, if requested.
Use his or her own clothing or possessions.	Make sure the person gets clean clothes every day. In a nursing home, make sure the person's possessions are marked with his or her name.
Be alone with his or her partner or spouse.	Provide privacy. Help the person plan visiting time.

ombudsmen are accidents, neglect of personal hygiene, lack of respect for residents, poor staff attitudes and resident requests that go unanswered. Complaints to ombudsmen are treated confidentially and can be made by the resident, the family or you, the nurse assistant. The resident, patient or family must give the ombudsman permission to investigate any concern or complaint regardless of who reported the complaint (Figure 3-3). After receiving permission, the

ombudsman talks with those involved to find out what happened and asks questions to find out what action the nursing home has taken to ensure that the incident does not happen again. After an investigation of a problem, the ombudsman informs the appropriate person or agency so that the problem can be resolved. The ombudsman has the same goal that you have: to make sure the needs and rights of the people in your care are met.

PROTECTING PATIENTS' HEALTH INFORMATION

Patients have the right to have their medical information kept secure and private. As a nursing assistant you play an important role in helping to ensure that a patient's rights are protected. As a nurse assistant you may have access to patient information about health status, provision of health care, or payment for health care that can be linked to an individual. This is protected

TABLE 3-2 RESOLVING COMPLAINTS

Informal Responses ...	Formal Responses ...
Listen to resident's complaint.	Discuss the resident's complaint with the charge nurse or your supervisor.
Ask questions, using good communication skills to find out exactly what the problem is.	Suggest that the resident discuss the complaint with the resident council.
Tell the resident exactly what you will do to find a solution to the problem. This might include any of the formal responses.	Assist the resident in writing a letter of complaint to the facility administrator. Be involved in setting up or attending a meeting between the staff and the resident to resolve the problem.

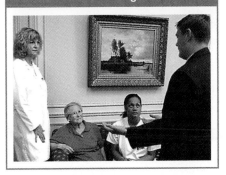

FIGURE 3-3 This ombudsman is helping to resolve a conflict about a room change.

healthcare information. This information is protected under the Health Insurance Portability and Accountability Act (HIPAA). In addition to rules covering how to protect patient information it includes rules covering administrative simplification, including making health care delivery more efficient. It applies to insurance companies as well—protecting patient's health care coverage for preexisting conditions and insurance underwriting. HIPAA also provides regulations for standardization of electronic transmittal of billing and claims information.

ETHICAL DECISIONS AND THE NURSE ASSISTANT

As a nurse assistant, you have a legal responsibility to protect a person's rights, which are guaranteed by law. If you do not protect these rights, you are breaking the law and may be sued or have other actions taken against you. When providing care for someone, you have another responsibility: to do what is right, meaning what is good or moral. As a caregiver, you must uphold the standards of healthcare workers, which are to help those in their care and to do no harm. Nurse assistants follow these standards when they practice the six principles of care. When you do what is right (that is, when you act in an ethical manner) and practice the six principles, you go beyond what is legally required.

Any behavior that could cause harm to a person, either physically or emotionally, is unethical. You may have to decide the right thing to do in situations involving people in your care. For example, one day Mr. Rivera is slightly injured when another nurse assistant accidentally catches Mr. Rivera's finger in the brake on his wheelchair. The

nurse assistant does not report the incident, so you have to decide whether to report it. If you do not report it, you may not be committing a crime. However, you will be acting in an unethical manner. Because you have witnessed Mr. Rivera's injury and the nurse assistant's failure to report it, you find yourself in an **ethical dilemma.**

Have you ever heard or read about an ethical dilemma in health care? Ethical dilemmas are problem situations in which health care workers must decide what solution is best for a person in their care (Figure 3-4). Some ethical dilemmas may have more than one good or moral solution. For example, ask yourself what you would do if Mr. Rivera's call signal came on 5 minutes before you had to leave for an inservice training. You know that he wants to use the toilet

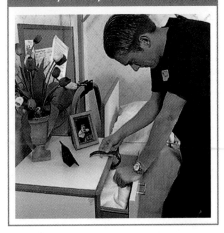

FIGURE 3-4 There are many possible reasons why this nurse assistant is taking Mr. Lightfoot's watch from his drawer. He may be taking it to the lock box for safekeeping; Mr. Lightfoot may have asked him to bring it to him in the dayroom; he may be stealing it. If you saw this nurse assistant taking someone's watch, what would you say to him?

and that it will take at least 10 minutes. One option is to ignore the light, but that would violate Mr. Rivera's safety, dignity and independence. Another option is to have him use the urinal. This would be a safe solution that also would allow you to get to the inservice training on time. The option Mr. Rivera prefers is using the bathroom toilet. This would provide for his safety, as well as his dignity and independence, but you would be late for the training. Another option is to ask a co-worker to take him to the bathroom. This option would provide Mr. Rivera with safety, dignity and independence and would also allow you to get to the inservice training on

time. In each option, you follow the six principles of care to help solve this ethical dilemma.

In your role as a protector of people's rights, you have both a legal and an ethical responsibility. Health care workers who do not act in legal and ethical ways may be held responsible for their actions in a court of law. Not only can they be prosecuted for illegal acts such as abuse, they can also be sued for **neglect** as well. To fulfill your legal responsibilities as a nurse assistant, you should know the legal rights of those in your care; to help make decisions about your ethical responsibilities, you should use your knowledge of the principles of care.

In Table 3-3 you can see examples of ethical situations that might arise. In each case, you can decide the right thing to do based on the principles of care.

Sometimes a situation will occur that is both illegal and ethically wrong. For example, you may see another nurse assistant pinch someone because he does not do what the nurse assistant wants. Not only is it ethically wrong to do anything to hurt a person intentionally, but this action also denies the person's right to be free from abuse and is illegal. It also is both illegal and ethically wrong to take anything that belongs to the person in your care, his or her family or your

TABLE 3-3 ETHICAL DECISIONS

Situation	What You Should Do	Principle
You are in a rush. Your hands are chapped, and you decide not to wash them just this once.	Always wash your hands. If your hands are chapped, use hand lotion and wear disposable gloves.	Infection control
Your friend Sue unintentionally drops Mrs. Compton's dentures. Only a small piece chips off one tooth.	Remind Sue to report every incident.	Safety, dignity
You would like to ask a person to use a bedpan instead of the bathroom because it is convenient for you.	Plan your care around the best interests of the person, not around your schedule or the amount of work involved.	Independence, dignity
A person tells you he hides his pills and does not take them. He shows you his stash because he trusts you.	Tell the person that you must report that he is not taking his pills and why. Tell him to discuss his medication with his doctor so that they can agree on what he needs and what he will take.	Safety, communication
Your day was busy, and several emergencies happened. You ran out of time to finish one person's exercise. You are new, and you do not want to admit that you did not finish that one task.	Report that you did not finish the person's exercise so that the nurse assistant on the next shift can finish it.	Communication
You are visiting a neighbor, who is also friends with a patient in the hospital where you work. The neighbor asks you what is wrong with her friend.	Tell your neighbor that you cannot give her this information.	Privacy

employer. In your job, you must protect the person in your care, as well as his or her belongings. What if you see someone else take something? If you do not report the incident to your supervising nurse, you may not be doing anything illegal, but you are doing something unethical, since your job also includes protecting the person in your care from other people's actions.

ABUSE, NEGLECT AND EXPLOITATION

One of a person's rights is freedom from abuse. It may be difficult for you to imagine that caregivers or family members would abuse someone who is dependent on them for care, but unfortunately, mistreatment occurs. When someone is hurt physically or emotionally by being treated unkindly, this action is called *abuse*. If someone is hurt because a caregiver fails to provide needed care, this lack of action is called *neglect*.

Abuse

Abuse happens in all parts of society. Abusers and victims of abuse can be male or female. They can be any age, be members of any race or practice any religion. Their families can have any cultural background, educational level or income. Residents in nursing facilities have the right to be free of all kinds of abusive treatment, from employees or other patients or residents. Residents experience **physical abuse** when their bodies are purposely hurt. **Emotional abuse** occurs when an employee teases a resident or when someone speaks to the person in a hurtful way. A resident experiences **sexual abuse** when anyone sexually molests him or her. Another type of abuse is **maltreatment,** which occurs when an employee provides poor or improper treatment or uses inappropriate responses; for example, isolating, confining or restraining a patient as a

disciplinary action. **Endangerment** results in a life-threatening situation caused by the inability of the threatened person to respond. For example, an employee gives a wheelchair-bound patient a shower in scalding water.

Anyone who depends on someone else for physical or emotional care is especially vulnerable, or open to being hurt. When you provide care for someone, you share the responsibility for keeping that person safe from abuse. If you are working in a hospital or nursing home, be alert for signs of abuse in patients or residents. As a nurse assistant, you have a legal responsibility to report abuse or neglect if you observe it or suspect that it is happening (Figure 3-5). States have laws that require you to report abuse that you witness or suspect. You are not responsible for investigating abuse; that is the responsibility of various state agencies, depending on the age of the person, where the incident took place and how serious the incident was. The name of the person making the report is kept confidential unless the person permits his or her name to be used or a court of law requires the person to testify. To be able to report it, you must know how to recognize the signs of abuse. Table 3-4 lists types of abuse, as well as signs that might tell you that someone is being abused.

Environmental Problems Leading To Abuse. A nursing home environment can contribute to abuse or neglect. Look out for things such as weak handrails, wet floors or missing floor tiles that can cause a resident to be injured. Seek out information and develop skills that will help you to recognize and deal with such situations, which, if overlooked, might lead to a charge of neglect. Other factors over which you may have less control, such as inadequate supervision and "short" staffing, can lead to increased frustra-

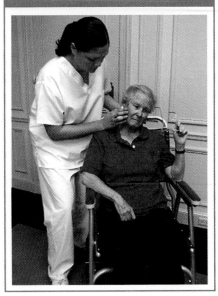

tion and stress; this, in turn, can lead to abusive behavior. Your personal stress may affect how you behave in certain situations. If you are able to control your behavior when you are under stress, and if you can recognize, report and correct environmental problems, you have taken steps to control and reduce the level of abuse in the facility where you work.

Neglect

Neglect is a specific form of abuse that can result in harm to the resident's health or welfare. Neglect is not something that someone *does* to a person. Instead, it is something that someone *fails to do* to or for a person. Neglect occurs when a person does not receive proper food, clothing, shelter, health care, supervision or human contact. Certain forms of neglect, such as ignoring someone or denying a person adequate food, can cause just as much physical and emotional pain as

TABLE 3-4 RECOGNIZING ABUSE

Types of Abuse	Signs of Abuse
Physical abuse Actions that include pushing, shoving, hair pulling, biting, kicking, choking and hitting.	A person who is physically abused may have burns, bruises, reddened areas that do not go away, scratches, cuts or bite marks. However, a person can be physically abused and *not* have any of these signs.
Emotional abuse Words and actions that lead to mental and emotional stress. These include verbal threats to harm or kill a person.	A person who is emotionally abused may not make eye contact; may be withdrawn, sad or fearful; or may shield himself or herself or become upset when the abuser enters the room.
Sexual abuse Actions that include rape; physical handling of the victim's breasts, buttocks or genitals; or forced sexual activity of any kind.	A person who is sexually abused may have bruises, scratches and cuts around the breasts, buttocks or genitals; may have vaginal or rectal bleeding; or may refuse personal care.

other forms of abuse. Neglect also occurs when a resident is restrained without a doctor's order. You must know how to recognize neglect. A person who is neglected may have poor personal care: dirty hair, body odor, dirty fingernails, crusty eyes, bleeding gums or lips or food in his or her teeth. His or her clothing or bedding may be dirty, he or she may be depressed and withdrawn, and he or she may refuse food or personal care.

Exploitation

When misuse of a resident's money or property occurs, this is called **exploitation.** For example, you are in the lunchroom listening to music on a radio. You ask another nurse assistant in the room about the radio. She says she borrowed it from Mr. Rivera's room while he was sleeping and intends to take it back. She is exploiting Mr. Rivera because she is using his property, not for his advantage but for her own. Using another person's money is

another form of exploitation. You might see or hear something that makes you suspect that a person in your care is being exploited. If you do, you should report your suspicions to your supervising nurse.

LEGAL DECISION AND THE NURSE ASSISTANT

Your Role in Reporting Abuse, Neglect or Exploitation

Whenever you see or hear something that makes you suspect possible abuse, neglect or exploitation, you must report it immediately to your supervising nurse. This is your legal and professional responsibility. Abuse and neglect are very disturbing situations. You may be afraid to report your suspicions about them, but it is important that you do. You may be helping the person in your care out of a dangerous situation. The abuser also needs help to learn not to try to control others by harm-

ing them. By reporting the abuser, you may be preventing future abuse of others. If you discover a situation similar to any of the ones described here, you might want to spend some time talking about your feelings with your supervising nurse or staff social worker.

You always want to do what is best for the person in your care. There may be times when you are unsure whether abuse has actually occurred; in these circumstances it is best to make the mistake on the side of reporting. Sometimes doing your best may mean waiting patiently while the situation is being investigated, and that may take a long time. Try not to be too frustrated by the amount of time it takes to find out what is really going on. Abuse and neglect are serious charges and must be investigated carefully. If you are aware of a situation, keep that information between you and the parties involved.

Circle the correct answers and fill in the blanks.

1. A privilege that belongs to a person and is protected by law is called a ___Right___

2. A person in your care says he does not understand the medical procedure he is supposed to have tomorrow. You should:
   a. tell him not to worry about it.
   b. tell him it will be painless.
   c. tell your supervising nurse about his concerns.
   d. tell your supervising nurse that he is afraid of the procedure.

3. When you bring mail to the person in your care, it should be:
   a. unopened.
   b. opened.
   c. read to him.
   d. tossed on the pile with other mail.

4. A ___health care proxy___ is a legal document in which a person names a friend or family member to make health care decisions for him if he becomes too ill to decide for himself.

5. The person who is charged with the responsibility to listen to, investigate and correct problems at a nursing home is an ___ombudsmen___

6. If you do what is right based on the six principles of care, you are acting in an ___ethical___ manner.

7. You notice that each time Jerry gets Mrs. Little ready for bed, he touches her breast. You mention this to another nurse assistant, who says, "Jerry is just friendly. He fools around with all of us." She also says, "Mrs. Little is so out of it she wouldn't notice it and I'm sure Jerry doesn't mean any harm." What should you do? ___immediatley report to nurse___

8. A person who is deprived of food, clothing shelter or human contact suffers from ___neglect___.

9. The identity of a person making a report is kept ___confidential___

1. *What would you do if you overheard another nurse assistant telling her friend about Mrs. Davis, for whom she is providing care?*

2. *You are providing care for Miss Eller. She is dying. She says she would like for you to have the expensive ring that is lying on her dresser. What should you say?*

3. *You see a co-worker slapping a person in her care. What should you do?*

4. *You meet some people in the grocery store who recognize you as the nurse assistant who is providing care for their aunt, Mary. They ask you specific questions about her medical condition. How do you reply?*

5. *Today, when you provide care for Mrs. Morelli, a patient who has multiple sclerosis, you notice that she is covered with bruises. When you ask her how she got the bruises, she begins to cry and begs you to promise not to tell anyone. What should you do?*

6. *You are providing care for a woman who believes it is wrong for anyone to view her unclothed body. She has the right to refuse a bath, but she needs one, and it is part of your job requirement. What would you do?*

7. *The person in your care is a vegetarian. A dish of beef stew is on his supper tray. What would you do?*

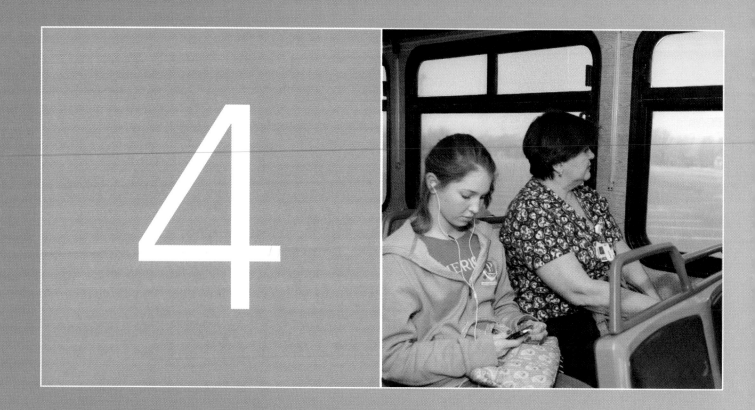

4

Chapter 4

Understanding People

GOALS

After reading this chapter, you will have the information needed to:

Recognize factors that can influence the way human beings behave.

Name four stages of the life cycle.

Describe one common behavior in each stage of the life cycle.

Identify three developmental tasks of aging.

Identify five basic human needs and give examples of each.

Describe one way a nurse assistant can meet each of the five basic needs.

Discuss the factors that make up human sexuality.

Develop strategies for responding to sexual behaviors.

Today you are on a crowded bus, riding home after a long workday at Morningside Nursing Home. You are surrounded by people you have never met, and you wonder what they're like. You watch what they're doing: Some are reading, some are dozing off to sleep, one woman is knitting, and two young people are kissing. You think: Why do people do what they do? You often ask this question about the people in your care: Why does Mrs. Wang look down when you enter the room? Why does Josie Miller insist that everyone call her by her first name? Why do Mr. Lightfoot and Mr. Wilson argue about when each will have time alone in their shared room? It seems you have to deal with someone's behavior every day. This situation reminds you of two residents arguing today about whose turn it was to buy the newspaper. They were arguing in the dayroom where everyone could hear them. You noticed that some people in the dayroom continued what they were doing as if nothing were happening, while others seemed to be embarrassed as they shifted uneasily in their chairs.

As you look around, you see many people who appear to have different ethnic backgrounds. You also see people wearing business suits, uniforms and jeans. Some people carry briefcases, tote bags and lunch boxes. Some wear wedding rings and some don't. Some look relaxed, while others look upset. You wonder what has happened in their lives that makes them who they are today. The people in your care also have different ethnic backgrounds and behave differently from one another. One woman likes to dress every day in her finest clothes and jewelry, while another woman refuses to wear anything but her nightgown and robe. One man has visitors several times each week, but his roommate has never had a visitor. Some people smile and talk pleasantly; others grumble or lie in bed and moan. You wish you knew more about why people do what they do.

KEY TERMS

adolescence: (add-uh-LES-ense) the period between the ages of 12 and 20 when a person becomes more interested in sex and begins to have relationships with other people.

adolescent: (add-uh-LES-ent) a person between the ages of 12 and 20.

behavior: (be-HAYV-yur) the way a person acts or conducts him- or herself. Anything a person does that can be observed and described.

body image: (IM-ij) a person's attitude toward his or her own body.

cognitive: (KOG-nuh-tiv) relating to thinking, understanding, remembering, believing, learning and creating.

demeaning: (duh-MEEN-ing) something that lowers someone's dignity.

emotional: (ee-MO-shun-uhl) relating to how a person feels and how he or she expresses him- or herself.

erection: (uh-REK-shun) a stiffening of the penis.

esteem: (es-TEEM) a high regard for someone.

frail: very slender and fragile.

gender: (JEN-der) view or perception of something as having masculine or feminine qualities.

genitals: (JEN-uh-tuhls) male and female external sex organs.

handedness: the tendency to use one hand more frequently than the other.

human development: (HUE-men/de-VEL-up-ment) the physical, social, emotional and cognitive changes a person experiences as he or she grows older.

human needs: basic requirements that enable a person to live healthfully and happily.

infancy: (IN-fan-see) the first stage of life. The word infant literally means "unable to speak."

intimacy: need and ability to feel closeness to another person and to have that closeness returned.

life cycle: (SI-kuhl) the stages of aging and development experienced as a person grows older.

masturbation: touching oneself to achieve an orgasm and release sexual tension.

physical: (FIZ-uh-kul) relating to the body.

sensuality: awareness and/or enjoyment in the way one's body looks, feels and behaves.

sex: being male or female.

sexual harassment: (SEK-shew-uhl/HAIR-as-ment or har-ASS-ment) purposely annoying or threatening someone by not respecting his or her sex or sexuality.

sexuality: (sek-shue-AL-uh-tee) a basic human need for sexual pleasure and sexual expression.

social: (SO-shul) relating to the way people interact with each other.

stage: (STAYJ) a defined and predictable period.

theory: (THEE-o-ree) an explanation based on observation and reasoning.

HUMAN BEHAVIOR

Have you ever asked yourself, "Now, why did I do that?" Or have you wondered why someone else did something? *Behind every behavior is a reason.* You may never know the exact reason why someone does something, but when you understand some general factors that can influence behavior, you will know how to respond appropriately and how to provide better care.

What is **behavior**? Behavior is what people do; it is how they act or conduct themselves. As a nurse assistant, you see different kinds of people who behave in many different ways. An example of simple behavior is a newborn baby sucking on a nipple or finger. A child who cries and asks for a peanut butter sandwich is behaving in a more complicated way. And a nursing home resident who steals money from his roommate's nightstand or wanders into another resident's room in the middle of the night is behaving in an even more complicated manner. What in a person's life might influence these various behaviors? Most factors that influence the way people behave can be categorized as either *physical, social, emotional* or *cognitive.*

First, let's look at behavior influenced by **physical** factors. Each person's body affects his behavior, and his behavior affects his body. (See Appendix B, "Body Basics.") Some behaviors are automatic, such as coughing, yawning and blinking. Others are responses to physical needs. For example, when a child cries and asks for a certain type of food, she may be responding to a physical need or desire for food (Figure 4-1). Other physical needs include sleep, air, water and exercise. A later section of this chapter describes these physical needs in greater detail. Biological factors such as heredity, **handedness** (the tendency to use one hand more frequently than the other) and gender are also physical reasons for behavior, as are certain ill-

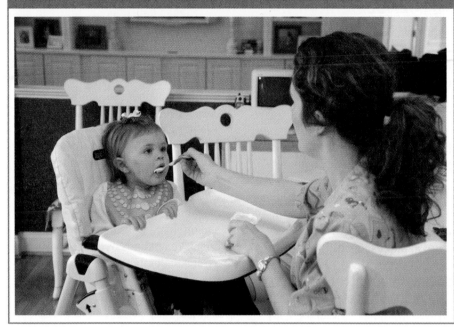

FIGURE 4-1 By offering a familiar food, this nurse assistant is comforting the child, as well as meeting her physical need for food.

nesses, which you will read about in Appendix B, "Body Basics."

Social factors also influence a person's behavior. A child who is a patient in a hospital may cry when his parents leave his bedside. Or a teenager may be hospitalized for an overdose of alcohol because his friends dared him to drink an entire bottle of vodka in a short period of time. Other people may behave in certain ways because they want approval from their parents, teachers or co-workers, or because they want to impress a spouse or life partner.

A strong social factor that influences a person's behavior is family. When Mr. Rivera lived at home, he and his family members ate large amounts of fried foods, which was not good for their health. But, even after the doctor told Mr. Rivera to change his diet, he continued to eat the same things because that's what his family had always eaten. A final social factor that influences a person's behavior is **gender.** Gender is different from **sex**: sex is a biological factor; gender is a

social classifying of certain behaviors as being "masculine" or "feminine."

A person's behavior also may be influenced by **emotional** factors (or the way he or she feels). The resident who stole money from his roommate may have felt upset because the next day was his grandson's birthday and he didn't have money or a gift to give him. Another person may feel angry and throw a plate of food on the floor, and still another may feel sad and curl up in bed.

When the resident stole the money, his behavior was also influenced by **cognitive** factors. He *remembered* that his grandson was coming to visit him. He may have *known* the roommate kept cash in the nightstand drawer. He may have *thought* no one was watching him. And he may have *believed* it was okay to take some of his roommate's money without asking.

These four factors can be looked at more extensively by exploring them in the following ways: *growth and development, needs* and *sexuality.*

HOW HUMAN GROWTH AND DEVELOPMENT INFLUENCE BEHAVIOR

All people move on the same basic track through life. They begin as infants, then grow into children, develop into teens, mature into adults and become old. The movement people make from one **stage** to the next is called the **life cycle,** and the changes they go through are called *human growth and development* (Figure 4-2).

Human growth refers to physical changes, such as growing bigger and cutting teeth in infancy or growing taller and developing breasts or a beard in **adolescence**. These physical changes occur along with changes in the size and structure of the human body as it ages. The endocrine and nervous systems regulate the body's growth. (See the sections on the nervous and endocrine systems in Appendix B, "Body Basics.")

Human development refers to all the changes that occur in the way a person looks, relates to others, feels and thinks as he grows from **infancy** to old age. These changes are called *social, emotional* and *cognitive*—we have looked at examples of these already. Social changes occur in the way a person relates to other people. Emotional changes occur in the way a person feels and how he or she expresses those feelings. Social and emotional changes are closely linked and often are considered together. Cognitive changes occur in the way a person understands the world: the way he or she thinks, remembers, believes, solves problems, learns and creates.

We can predict differences in behavior that occur at certain stages in a person's life and recognize the differences in the things she or he does. For example, adult women ages 50 to 60 differ from teen and young adult women in many ways. One of the most notable differences is that they generally do not have babies. Physically most women are not capable of becoming pregnant after about age 55 because they no longer menstruate. Emotionally, socially and cognitively they focus on other things, such as careers, volunteer interests, friends, older children and grandchildren and leisure activities. However, this behavior is not set in stone.

How Do Growth and Development Occur?

Certain things about human growth and development apply at every stage in the life cycle. Human growth and development are continuous processes that occur in the same order and follow the same pattern for all human beings. All people must go through each stage in the same order because each stage includes progress that is needed for the next stage. However, people may go through stages at different ages because people grow and develop at different rates.

Human growth and development move from head to foot. Newborn babies' heads, for example, are much larger than any other part of their bodies. Later, their bodies begin to grow faster than their heads. Growth and development also move from the simple to the complex. Preschoolers learn to jump with both feet before they can hop on one foot alone. When developing language, they use one word by itself at first, then put two words together, and then speak in whole sentences.

Human *growth* is influenced by physical changes inside the body, whereas human *development* is influ-

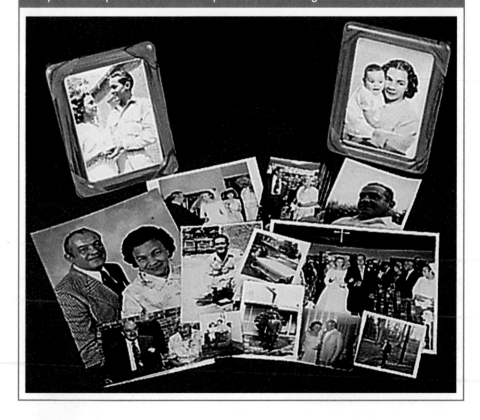

FIGURE 4-2 When you provide care for older people, remember that they have experienced all the previous life stages.

enced by conditions in which people live. These physical and external factors frequently work together. For instance, the process of learning to walk is influenced by both growth and development. Some of the major physical factors that must be present before a person can walk are a functioning nervous system, adequate muscle strength in the lower body and well-formed spine, legs and feet. The increasing need to be independent, the encouragement of caregivers and other external factors also contribute to a person's developmental readiness to walk.

Each stage of human development emphasizes a particular type of behavior. For example, schoolage children seem to spend most of their time and energy practicing physical skills, such as building, playing sports and making crafts. Young **adolescents,** on the other hand, are much more focused on practicing social skills, such as dancing, talking with their friends and getting into, or out of, relationships (Figure 4-3).

Scientists who study human growth and development divide the process into eight separate stages: *infancy, toddlerhood, preschool age, school age, adolescence, young adult years, middle adult years* and *older adult years*. They define each stage of growth and development by certain distinctive characteristics. These characteristics are guidelines to help you understand a little about each stage in the life cycle. Depending on where you work in the health care system, you may provide care for people of all ages, for adults only, or mostly for very old people. It is important not to confuse *ages* with *stages,* because *there is no definite time when someone can or should be able to do something.* Box 4-1 provides a description and the basic characteristics of each stage according to the kinds of changes that occur—physical, social/emotional and cognitive. It is important to remember that these

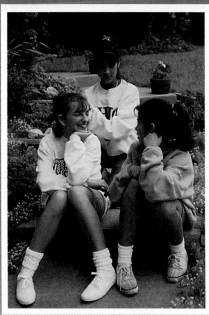

FIGURE 4-3 To a young adolescent, acceptance by her friends is so important that she may go to great lengths to look, act and talk the same way they do.

characteristics are general guidelines, not rules.

For the most part, this book focuses on older adults. The "older adult years" is a normal stage in the life cycle, and it is the last stage. As people move through their older adult years, they typically wrestle with certain necessities as the end of life approaches. If you work with this age group, it is important for you to know that older adults struggle with accepting the reality of being old, fulfilling their responsibility to themselves and others as they approach the end of life and exercising their rights in spite of their age.

In accepting reality, an older adult such as Mr. Rivera struggles as he gets used to his physical limitations, develops new relationships when his loved ones die, asks for and accepts help and prepares for death. He fulfills

responsibilities by planning for his survivors, budgeting his income and energy to meet everyday needs, choosing how to spend the rest of his life, and assuming as much responsibility for his own care as possible. At the same time, Mr. Rivera must exercise his right to move at his own pace, have privacy (even when he is being cared for by another person), be treated with respect and dignity, refuse certain kinds of care or treatment and participate in plans and decisions about his life.

Why Nurse Assistants Must Understand Human Growth and Development

As a nurse assistant, you come into contact with people at all ages of life and all stages of growth and development. You may respond differently to someone's behavior when you understand what stage of development may be influencing that behavior. For example, you are not surprised when a 2-year-old child occasionally throws temper tantrums and shouts "No" when you try to do something for him. You also expect an adolescent to be very concerned about what his friends will think, and you will take these feelings into consideration when providing care. Because a 30-year-old husband and father has different responsibilities from those of an 85-year-old man, you might anticipate the younger man to react differently to a diagnosis of chronic arthritis and foresee a need for special services and counseling for him.

HOW BASIC HUMAN NEEDS INFLUENCE BEHAVIOR

Now that we have a clear idea of the effects of human growth and development on behavior, let's turn our attention to the basic human needs. To live and to be healthy and happy, people

BOX 4-1

CHARACTERISTICS OF THE EIGHT STAGES OF HUMAN GROWTH AND DEVELOPMENT

Infancy (birth to 1 year).

When babies are born, they have been growing and developing since conception, about 9 months. At birth babies are called *neonates*, and by the time they are 1 month old, they are called *infants,* which describes this first official stage of growth and development—infancy.

Areas of Change	During Infancy a Person...
Physical	Triples weight and increases length by 10 inches at 1 year. Begins to control body movement: Lifts head at 1 month; holds and throws objects and puts them in mouth; rolls over, sits up, crawls, climbs, takes first steps with assistance; and stands at 1 year. Begins cutting teeth and taking solid food at 6 months.
Social/Emotional	Cries to communicate. Smiles by 3 months. Trusts caregivers at 6 months. Cries at sight of strangers at 7 months.
Cognitive	Uses senses to explore the world. Sees well at 2 months. Explores with fingers and mouth at 5 months. At first, knowledge of the world is based on physical interactions/experiences. Symbolic abilities are developed at the end of this stage. Can say a few short words at 1 year.

Toddlerhood (1 to 3 years).

Toddlers are children who, at the beginning of this stage, are not very steady on their feet. By their first birthday many young children are not yet able to stand alone. However, by age 3, these same children are climbing, running and jumping, feeding and dressing themselves and talking in sentences.

Areas of Change	During Toddlerhood a Person...
Physical	Usually walks alone by 15 months. Does many things that require coordination of large muscles in arms and legs: runs, jumps and climbs. Plays with toys. Has 6 to 12 baby teeth and eats regular table food. Learns to use the toilet and eats, drinks and dresses with little or no help. Needs to rest frequently during the day.
Social/Emotional	Does not share toys. Likes to play alone or side by side with another child. Does not like to take orders. Learns to be independent. Throws temper tantrums when desires are not met. May be afraid when left alone.
Cognitive	Responds fairly well to adult language. Points to objects named by adults. Beginning to understand symbols. Has a strong, self-oriented point of view and is unable to understand others' points of view. Follows simple instructions when given slowly and clearly. Begins to put words together to make short sentences. Understands that objects taken out of sight still exist. Likes to choose own activities and toys.

BOX 4-1

CHARACTERISTICS OF THE EIGHT STAGES OF HUMAN GROWTH AND DEVELOPMENT (continued)

Preschool Age (3 to 5 years).

Preschool children seem like miniature adults at times. They can do most things for themselves, have friends, may go to nursery school or kindergarten, can hold very interesting conversations and spend a great deal of time "pretending" to be grown-ups. However, they still see the world through young children's eyes and imagine and fear things adults know cannot be possible.

Areas of Change	During Preschool Age a Person...
Physical	Has improved large-motor skills. Has more control over small-motor skills such as drawing and writing. Combines several motor skills into one project or activity. Does many things to take care of self such as dressing, eating and using the toilet.
Social/Emotional	Has a strong sense of identity. Responds to messages about self received from parents and other adults. Is more independent than a toddler. Makes own choices. Plays easily with other children and enjoys games involving sharing and taking turns. Looks up to and imitates adults. Likes routine and may feel insecure if schedule is changed too often.
Cognitive	Knows many words and names of people, places and things. Learns new words quickly. Begins to read some words before age 5. Counts and enjoys learning things with numbers. Groups objects that are alike. Picks out objects that do not fit with others. Follows directions. Has strong curiosity and imagination. Asks many questions. Has a strong, self-oriented point of view and sometimes is unable to understand others' points of view.

School Age (5 to 12 years).

School-age children come in all sizes and shapes and behave in many different ways. During school years children develop skills and grow at different rates. Because no two children have the same experiences, they behave differently.

Areas of Change	During School Age a Person...
Physical	Grows steadily. (Females usually reach adult height by age 12.) Is physically well coordinated. Uses large muscles for games and sports, cycling and dance. Develops muscle tone, balance, strength and endurance. Uses small muscles to write, draw and do crafts. Enters puberty at about age 10 to 12 for girls and age 12 for boys.
Social/Emotional	Begins to form lasting relationships with friends. Spends more time away from parents. Forms small, close-knit groups that exclude other children, especially those of the opposite sex. Begins to understand that other people also have feelings. Has many emotions and sometimes has difficulty expressing them. May have dramatic mood swings that accompany hormonal changes when going through puberty.

Continued

BOX 4-1

CHARACTERISTICS OF THE EIGHT STAGES OF HUMAN GROWTH AND DEVELOPMENT (continued)

Cognitive   Pays attention longer, remembers longer, and follows more complex directions. Thinks logically and makes decisions about the "real" world. Operational thinking develops (mental actions that are reversible). Starts to organize new information in meaningful ways. Behaves more responsibly. May question and resist adult decisions.

Adolescence (12 to 20 years).

During adolescence, children leave their childhood ways behind and gradually move into adulthood. Their bodies reach full size during these years, and their minds begin to work like those of adults. Social and emotional experiences are intense because this is a time to deal with strong friendships and early love relationships. Some adolescents begin parenting children of their own.

Areas of Change   *During Adolescence a Person...*

Physical   Reaches reproductive maturity. In the female, breasts develop, hips widen, pubic and underarm hair appears and menstruation begins. In the male, penis and testes grow to adult size, ejaculations begin, pubic and facial hair develops, voice deepens and neck and shoulders grow. Girls tend to be taller than boys of the same age at the beginning of this age range and tend to be shorter at the end.

Social/Emotional   Feels awkward around adults and strangers because of recent changes in his or her body. Gets embarrassed easily if he or she has to undress in front of an adult or talk about body, growth or sexual development. Assumes more responsibility for own behavior. Often rebels against adult authority.

Cognitive   Thinks logically. Learns about and deals with the abstract or possible. Thinks about himself or herself privately. Plans for the future. Imagines alternatives when making a decision, which makes decision making more difficult. Becomes more self-conscious. Tries to change physical image. Imagines an ideal world and ideal self. Is easily disappointed and discouraged. May set unreasonable goals.

Young Adult Years (20 to 45 years).

For most people, the young adult years are years filled with beginnings: living on one's own away from parents, starting a career, beginning a sexual relationship with someone who may be a life partner and marrying or living with one person. Many adults begin a family by conceiving or adopting children.

Areas of Change   *During the Young Adult Years a Person...*

Physical   Has all body functions fully developed by age 23. (Most women are fully grown by age 17; about 10 percent continue to grow until age 21. Most men are fully grown by age 21; about 10 percent continue to grow until age 23.) Reaches peak of muscular strength between ages 25 and 30 and then strength begins to decrease. Has

BOX 4-1

CHARACTERISTICS OF THE EIGHT STAGES OF HUMAN GROWTH AND DEVELOPMENT (continued)

	best small-motor skills until about age 35, then these skills decrease. Has sharpest senses at about age 20, then senses gradually decrease. Is healthiest of population. Gets sick infrequently. Recovers more quickly. Continues to menstruate and may bear children, if female.
Social/Emotional	Establishes lasting and intimate relationships with friends and partners. Makes commitments. (Most men and women marry by age 30. Many adults become parents. Some struggle with infertility. Some voluntarily choose not to become parents. Still others choose celibacy.)
Cognitive	Functions at higher level than children and adolescents, although some young adults continue to think and reason much like adolescents and children. Is able to put self in another's place and imagine how the other feels. Has better-developed moral reasoning.

Middle Adult Years (45 to 65 years).
Middle-aged adults experience the satisfaction of enjoying what they began in their 20s and 30s. Their careers are often at their peak, children are growing or grown, finances may be secure enough to allow for more leisure time and health and vitality have not yet begun to fade. For many people, the middle adult years are the "prime" years of their lives.

Areas of Change	During the Middle Adult Years a Person...
Physical	May develop chronic illnesses. (Some find that existing health conditions disappear or become less problematic.) Has slight sensory ability loss. Has slight loss in physical strength and coordination. Has occasional difficulty sleeping and eating certain foods. Goes through menopause between the ages of 45 and 55, if the person is female.
Social/Emotional	Begins to feel anxious about aging. Begins to become aware of mortality and death. Feels more satisfied by work. May become depressed as children grow up and leave or may delight in the new freedom.
Cognitive	Increases in mental growth and has high levels of intellectual performance. Can learn new skills. Finds this is often the most creative time of life and may pursue adult education.

Older Adult Years (65 years and older).
In our society, older adults often are called *senior citizens, golden agers* or *the elderly* in an attempt to avoid calling them *old*. Even though most older adults still lead healthy, productive lives, being old often is seen as a negative experience, and few people want to admit to being old.

Continued

BOX 4-1

CHARACTERISTICS OF THE EIGHT STAGES OF HUMAN GROWTH AND DEVELOPMENT (continued)

Areas of Change	During the Older Adult Years a Person...
Physical	Is likely to experience more chronic illnesses, such as high blood pressure. Is generally healthy enough to continue normal physical activities. Has decrease in vision, with loss of night vision and less depth and color perception. Experiences some hearing loss and a decreased sense of smell and taste. Has less strength and balance and is prone to accidents and falling. Is noticeably shorter because of spinal column shrinkage. Adjusts less quickly to cold.
Social/Emotional	May experience old age as positive and feel increased energy, productivity and creativity, although the negative attitudes of younger generations can make this stage less than pleasant. May have strong desire to make a will and have strong attachment to familiar objects. May have increased awareness of time and life cycle. May be less confident and have lower self-esteem because of loss of loved ones, work roles, and physical and sensory capabilities. May have more clearly defined personality and values. Has continued need for friendships and other relationships. May have a need for the companionship of a pet. Continues sex life if he or she was sexually active earlier.
Cognitive	Generally maintains intellectual abilities, although may not process information as quickly. Makes decisions with less speed. Is able to learn new information and skills but needs more time to learn. May experience some memory loss as a result of external conditions, such as medication or the need to move to a new residence, or because of physical or emotional reasons, such as poor nutrition, depression or illness.

need certain things, such as food, sleep and air. These things are called **human needs.** How these needs are met varies from person to person.

Mrs. Ryan is one of the easiest residents to provide care for, even though she is one of the oldest. Her health is good and she eats well, drinks a lot of water, uses the bathroom regularly, exercises, gets lots of fresh air and rests and sleeps well. She enjoys living at the nursing home, dresses and grooms herself every day, socializes with the other residents and enjoys talking with several friends and

relatives who visit her each week. She also prides herself on her quiltmaking, as well as on the number of books she reads each month. She may be older, but she still enjoys life.

On the other hand, Josie Miller, who is 9 years younger than Mrs. Ryan, is very **frail.** Some days she refuses to eat because she says she is too tired. Yet, at night, she doesn't sleep well. Because she is frail and often tired, she doesn't exercise much and seldom goes outside for fresh air. She spends much of her time in her room or dozing off in the dayroom.

She doesn't socialize as much with the other residents as she once did, except for Jack Williams, who has become her special friend. When Josie's friends and relatives visit, she often dozes off, so now they don't come as often as they once did (Figure 4-4).

There are other differences in these two patients as well. Look closely at how each responds to some of the basic human needs. Both Mrs. Ryan and Josie need food, but each responds differently when you bring her food tray. Mrs. Ryan

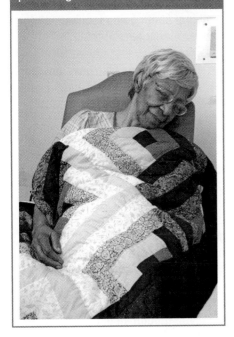

FIGURE 4-4 Josie uses all her energy just to try to manage her activities of daily living—eating, bathing, dressing, moving and using the bathroom—so she has little energy left for socializing or pursuing other interests.

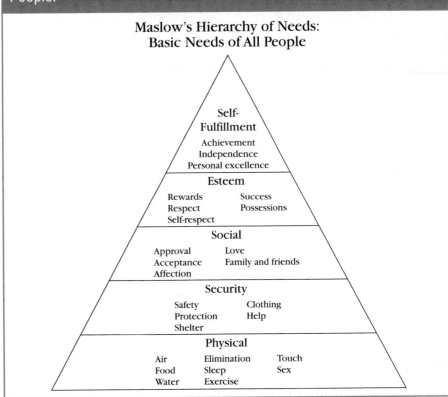

FIGURE 4-5 Maslow's Hierarchy of Needs: Basic Needs of All People.

smiles, says, "Thank you," and begins to eat with enthusiasm. Josie turns her head away and says, "I just want to sleep." Mrs. Ryan eats her full meal, and Josie usually picks at her food. Both are responding to their need for food, but in different ways.

Many years ago, Abraham Maslow, a famous psychologist, studied how people feel and behave. He spent many years trying to find out what people need to live and be happy and to grow in a healthy way. He developed a **theory** about people and their needs. *Maslow's theory is only one theory on human needs*, and it focuses on what motivates people. Some of what he learned appears in Figure 4-5.

Maslow learned that people have needs on different levels, beginning with physical needs and moving to self-fulfillment needs. People need to have the lower-level needs met before they can think about higher-level needs. When people struggle to have their physical needs met, they put their higher-level needs in the back of their minds. For example, you may come to class one day feeling very tired. If the need is great enough, you might fall asleep. You may be somewhat concerned about whether your action upsets your instructor or classmates, but your basic physical need is more important at that time than your social need.

The people in your care have physical needs. They, too, do not concern themselves with higher-level needs until their physical needs are met. For example, a person who needs

to use the toilet immediately may not worry about being polite to others. A person who feels nauseated probably does not care about going to physical therapy.

As a nurse assistant, you play a large role in helping people meet their physical, security, social and esteem needs. As these needs are met, the person turns inward to meet the self-fulfillment need on his or her own.

Physical Needs

Physical needs are a person's most basic bodily needs and are what he or she needs to be able to live. The most important physical needs are air to breathe, food to eat and water to drink. Everyone also needs to sleep, exercise, eliminate body waste and experience human touch.

If you stay up late several days in a row, you know how much you need sleep and rest. And if you have ever been sick in bed for a week or more, you know how hard it is to begin to move around and exercise when you get better. The people in your care also need exercise, rest and sleep. As a health care worker, you can help those in your care meet these needs by making sure that they exercise and participate in activities during the day and by providing them with quiet time in the evening. You can provide a person with a comforting item, such as an afghan or pillow, or a favorite teddy bear for a child. You can further enhance a person's sleep time by giving a back massage, turning lights down or off and creating a quiet environment with closed doors and limited noise and discussion at the nurse's station.

Another basic human need is going to the bathroom or eliminating wastes from the body. Satisfying other basic needs may be put off for a day or longer, but eliminating body wastes cannot be put off for a long time.

Being touched by another person is also a physical need. Think of a time when you had a bad day. Nothing went right. You were feeling really bad. Then a friend came along and gave you a big hug. How did you feel then? The people in your care also need to receive a hug, a pat on the arm or a squeeze of the hand. This physical need for touch is one that people often forget about. To live and to be well, people need the touch of others.

Health care workers know that, even if healthy babies get enough food, water, rest and exercise, they get sick and eventually die if they are left alone and not held. Babies need to be held and touched. Sick people in hospitals and older people in nursing homes also get well sooner and stay healthier when they are touched by other people. They have a need to be touched by health care workers, family members and friends (Figure 4-6).

Touch is important, but it is also very personal. Some people do not

like to be touched by anyone outside their families or circles of close friends. People from certain cultures may have strong feelings about being touched. For example, in Southeast Asia, touching a child on the head is a **demeaning** act, while in the United States such an act can be a sign of affection or approval. When you provide care to people, ask them how they feel about being touched, and then ask what kind of touch is acceptable.

Human beings also have another physical need—a sexual need. Even sick, disabled, old and dying people have sexual needs. Sexual needs do not end when people reach a certain age. They do not end when people lose the use of their legs or develop illnesses. People do not need to express their sexual feelings daily, but, like the need for food and water, sexual needs are always there. The best way you can help people in your care meet their sexual needs is to provide privacy and have an accepting attitude.

Even though all people have the same physical needs, they do not have them at the same times. One person may be hungry and need to eat, while someone who feels nauseated may need to eat but does not want to. One person may need to go for a walk, while someone else may need to sleep. It is part of your job to find out the physical needs of each person in your care. Table 4-1 contains examples of ways you can help people in your care meet their physical needs.

Security Needs

People whose basic physical needs are reasonably well met begin to want their needs for security met. For most people, security means feeling safe and comfortable. We all need shelter, clothing, safety and someone who can help when we need assistance. What would make you feel more secure in

FIGURE 4-6 This nurse assistant knows how important touch and affection are.

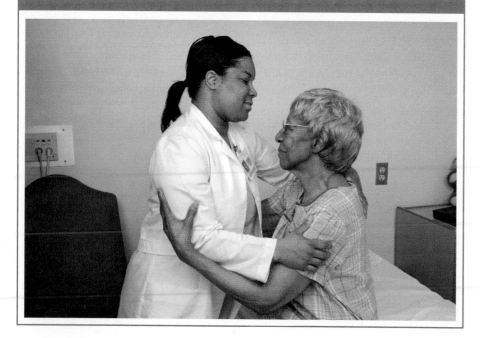

TABLE 4-1 MEETING PHYSICAL NEEDS

To Help Meet the Need for...	You can...
Air	Tell your supervising nurse if a person is having trouble breathing
Food	Serve a person's meals. Check food's temperature.
Water	Refill a water glass.
Elimination	Answer call signals immediately.
Sleep	Report any sleeping troubles.
Exercise	Help a person with prescribed exercises. Help someone walk.
Touch	Touch someone's arm and make eye contact as you pass. Encourage family members to touch and hug the person.
Sex	Provide privacy.

TABLE 4-2 MEETING NEEDS FOR SECURITY

To Help Meet the Need for...	You can...
Safety	Lock wheelchair brakes when chair is still. Answer call signals quickly. Make sure eyeglasses are used, if needed.
Protection	Check often on someone who cannot get around independently.
Shelter	Close someone's door if privacy is requested. If someone's home has no heat or cooling, report this to supervising nurse.
Clothing	Make sure clothing is suitable to the weather.
Help	Keep room door open if the person wants to be able to call for you.

your own life? Table 4-2 contains some examples of ways you can help people in your care meet their needs for security.

You must find out what makes each person in your care feel secure. For example, Mrs. Garcia may want to keep her door closed so that strangers do not look in. Mr. Rivera may want his door open so that people can hear him if he calls. Each person feels more secure when you provide what that person needs. When you help a person meet his individual security needs, that person begins to trust you. To find out what makes a person feel secure, ask the person, his or her family, or your supervising nurse.

Social Needs

When their needs for security are fairly well met, people become interested in meeting their social needs. Even as people are seeking to have their social needs met, however, they still need to have their physical and security needs met.

What are social needs? Think for a moment about the people in your life. Think about family members, friends, a special person you love and people you work with. What things do you need from them to feel good? Most people need to be liked, loved and accepted by individuals and groups. These are social needs. No one wants to be ignored, to feel left out or to feel unloved or lonely. As a nurse assistant, you can help meet the social needs of people in your care many times each day. You can be especially helpful when a person's family and friends cannot be with her (Figure 4-7). Budgeting your time will help you divide your time among the persons in your care.

Being sick, disabled or elderly can be lonely. To people who are old or ill, it often seems as if everyone else is healthy, able-bodied and young, which may make it difficult for them to seek out new friendships and social oppor-

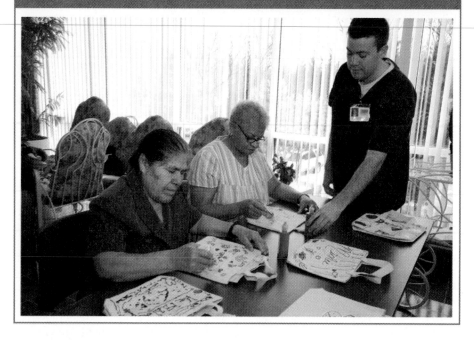

FIGURE 4-7 Taking an interest in a resident's activities helps meet her social needs.

TABLE 4-3 MEETING SOCIAL NEEDS

To Help Meet the Need for...	You can...
Approval	Show interest when someone talks about past accomplishments.
Acceptance	Introduce people.
	Talk in a friendly way.
	Listen in a way that shows you care.
Affection	Give people smiles and hugs.
Love	Tell a person you care.
Family and friends	Encourage family and friends to visit as often as they can.
	Help someone dial a friend's number.
	Help someone spend time with favorite people.

tunities. Your role in meeting the social needs of the people in your care is very important. You can reach out to them in a friendly way and encourage them to engage in social interaction. This will help prevent loneliness and produce friendships. Table 4-3 contains examples of small but important things you can do to help people meet their social needs. What other things can you do to help meet someone's social needs?

Esteem Needs

People whose social needs are met may be interested in having their needs for **esteem** met. They need to feel good about themselves and also to feel that others respect them. At the same time, they still need to have their physical, security and social needs met.

What do you do that makes you feel good about yourself? What do you do so that others respect you? Your answers to these questions show how you meet your needs for esteem. What do your family and friends do to help meet your needs for esteem? Do they compliment you, encourage you and say you are important to them?

Some people who are sick, old or disabled feel that they are no longer important. They do not feel good about themselves because they cannot do what they once were able to do.

People who are ill, disabled or old often do not have the opportunity to reap the pleasures of success. As a nurse assistant, you can increase their opportunities by noticing small accomplishments and mentioning them. Your role in meeting the needs for esteem of the people in your care is very important. Table 4-4 contains examples of ways you can help people meet their needs for esteem and let them know that you think they are important. What other things can you do to help meet these needs?

Self-Fulfillment Needs

People whose basic four needs are met satisfactorily can seek self-fulfillment. Self-fulfillment means that a person feels satisfied with himself. Each person needs to strive to satisfy his own self-fulfillment needs. The only way you can help is by helping to meet the other four needs.

Maslow, who talked about the levels of needs, explained self-fulfillment as the highest level of human need. He said that when people satisfy their self-fulfillment needs, they believe that they are doing what they are best suited to do. For example, a person may experience self-fulfillment by writing a great book, working toward finding a cure for a disease, becoming a terrific parent, or working to provide good care for the elderly. Because each person excels in

different areas of life, each person's self-fulfilling experience will be different. When you talk with the people in your care, you can help by encouraging them to talk about their needs for self-fulfillment.

Why Nurse Assistants Must Understand Human Needs

When you work as a nurse assistant, you provide care for many people with many different needs. When you understand the levels of needs, you can provide better care. For example, Mrs. Ryan looks forward to dressing every day. If she says she doesn't want to get dressed today, this statement is a clue for you that something may be wrong. A change in a person's usual pattern of behavior may mean that one or more of her needs have not been met.

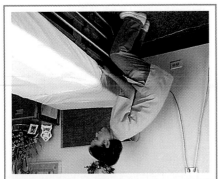
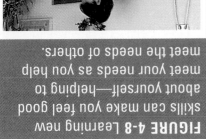

FIGURE 4-8 Learning new skills can make you feel good about yourself—helping to meet your needs as you help meet the needs of others.

THE NEEDS OF A NURSE ASSISTANT

Did you spend some time thinking about your own needs as you read about other people's needs? Just like them, you also have human needs. For example, one of the reasons you work is to help meet your own physical survival needs. The air is free, but many other things you need and want to live and be happy cost money. You also may work because being in the workplace meets a social need for you.

Many people choose to be nurse assistants because they need to help others and provide care for them. Think about your needs for social belonging, esteem and self-fulfillment. You may feel as if you are part of something important as you learn to become a nurse assistant. How do you feel about becoming part of the health care system that is responsible for the lives and well-being of so many people in hospitals, nursing homes and their own homes? Do you feel as if what you do is important? Are you doing the best you can do? Are you learning to be the best you can be? (Figure 4-8)

When you work hard, it may be difficult to have your own needs met, especially if you also are trying to help meet the needs of others in your life. It

TABLE 4-4 MEETING NEEDS FOR ESTEEM	
To Help Meet the Need for...	**You can...**
Rewards	Give recognition in hugs, handshakes, or any physical touch that is appropriate and acceptable to the person.
	Congratulate someone on accomplishments.
Respect	Use a person's correct name and title.
	Listen in a way that shows that this person matters to you.
Self-respect	Help a person do what he or she can to feel more independent.
	Encourage a person to talk about times he or she was held in great esteem.
Success	Help a person share successes with others.
	Praise someone when you notice improvement.
Possessions	Compliment someone's clothing when you know it is something the person is proud of.

may be difficult some days to find time to eat breakfast before coming to work. Then you may have an unmet need for food. It may be difficult to buy a comfortable pair of shoes. Then you may have a need for physical comfort. You may forget to lock your door at home one day. Then you worry about your security. Remember that if your needs are not met, you may have a hard time doing your job well.

HOW HUMAN SEXUALITY INFLUENCES BEHAVIOR

What do you think of when you hear the word **sexuality**? As with most peo-ple, you may be more familiar with the word *sex*. To many people, sex means having sex, or sexual intercourse. But *sex is only part of the word sexuality,* only the first three letters of a larger and more complicated term. Sexuality includes sensuality, intimacy, sexual identity and sexualization.

Sensuality

The part of people that lets them feel pleasure from the way their bodies look, feel and behave is called their **sensuality**. Sensuality enables people to feel attractive when they look at their bodies in the mirror (Figure 4-9). It allows them to experience pleasure when they touch or rub certain parts of their bodies. It also makes it possi-ble for them to enjoy the release of sexual tension known as sexual cli-max, or orgasm.

Sensuality lets people feel good about other people's bodies, too. It is what makes one person feel attracted to another person. Sensuality lets each person feel pleasure when he or she is touched by a special person. It also makes people want to be touched and held by other people they know, not just in a sexual way but in loving, caring ways.

Knowledge of sensuality is impor-tant in your work. As a nurse assistant,

you help people with their personal care. You help them bathe, dress and comb their hair. They may behave dif-ferently, depending on how they feel about themselves. Part of a person's healthy sexuality is having a good **body image**. When you provide care for a person, it is important that you:

• Notice some small difference—a new shirt or hair cut—and com-ment on it, complimenting the per-son on his or her appearance.
• Ask the person what he or she wants to wear, encouraging him or her to make choices.
• Focus on the positive things about a person's appearance—his or her smile or sparkling eyes—things that do not degenerate with disease or age.

You must be sensitive to someone who does not feel comfortable with his or her body image because of a dis-ease, disability or disfigurement or because he or she is very old. You help this person by looking beyond the physical features and seeing the per-son inside.

You also have to be aware that any person you provide care for may get pleasure by touching and rubbing his or her **genitals**. This person may be a baby, teenager, adult or older person. Many people touch themselves to achieve an orgasm and release sexual tension. This touching is called **masturbation** (măs´tər-bā´shən). Some people have been taught by parents or their religion that masturba-tion is a wrong way to behave. If that is what you were taught, it's okay for you to have that belief. However, you must remember that some people in your care may believe that masturbation is an acceptable action. They may want privacy to engage in masturbation. No matter how you personally feel about masturbation, every person in your care has a right to privacy when they want it.

There may be times when a per-son who is in your care may be physi-cally, or sexually, attracted to you. You may even be attracted to someone in your care. Feelings of sexual attraction for someone, even for the person in your care, can happen any time. It is okay for you to acknowledge these

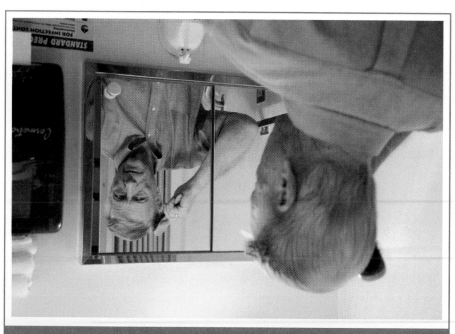

FIGURE 4-9 This resident feels more confident when he is pleased with his appearance.

feelings to yourself, but you should not act or comment on these feelings when you are with the person. Likewise, if a person in your care is attracted to you, he or she should not act on these feelings. If a person in your care makes sexual advances toward you, you should refuse them firmly but gently. You can say something such as:

"I really like you as a person, but I don't like it when you touch me that way."

"I really enjoy providing care for you, but I feel uncomfortable when you talk to me that way."

"I want you to stop touching me like that. Please do not do that again."

Let the person know that you do not want the sexual behavior but that you still like him or her.

At the same time, you must be careful not to misread something that may look like sexual attraction. For example, when you are bathing or washing a male, he may have an erection. When a male has an **erection**, this physical change does not necessarily mean that he is attracted to you or that he is thinking about you sexually. Erections are normal and happen to teenage boys and men for many different reasons. An erection may mean the person has a full bladder, is thinking about something that is sexually exciting, is feeling pleasure. You may feel embarrassed if someone in your care has an erection, but he also may feel embarrassed. To make the situation more comfortable, you may want to talk about something unrelated or simply continue the task without talking.

Intimacy

The need and ability of a person to feel close to another human being and to have that closeness returned is called **intimacy**. Intimacy includes all those good feelings that people have for one another, such as liking, loving, sharing and caring (Figure 4-10). To express their feelings of intimacy, people may kiss, hug, touch or hold hands. Intimacy may include a sexual relationship, or it may not.

Intimacy can affect your job as a nurse assistant. For example, in your relationship with someone in your care, you can be emotionally close even if the person does not respond to you at first. You can decide to make an emotional investment in that person and to show how much you care for him or her. You can let a person know that you like him or her. Your emotional investment may or may not lead to an intimate relationship in which the person also makes an emotional investment. However, it is not appropriate to have intimate relationships with residents, patients or clients.

In addition, you can respect the person's intimacy with a partner or spouse, family members and friends. Be accepting of behaviors such as holding hands, touching, kissing and hugging. Romance or sex may or may not be part of this intimate relationship. Since many people might be embarrassed to ask the nurse assistant to provide privacy for themselves and their partner, you must look for cues that a couple may want to be alone. When a couple is together, you

FIGURE 4-10 To help nursing home residents become intimate with one another, you can encourage them to sit together at a meal or special activity.

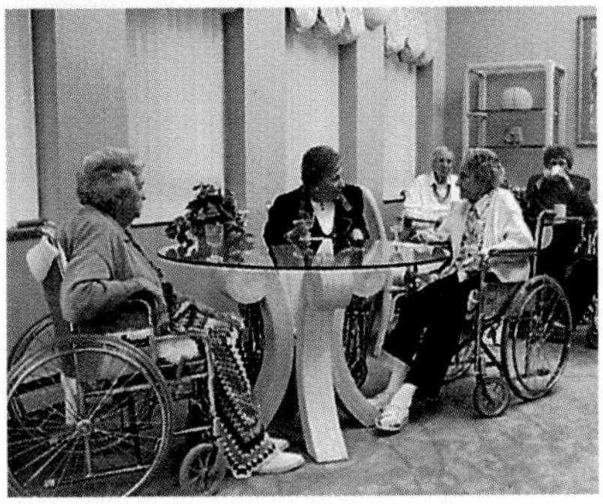

should excuse yourself and say what time you will be back. As always, you should knock on the person's door and wait for a reply before entering.

Sexual Identity

The way a person feels about who he or she is sexually, including his or her maleness or femaleness, is called *sexual identity*. Sexual identity may seem complicated. But, if you think of it as three pieces of a puzzle that fit together, it makes more sense. The three pieces of sexual identity are (1) recognizing that we are male or female; (2) learning how males and females are expected to behave; and (3) knowing whether we are attracted to the other sex, the same sex or both.

Most children recognize whether they are male or female by the age of two. They know by looking at their bodies whether they are girls or boys. People learn how men or women should behave by watching the groups in which they grow up. Families and cultures have strong opinions and have made "rules" about what men and women can and cannot do. For example, some people have rules about whether women with children should work, whether men should cry, whether women should play certain sports and whether men or women should hold certain jobs. Some people learned the "rule" that only women, and not men, should have jobs as nurse assistants (Figure 4-11). How do you feel about this idea? What rules about being men and women did you hear when you were growing up?

A person can be attracted to someone of the opposite sex, the same sex or both. A person who is mostly attracted to a person of the opposite sex is called *heterosexual* (some people say "straight"), and a person who is attracted to someone of the same sex is called *homosexual* (some people say "gay" when they refer to a man who has sex with a man or "lesbian" when they refer to a woman who has sex with

active. It may be even more difficult to think about older people being sexually active. Sometimes it is difficult to think about an older homosexual couple. Providing care to an older homosexual couple often lasts a lifetime, you may be providing care to an older homosexual couple. Sometimes it is difficult to think about older people being sexually active. It may be even more difficult to

The person in your care may have a partner of the same sex. Whether you believe that homosexual relationships are right or wrong, you may feel uncomfortable observing intimate behavior, such as hugging and kissing, between people of the same sex. And, because a person's attraction to other people of the same or opposite sex often lasts a lifetime, you may be providing care to an older homosexual couple. Sometimes it is difficult to think about an older homosexual couple. Sometimes it is difficult to think about older people being sexually active. It may be even more difficult to

The person in your care may have when you provide care. Regardless of what you feel, you must treat all people with the same respect and consideration when you provide care.

As a nurse assistant, you provide care for all people, including homosexuals. It is important to think about what you have been taught about homosexuality and how you feel about gay and lesbian people. Regardless of what you feel, you must treat all people with the same respect and consideration when you provide care.

They may not want to associate with them, and may even want to harm them. This kind of fear and harm is called *discrimination*. Have you ever been discriminated against or mistreated because of something special or different about yourself? How did you feel?

As a nurse assistant, you provide care for all people, including homosexuals. It is important to think about what you have been taught about homosexuality and how you feel about gay and lesbian people. *Regardless of what you feel, you must treat all people with the same respect and consideration when you provide care.*

Some people may not understand homosexual people. Just as they may not understand other minority groups, they may be afraid of homosexuals. They may not want to associate with them, and may even want to harm them. This kind of fear and harm is called *discrimination*. Have you ever been discriminated against or mistreated because of something special or different about yourself? How did you feel?

a woman). A person who is attracted to people of both sexes is called *bisexual*.

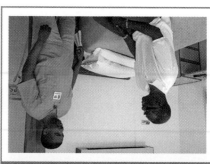

FIGURE 4-11 In the past, few men worked as nurses and nurse assistants. Today that has changed.

think about the sexually active couple being homosexual. No matter what you feel about the couple's relationship, you must respect the right of the partners to be together, provide them with the privacy they may want and provide them with the best possible care.

Some situations in your job as a nurse assistant also may be affected by sexual identity. For example, you may provide care for people who have very different ideas about the roles that men and women should play. A man in your care may believe that only a male nurse assistant should give him a bath. A person in your care may believe that only males should take charge in an emergency. You, too, may have your own ideas about male and female roles, but you must put these ideas aside so that you can fulfill the responsibilities of your job as a nurse assistant.

Sexualization

Using sex or sexuality to control other people is called sexualization. Some people use sexuality to get other people to do what they want. For example, a teenager may say to a date, "If you really loved me, you'd have sex with me." Or an adult who is upset with a spouse or sexual partner may respond to sexual advancements by saying, "Not tonight. I have a headache." Sexual abuses, such as rape and incest, are extreme forms of sexualization.

Another form of sexualization that happens on the job is called **sexual harassment**. Sexual harassment often happens to women and sometimes to men. Read more about this topic in Chapter 17, "Providing Care for People with Specific Illnesses." Report sexual discrimination and sexual harassment to your supervising nurse.

Sexualization also affects the elderly and disabled when others deny them their right to sexual expression. This denial is called *sexual oppression*. For example, someone may refuse to close the door to provide privacy for a person's sexual activities.

Situations in your job as a nurse assistant might involve sexualization. For example, you may provide care to a person who has been sexually abused, such as an adult or a child who has been raped. Although you may feel angry about the abuse, you must provide care for this person in the same way that you provide care for anyone, with kindness and gentleness. Often a social worker is assigned to talk with someone who has been abused. You can talk with the social worker about your own feelings about the person's abuse. There may be a time when you suspect that someone has been sexually abused. You must report your suspicions to your supervising nurse. (Refer to Chapter 3, "Protecting People's Rights.")

Why Nurse Assistants Must Understand Human Sexuality

Learning about and understanding human sexuality is important to you as a nurse assistant, because you have to deal with sexual behaviors and feelings in your work. For example, when someone in your care makes hints about wanting to be alone in his or her room, because you know about and understand human sexuality, you will respect that need. Or, when someone in your care is sexually attracted to you, you will know how to respond to his or her behavior in a professional way.

You may want to spend some time thinking about what you have just read about human sexuality. Talk about these ideas with friends and family members. Much of this information may be new to you. Since we all learn many myths about sex and sexuality when we are growing up, it is sometimes hard to sort the facts from the fiction. But what you have learned can be useful in your everyday life. If you have children, you can help them learn about their sexuality in a positive way. And, if you have a sexual partner, you may discover a new understanding of him or her.

Circle the correct answers and fill in the blanks.

1. Four factors that influence how a person behaves are _physical_, _social_, _emotional_ and _cognitive_.

2. Human development occurs in the same _order_ and follows the same _pattern_ for all human beings.

3. You are providing care for 13-year-old Kathy Harrison at her home while she is recovering from injuries caused by a car crash. She has stitches along her forehead and across one cheek and sits in a wheelchair for much of the day. Her friends call, but she doesn't want to see them. She may be worrying that:
   a. her friends want her to go to the mall.
   b. her friends will think she is ugly.
   c. her mother won't let them come over.
   d. her friends will bring her schoolwork.

4. Mrs. Wang's niece is discouraging her aunt from learning how to knit. She tells you that her aunt is too old to learn anything new. You could tell the niece that:
   a. older people can still learn things, but it may take a little longer than it once did.
   b. she is right, and you will take the knitting needle from her aunt so that she won't frustrate herself.
   c. she is right. Knitting is too complicated for an older person to learn.
   d. she should not be concerned about what her aunt wants to learn.

5. Mr. Jameson always talks about his days as a leader in his union but he hardly ever talks about the present. When he starts to talk about the past, you could:
   a. tell him not to dwell on the past.
   b. tell him how interesting it must have been in those days and ask him some questions about it.
   c. change the subject by asking him what he would like to do today.
   d. ignore him.

6. According to Abraham Maslow, the five basic needs are _physical_, _security_, _social_, _esteem_ and _self-fulfillment_.

7. If your _needs_ are not met, you may have a hard time doing your job as a nurse assistant.

8. Having a good body image is part of a healthy person's _sexuality_

1. *What are the care needs of an 80-year-old woman? Of a 30-year-old woman? Which needs are the same? Which are different?*

2. *How can you find out exactly what a person needs? What can you look for? What can you do?*

3. *Think of a time when you had a special need that was met. How did you feel when that need was met?*

4. *How can you help a very shy woman become less embarrassed about having her genitals washed?*

5. *If you found a nursing home resident masturbating in the dayroom, how would you feel? What would you do?*

6. *Have you taken time to think about your own needs as you prepare to help others?*

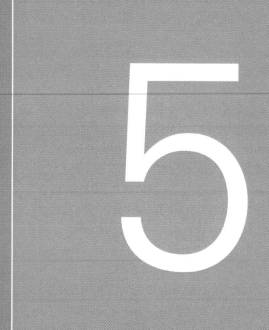

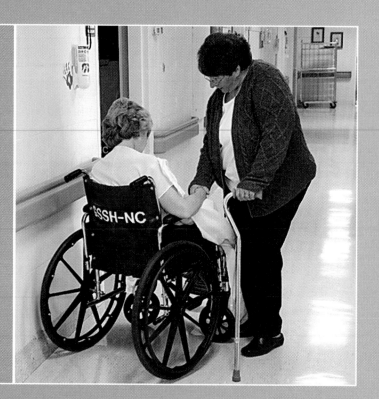

Chapter 5

Communicating with People

GOALS

After reading this chapter, you will have the information needed to:

Understand communication and how it works.

Use communication skills to interact with all people in your care, influence a person's behavior, interact with families and teach.

Describe cultural diversity and how culture may influence behavior.

Recognize and respect differences among people in your care.

When you knock on Rachel Morgan's door, you brace yourself to deal with this new resident, who has not spoken to you since she was admitted yesterday to Morningside Nursing Home. Mrs. Morgan is just 45 years old, but as you read on her chart, you see that she often has double vision, weakness and loss of balance caused by multiple sclerosis. Sometimes her hands shake and often she has sudden, uncontrollable outbursts of anger or crying. She can no longer live alone safely.

You are surprised when Mrs. Morgan says, "Come in," and are even more surprised when she looks up at you and smiles.

You say, "Hello, Mrs. Morgan," introduce yourself and check her name band as you give her a firm, but gentle, handshake. "I've come to help you get ready for bed."

"Thank you," she says, "for introducing me to Agnes Ryan. She is such a dear woman. I was sitting in this chair, thinking how I don't belong in a nursing home with a bunch of old people—I'm too young and I should be in my own home, with my own friends, surrounded by my own things. At that point, I had never felt so alone. I was crying, when I felt a gentle touch on my hand. I looked up and saw Agnes.

"Then she explained that you had introduced us yesterday when I was coming in. She said she'd stopped by to see how I was doing and to let me know that everyone missed seeing me at dinner.

"I was amazed. I wasn't seeing too well when I came in yesterday. And I didn't go to any meals today because I'm embarrassed about my weak, shaky arms. But I just couldn't believe what I was hearing: They missed seeing me at dinner!"

You tell Mrs. Morgan you're glad to hear that Mrs. Ryan stopped in to see her. You mention that Mrs. Ryan makes beautiful quilts.

"Do you think she would show me one?" Rachel asks.

You tell her "yes" and suggest that Mrs. Morgan ask her during lunch tomorrow in the dining room. "I think I *will* talk with her tomorrow at lunch," Mrs. Morgan says, and smiles.

USING COMMUNICATION TO INTERACT WITH OTHERS

As you read in the previous chapter, people can be hard to understand. But they do not have to be a mystery if you talk with them and listen to their stories. When you interact with the people in your care, you learn many things about them that help you understand them better. To do this well, you must understand **communication**, how it works, and how you can use it effectively in your work.

Communication is the principle of care that you use when you follow all the other principles. You communicate to help keep people safe, to respect their privacy, to give them dignity, to

promote their independence and to help maintain infection control.

Your ability to send and receive messages helps other people understand you and makes it possible for you to understand others. You may think that communication takes place only when you talk or write, but much communication takes place in the expressions on your face, the grip of your handshake or the tilt of your head.

HOW COMMUNICATION WORKS

You probably know from personal experience how common it is for people to misunderstand one another. When you talk and someone misunderstands you, you may react by thinking, "What's wrong with her? Why didn't she understand me? What I said was so clear!"

Effective communication requires more than just one person talking or providing information. Table 5-1 shows how five important parts or elements of communication work together to get a message across. Look at how these five elements worked together when Mrs. Morgan talked with you about Mrs. Ryan.

You tell Mrs. Morgan that she could ask Mrs. Ryan about her quilt-making tomorrow during lunch. Mrs. Morgan says she thinks she will do that. You are the *sender*. The suggestion to talk with Mrs. Ryan at lunch is

---

KEY TERMS

ancestry: (AN-ses-tree) A family's history.

appropriate: (ah-PRO-pree-it) Right or correct for a given situation.

closed-ended question: A question that requires only a simple "yes" or "no" answer.

comfort zone: (KUM-fert) The distance between one person and another that feels comfortable when communicating.

communication: (kuh-myou-nuh-KAY-shun) The process of giving and receiving information.

heritage: (HAIR-uh-tij) The culture passed on to a person through birth.

open-ended question: A question that requires more than a simple "yes" or "no" answer. An open-ended question encourages a person to talk.

TABLE 5-1 FIVE ELEMENTS OF EFFECTIVE COMMUNICATION

Communication Element	Description of the Element
Sender	The person who wants to communicate information
Message	The information the person sends
Channel	The way the message is sent—verbally (talking), nonverbally (facial expressions, body movements) or in writing
Receiver	The person to whom the message is sent
Confirmation	The way the receiver lets the sender know that he has received the message

the *message*. You use verbal communication as the *channel*. Mrs. Morgan is the *receiver*. *Confirmation* occurs when Mrs. Morgan says that she thinks she will talk with Mrs. Ryan tomorrow.

If these five elements work together for clear communication, why do people misunderstand one another? Sometimes the message itself may not be clear. Other times the sender may be using the wrong channel. For example, a man who talked to a nurse about the care his mother received became so upset that he didn't make sense when he spoke. His message might have been understood better if he had calmed down before he spoke or if he had communicated through a different channel, such as a letter.

Other times, misunderstanding occurs when the receiver does not confirm the message to the sender by telling the sender what she thinks the message means. If you are the receiver, confirm the message by repeating, in your own words, what the sender said. If you are the sender and you have to ask the receiver for confirmation, ask an **open-ended question,** not a **closed-ended question.** For example, the man who was

talking to the nurse about his mother could have said, "Do you understand?" (a closed-ended question) and the nurse could have said, "Yes," even if she didn't understand. However, if the man had said, "What do you understand about the situation that I just explained?" (an open-ended question), the nurse would have answered by repeating the man's message in her own words if she understood him.

Good communication requires much thought, careful attention, skill and cooperation. It also has many benefits, including increased understanding among people.

CHOOSING COMMUNICATION CHANNELS

As a nurse assistant, you use three channels of communication: *Verbal communication* is words spoken for the receiver to hear, *nonverbal communication* includes actions and expressions for the receiver to observe, and *written communication* consists of words or symbols written on paper or some other medium for the receiver to read. The channel that you choose to send your message

depends on the message and the receiver. For example, you would choose verbal communication to send a message to someone who cannot read or who is blind. In certain situations, you might use more than one channel to send your message. For example, you could explain something (verbal communication) and then write it down (written communication) as a reminder (Figure 5-1). Or you could demonstrate a skill (nonverbal communication) and describe what you are doing (verbal communication) at the same time.

Verbal Communication

Verbal communication has two important parts: (1) what you say and (2) how you say it. Effective verbal communication requires that you have useful information to share, speak clearly and express your thoughts well. When you talk with a person in your care or with your co-workers, use the following verbal communication skills:

Get the Receiver's Attention Before You Start Talking. If the person is doing something, and your message is not urgent, it may be better to talk with her later.

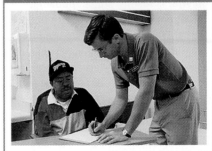

FIGURE 5-1 A written reminder can be especially helpful if your message is complicated or if the person in your care has trouble remembering things.

Use Words That the Receiver Understands. When communicating with people in your care, be careful about using medical terms that may not be familiar to them. Because some people may feel shy about asking what you mean, they may not get the message.

Choose the Right Volume. Speak loudly enough to be heard but not too loudly. How loudly you speak depends on how well the receiver can hear, how much noise is around you and whether you are discussing personal information. If a person is having trouble hearing you, move closer to her.

Speak Slowly and Clearly. Talk slowly enough to express your thoughts clearly and to give the receiver time to hear and think about what you are saying, as well as the opportunity to respond or ask questions.

Be Aware of Your Tone of Voice. Listen to how you sound to be sure that your tone of voice matches what you are trying to say. Sometimes, when you are in a hurry or have something else on your mind, you say things in a tone of voice that is not **appropriate** for the situation. For example, if you are thinking about an unpleasant conversation you experienced with the bus driver today, you may inappropriately reflect your anger at the bus driver when you speak to the person in your care.

Listen to the Receiver. By asking receivers to respond and by listening to what they say, you receive confirmation that they understand your message. If they do not understand, you may have to send the message again in a different way. Wait until the person who is talking stops speaking, then begin to speak. If they do not stop, politely say excuse me and wait one minute so that they may respond.

Nonverbal Communication

A performing mime never speaks. He or she uses only actions—nonverbal communication—to send a message.

Information and feelings often are shared through body movements and facial expressions. Sometimes these actions are called *body language*.

To communicate effectively, you need to understand two different elements of nonverbal communication: receiving information and sending information. When you look at people, you notice their facial expressions and how they hold their bodies. The information you receive from their faces and bodies affects how you interpret their messages. If you talk to a woman whose arms are folded tightly across her chest, you may think she is angry or upset. You interpret this message not by what she says, but by how she holds her body. However, her arms may be folded because she is cold. A person's background and culture also can affect nonverbal expression. For example, looking a person in the eye is a form of respect in some cultures, but it is considered offensive in others.

When you receive information through nonverbal communication, ask the sender whether you are interpreting it correctly (Figure 5-2).

On the other hand, you must be careful about the information you send. Sometimes you have to keep your feelings inside so that they do not show on your face. For example, when you provide care to someone who has an infection that neither looks nor smells nice, you must keep a calm look on your face so that the person does not feel afraid or rejected. If a situation really bothers you, you may need to excuse yourself, get a breath of fresh air and return. Be aware of how you hold your body and what you are doing so that you communicate the right message. For example, if you are pleased about something, make sure your facial expression (perhaps a smile) and body (standing erect), as well as your words, communicate your pleasure.

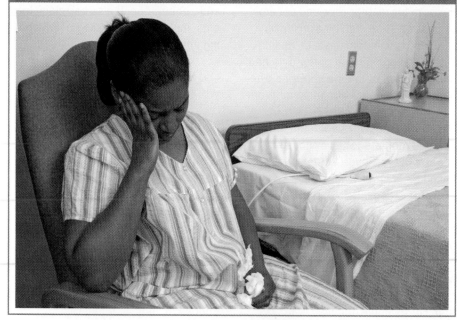

FIGURE 5-2 You have already read some things about nonverbal communication. If you saw this resident sitting alone and crying, you might conclude that she is sad and wonder what you could do to make her feel better. In response to what you see, you can approach her and offer help.

The same nonverbal clue can signal many possible messages, which the receiver needs to check out. Consider the following aspects of nonverbal communication.

Personal Appearance. When you look professional—by wearing clothing without stains, wrinkles or holes and by polishing your shoes, keeping your hair clean and neat and trimming your nails—you send the message that you care about yourself and the people you are with (Figure 5-3).

Facial Expressions. The meaning of facial expressions can vary. For example, a smile can be a sign of welcome or a sign of approval. A frown can suggest unhappiness or annoyance. The look in a person's eyes can show understanding or confusion. Keep in mind, however, that a facial expression can be affected by specific developmental disabilities where the person does not look at the person to whom he or she is speaking. In this circumstance it is best to use other means to confirm the listener's understanding or feelings.

Touch. A caring touch, such as a hand on a shoulder, a pat on the back or a hug, is often a good way to make someone feel special or emphasize what you are saying. However, as you know, touching is not considered appropriate in all cultures, and some people simply do not like to be touched (Figure 5-4). It is important to remember that physical touch can be very disturbing to individuals with specific neurological disorders or conditions. This is called tactile sensitivity, and should not be taken personally by the caregiver.

Sometimes, because of how you feel, it is not appropriate to send a message by touch. If you feel angry, tense or impatient, you may want to grab, slap or shake a person, but you must never touch a person in this way. If something is bothering you, talk about it right away with your supervising nurse or with someone else you trust.

Body Position and Movement. People in your care communicate how they feel physically and emotionally by the way they move, stand and sit. For example, a person who usually sits up straight may be slouching in his chair today. His slouched position may indicate that he is in pain, tired or feeling depressed.

You also send messages when you move, stand and sit. Move toward people slowly so that you do not startle them and so that they do not think that you are in a hurry or that you do not want to be bothered with them. *Where* you stand or sit in relation to another person also is important. Every person has a **comfort zone.** Your own comfort zone may allow you to stand very close to others, but some people in your care may find your closeness uncomfortable and back away. Or you may need a lot of personal space, but someone in your care may think that the distance means you do not like her. Be aware of each person's comfort zone, and

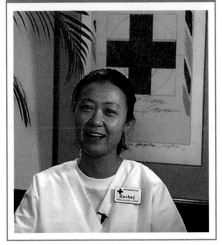

FIGURE 5-3 It takes effort to present a neat, professional appearance on the job. Having a good personal appearance is important to your own self-esteem and also sends a positive message to others.

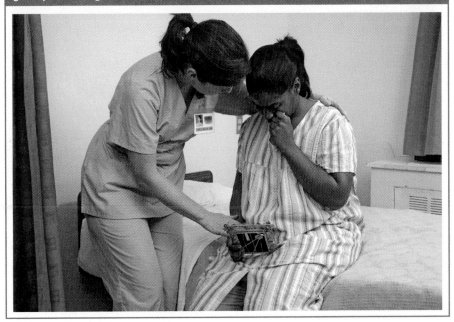

FIGURE 5-4 This resident has recently arrived at the nursing home. Since you don't know her very well, before touching her, ask, "Can I give you a hug?"

find a distance that feels right to you and the other person.

Written Communication

In your work, you often communicate by writing telephone messages for co-workers, reminders for people in your care and information for your co-workers about the people in your care. Before you write a message for someone in your care, find out whether she will be able to read it. Her ability to read may be a source of pride or embarrassment. Although she communicates well verbally, she may not be able to read because she never learned, she does not read English, or she has problems with her eyesight. To find out about her reading ability and protect her dignity, talk to her or her family members. Then, when you do communicate in writing, use the following written communication skills:

- Write neatly. If your handwriting is hard to read, print instead.
- Choose the best size and colors for your letters. If you write something for a person with limited eyesight, use large letters and a black or dark blue pen or crayon on white paper.
- Draw pictures. Sometimes a picture says more than words, and it communicates well to a person who cannot read.
- Choose simple words. Use the simplest words you can to get the message across.
- Be specific. For example, if you are noting the time, be sure to write A.M. or P.M. If two people with the same last name are in your care, provide additional information, such as their first names or their room numbers.
- Be thorough. Make sure that your message is complete.
- Spell correctly. If you are not sure of the spelling, look it up or ask.
- Include your signature. Always sign your note so that people know who wrote it.

- Double-check your message. To make sure that you have not made any mistakes, check over what you have written before you deliver the message.

Computers. Computers may be used to communicate information about the person, to obtain your assignment or to record observations or tasks that you have performed, or even to take a nurse assistant examination. As with any piece of equipment, the more familiar you become with it, the easier it is to use. If you do not own a computer, you may be able to go to your local library to practice. If you feel uncomfortable, ask for assistance, and remember: the more you practice, the easier it will become.

Whether you use verbal, nonverbal or written communication as the channel for sending a message, you want to do your best to make sure the message that you intend is the message that you send.

USING CLEAR COMMUNICATION WHEN PROVIDING CARE

In your work as a nurse assistant, your ability to communicate can have a positive impact on the health and well-being of the people in your care (Box 5-1). At the beginning of the chapter, when you went to Mrs. Morgan's room to help her get ready for bed, you used verbal and nonverbal communication as you interacted with her. Look at Table 5-2 to see the positive meaning that your messages carried.

BOX 5-1

CHANGING RAZORS

Mr. Rivera, the 78-year-old man in your care who had a stroke, takes medication that increases the amount of time it takes for blood to clot. Because even a small cut may bleed a long time, Mr. Rivera has to avoid any skin injury. Your supervising nurse has alerted you to watch for any signs of bleeding during personal care. She has also instructed you to have Mr. Rivera switch from shaving with a safety razor to shaving with an electric razor to help prevent nicking his skin. One morning, while helping Mr. Rivera shave, you have the following conversation with him.

Mr. Rivera: "I don't see why I have to use this electric razor. I've been shaving with my safety razor for years, and I never had a problem."

You could say: "I know you like the safety razor better, Mr. Rivera, but because of the kind of medication you are taking, it is important that you don't cut yourself. The electric razor doesn't nick your skin. It is better for you to use."

Mr. Rivera: "I don't like electric razors, but I don't like bleeding either, so I guess I'd better try it."

TABLE 5-2 CLEAR COMMUNICATION IN CAREGIVING

Your Message	Channel	Positive Meaning
Knock on the door.	Nonverbal	You show respect for Mrs. Morgan and her privacy.
Greet her and call her by her title (Mrs.) and last name.	Verbal	Your greeting is friendly, and you show respect for her dignity.
Introduce yourself.	Verbal	You help Mrs. Morgan to remember your name by introducing yourself each time you see her.
Check her name band.	Nonverbal	You care about her safety.
Shake her hand firmly yet gently.	Nonverbal	You care about her and are sensitive to her needs; you also are confident about yourself and your work.
Ask permission to help her get ready for bed.	Verbal	Mrs. Morgan still has control over her life.
You tell Mrs. Morgan that Mrs. Ryan makes quilts.	Verbal	You confirm that you listened to Mrs. Morgan's story.
You suggest that Mrs. Morgan talk with Mrs. Ryan at lunch.	Verbal	You want to help Mrs. Morgan make friends and be happy at the nursing home.

USING COMMUNICATION IN SPECIAL SITUATIONS

As a nurse assistant, you provide care to people who are different from you, and you may not feel comfortable talking with them about some things. You may also communicate with people who cannot see or hear well, people who speak different languages, children, people that have neurological disorders or with people that have mental illness that affects communication. In addition, you use the telephone, which requires you to use your best verbal skills.

Communicating About Difficult Subjects

The people in your care and their families look to you for answers to their questions and talk to you about difficult situations. Most of the time you probably can provide answers. Sometimes, however, you may not know

how to respond. These situations happen to everyone.

When you have a good relationship with the person in your care, as you hope to have with Mrs. Morgan, she trusts you enough to express private and personal thoughts. For example, a person might say, "My family doesn't care about me anymore." A family member might say, "I wish she would just die." These messages may make you feel uncomfortable.

When a person says such things, you may feel afraid, nervous or unsure about how to respond. You may have the same uncomfortable feelings about messages that a co-worker might send when he or she confides in you about problems at work or at home. Sometimes you may feel so uncomfortable with such messages that you may want to do things to get out of the conversation, such as leave the room quickly, change the subject, tell a "little white lie" that might help the per-

son feel better or make a comment such as, "You don't really mean that," or "Don't be silly."

While these responses may get you off the hook, they cut off communication with the person who is sending the message. Because part of your job is to listen and talk with the person in your care, it is important to keep lines of communication open (Figure 5-5), even when you feel uncomfortable with the message.

The suggestions explained below may help you handle difficult messages better.

Pause for a Few Moments. To calm yourself, stop to figure out how you feel and why you feel that way. Then, instead of focusing on your uncomfortable feelings, think about the feelings of the sender and how she is trying to communicate with you. Taking slow, deep breaths will help reduce anxiety and allow you to focus more clearly.

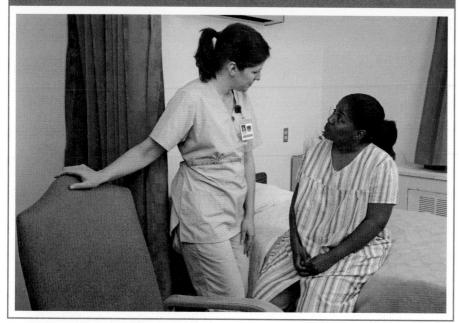

FIGURE 5-5 Often when a person is upset she doesn't want to be cheered up or offered advice or solutions. She may just want you to listen to her.

Nonverbally Show Your Interest. Show the person that you care about her feelings by stopping what you are doing, paying full attention and making eye contact. If it is appropriate, hold or gently squeeze her hand or touch her on the shoulder. If she feels your interest and concern, your silent support can sometimes help more than words.

Verbally Encourage the Person to Talk. Ask a question that focuses on what is happening. Avoid questions such as, "How do you feel?" You might ask a question to confirm the person's message: "Are you saying that you miss being close to another person?" Or confirm the message by repeating it in your own words: "It sounds like you are saying that you miss seeing and hearing from your family."

Listen. Sometimes all a person needs is someone who listens. Don't "talk over" a person. Let him or her finish their thoughts, then answer. If she or he needs answers that you are unable to provide, let another member of the

health care team handle the situation or concern. Tell the person that you will talk with someone who may be able to help. *Then be sure to follow through*.

Talk About Your Feelings. To help you understand your feelings, to clear your mind and to gain confidence in handling a similar situation, talk with your supervising nurse or someone else you trust.

Communicating with Families
When you communicate well with the person in your care, you learn a great deal about her. She is your primary source of personal information. You also can learn more about her from her family members, who are important to her and to you. By asking them questions, you can learn more about her food likes and dislikes, clothing preferences and family and cultural traditions that may affect her care. They can tell you about the work she has done and the hobbies she enjoys.

In this way, you are involving the family as part of the health care team.

You can encourage families and help them feel more comfortable by getting to know them, learning about their family history, talking with them and listening to them (Figure 5-6). You also can learn a great deal about the person in your care by observing how her family members relate to one another. At the same time, you must stay on the outside of their family circle and avoid making judgments, expressing opinions or taking sides when there are disagreements, because these actions may add to stress or unresolved family problems.

Family members also may want to learn things about the person from you. For example, Mrs. Ryan's family may want to know how well she is eating, sleeping and getting along with other people. Families want to know whether their loved ones are getting better or worse. Be sure to answer questions about her activities of daily living. Share only information you are authorized to share.

If a family's question needs a medical answer, refer the family to the doctor or nurse.

Use your communication skills to help family members. Listen to them and inform your supervising nurse if someone in the family has questions about the condition of the person in your care, or if someone has a complaint.

Families can feel reassured by your skilled caregiving, but they also may feel resentful or guilty because they can no longer provide care for their loved one or because she became ill or her condition got worse while they were taking care of her.

Family members generally want to continue to be involved with caregiving. They may continue this involvement by trying to make sure their loved one receives the best care possible (Box 5-2). To put the family at ease, be sure to talk with them about

FIGURE 5-6 You can learn family members' names and find out when they like to visit. Then you can let them know that you are expecting them by planning your caregiving around their visits, bringing extra chairs to make them comfortable and providing privacy for them.

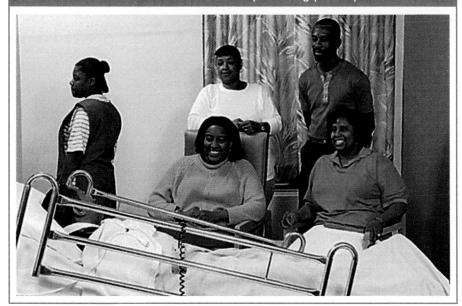

your role in providing care for their loved one and explain why you do things in a certain way. When talking with family members, be kind and respectful. When possible, encourage families and friends to participate with the resident in activities, use their caregiving suggestions, but make sure that these recommendations support the principles of care. Communication is of course the best way to get information, but it is also the best way to get people to cooperate with you.

Communicating with People of Different Cultures

The culture that people are "born into" is their **heritage**, or inherited culture. All people have a national, racial or tribal heritage that connects them by a shared language, **ancestry** and religion, and often by physical characteristics, to other people with the same heritage.

Our inherited culture helps us understand who we are and how we fit into our society. Together with our environment, it tells us how to think about being male or female, being young, growing up, marrying, aging, becoming ill and dying. These ways of thinking feel natural, comfortable and "right" to us. Problems may arise when we experience the differences of other people's inherited culture. We sometimes fear these differences and decide that our way is right and their way is wrong. You provide nursing care for people who may have inherited a culture that is different from yours. Two important things to remember are that our world is a diverse place made up of many peo-

---

BOX 5-2

HOW FAMILIES CAN HELP

Give the nurse assistant information:	Likes and dislikes (activities, food, colors), habits (sleeping, bathing, elimination), feelings and fears, past history (career, children, hobbies)
Play a role in caregiving:	Feeding, ambulation (walking), hair care, nail care, bathing and backrubs
Play a role in decision making:	Care planning and levels of care, restrictions on movement, maintaining household, discharge planning, needed support services
Give emotional support:	Visiting or phoning; sending cards, letters and photos; listening and talking; showing affection (hugging, touching)
Give financial support.	

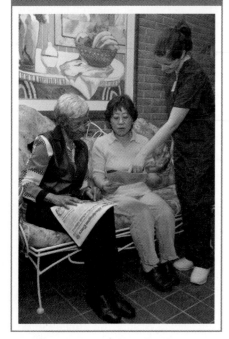

FIGURE 5-7 Working with people of different cultures gives you an opportunity to learn about their customs and traditions.

ple and many cultures and that each person's culture is important to him or her (Figure 5-7).

Communicating with People Who Speak a Different Language

People who speak a language other than English have the same needs and desires for communication as anyone else. In fact, in a nursing home or hospital, their needs may be greater because they have fewer people to talk with. In addition, they may not have materials written in a foreign language that they can read. You can improve communication with a person who speaks another language by building trust and sending nonverbal messages.

Build the Trust of a Person Who Speaks a Different Language. Try to find out how much English the person speaks. Be sensitive to her possible embarrassment about making mistakes; she may not want to try speaking. When she does speak English, praise her efforts.

Send Nonverbal Messages. Draw pictures, point and use facial expressions. Encourage her also to use nonverbal communication so that she can point to what she wants or show you the location of her pain.

If a language barrier makes it seem impossible to get important information across, try to find someone who speaks and understands both English and the language of the person in your care. Ask this person to serve as a translator. This person may be a family member, a friend or someone who works for your employer. When you communicate through a translator, make sure that both the translator and the person in your care understand your message.

Why Nurse Assistants Must Understand Cultural Differences

When you work as a nurse assistant, it is important to understand how culture influences behavior and to respect each person's culture and individuality. You have your own cultural background that influences your actions on the job. You need to be aware of your feelings and how they may affect the person in your care.

If at any time you believe you may have offended someone by something you said or did, ask and apologize. Asking about the person's traditions or preferences not only will help prevent this situation, but it also shows the person you are interested in him or her.

Table 5-3 lists some areas in which you may see cultural differences among the people in your care. Next to the differences is a list of suggested actions you can take when you help plan the care for these people.

To provide the best care possible for people, you must learn to see the beauty of each person, each family and each culture.

Communicating with People Who are Visually Impaired

You may provide care for people who have impaired sight. Some people may need only reading glasses, whereas others may be blind. Visual impairment may be caused by many factors. For example, Mrs. Andrews has cataracts, a clouding of the lens of the eye that causes a gradual decline of sight. Cataracts may be caused by aging, injury, or other diseases and may develop in one eye or in both eyes. Mrs. Andrews, whose vision is blurred, says she feels as if she has a film over her eyes. Another resident in your care has diabetes, which caused changes in his eyes, resulting in blurred vision.

Imagine what it must be like for these residents. They cannot move around at will because they cannot see clearly what is in front of them. They are unable to read a newspaper or watch television comfortably. When planning care for a person with vision problems, the important points to consider are safety and communication. You can improve safety and communication by remembering that he may not see you, by being sensitive to his surroundings and by using your voice, words and touch to help him see.

Remember that a Person with a Visual Impairment May Not See You. Knock on the person's door or tell him right away that you are there so that you don't startle him. Stand where he can see you, and call him by name: "Good morning, Mr. Wilson." Then tell him who you are.

Be Sensitive in Arranging and Managing His or Her Surroundings. If a person with a visual impairment wears eyeglasses, keep them clean and within his reach. Keep the room well lighted by opening the curtains to let in

TABLE 5-3 HANDLING CULTURAL DIFFERENCES

To Help Bridge the Cultural Difference Gap...	You Can...
Language	Ask clear, short questions.
	Point to pictures or use flash cards.
	Watch facial expressions and nonverbal language to understand what the person may be feeling, understanding or trying to communicate.
Diet	Gather information about the person's likes and dislikes. (Some cultures or religions have rules about food. This information needs to be part of the person's care plan. See Chapter 14, "Healthful Eating.") Ask whether the person has a special diet.
Religion	Ask whether the person would like to see clergy.
	Report a request to see clergy to your supervising nurse.
	Provide privacy for visiting clergy, as well as for religious practice, such as prayer.
Illness	Respect rituals as long as they do not interfere with the care plan or anyone else's well-being.
Death	Ask the family if they want a special ritual before death or immediately after.
	Ask them if special treatment of the body is required.

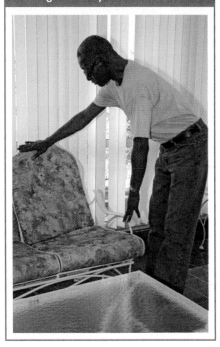

FIGURE 5-8 Mr. Wilson has impaired vision. He knows that this chair is always in the same place and has no trouble finding his way around it.

daylight and turning on the lamps in early evening. Describe his surroundings and tell him what is going on. Describe the people or events in a way that helps him create a picture: "Mr. Wilson, your daughter Susan is here, and she's wearing a beautiful red dress." Or "It's sunny today, and the patio door is open if you would like to go outside." Keep furniture and belongings in the same place all the time to help him keep a mental picture of where things are and to avoid mishaps (Figure 5-8). If he is in a hospital or nursing home and if the facility has raised numbers or symbols on the doors, help him find them.

Use Your Voice, Words, and Touch to Help a Person with a Visual Impairment See. Describe what you are going to do: "It's time for dinner, and I'm going to help you get to the dining room." When serving food, describe the items on the table or tray by location, using a clock as a reference point: "Your meal is chicken, green beans and potatoes. The chicken is at 12 o'clock on your plate, the potatoes are at 4 o'clock and the beans are at 8 o'clock." Identify the placement of food or drinks that are not on the plate: "Here is your hot tea. I'm putting it at the top of your plate at 1 o'clock."

When helping a person move around, encourage him to hold your arm just above your elbow for support, describe where you are going, and mention things that are in your path: "We're going up three steps now." When using a piece of equipment, describe it to the person. If it doesn't cause an infection control risk and if he is interested, let him touch what you are holding. Check with your supervising nurse about available aids for people who are visually impaired.

A vision problem is often a chronic condition that doesn't go away. Therefore, keep your focus on safety and on how well you communicate so that the person's life is as pleasant and safe as you can help to make it.

Communicating with People Who are Hearing-Impaired

You provide care for a resident, who is hearing-impaired and wears a hearing aid. Sometimes he becomes depressed about losing his hearing. His speech has changed because he cannot hear himself talking. He often appears self-conscious or embarrassed and doesn't want to be around other people. Sometimes he tries to dominate the conversation to avoid the embarrassment of giving the wrong answer to a question. As you help plan care, you concentrate on how to communicate effectively with him.

Some people who are hearing-impaired may be deaf, whereas others may have problems hearing certain sounds. Hearing aids improve some hearing problems, as with Mrs. Wang, but just because someone has a hearing aid does not mean she can hear well. Because people with hearing impairments still need to communicate, learn what the people in your care can and cannot hear. You can improve communication by remembering that she may not hear you, by being sensitive to her surroundings, and by using your face, hands, body and words to help her hear.

Remember that a Person with a Hearing Impairment May Not Hear You. Gently touch him on the hand or arm to gain his attention before speaking. Always approach him from the front, and face him so that he can

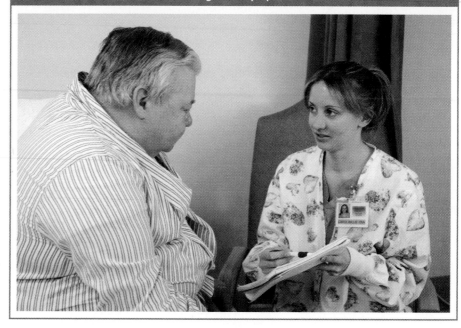

FIGURE 5-9 If a person in your care is hearing-impaired, adjust your position so that you are face to face with him, not standing over him. Or if he can read, write messages on paper.

see your moving mouth and facial expressions (Figure 5-9). If he has a hearing aid, encourage him to wear it whenever he is awake, and ask him from time to time whether it is working well. Help him use the hearing aid properly, care for it according to the manufacturer's directions and store it in the same place when he is not using it.

Be Sensitive in Managing the Surroundings of a Person with a Hearing Impairment. Reduce background noise as much as possible, because television or radio sounds can be very distracting to the person with a hearing impairment during conversation. Avoid talking and laughing in front of him unless you include him in the conversation, because he may think that you are talking about him or laughing at him.

Use Your Face, Hands, Body and Words to Help the Person Hear. If the person doesn't seem to under-

stand what you say, change your words, not the volume of your voice, unless you may have spoken too softly. Shouting sometimes creates more distress for the person, and she still may not understand what you are saying. Don't cover your mouth while speaking, because hearing-impaired people often learn to read lips and rely on watching your mouth move. Pronounce your words slowly and clearly, without saying words unnaturally, exaggerating syllables or shouting. Speak in short sentences.

If someone with a hearing impairment hears more clearly in one ear than the other, find out which ear is better, and position yourself near that ear when you talk. Use gestures and body movements to help explain what you are saying. Or, if he can read, write messages on paper. When you have important information to get across, make sure that he understands you by asking for confirmation. Ask your supervising nurse about available special devices that can help some hearing-impaired people.

When you make the effort to communicate with a person who has a hearing loss, he may feel more comfortable about communicating his needs and feelings to you.

Communicating with People Who have Specific Developmental Disabilities

We are seeing more and more people with specific learning disorders such as Autism, or Asperger's Syndrome. Although we have often heard Autism connected with mental retardation, these disorders do not necessarily mean the person has mental retardation. In the same way that a person who is hearing-impaired does not have that input, a person who is visually impaired does not have that input. People with these disorders do not have the benefit of the "shortcuts" to emotions that are available through the right hemisphere of the brain. People with these disorders interpret the world only through verbal reasoning. We also see this response when people have traumatic brain injury that has affected the right hemisphere. Imagine what it must be like to not understand what the facial expression we know as smile or frown "means." Imagine how it must feel to have to evaluate all nonverbal or emotional expressions with verbal logic only. It is important to remember that the person might not look at you directly. Physical touch may also be very disturbing to individuals with specific neurological disorders as well. It is also important to avoid interpreting the mannerisms or responses as being unsociable.

When communicating with people that have these neurological disorders, you may find it helpful to use verbal explanation of emotions.

INFORMATION REVIEW

Circle the correct answers and fill in the blanks.

1. The five elements of communication are __sender__ , __message__ , __channel__, __receiver__ and __confirmation__

2. When you communicate a message to someone, what should you do after you deliver it?
    a. Expect the person to do what you told him.
    (b.) Ask for confirmation that the message was understood.
    c. Communicate the next message.
    d. Look for written communication.

3. When entering the room of a person who is blind, you should:
    a. walk up quietly and touch the person on the back.
    (b.) knock on the door, wait for a response and introduce yourself.
    c. knock on the door and go in.
    d. talk in a low voice.

4. What two channels of communication could you use to communicate with someone who is deaf?
    (a.) Nonverbal and written
    b. Verbal and confirmation
    c. The sender and receiver
    d. Written and verbal

5. Several days ago you taught Mr. Rivera to shave with an electric razor instead of a safety razor. He needs to use an electric razor for medical reasons. Today he gets his electric razor out without making the usual comments about how he dislikes shaving this way. You want this behavior to continue. What should you do? You should:
    a. ignore the situation because he has already changed his behavior.
    b. tell him you're surprised that he didn't complain today.

Continued

  c. tell him he probably will be able to go back to his old razor in a few months.

  d. give his shoulder a squeeze and tell him that he is doing a great job.

6. Mrs. Morgan's daughter always asks you what you are doing and tells you how she provided care for her mother when Mrs. Morgan was at home. The daughter often goes to the nurses' station to ask questions or complain about her mother's care. What could you say to help the daughter feel more comfortable?

  a. ask Mrs. Morgan to tell her daughter that she likes the care you provide.

  b. tell the daughter that her mother likes the care she is receiving.

  c. tell the daughter that what you are doing is the right and only way to provide care.

  d. tell the daughter what you are doing and why you are doing it, and ask her to help with her mother's care.

7. Mrs. Goldstein has recently been diagnosed with diabetes and must eat meals at regular intervals. Today is a fasting day in her religion. She knows that she needs to eat because of her disease, and she knows that her religion says that sick people don't have

to fast. Yet, when you serve her food, she tells you that she feels funny about eating. You could:

  a. tell her that she shouldn't feel bad.

  b. avoid talking about religion and serve her food without saying anything.

  c. tell her that she doesn't really have to eat if she doesn't want to.

  d. tell her that you can understand that it must feel strange to eat on a fasting day and encourage her to talk about it.

8. Mr. Smith never looks at you when you speak to him. You are getting really annoyed by this because you think that he is not listening to you. He tells you that he has a diagnosis of Asperger's Syndrome. You could:

  a. Tell him to look at you when you are speaking because he is being rude.

  b. Continue with your communication even without eye contact, but get verbal feedback from him to be sure he understood what you said.

  c. Talk to him in simpler terms because this behavior means he must be mentally retarded.

  d. Draw pictures to make the directions more clear.

1. Mrs. Alvarez is getting better after suffering a stroke but wants you to do everything for her. How can you encourage her to start taking care of herself again, and how can you reinforce her efforts?
2. What subjects would you find difficult to discuss with a person in your care? How would you respond if someone started to talk with you about these subjects?
3. How would you feel if a person in your care cursed and threw a glass at you? How would you respond to that person? How would you handle your feelings?
4. Mr. Chin's adult son doesn't visit his father at the nursing home very often. You know that the father would like to see his son more often. What could you do?
5. Mrs. Cohen's two daughters argue loudly in their mother's room about the kind of care each one thinks her mother should be receiving. Their voices get louder and louder, and you see that Mrs. Cohen is getting more and more upset. What could you do to ease the situation?
6. Mr. Dutta believes that a special ointment from a "healer" can cure his open sore, and he uses it, even though his doctor instructed him not to. What should you do?

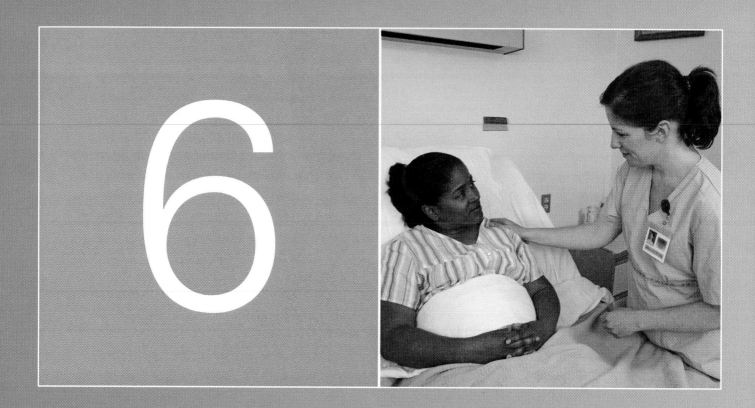

6

The Language of Caregiving

GOALS

After reading this chapter, you will have the information needed to:

Reduce inappropriate behaviors.

Teach people in your care effectively.

Use medical terminology, including abbreviations.

Use your senses to make observations.

Communicate accurate observations about people to other health care workers.

Your co-worker Tara sighs as she sits down beside you in the lunch room and unwraps a tuna sandwich. She laughs wearily and holds up the sandwich. "My bread got soggy. But that's about right, I guess. I feel about as limp and useless as this sandwich!"

Tara has been a nurse assistant at a rehabilitation center for six months, but, she tells you, "I have *never* had to care for someone like Mrs. Jones. I always thought I was so good with people—good at calming them down, good at listening, good at encouraging. But Mrs. Jones just doesn't seem to like me."

Mrs. Jones is a woman in her mid-thirties who was moved to the rehabilitation center from the hospital, after recovering from surgery after a terrible car accident. Mrs. Jones lost a family member in the accident, and her pelvis was crushed. For a while, no one knew if Mrs. Jones would live. Now, she is on the road to recovery, but she still will face numerous surgeries down the road. For right now, her surgeon wants her to concentrate on learning to walk with an artificial hip replacement.

"But Mrs. Jones has fought me from the beginning," Tara says, "about even sitting up in bed and facing the day—let alone doing her exercises. Usually by the end of a few days, I can rally a person to at least begin trying

something, even if it's just washing their faces or combing their hair. At least that's a start. But Mrs. Jones has been here for almost a week, and she still refuses to let me help her with anything."

However, Tara does not give up. One morning, with her supervisor's permission, Tara stops trying to "make" Mrs. Jones do anything. She enters her room with a cheerful "good morning," and asks Mrs. Jones if she'd like to start "getting ready for the day." But this time, when Mrs. Jones doesn't respond, Tara does not try to coax her or do anything for her. Instead she sits down where it is easy for Mrs. Jones to see her.

"Recovering from surgery is very hard, isn't it," she says softly. "But I'm so glad you're going to be all right." She brushes Mrs. Jones's hair and talks about what has been scheduled for the day—including what's for breakfast and lunch. Mrs. Jones doesn't say anything, but she listens. Tara does this for several days. She offers assistance, asks Mrs. Jones if she needs anything, and sometimes, as she quietly relates what's going on in the center for the day, Mrs. Jones begins to respond. First, she begins to cooperate with her care more, and then she begins to participate more actively in her range-of-motion exercises.

Finally, one day, when Tara is brushing her hair, Mrs. Jones begins to cry.

At first Tara is afraid she has done something wrong, but Mrs. Jones takes her hand and says, "My daughter used to love to brush my hair."

Tara stops brushing and sits down to listen.

"My daughter was killed in the car crash," Mrs. Jones says, looking into Tara's eyes, still holding her hand.

And Tara finds the key—Mrs. Jones needs someone to just listen.

USING EFFECTIVE COMMUNICATION TO INFLUENCE BEHAVIOR

Many factors influence behavior. What you say and do can influence other people's behavior in either a positive or negative way. At times, you may influence the people in your care to increase appropriate behaviors that improve their health and well-being. When you do you are providing **restorative care**. At other times, you may influence them to stop or reduce **inappropriate** behaviors that may be harmful.

Communication sends messages to let people know whether their behaviors are liked or disliked. Sometimes people respond to these mes-

---

KEY TERMS

abbreviation: (uh-bree-vee-AY-shun) a shortened version of a word. An abbreviation is often made up of the first letters of several words.

adapt: (uh-DAPT) to change a behavior to adjust to a certain illness or condition.

care plan: a form used to record overall health care information.

flow sheet: a form used to record health care information and track changes in a person's condition over a period of time.

inappropriate: (in-uh-PRO-pree-it) not right or correct for a given situation.

nursing notes: information documented by the supervising nurse on a health care record or chart.

precise: (pree-SISE) another term for exact.

prefix: (PREE-fiks) the first part of a word, which comes before the root word and changes the meaning of the root.

root: the middle part, or base, of a word.

restorative care: care that helps rehabilitate the person, bring back the person's health, maintain functionality and maximize their independence.

social reinforcement: encouragement that emphasizes appropriate attitude and behavior.

suffix: (SUH-fiks) the last part of a word, which comes after the root word and changes the meaning of the root.

sages by continuing behavior that is liked and stopping behavior that is not liked. Your messages may help influence the behaviors of the people in your care.

Increasing Appropriate Behaviors

Each person in your care needs to accomplish what is specified in his or her individual **care plan.** In addition restorative care—helping the person to maintain their functionality, independence and to improve their health is also part of your job in many states. Restorative care includes helping people do the things called for in the care plan correctly and regularly. One of the items in the care plan may be the encouragement of certain appropriate behaviors, such as eating without assistance and taking walks. **Social reinforcement** helps increase the likelihood that people repeat these appropriate behaviors (Table 6-1).

Each type of verbal social reinforcement helps people increase their appropriate behaviors, especially if you combine the reinforcement with a physical expression of approval, such as a hug, handshake or touch on the shoulder. Look at the following formula for increasing appropriate behavior to see how verbal and nonverbal reinforcement work together to influence behavior:

Verbal Social Reinforcement + Nonverbal Physical Reinforcement = Increase in Appropriate Behaviors

No single type of reinforcement is always successful with the same person or in the same situation, because people behave in certain ways for many reasons. For example, a person may not try to walk with a walker because she does not understand or is afraid. If what you are doing to reinforce a positive behavior is not working, try to figure out why the person is not responding, and with the rest of the health care team, try a different approach.

Reducing Inappropriate Behaviors

Most of the people in your care appreciate what you do for them and try to cooperate. At times, however, a person may yell, spit or curse at you, or make a racist or sexist remark.

These inappropriate behaviors could be harmful and difficult to handle. Some people think that those who behave in such inappropriate ways should be punished. However, it is *never* acceptable for you, as a nurse assistant, to punish people in your care. Your response, even to inappropriate behaviors, must uphold the six principles of care. An appropriate response to an inappropriate behavior always allows for safety, privacy, dignity, communication, independence and infection control. An appropriate response never violates a person's rights. When a person in your care behaves in an inappropriate way, it is natural for you to feel upset, angry, embarrassed or frustrated. It is understandable that you feel this way, but it is never all right to *act* the way you feel if that action is not an appropriate response.

If it seems appropriate, you may leave a negative situation and come back when you and the person feel calmer. When you return, tell the person that you noticed that she seemed upset about something. By communicating in this way, you make it possible for her to talk about what is troubling her, which may stop or reduce negative or harmful actions.

TABLE 6-1 VERBAL SOCIAL REINFORCEMENT

Type of Verbal Social Reinforcement	You Can Say . . .
Praise	"Mrs. McDay, I really like the way you styled your hair." "Congratulations, Mrs. Garcia. The physical therapist said you walked 10 feet farther than you did last week."
Appreciation	"Thank you, Mr. Lightfoot, for helping me." "Mrs. Ryan, thank you for helping Mrs. Morgan feel more at home here."
Encouragement	"Keep trying to touch your shoulder, Mr. Rivera. You're doing a little better every day!" "You're doing a great job walking today, Mrs. Wang. I know you can make it another 2 feet to the dayroom."
Approval	"That's right, Josie. You're doing it exactly right." "I think that was a good choice, Mr. Rivera."
Recognition	"Everyone, Mrs. Morgan has joined our group today. Let's welcome her." "Let's all thank Mrs. Ryan for the beautiful wall hanging she quilted for our dayroom."

When a person in your care behaves in an inappropriate way, try to ignore the behavior. Sometimes a person uses inappropriate behavior to attract attention. If you pay much attention to these behaviors, she may repeat them. If you think someone in your care is trying to attract attention through inappropriate behavior, pay more attention to her when her behaviors are appropriate.

When a person in your care behaves in a harmful way, report his actions to your supervising nurse. Be as specific as you can. For example, if you say, "Mr. Lightfoot was a pain in the neck today," or "Mr. Lightfoot is so messy," you are communicating only your judgments rather than facts. A more useful way to report the behavior would be, "At 9 A.M., when I was helping Mr. Lightfoot shave, he suddenly grabbed the razor out of my hand and threw it on the floor, barely missing my foot, and said

he wanted me to go away and leave him alone."

You may have many feelings to sort out after someone behaves in an inappropriate way. If you keep your feelings bottled up inside, they can create stress and cause you to act in inappropriate ways with other people. To help you deal with the feelings that you have with difficult situations, try some of the following suggestions.

Try Not to Take Inappropriate Behaviors Personally. A person sometimes directs inappropriate behaviors toward the people he sees most often. He may really be upset with something or someone else. If you try not to take his behaviors personally, it will be easier for you to handle the situation (Figure 6-1).

Breathe Deeply. Take deep breaths and count to 10 or 20. Keep taking deep breaths until you feel that you are calm and in control.

Leave the Room. If you can, go on with your duties. If you are afraid you may say or do something that is not appropriate in your role as a nurse assistant, leave the room, providing that the person is safe. If you are too upset to work effectively, you may need a few minutes to yourself.

Take a Break. Ask your supervising nurse for permission to take a break so that you can take a brisk walk, get a drink of water or breathe in fresh air.

Talk to Someone. Tell your supervising nurse or someone else you trust about your feelings. When you are talking, always respect the privacy of the person you are talking about, even if he or she did not treat you with respect.

Develop a Plan. Work with other members of the health care team to develop a plan of response to the person's inappropriate behaviors. You might be able to influence his or her behavior and also help prevent a co-worker from being faced with a similar situation.

Talk with the Person. Let her know that you are unhappy with her behavior but that you still care about her.

COMMUNICATING WITH PEOPLE WHEN TEACHING

The people in your care need to learn about their illnesses, injuries, disabilities or medical conditions. As a nurse assistant, providing restorative care, you can help these people learn how to **adapt** their lives so that they can stay healthy or comfortable. To help them, you must know how people learn and how to teach. When you teach, your communication skills become very important.

Your Role as a Teacher
Teachers from your school days probably talked in front of their classes, wrote on chalkboards and gave struc-

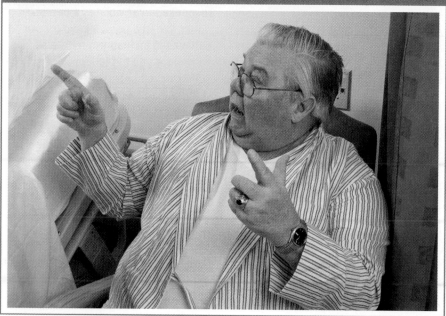

FIGURE 6-1 It is not unusual for someone who is sick or in pain to feel frustrated, angry or afraid. Although your natural response to inappropriate behavior may be anger, you must try to understand the cause of the person's behavior. If it is safe try saying, "You seem to be very upset about something. Would you like to talk about it?"

tured tests. They taught formally. But teaching is also an ongoing process that often happens informally through conversations or as one person watches another person do things.

You may intentionally teach people new activities or new ways of doing familiar activities because it is part of the care plan. Or you may teach informally by performing your daily tasks, talking with people about their concerns and giving them new information so that they can make correct choices. Through all these ways you help people understand how to adapt to the changes in their lives (Figure 6-2).

You can be a good teacher by practicing three roles: reinforcing, teaching and observing and reporting.

Reinforcing. Your supervising nurse may ask you to reinforce, or strengthen, the teaching that another

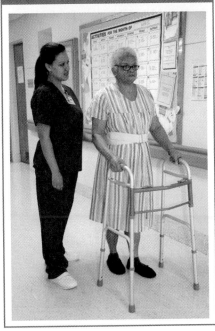

FIGURE 6-2 By reinforcing what the physical therapist taught, this nurse assistant helps Mrs. Garcia adapt to her condition and maintain her independence.

health care worker has begun. Perhaps the physical therapist taught Mr. Wilson how to move and walk with a cane. You can reinforce these lessons by observing his use of the cane when you help him get from one place to another.

Teaching. Your supervising nurse may ask you to teach a person how to do certain things that are within the scope of your job responsibilities. For example, she may ask you to teach someone who has a weak arm how to dress him- or herself or how to use a special fork or spoon.

Observing and Reporting. Your supervising nurse may also ask you to observe and report on how well someone is doing, as well as on areas in which the person needs additional teaching. You may see Mr. Wilson using his cane incorrectly. You would first correct the situation if it was unsafe, and then you would report this observation to your supervising nurse.

The Learning Process

To communicate effectively through teaching, you must understand how people learn and how you can help in their learning process.

How People Learn. The people that you teach, as well as their family members and friends, learn better when *they:*

- Can practice what they are learning.
- Can associate new information with their experiences and with something they already know.
- Can clearly see a reason or purpose for their learning.
- Are treated with respect.
  They also learn better when *you:*
- Listen to what they are saying or asking.
- Have patience.
- Give encouragement and feedback.
- Take time out if they are not feeling well or are upset.

How the Learning Process Works. Learning is an ongoing process, during which a person's knowledge, attitudes and behaviors change. Learning is not restricted to the classroom. Every day you learn by reading, working, communicating with your friends and family, listening to the radio and watching television. Just as you learn from other people and experiences, the people in your care learn from you.

When you were a child in school, you learned what your teacher and school chose to teach you. As an adult, you make choices about what you learn, based on what is important to you. Just as you chose to learn to become a nurse assistant, the adults in your care choose what they want to learn. What they learn and how they learn are affected by many things, including knowledge, attitudes or feelings, and experience.

Knowledge. A person's learning is affected by what he already knows. For example, if a resident already knew how to plan nutritious meals when he changed to a diabetic diet, he probably had an easier time learning to plan and prepare a new diet than someone who does not know anything about meal planning. However, he may have had a harder time learning if the information he received was different from what he already knew (Figure 6-3).

Attitudes or Feelings. The person's learning also is affected by how he feels about what he needs to know. For example, if a man believes that cooking is "woman's work," he may not want to learn about nutrition and meal planning.

Experience. The person's past experience affects how he learns. For example, if someone with high blood pressure tasted a few meals with less or no salt and liked them, it is easier to teach him how to prepare foods with less salt. On the other hand, if he did not like the way low-salt meals tasted, he might find it harder and need more

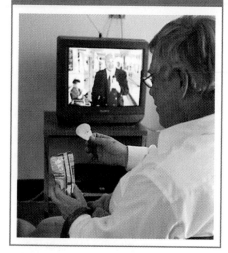

FIGURE 6-3 For many years, this man snacked on potato chips and peanuts, thinking they were good for him. He may have a hard time accepting his new diabetic diet, which eliminates or reduces these foods.

encouragement to learn how to cook with less salt.

How might you use knowledge, experience and attitude to help Mr. Rivera switch from a safety razor to an electric razor? Look at Box 5-1, page 60, for one answer. By talking with Mr. Rivera, you discover his knowledge level, his attitude and his behavior. You learn that he may need more information about his disease and its conditions, because he doesn't seem to understand how his medication affects bleeding. You supply some information and report your observation to your supervising nurse so that she can provide Mr. Rivera with more information. You may find that, even though Mr. Rivera still prefers his safety razor, he is willing to try a new behavior.

The Teaching Process

During Mr. Rivera's morning shower, you try to help him transfer himself from his wheelchair to a shower chair. During the past few days, your super-

vising nurse and the physical therapist have been teaching him how to do the transfer. You have been told to provide restorative care by reinforcing the instructions and to encourage Mr. Rivera to do as much of the transfer by himself as possible. Mr. Rivera makes several unsuccessful attempts. After his third try, he mumbles, "Oh, forget it. I'm sure my wife knows how to do this. I don't."

You can help Mr. Rivera learn to do the transfer if you understand the four steps of the teaching process: *assessing* the person's knowledge, *planning* what you have to teach and how to teach it, *implementing* your teaching plan, and *evaluating* the impact of your teaching.

Assessing. Before you begin to teach your supervising nurse will assess what the person already knows and feels about the information he needs to learn. First, your supervising nurse makes a formal assessment by looking at several different factors, including age, past education and knowledge, present health status and illness. She takes into account that certain disease conditions have very specific learning needs. For example, she knows that Mr. Rivera has weakness and some paralysis on his left side as the result of a stroke. She knows that he needs to learn to move around by himself but also that he depends on his wife to help him.

After your supervising nurse completes the formal assessment, she tells you what she thinks the person needs to learn and how you can help. She may ask you to repeat or reinforce certain points while you provide care. Then, every day as you provide restorative care for the person, you continue to observe what he does or does not know and to help your supervising nurse understand more about his needs. You look for any hints or clues from the person that may suggest he needs more information. For example, Mr. Rivera may say, "I know the nurse

and physical therapist showed me how to do this, but I keep forgetting. Besides, my wife knows how to do it." Some clues are not this obvious. Mr. Rivera's statement about his wife knowing how to do it may have been a message that he needs more information or that he is frustrated. You report this observation to your supervising nurse. As you develop relationships with your residents, you will be able to know their needs and wants through your listening abilities.

Planning. When your supervising nurse knows what the person needs to learn, she usually plans what needs to be taught and how it should be done. When she tells you what to teach, first review the information and skills before planning how to present them to the person. Plan how to fit the teaching into the time that you spend providing care for the person. For example, you might plan to help Mr. Rivera learn to dress himself during his personal care times. And you might plan to bring a long-handled shoe horn so that he can put on his shoes without bending over and getting dizzy as you learned he had done before. First, you plan to teach him how to put on his pants. When he does that well, you plan to teach him how to put on his shoes. You save teaching him how to button his shirt until last because he thinks this will be the hardest task. This teaching plan becomes a guideline to make sure you communicate the information he needs.

To make sure that your plan is what your supervising nurse wants, discuss it with her and ask any questions that you may have about the procedures you will teach.

Implementing. Once you have an assessment and a plan, implement your plan—that is, put it into action. An important part of implementing your plan is choosing when to teach. Teach only when you have enough time, when the person is feeling well and when his surroundings are quiet and private. Otherwise, postpone or adjust your teaching plan until conditions are more favorable for learning.

For example, Mr. Rivera has repeated difficulty with putting on his shirt. He makes several attempts but just can't get the arm through the sleeve. After his fourth try, he says angrily, "I just can't do it! I'll never be able to do it! It's hopeless." You could say, "I know you must feel frustrated, but I'm sure you'll get it. Why don't you take a little break right now?"

By recognizing that Mr. Rivera is upset and suggesting that he wait, you are communicating your calmness and patience. You may know from your own experience that trying to do something difficult when you are frustrated is almost impossible (Figure 6-4). What Mr. Rivera really needs to do is to take a break and relax.

Evaluating. After assessing, planning, and implementing your teaching plan, you must test, or evaluate, how effective the teaching was by observing the person and asking questions to find

out how much he learned. For example, all week you and Mr. Rivera have worked together on dressing. Today, when you come in to help him with his personal care, he has already eaten his breakfast and is in the process of getting dressed. You notice that he is able to put on his shirt and button it with only a little difficulty.

Evaluating shows you how effective your teaching is, whether the person understands and whether you need to repeat anything. Ask the basic evaluation question: Is the person willing and able to do the task or use the information that I have been teaching him? To find the answer to this question, you should ask the person to demonstrate what he learned. After you evaluate, you should give prompt, helpful and realistic feedback on how the person is doing. You also must report your evaluation to your supervising nurse.

Reinforcing What You Teach

If people in your care are overwhelmed by the amount of information you give them, use teaching skills to help them remember what you teach

and use communication skills to find out what they did not understand.

Help the Receiver Remember the Message. If you have a great amount of information to teach, separate the message into several parts, ask the person for confirmation from time to time, and give a summary of all the information when you are finished.

Encourage the Person to Ask Questions. To find out whether the person understands the information, encourage him to communicate by regularly inviting questions. To let him know that others also may have the same questions, you might say, "Many people ask me questions about this." To encourage questions, praise him when he asks, by saying, "That's a good question. I'm glad you asked!" If a person asks a question that you do not know how to answer, say that you do not know the answer and that you want to check with your supervising nurse. Write down the question, find out the answer and then give the information to the person as soon as you can.

Communicating by Telephone

In your work, you may talk on the telephone with many different people, such as the family and friends of people in your care, doctors and other health care professionals. Because the person on the other end of the telephone cannot see you, you must speak clearly and choose your words carefully. Most employers have strict rules about what you can and cannot tell various people. If you are unsure about what to do in a specific situation, ask your supervising nurse. In all situations, use professional manners, common sense and the following suggestions for talking on the telephone.

Be Professional. Know how to use the telephone system to make outgoing calls, answer incoming calls, put someone on hold, transfer a call and use any other features. If you make a professional call, identify yourself as soon as

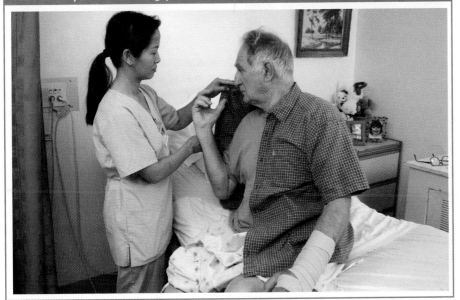

FIGURE 6-4 The nurse assistant notices that Mr. Rivera is becoming frustrated while trying to learn a dressing task. She will reevaluate and modify her teaching plan for him.

someone answers the telephone. For example: "This is nurse assistant Anna Li calling from Metropolitan Hospital Center. May I speak with Mrs. Jones?"

Be Courteous. Answer the telephone as soon as you hear it ring. Speak slowly and clearly. In a hospital or nursing home, tell the caller your location, your name and your position. For example: "Metropolitan Hospital Center, 3rd floor. This is nurse assistant Greta Casey speaking. How may I help you?" (Figure 6-5). In someone's home, you might say, "This is the Garcia residence." Check with your supervising nurse to find out if there are any additional rules to follow when answering a client's phone.

If you have to put a caller on hold, do it for only a short time. If the wait is going to be longer than a minute, get back on the line to let the caller know. Offer to take a message.

Take Accurate Messages. If you are asked to take a message, write it down carefully and repeat it to the caller to make sure the information is correct. Include the date and time of the call

on the message, and sign your name. Put the message where the receiver is most likely to find it.

Respect Privacy. Callers may ask questions about someone's health or may request other personal information. Do not provide any information unless you are sure that your employer permits it, and be sure that any information you provide is correct. If you are unsure about what information to provide to the caller, ask your supervisor.

LEARNING THE LANGUAGE OF CAREGIVING

One day after work, you and a co-worker go to a restaurant for dinner. As you walk into the restaurant, you hear the waitress yell back to the short-order cook, "BLT on white! Hold the mayo!" You may wonder what language she is speaking. To some people, these words may not sound like any English words they have ever heard before. But these words are restaurant "lingo" for "a bacon, lettuce, and tomato sandwich on white bread, without mayonnaise."

People who provide health care also use a special language that everyone "on the inside" knows. This language helps them to communicate more effectively. For example, when a nurse says that Mrs. Wang needs "ostomy" care, most people do not know what she is talking about, but the people on her health care team know that she is referring to a surgical opening in Mrs. Wang's body that needs care.

As a nurse assistant, you learn this special medical language, or terminology, so that you can communicate effectively with others on your health care team. Learning basic medical terms will help you understand the directions that your supervising nurse gives. Using the appropriate terminology will help other nurse assistants understand what you need when you ask for their help, and it will help other members of the health care team understand what you have observed and reported.

In the medical setting, it is important to be clear and **precise** in describing behavior, illness and treatment. Medical terms are precise: They mean the same thing to the person who is hearing or reading the terms as they do to the person who is speaking or writing them.

How Small Words Make Large Words

Many medical words seem to be a mile long and impossible to pronounce, but they really are just many small words that are hooked together. Many words in the English language have a beginning, a middle and an end. The beginning is called a **prefix,** the middle is called the **root,** and the end is called the **suffix.** For example, an everyday word that has these three parts is *preschooler.* The prefix *pre-* means "before." The root *school* means "a place for teaching and learning." And the suffix -*er* means "a

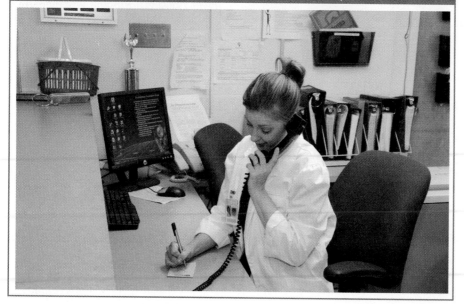

FIGURE 6-5 Callers often make judgments about a health care facility based on the way staff members answer the phone.

person or thing that . . ." When you put these three meanings together, you have the definition of *pre-schooler:* a person who is "before learning," or someone who is not old enough to be in school. The root word can be a word that stands by itself, such as the word *school.* Prefixes and suffixes, on the other hand, cannot stand alone. They always are attached to root words. *Pre-* and *-er* are not strong enough to stand by themselves. However, when you attach them to a root word, they are powerful enough to change the meaning of the word.

Most words do not have all three parts. A word may have a prefix and a root, such as *replace,* which has the prefix *re-* (again or back) and the root *place* (put or position). For example, "After the floor dries, the man replaces the furniture." Together, the prefix and the root of *replace* mean "put back."

Other words have a root and a suffix, such as *alcoholic,* which has the root *alcohol* (an intoxicating liquor) and the suffix *-ic* (having to do with). The root and the suffix together mean "having to do with alcohol." For example, "Only one bowl of punch was alcoholic. The other one was just fruit juice. So the recovering alcoholic took his drink from the nonalcoholic punch bowl."

Box 6-1 contains some familiar everyday English words and some medical words that give you an idea of how roots, prefixes and suffixes are combined to form longer words with specific meanings.

In addition, words created from prefixes, roots and suffixes may leave out, change or add certain letters so that they conform to general rules of spelling and pronunciation. That is what happened with the last word in Box 6-1, *physiology.* The root is *physio,* but the *o* was cut out when it was combined with *-ology,* so the word is not *physioology* but *physiology.* This change also happens with the word *ejaculate,* which is combined from the prefix *ex-* (out or out

of) and the root *jaculor* (throw) to make the word that means "to discharge suddenly and briefly."

Using Medical Terminology

As a nurse assistant, you must know the meanings of prefixes, roots and suffixes and how to combine them to understand the longer words. For example, Box 6-2 contains words that relate to the heart. From this list, you can see how knowing just one word gives you a clue for understanding many other words. When you know the meaning of the different parts of a word, you can identify each piece and then figure out what the whole word means.

Using Medical Abbreviations

Remember at the beginning of this section how the waitress yelled back to the cook for a BLT? *BLT* is an **abbreviation** for *b*acon, *l*ettuce and *t*omato. *BLT* is made up of the first letters of the three things that are on the sandwich. An abbreviation that we often use is *USA,* which is an abbreviation for the *U*nited *S*tates of *A*merica. *USA* is made up of the first letters of the three most important words in the phrase.

In the language of medicine, members of the health care team use abbreviations to save time and space. For example, when a doctor surgically removes the tonsils and adenoids of a patient, he performs a *t*onsillectomy *and a*denoidectomy. However, when he records information about the procedure, he writes *T and A.* Likewise, on a person's chart you may see that he had a *CBC,* which is the abbreviation for *c*omplete *b*lood *c*ount.

Not all abbreviations stand for the first letters of the words in a phrase. For example, *no.* stands for "number," and *fld.* stands for "fluid." Some abbreviations used in medical settings do not seem to relate to the words they stand for. For example, *q* stands for "every," *qd* stands for "every day," and *q2h* stands

for "every 2 hours." You must memorize abbreviations like these, because they may not look like the words they represent. If you are not sure about an abbreviation, look it up before you use it.

As a nurse assistant, you use these abbreviations in your daily work, but you must use only the abbreviations that everyone else in your health care setting uses.

COMMUNICATING ABOUT THE PEOPLE IN YOUR CARE

When you use medical terminology, you communicate about the person in your care with other caregivers on that person's health care team. Every day, health care workers must pass information from one group of caregivers to another so that all caregivers can provide coordinated, high-quality care. For example, the caregivers who work at night must give information to the people who provide care during the day. They must write down the information so that it is not forgotten.

Suppose your supervising nurse gives you a lot of information about a new person in your care: For example, "Mr. Chalmers was admitted from the emergency room last night complaining of chest pain and shortness of breath. He has no known allergies. He is on bed rest but can get out of bed to use the bathroom. He can have nothing by mouth now, but after blood is drawn for the lab, he can have fluids as desired. He can have nothing by mouth after midnight tonight. He is on oxygen at 2 liters and is on intake and output. Today he is scheduled for a complete blood count, a 6 A.M. fasting blood sugar, an electrocardiogram and urinalysis. Get a urine specimen. Take his vital signs four times a day. Mr. Chalmers has an order for pain medication every 3 hours as needed and a sleeping pill at bedtime if he needs it."

To make sure you remembered everything she said, you would take

BOX 6-1

FORMING WORDS

Prefix	Root	Suffix	Word	Meaning
re- (again or back)	use (to put into action or service)	-able (that can be)	reusable	that can be used again
Example: The blanket and spread may be reusable linens.				
ab- (away; from; away from)	use (to put into action or service)	-er (a person or thing that)	abuser	a person who uses or treats someone or something in a way that is different from the acceptable way
Example: The abuser is often someone the victim knows.				
ab-	norm (standard; pattern)	-al (pertaining to)	abnormal	not as it should be; not in the usual pattern
Example: The person's bowel elimination pattern has become abnormal.				
ab-	norm	-ality (the condition of being)		a condition in which things are not as they should be
Example: The test on the specimen shows whether there is an abnormality.				
co- (with)	operate (work)		cooperate	to work together with someone
Example: When people on the team cooperate, the work is more easily done.				
	trachea- (tube that carries air to the lungs; wind-pipe)	-tomy (cutting into)	tracheotomy	surgical operation of cutting into the trachea
Example: A nurse assistant must provide special care to someone who has had a tracheotomy.				
ana- (living)		-tomy (cutting into)	anatomy	study of a living body based on dissection or cutting open
Example: When you study anatomy, you learn about the separate parts of the body.				
	physio- (of the body)	-ology (a science or knowledge of)	physiology	science of the normal function of a living body or its parts
Example: We must know about the kidneys, heart, lungs, and blood vessels to understand blood physiology.				

BOX 6-2

FORMING MEDICAL WORDS

Cardio is a root word that means "heart." If you add different prefixes and suffixes to cardio, you get a variety of terms to use when communicating about the heart. For example:

Prefix	Root	Suffix	Word	Meaning
	cardio	-ology	cardiology	science of heart function and disease
	cardio	-ologist	cardiologist	specialist who studies and treats heart disease
	cardio	-vascular	cardiovascular	having to do with the heart and blood vessels
	cardio	-pulmonary	cardiopulmonary	having to do with the heart and lungs
myo-	cardium		myocardium	heart muscle

notes, using the abbreviations you learned, while listening to her report: "Mr. Chalmers was adm. from ER last noc c/o chest pain and SOB; NKA. Bedrest c̄ BRP, NPO til lab draws blood; then fld. ad lib; NPO after midnight; O2 at 2 L; I&O; CBC, 6 a.m. FBS, EKG, U/A (get spec.) today; VS q.i.d; pain medication q3h, prn; sleeping pill q.h.s., prn."

Communicating in Three Documents

Your supervising nurse must have written records of the care a person receives. Because you are responsible for contributing information and observations to one or all of these documents—the care plan, the flow sheet and nursing notes—and because you have to read and use the forms, you must be familiar with all three of them. While providing care you may have to record your observations. When recording, communicate your findings clearly and completely. If you make a mistake in your recording never erase or use correction fluid. Cross out the incorrect statement and initial it. Rewrite the statement correctly. Follow your facilities on any additional procedures concerning recording observation.

Care Plan. Each day, the first documentation tool you use is a care plan. Care plans often are kept in a card file, and each person receiving care has a separate card in the file. A nurse obtains information from the doctor's orders and writes it on the care plan. Like other documentation tools, care plans may be kept on a computer. In place of a card, each person has a computer printout. You read the care plan every day to obtain information for providing care. The following list includes some of the information you may find in each person's care plan:

- The person's name, age, religion and date of admission
- Diagnosis
- Diet
- Activity level
- Special procedures and dates
- Treatments, such as dressing care, intravenous therapy, respiratory therapy and intake and output recordings
- Special equipment, such as an air mattress, a Foley catheter and traction devices

Flow Sheet. Caregivers use a **flow sheet** to track a person's changes over a period of time (Figures 6-6 and 6-7).

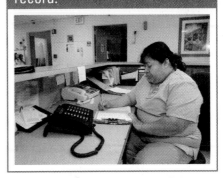

FIGURE 6-6 Other caregivers rely on information that you record.

The flow sheet often is kept in a person's room or at his bedside for immediate recording. Documentation on a flow sheet also may include vital signs, intake and output recordings, weight, measurements, treatments and procedures. For example, Grace Smyth's flow sheet shows that on her first day in the hospital, she ate 100 percent of her diet at breakfast, 80 percent at lunch and 80 percent at dinner.

Nursing Notes. Members of the health care team read another form of communication called **nursing notes.** The supervising nurse writes nursing notes in the medical chart to record the person's condition, the care pro-

Activities of Daily Living (ADL) Flow Chart

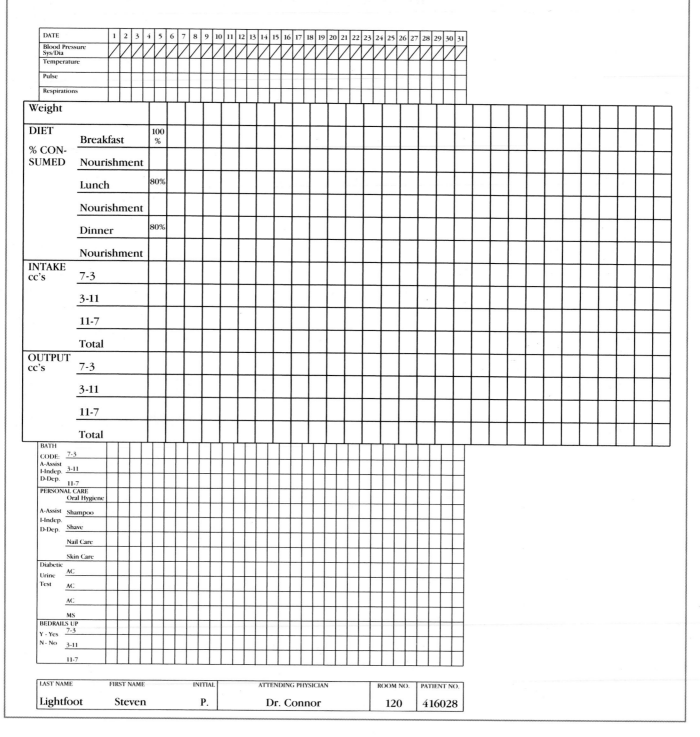

LAST NAME	FIRST NAME	INITIAL	ATTENDING PHYSICIAN	ROOM NO.	PATIENT NO.
Lightfoot	Steven	P.	Dr. Connor	120	416028

vided to him or her, and significant events that took place during the shift or visit. You contribute information to your supervising nurse, which she writes into the nursing notes.

Observing

As a nurse assistant, one of your biggest jobs is to be the eyes, ears, nose and fingertips for the rest of the health care team. You spend much time with the people in your care, and you have to communicate when something changes. To communicate changes, you must observe carefully with your senses, and you must report these observations to your supervising nurse. A person may not tell you if they have a problem. You will have to observe for nonverbal signs of communication. Table 6-2 contains examples of how to use your senses of sight, sound, smell and touch to learn about a person's condition.

Assessing for Pain in Older Adults

There are many barriers to identifying and managing pain in the nursing home resident. Many people, often including the resident and family members, believe that pain is a natural side effect of getting older. To some extent, residents often underreport pain because they do not want to "give in" to pain. Some residents just "don't want to bother anyone." Some may feel that they won't be believed; others may feel that the increase in their pain means that their condition is getting worse.

As a nurse assistant, you are with the person more and can give your supervising nurse useful information.

The Assessment Process. If the person is having pain, find out:

- How long the pain has lasted.
- Where the pain is located.
- Nature of the pain (constant, intermittent, sharp, burning, aching, heavy, stabbing?).
- Rate the pain (on a scale from 1–10, 10 being the worst)

Sense	Common Observations
Sight	**You See . . .** that the person's skin looks pale or red open areas on the person's skin sores in the person's mouth that the person's hand shakes or that the person is too weak to hold a glass that the person limps or cannot stand alone that the person's urine, stool or sputum has an unusual color that the person's emesis (vomit) has an unusual color that the person is not eating or is having trouble eating that the person squints or bumps into things and people that the person's usual facial expression has changed (for example, he smiles less often) that the person sleeps a lot or does not make eye contact that the person's breathing is different, labored or slow, or the person gasps for breath that a part of the person's body looks different or abnormal to you (for example, one limb is larger than the other) that there is blood or other leakage coming from some part of the person's body or medical device, such as a drain or IV
Sound	**You Hear . . .** the person coughing the person making a noise when breathing the person complaining of a change in his condition (for example, pain, numbness or swelling) the person crying no response from the person when you talk to him or her that the person does not speak clearly
Smell	**You Smell . . .** that the person's breath has an unusual odor that the person's emesis (vomit) has an unusual odor an unusual odor in the person's urine or stool that the person's dressing or wound has an odor
Touch	**You Feel . . .** that the person's pulse is strong that the person's pulse is weak that the person's skin is warm, cool or moist a lump under the person's skin

TABLE 6-2 USING YOUR SENSES TO OBSERVE

To further assess the person for pain, you can ask the following questions:

- Does the pain radiate?
- What makes pain better or worse (food, rest, cold, heat)?
- Is there nausea, vomiting, urinary burning or retention?
- Is the person coughing more than usual?
- Are symptoms new or increased?
- Does the person look ill?

Try to get specific information but do not lead the person to give the answers you are looking for. After you have made your assessment, record the results on the proper form. Anything abnormal or out of the ordinary should be reported to your supervising nurse.

Reporting Your Observations

When you use your senses to observe the people in your care, you must know which observations are important to report, what is the best way to report the observation and when is a good time to report it.

What to Report. As you make observations, assess the person's condition and decide what information to pass on to other members of the health care team. A rule of thumb to use when deciding what information to report is, "When in doubt, report." It is best to tell your supervising nurse and let her or him determine whether something needs to be done. When deciding what to report, focus on the word *change*. Report observations that indicate changes in:

- Mood, mental awareness and level of independence.
- Vital signs.
- Elimination.
- Skin condition and color.
- Appetite (Figure 6-8).
- Sleep habits.

How to Report. After you decide what needs to be reported, the next step is to communicate. Give your information and assessment to others by telling or writing what you observed. Your observations of a person's condition contribute important information to the care plan. For the information to be helpful to those who use it, it must include as many accurate details as possible. Be objective by reporting clear, accurate information and by paying attention to the facts and not to your personal opinions. Table 6-3 contains examples of differences between facts and opinions.

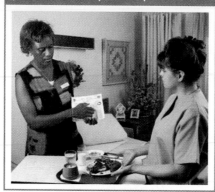

FIGURE 6-8 Monitor and report leftover food portions and discuss changes in eating patterns with your supervisor.

The following examples demonstrate helpful ways of reporting information that is very important and reporting information that is less helpful:

Example 1. After Mrs. Garcia broke her hip, she used a wheelchair to get around in the hospital. Her physical therapist worked with her to improve her strength so that she could stand up. The care plan said that you should help her stand three times a day. You knew that she usually stood for 2 or 3 minutes each afternoon. One day, using your arm for support, Mrs. Garcia stood for 5 minutes.

> *Helpful:* "Mrs. Garcia stood for 5 minutes this afternoon. She leaned on my arm."
> *Less helpful:* "Mrs. Garcia stood for longer than usual."

Example 2. Since his stroke, Mr. Rivera has been working with an occupational therapist to relearn how to shave himself using an electric razor. When he started therapy last week, he had a hard time holding the razor and making his hand move the right way. He got frustrated and asked you to finish the job. Today you notice that he shaved his whole face.

> *Helpful:* "Mr. Rivera has made progress with his shaving skills. He is able to shave his whole face."
> *Less helpful:* "Mr. Rivera is doing better holding the razor."

When to Report. Two regular times for reporting are when you begin to provide care for a person and when you complete it. In some settings, especially hospitals, there is a meeting called *shift report* or *shift change*. During report, you *receive* information about each person in your care from your supervising nurse. At the end of your caregiving or shift, you *give* a report and share information about what you observed and what you did for each person in your care.

Also, report to your supervising nurse right away whenever you think it is necessary. Use the guidelines in this chapter, information throughout this book and the six principles of care to guide you as you decide what to report and when to report it.

TABLE 6-3 FACT AND OPINION

Fact	Opinion
The person is not putting his full weight on his left foot.	The person walks funny.
She is crying.	She must miss her dog.
He weighs 250 pounds.	He is overweight.
The person has a dry cough.	I'll bet he smoked a cigarette.
She did not eat any of her dinner.	She must be sneaking candy.

Circle the correct answers and fill in the blanks.

1. When the care you provide is contributing to the health care team's plan to rehabilitate the person, it is called _restorative_ care.

2. Before you teach Mrs. Ryan about her skin care, you must first learn:
   a. nothing; just teach her what she needs to know.
   b. what she knows and how she takes care of her skin.
   c. how she takes care of her hair.
   d. what her favorite brand of soap is.

3. You see a new medical word and are not sure what it means. There is no dictionary available. How do you try to figure out its meaning?
   a. Look at the different parts of the word, especially the root, to see whether you know the meaning of any of the word's parts.
   b. Look at the suffix to see what the word means.
   c. Say the word out loud.
   d. Ignore it.

4. Three documents that health care workers use to communicate about the people in their care are the _care plan_, _flow sheet_ and _nursing notes_

5. When deciding what to report to your supervising nurse, you should focus on:
   a. any change in a person's behavior or condition.
   b. the person's appearance.
   c. what the person does from moment to moment.
   d. whom the person talks with during the day.

1. While you help Mr. Rivera transfer himself from the bed to the wheelchair, he says that your directions don't match the way he learned to do it. What should you do?

2. You notice that Mrs. Roth's daughter often brings a box of chocolate candy when she comes to visit her mother. Both you and Mrs. Roth know that candy is not permitted on her diet, but she eats it anyway because she says she doesn't want to hurt her daughter's feelings. What should you do?

3. Mrs. Wang normally greets you with a smile and pleasant conversation. Today she doesn't. Also, she seems to be sleepy and says she isn't hungry. You remember that she had many visitors yesterday, but you also know that several people in the unit have colds. What additional observations could you make to help your supervising nurse or the doctor assess her condition? How do you record/report your observations?

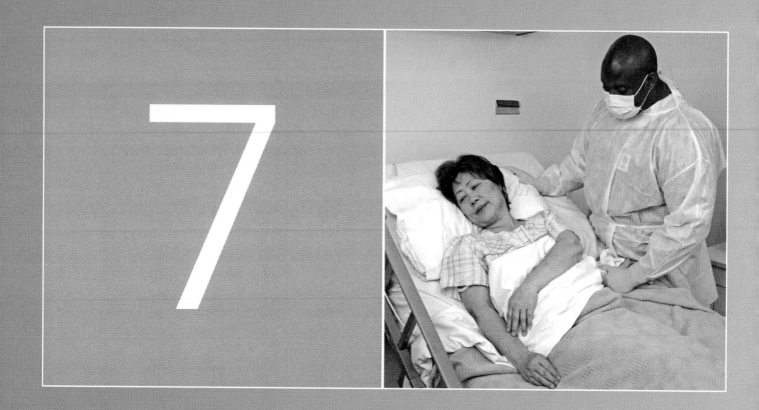

7

Controlling the Spread of Germs

GOALS

After reading this chapter, you will have the information needed to:

Apply general infection control measures to control the spread of germs.

Clean, disinfect and sterilize objects.

Use Standard Precautions when necessary.

Use Isolation Precautions when necessary.

Explain Isolation Precautions to someone in isolation.

After practicing the corresponding skills, you will have the information needed to:

Wash your hands in a way that controls the spread of germs.

Put on and take off protective clothing correctly.

Open and close a trash bag correctly and double-bag contaminated trash and laundry.

During morning report at Metropolitan Hospital Center, your supervising nurse tells you about your new patient, Louise Wang, an 53-year-old woman who was admitted through the emergency room from Morningside Nursing Home last night. Because she was diagnosed with highly contagious staph pneumonia, she is in isolation in Room 117. Last year, she had part of her intestines removed because of colon cancer. A colostomy was performed, which means that you will have to provide care for the stoma, the surgical opening in her abdomen that allows feces from her intestines to empty into a bag rather than through her rectum. In addition to colostomy care, Mrs. Wang needs help with a complete bed bath and with transferring from the bed to the chair, because she is very weak. Your supervising nurse also tells you that Mrs. Wang is originally from China but speaks and understands English very well.

You decide to visit Mrs. Wang immediately because you think she might be afraid. Before going into her room, you wash your hands and using isolation precautions; put on a gown, mask and gloves. Outside her room, you notice the sign posted on her closed door. The sign requests visitors to report to the nurses' station.

You knock gently, then a little louder when you hear no response. When you finally hear a faint "Come in," you open the door to see the back of a small woman lying in bed. You walk toward the bed, gently calling Mrs. Wang's name and telling her who you are. When she turns toward you and sees your masked face, her eyes open wide before she turns back to face the wall.

KEY TERMS

acquired immunodeficiency syndrome (AIDS): (uh-KWY-erd/im-MYOUN-o-duh-FISH-uhn-see/SIN-drohm) a condition caused by the human immunodeficiency virus (HIV) that results in a breakdown of the body's defense systems.

airborne germs: germs that are carried in the air by breathing, coughing or sneezing.

antimicrobial: (an-ti-my-CROW-bee-uhl) capable of killing or slowing the growth of pathogens.

body fluids: liquid substances produced by the body.

contaminated: (kun-TAM-in-ay-tid) containing dirt or disease-causing germs.

disinfect: (dis-in-FEKT) to remove disease-causing germs.

disinfectant: (dis-in-FEK-tunt) a substance that destroys disease-causing germs.

HEPA: an abbreviation for high-efficiency particulate air filter mask that filters out contaminates in the air.

hepatitis: (heh-puh-TY-tis) a disease or condition marked by an inflammation of the liver.

human immunodeficiency virus (HIV): (im-you-no-duh-FISH-uhn-see) the microscopic organism that causes AIDS.

infection: (in-FEK-shun) a harmful condition caused by the growth of pathogens in the body.

infection control: action taken to control the spread of germs. Infection control is one of the six principles of care.

infectious: (in-FEK-shus) spreading or capable of spreading rapidly. Infectious germs are also described as communicable and contagious.

Isolation Precautions: practices used to separate a person from others and prevent the spread of infection.

microorganism: (my-crow-OR-guh-niz-um) tiny living thing that can be seen only through the magnification of a microscope.

mucous membrane: (MYOU-kus) a thin layer of body tissue that lines the inside of body passages and cavities, such as the inside of the mouth, nose, eyes, vagina and rectum.

pathogen: (PATH-o-jen) a harmful germ or microorganism that causes disease.

sharps container: a sturdy box with a tight-fitting lid that cannot be punctured by sharp objects such as needles or razors. Use of a sharps container protects health care workers from injury and exposure to contaminated items.

sign: any thing that you see, hear, feel or smell during your observation of a person in your care.

speculum: (SPEK-you-lum) an instrument used to examine a body passage or cavity.

Standard Precautions: (also known as universal precautions) practices used by caregivers when providing care to a person, regardless of the person's condition or injury, to minimize the spread of germs.

sterilize: (STAIR-uh-lize) to destroy all germs.

symptom: (SIMP-tum) anything that the person in your care tells you about how they are feeling. You cannot observe this change within a person's body.

GERMS AND INFECTION

Louise Wang is in a room by herself because she has *Staphylococcus pneumonia,* also called staph pneumonia, a disease that other people could catch from her. Colds and flus also are diseases that people can get from one another. Have you ever caught a cold or flu from someone? You can lessen your chances of getting sick and avoid passing on an illness to someone else by learning about germs, how they can cause illness and how you can help control their spread.

Germs is the word that most people use to describe tiny living things that are too small to see but are all around us and can cause disease. Scientists call them **microorganisms.** Microorganisms, such as bacteria, viruses, fungus, yeasts and molds, can be seen only with a microscope. Some microorganisms are harmful to humans and some are not. Harmful microorganisms that cause disease are called **pathogens.**

Sometimes pathogens move from place to place and may spread disease from one person to another. These diseases are called **infectious.** **Infection** is a general term for a disease caused by bacteria, viruses or other germs that enter and infect the body in a variety of ways.

You use specific precautions and take certain actions to control the spread of germs that cause different infectious diseases. This practice is called **infection control,** which is one of the six principles of care. You probably already use some of these precautions in your daily life without thinking much about them. If you cough or sneeze, for example, do you cover your mouth with a tissue or turn your head to control the spread of germs? If someone you know has a cold or flu, do you try to keep your distance from that person so that you will not catch these germs? (Figure 7-1) Do you always wash your hands after using the bathroom? If you do these

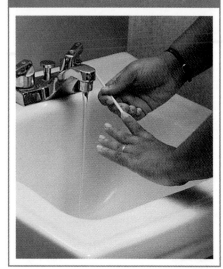

FIGURE 7-1 You probably already practice some common methods of infection control.

things, you already are controlling the spread of infection.

Practicing infection control is especially important when providing care for people of all ages, especially if their health condition is compromised.

When you work in any health care setting, you can help control the spread of infection if you understand exactly what is meant by *clean* and what is meant by *dirty.* Clean items or surfaces are considered to be free of dirt and pathogens, or disease-causing germs. Dirty items or surfaces are considered to be **contaminated** because they contain dirt or pathogens. An unused item is considered to be clean until it comes in contact with a person or his or her environment. It is then considered to be dirty and cannot be reused for another person.

In a hospital or nursing home, the clean utility room has clean, unused supplies, such as linens and dressings. The dirty utility room has trash containers and reusable supplies that must be cleaned or laundered.

How to Recognize an Infection

In addition to practicing the everyday control of spreading germs, you must

know how to recognize infection. For example, germs live and multiply on and in your body. They grow rapidly wherever they have warm temperatures, moisture, darkness and food. Think of an area of your body that is dark and moist. That is a place where germs live, grow and multiply fast. That is a place where an infection might occur.

Although some germs are useful and necessary in certain areas of the body, these same germs may cause disease if they spread to another part of the body. For example, certain bacteria in the stomach and intestines help to digest food. But, if these same bacteria are present in the kidney or bladder, they can cause an infection.

An infection occurs when pathogens grow inside the body; almost any part of the body can become infected. You can recognize a possible infection in a person's body by certain **signs** and **symptoms.** The signs and symptoms are not always the same because they vary according to the kind of germ and the place in the body where the infection is occurring. Box 7-1 contains some of the common signs and symptoms that help you recognize an infection.

If you observe that someone in your care has one or more of the signs and symptoms in Box 7-1, report it to your supervising nurse, just as you report any changes that you observe with your senses. (Read Table 6-2 in Chapter 6 again.) By recognizing infections early, you increase the chances of treating them and preventing their spread to other people. Although it is important to know the signs and symptoms of possible infection, you must always practice infection control, even when you do not observe any signs or symptoms.

How Germs Spread

To control the spread of germs, you need to know how germs move from one place to another. Germs are most commonly spread through direct and indirect contact.

BOX 7-1

COMMON SIGNS AND SYMPTOMS FOR RECOGNIZING AN INFECTION

High body temperature
Red or draining eyes
Stuffy nose
Coughing
Headache
Sore throat
Flushed face
Loss of appetite
Nausea
Stomach pain
Vomiting

Diarrhea
Cloudy or smelly urine
Joint pain
Muscle ache
Skin rash
Sores
Redness around a wound or incision
Drainage from a wound or incision
Swelling

Direct Contact. If you are not protected by gloves while you provide care for Mrs. Wang's stoma, you can get bacteria directly from her feces onto your hands. If you do not wash your hands and you eat a snack, these germs will spread to you. *Direct contact* means that germs spread from one living thing to another living thing through the skin or an opening in the body. If you kiss a person who has a cold, you can catch the cold. The germs will spread by direct contact.

Indirect Contact. If Mrs. Wang drinks from a glass, some of the pathogens that caused her illness are transferred to the glass. Then, if you handle the glass without gloves, you can get these same germs on your hands. If you then touch your eyes or mouth, or if you have a crack in your skin, you can develop the infection. The germs will spread by indirect contact.

Indirect contact means that germs are spread by way of an object. Usually this situation occurs when an infected person touches something and then someone else touches that same object (Figure 7-2). For example, if you have a cold and blow your nose

into a tissue, and someone else picks up the tissue to throw it away without wearing gloves, that person can get your cold by indirect contact. The germs will spread from your nose secretions to the tissue to the other

FIGURE 7-2 Sharing items can spread germs because commonly borrowed items, such as pens, often are contaminated with harmful microorganisms.

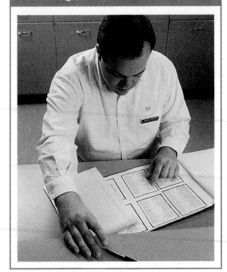

person's hand. You can get other infections by indirect contact if you:

- Eat contaminated food such as a custard that has been left out of the refrigerator overnight.
- Use contaminated water for cleaning or drinking.
- Handle dirty equipment without gloves.
- Handle soiled linens without gloves.
- Handle dressings that are contaminated with wound drainage without gloves.
- Do not perform proper handwashing technique.

How to Control the Spread of Germs

When you understand what germs are and how they spread, you can use precautions to keep them from spreading. In addition, if you are always ready to recognize potential infection and take positive actions, such as washing your hands, you can control the spread of germs and infection every day.

Taking Precautions Every Day. You can control the spread of germs 24 hours a day by taking the following actions:

- **Wash your hands.** Read the next section on handwashing to know the appropriate times for washing your hands.
- **Use an antimicrobial soap.** If possible, use **antimicrobial** soap from a liquid soap dispenser, rather than from a bar that is used by others.
- **Eat well and exercise.** Select a well-balanced diet to stay healthy.
- **Discuss any illnesses.** Before doing any personal care, discuss any illness you may have with your supervising nurse.
- **Stay home if you are sick.**
- **Keep things clean.** Keep yourself, the person in your care and the person's space clean. You can remove dirt and some germs from

an object if you clean the object with soap and water. Or you can **disinfect** the object to remove disease-causing germs by soaking it in a **disinfectant** solution. To destroy all germs, **sterilize** the object by treating it with gas, liquid, dry heat or pressurized steam. A special department of the hospital or nursing home, often called Central Supply, usually sterilizes objects. In a person's home, you can sterilize durable objects by boiling them in water for 20 minutes. Or you may clean them with a fresh mixture of 1/4 cup bleach to 1 gallon of water and let them air dry.

- **Keep dirty linens away from your uniform.**
- **Avoid shaking dirty linens or clothing to prevent spread of germs.**
- **Bag dirty linens.** Place dirty linens in the laundry bag in the person's room before you carry the bag to the laundry hamper outside the room. Place wet and soiled linens in a plastic or leakproof laundry bag.
- **Clean, dry and store utensils.** Follow your employer's policy for cleaning, drying and storing utensils after you use them.
- **Ensure single use of personal equipment.** Make sure each person in your care has their own personal items such as bedpans, urinals, washbasins, emesis basins, toothbrushes, toothpaste, lotion and soap. These items should never be shared.
- **Cover bedpans and urinals.** To contain fluids when carrying them from one place to another, always cover bedpans and urinals.
- **Recognize and report signs and symptoms of infection.** Be on the lookout for any signs of infection and report any findings immediately to your supervising nurse.

- **Prepare food carefully.** When preparing food for yourself or for your client:
  - Wash your hands first.
  - Rinse off the tops of cans before opening them.
  - Wash fruits and vegetables before using them.
  - Cook food properly; cook chicken and pork thoroughly.
  - Clean dishes and utensils after each use.
  - When using cutting boards to prepare chicken, pork or other meats, wash them thoroughly with hot soapy water immediately after use. Use separate cutting boards for cutting meat and for cutting vegetables that are not going to be cooked.
- **Serve meals immediately.** After food arrives from the dietary department of a hospital or nursing home, or as soon as you prepare food in a client's home, serve it immediately.
- **Store foods carefully.** Make sure residents do not store food in their rooms, unless the food is nonperishable and is stored in a tightly sealed container. For example, if Mrs. Wang does not finish her lunch but wants to keep a cup of chocolate pudding to eat later, explain to her that unrefrigerated food can grow bacteria that could make her ill if she eats it several hours later. If she is hungry later in the day, bring her a fresh serving of pudding.

Washing Your Hands. Washing your hands is *the most important thing* you can do to control the spread of germs. As a nurse assistant, you wash your hands in a special way so that they are free of germs. The specific procedure for handwashing is explained step by step in Skill 1. As you practice the handwashing procedure, remember the additional tips about infection control in Box 7-2, and look at Box 7-3 to make sure you are using every possible opportunity to keep your hands clean.

Sometimes you may think that handwashing is a "pain in the neck" when you have so much else to do. But the one time you say, "I'll skip it. I'm too busy," may be the time you infect yourself or someone else with germs from another person.

BOX 7-2

HANDWASHING PRECAUTIONS

- Keep your fingernails trimmed short and use a nail-brush or orangewood stick to remove any dirt underneath them.
- Do not wear rings to work, except for a simple wedding band. The tiny spaces in jewelry provide a good place for breeding germs, which may spread from one person to another.

- Because you must wash your wrists along with your hands, push your watch above your wrist, put it in your pocket or pin it to your uniform.
- If antimicrobial soap is not available from a dispenser, rinse the bar of soap before and after you use it.

BOX 7-3

WHEN TO WASH YOUR HANDS

As a Nurse Assistant, You Should Wash Your Hands:
As you are coming on duty.
Before and after contact with a person in your care.
Each time you remove your gloves.
After using the bathroom.
After coughing, sneezing, or blowing your nose.

Before handling food.
After smoking.
Before handling clean linens.
After handling dirty linens.
Before going home.
Any other time you think it may be important

STANDARD PRECAUTIONS AND ISOLATION PRECAUTIONS

Health care workers control the spread of germs by always practicing **Standard Precautions (also known as Universal Precautions)** and by following **Isolation Precautions** when they are necessary.

As a nurse assistant, you come in contact with many different substances that are produced by and released from a person's body, such as blood, vomitus, tears, semen, vaginal secretions, saliva, urine, feces and sweat. These substances are called **body fluids.** If a person has an infection, these body fluids can contain pathogens. Some serious pathogens, such as **human immunodeficiency virus (HIV)** and those that cause **hepatitis (HBV),** may be spread when a person comes in contact with an infected person's body fluids, especially blood. HIV, which is carried in the blood and in some other body fluids, causes **acquired immunodeficiency syndrome (AIDS).** You will learn more about providing care for people with these conditions in Chapter 18, "Providing Care for People with HIV/AIDS, Hepatitis and Tuberculosis."

Bloodborne Pathogen Standard

In 1986, at the request of the American Federation of State, County, and Municipal Employees (AFSCME), the Occupational Safety and Health Administration (OSHA) passed a regulation to protect workers from exposure to HIV, hepatitis and other diseases. The Bloodborne Pathogens Standard was issued in 1991 to prevent on-the-job needlesticks and other exposures to blood and other body fluids that contain blood. The regulation requires that an exposure plan be developed and implemented in the workplace, where exposure to blood or other potentially infectious material exists. Workers who are at risk must be identified, and the plan must be reviewed at least yearly. The employer must also offer workers who have a risk of exposure to blood an opportunity to receive the hepatitis B vaccination at no cost. All nurse assistants should take advantage of this and receive the vaccination.

Practicing Standard or Universal Precautions

You must practice Standard Precautions or Universal Precautions when-

ever you come into contact with body fluids, such as when assisting with a medical procedure or when providing personal care—even if you think the person in your care is not infected. Box 7-4 contains a list of the ten precautions you must follow when you might come into contact with all human blood and certain

BOX 7-4

TEN STANDARD PRECAUTIONS

1. Wear disposable gloves.
2. Wash your hands and other skin surfaces immediately and thoroughly if contaminated with body fluids or if you have handled potentially contaminated articles.
3. Wear protective clothing, such as a gown and a mask, when required.
4. Dispose of sharp objects by placing them into a biohazard container.
5. Wear gloves if you have open cuts or oozing sores.
6. Clean up blood or body fluid spills promptly.
7. Handle linens carefully.
8. Bag contaminated articles carefully.
9. Put waste in a leakproof, air-tight container.
10. Keep resuscitation masks and/or bags on hand in a hospital or nursing home setting.

human body fluids. Read about the precautions in the following paragraphs, memorize them and make them a way of life as you work as a nurse assistant.

Wear Disposable Gloves. Wear gloves when:

- You touch blood.
- You touch semen and vaginal secretions.
- You touch **mucous membranes.**
- You touch any body fluids that may or may not contain visible blood.
- The person in your care has broken skin or you have broken skin on your hands.
- You must handle items on surfaces soiled with blood or other body fluids.

Example: You wear gloves when you provide oral hygiene care, perineal care or care for someone who has a draining wound or open sores on the skin. You also wear them when you touch a contaminated dressing.

Change gloves and wash your hands after each contact with a person. Wear disposable gloves, such as vinyl or nitrile.

If while wearing gloves you or the person you are providing care for starts experiencing skin redness, rash, hives, itching, runny nose, sneezing, itchy eyes, scratchy throat or signs of asthma, wash hands immediately. If conditions persist or you experience a severe allergic reaction, contact the nurse in charge.

Wash Your Hands and Other Skin Surfaces. Wash your hands and other skin surfaces immediately and thoroughly:

- If you are contaminated with blood or other body fluids.
- If you have handled potentially contaminated articles.
- After removing gloves.
- Before putting on new gloves.

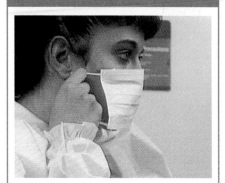

FIGURE 7-3 Use personal protective equipment whenever you are likely to be exposed to blood or other body fluids.

Wear Personal Protective Equipment. Wear personal protective equipment, such as:

- A gown or apron when your clothing might become soiled with body fluids or excretions.
- A mask, goggles or face shield if you think blood or other body fluids might splash into your mouth, nose or eyes (Figure 7-3).

Example: The nurse asks for your help to position a person on his side. The person has a large, open draining wound that needs cleaning. The nurse explains to you that a great deal of solution will be used to clean the wound and that it is likely to splash. You must put on a gown to protect your clothing and a mask and protective eyewear to protect your mouth, eyes and nose.

Handle Sharp Objects Carefully. To avoid wounds from sharp objects contaminated with blood or body fluids:

- Immediately dispose of sharp objects (such as razors) without recapping them, because you may cut or injure yourself if you try to recap a sharp instrument.
- Put all sharp objects in a **sharps container** (Figure 7-4).

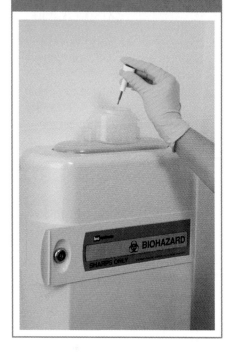

FIGURE 7-4 Use a sharps containers, such as this one, to dispose of razors and other sharp items without recapping them.

Wear Gloves When You Have Cuts or Sores. Wear gloves when giving care if you have an open cut or oozing sore. Make sure you:

- Wear gloves when giving direct care and handling equipment.
- Examine yourself daily, because scratches, cuts and breaks in the skin often occur without your knowledge.
- Discuss precautions with your supervising nurse before assisting with care.

Clean Up Blood or Body Fluids Promptly. Clean up blood or body fluid spills promptly by using a freshly mixed disinfectant solution, such as household bleach and water ($1\frac{1}{2}$ cup of bleach to 1 gallon of water), or any other approved disinfectant. Mix a fresh solution of bleach daily.

Handle Linens Carefully. Handle linens carefully and be sure to:

- Wear gloves when you touch linens soiled with body fluids.
- Keep linens as still as possible to prevent contaminating yourself or putting germs into the air.
- Bag all soiled linens where they were used. Do not sort or rinse them in areas where you provide care.
- Put wet linens into leakproof bags, carry linens in these bags and *never put soiled linens on the floor.*

Bag Contaminated Articles Carefully. Bag contaminated articles carefully and be sure to:

- Put articles that have been contaminated with germs or body fluids, such as emesis basins and **speculums,** into a puncture-proof, labeled biohazard bag.
- Put a second bag over the first bag if the first bag may have been contaminated.

Put Waste in a Leakproof, Air-Tight Container. Put waste in an air-tight container that:

- Does not leak and may be thoroughly cleaned.
- Has a tight-fitting cover (unless it can be maintained in a sanitary condition without a cover).

Keep Resuscitation Masks or Bags on Hand. In a hospital or nursing home, resuscitation masks or bags are used for helping a person breathe again during cardiopulmonary resuscitation (CPR). CPR breathing barrier devices protect both the person being resuscitated and the rescuer from the spread of germs from saliva, blood or other body fluids. When a person stops breathing and needs rescue breathing or CPR, the nurse or doctor will give oxygen to the person by applying a mask or bag over the person's mouth and nose (Figure 7-5). Know where these are kept so you can get them in a hurry.

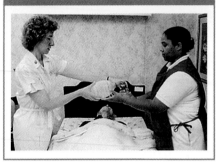

FIGURE 7-5 A bag valve mask may be kept on hand to help protect against the spread of germs if CPR is needed.

Following Isolation Precautions

You know from your supervising nurse's report that Mrs. Wang is in respiratory isolation because her staph pneumonia is contagious. In addition to following the general principles of infection control and Standard Precautions when you provide care for Mrs. Wang, you focus on the Isolation Precautions you must follow to protect yourself and others from her contagious disease. Before serving her breakfast, you check the supply table outside her private room to make sure everything you need is there: masks, gloves, a container for soiled linens, plastic bags and a container for contaminated trash. If disposable plates and utensils are required as a precaution, you must also check to make sure her breakfast is served on them, and you remind yourself to close her door after you enter her room.

If someone is placed apart from other people, we say that person is in isolation. If you had chicken pox as a child, you may remember that your mother kept you in your room and did not let your playmates visit. She may have used paper plates and plastic utensils that she could throw away after you used them. By doing these things, your mother practiced methods of isolation at home. A person may be isolated from other people if he or she has a contagious disease. Examples of contagious diseases that often are cared for at home are measles, chicken pox, hepatitis, tuberculosis, conjunctivitis, infected sores and some kinds of diarrhea. What are some other contagious diseases that you or your family members may have had?

When a doctor suspects or confirms that a person has a contagious disease, you must take additional precautions and follow additional procedures to control the spread of the disease to other people. These precautions are referred to as transmission-based precautions. The health care provider who writes the orders for the person's care decides which of three isolation categories to specify. This decision is based on *two things: the type of germ* that causes the person to have a contagious disease and *how that type of germ spreads.* When a person is placed in isolation in the hospital or nursing home, a sign is posted outside the room. Box 7-5 contains the kind of information that may be posted outside an isolation room. Check with your facility for its policy on notifying other health care workers of Isolation Precautions.

When a person is in isolation, you must:

- Make sure the person knows why she is isolated.
- Check on her often and listen to her concerns. Try to understand her feelings and help provide care for her needs. Stress to her that isolation helps speed her recovery and prevents others from getting sick.
- Make sure that visitors (if permitted) follow the nurse's instructions.
- Keep clean items separate from dirty items.
- Know your employer's specific precautions for isolation.

BOX 7-5

ISOLATION SIGN

Visitors—Report to Nurses' Station Before Entering Room
1. Private room indicated?
   ____ No
   ____ Yes
2. Masks indicated?
   ____ No
   ____ Yes, for those close to patient
   ____ Yes, for all persons entering room
3. Gowns indicated?
   ____ No
   ____ Yes, if contamination is likely
   ____ Yes, for all persons entering room
4. Gloves indicated?
   ____ No
   ____ Yes, for touching infectious material
   ____ Yes, for all persons entering room
5. Special precautions indicated for handling food?
   ____ No
   ____ Yes
6. Hands must be washed after touching the patient or potentially contaminated articles and before taking care of another patient.
7. Articles contaminated with _____ should be discarded or bagged and labeled "Infectious material(s)" before being sent for decontamination and reprocessing.

Contagious diseases can be sorted into categories that then determine the type of isolation that is used. The three isolation categories are explained below.

1. *Airborne:* Airborne precautions are used when caring for a person who is known or thought to have an illness that is transmitted through the air. The **airborne germs** can travel a long distance from the source by air currents and ventilation systems. Tuberculosis and measles are spread in this manner. Nurse assistants must wear a high-efficiency particulate air filter (**HEPA**) mask when caring for a person with this type of infectious disease.

2. *Droplet:* Droplet precautions are used when caring for a person who is known or thought to have an illness that is transmitted by large droplets in the air. These droplets are spread by sneezing, coughing, laughing, singing and talking. The droplets do not travel far. Flu and mumps are spread this way. Nurse assistants can wear a surgical mask when caring for this person.

3. *Contact:* Contact precautions are used when caring for a person who is known or thought to have an illness that can be spread by direct contact (by someone touching the contaminated area). The germs may also be spread by indirect contact (by someone touching an item contaminated by the germ). Some of the illnesses included in this category are wound infections, as well as skin infections such as scabies and impetigo. A gown and gloves should be worn by the nurse assistant when providing care.

Table 7-1 shows the similarities and differences in the precautions and equipment used in each isolation category. To practice Standard Precautions and Isolation Precautions for controlling the spread of germs, you must know what equipment to use and how to use it properly.

Equipment for Practicing Standard Precautions and Isolation Precautions

When practicing Standard Precautions and following Isolation Precautions, you must know how to use required equipment: gowns, masks, eyewear, gloves and plastic bags. When putting on protective clothing, follow the specific precautions that are explained step by step in Skill 2.

Gowns. Wear a gown when required by Standard Precautions and Isolation Precautions to provide a barrier against germs. They protect your clothes and body from splashes and sprays of blood and body fluids. Gowns must completely cover you from your neck to your knees. A gown is worn only one time by one person

TABLE 7-1 ISOLATION PRECAUTIONS AND CATEGORIES

Precaution	Airborne	Droplet	Contact Isolation
Keep door to private room closed	Yes	Yes	Yes
Wash hands when entering and leaving the room	Yes	Yes	Yes
Wear gown	Yes	Only if specific tasks require its use	Yes (when in contact with a wound)
Wear mask	Yes (HEPA mask)	Yes	Yes (for close or direct patient contact)
Wear gloves	Yes	Only if specific tasks require their use	Yes (when in contact with a wound)
Bag linens and contaminated articles	Yes	Yes	Yes
Disinfect or throw away articles from the room after use	Yes	No	No

Note: Wear protective eyewear when the possibility exists for blood or other body fluids to splash into your eyes.

and then is placed in a laundry hamper or is thrown away. Because a damp or wet gown is a breeding place for germs and will not protect you, wear only a gown that is dry. Follow your employer's precautions for wearing gowns that are appropriate to the type of anticipated exposure.

Masks. Wear a mask to keep from inhaling infectious germs into your lungs. Use a mask only once. Change your mask if it becomes moist, because moisture makes it easy for bacteria to enter your mouth and nose. The mask should fit snugly over your nose and mouth. Also change the mask after you have worn it for 20 minutes, because it will be moist from exhaled breath.

Protective Eyewear. Wear protective eyewear to keep splashes of body fluids from contacting the mucous membranes of your eyes when cleaning items or disposing of fluids (Figure 7-6). Protective eyewear is either reusable or disposable.

Gloves. Wear disposable gloves such as vinyl or nitrile when you practice Standard Precautions. *Never* wash or disinfect these gloves for reuse. Always discard them. Do not use gloves that are peeling, cracked or discolored or that have punctures, tears or are deteriorating. In the home, you may decontaminate and reuse general-purpose utility gloves worn for housekeeping and laundry.

Be sure to wear the appropriate gloves for the appropriate tasks. Do not wear gloves as a "second skin" throughout the day. Put them on and remove them after contact with a potentially contaminated object or person.

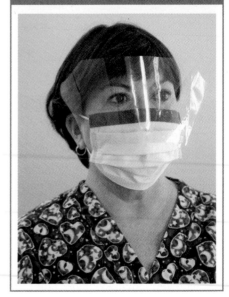

FIGURE 7-6 Protective eyewear that includes a face shield will help protect you from body fluid splashes.

Plastic Bags. Use leakproof plastic trash bags to provide protection from wet items. When closing a used trash bag, touch only the outside of the bag. When a bag contains items contaminated with body fluids, label it as contaminated or put it in a red isolation or biohazard waste bag. When handling plastic trash bags, follow the specific precaution that is explained step by step in Skill 3.

PREPARATION AND COMPLETION STANDARDS

In addition to Standard Precautions and Isolation Precautions, you can help control the spread of germs in the most routine, everyday procedures. We do this in caregiving by using the same procedures both in preparing for and completing each skill. These uniform steps are called Preparation Standards and Completion Standards. By repeating these same steps before and after each caregiving skill, we can help good precautions to become good habits.

Keep in mind that both lists may differ from one institution to the next. It is important to follow the procedures preferred by your employer. The Preparation Standards and Completion Standards you will use for each skill in this course are listed below. Your instructor will give you a handout with these that you can keep with you when performing skills in this course.

Preparation Standards

1. Wash hands.
2. Gather supplies.
3. Focus on task.
4. Knock and wait.
5. Introduce and identify.
6. Explain the procedure.
7. Place supplies.
8. Gather and prepare.
9. Put on disposable gloves.
10. Lock brakes on equipment (BED).
11. Adjust bed.
12. Provide privacy.

Completion Standards

1. Ensure safety, comfort and body alignment.
2. Put disposables in trash bag and laundry in laundry bag.
3. Clean and put away equipment.
4. Put call-light in reach.
5. Put bed in proper position.
6. Remove privacy curtain.
7. Say good-bye.
8. Dispose of trash bag.
9. Put laundry bag in hamper.
10. Dispose of gloves and wash hands.
11. Note, record, report.

RESPONDING TO THE PERSON'S NEEDS

As you enter Mrs. Wang's room, she turns her face away and covers her eyes so that you can't see her tears.

"Good morning, Mrs. Wang," you say and then introduce yourself. You explain that you will be taking care of her today. When you suggest that she seems upset and you offer to help her, Mrs. Wang shakes her head and looks out the window. You suggest that it must be hard to be cooped up in her room by herself on such a nice day.

"At the nursing home I like to sit on the sun porch with my roommate Agnes," she replies.

You suggest that she must feel very lonely in her isolation room and offer to tell her why she has a private room and why you are wearing a mask. She looks at you and smiles sadly.

Even though you must practice infection control, you have to be sensitive to Mrs. Wang's needs. How would you feel if the door to your room had to be closed all the time for isolation? Perhaps you would feel as if no one wanted to be near you or that no one liked you. How would you feel if the people providing personal care for you wore gloves? How would you feel if they were completely covered with gowns, masks and gloves? (Figure 7-7)

Try to imagine what it would be like to be in isolation. How do you think you would feel? Lonely? Angry? Depressed? Maybe embarrassed or afraid? You can be more sensitive to the person's needs if you try to imagine what it would be like to be in her or his situation.

In this chapter you read about germs and how they spread. You also read about Standard Precautions and Isolation Precautions, and you now know when to follow these practices to protect yourself and others. In addition, you now know what equipment you need and how to use it. You understand the important role you play in controlling the spread of germs and in meeting the needs of the people in your care, not just physically, but emotionally as well.

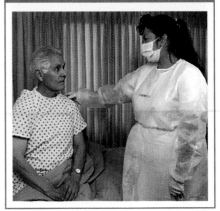

FIGURE 7-7 By explaining why you are wearing a gown, mask and gloves, you can help a person in your care get used to seeing you in protective clothing.

Circle the correct answers and fill in the blanks.

1. The three categories of Isolation Precautions used to control the spread of contagious disease are _airborne_, _droplet_ and _contact_ precautions.

2. Three ways for removing germs from a contaminated object are to _____, _____ and _____.

3. When you take dirty linens to the laundry hamper you should:
   a. shake them first.
   b. hold them away from your uniform.
   c. take only one sheet at a time to prevent contamination.
   d. save steps by tossing them into the laundry hamper from a short distance.

4. What is the most important thing you can do to control the spread of germs?
   a. Bag all contaminated linens.
   b. Wash your hands.
   c. Always cover bedpans and urinals when carrying them from place to place.
   d. Eat a well-balanced diet and stay healthy.

5. You should practice Standard Precautions:
   a. when you provide care for any person.
   b. only when you provide care for people infected with HIV or HBV.
   c. only when a person is in isolation.
   d. only when you need to wash your hands.

6. What is one time when you must wear disposable gloves?
   a. When you give someone a backrub
   b. When you cough or sneeze
   c. When you serve meal trays
   d. When you touch blood or other body fluids

7. When handling sharp items, dispose of them in a _____ _____.

8. If you have a cut or open sore on your hand, what must you do to protect yourself from infection?
   a. Avoid providing care for people with infections.
   b. Stay away from work until the wound heals.
   c. Wear disposable gloves while providing care.
   d. Handle only clean items.

9. Which of the following is a reason to place someone in isolation?
   a. The person has a contagious disease.
   b. The person had surgery.
   c. The person has germs.
   d. The person wants the privacy of a single room.

10. Four items of protective equipment that you may wear when practicing Standard Precautions and Isolation Precautions are _____, _____, _____ and _____.

1. How can you control the spread of infection when you provide care for a person with an open wound?

2. How can you spread infection if you have a cold?

3. In the past, how have you spread germs through direct and indirect contact? Think of three ways.

4. What will you do in the future to avoid spreading germs by direct and indirect contact? Think of three ways.

5. You are changing the linens in Mrs. Wang's isolation room when you realize that you brought only one sheet instead of two. How would you handle this problem? What would you do first?

6. How can you help Mrs. Wang get the information she needs about isolation and infection control? How can you help her with her feelings of loneliness?

7. When you put on gloves to help Mr. Wilson with mouth care, he eyes the gloves and says, "I don't have AIDS, you know. Why are you wearing those things?" How should you respond?

8. Emma Jones, who works as a nurse assistant, became engaged over the weekend. She wants to wear her new engagement ring to work on Monday so that she can show it off. What does she need to consider when deciding whether to wear the ring?

Skill 1: Handwashing

PRECAUTIONS

- Do not wear rings to work, except for a simple wedding band.

WHY? *The tiny spaces in jewelry provide excellent breeding places for germs, which may spread from one person to another.*

- Keep long fingernails trimmed.

PREPARATION

1. Gather supplies:
   - Soap
   - Paper towels. ☐ ☐
2. Remove your watch, or push it up on your forearm, and roll up your sleeves. ☐ ☐

PROCEDURE

1. Turn on the water and adjust the temperature until it is comfortably warm. ☐ ☐
2. Put your hands under the running water to wet your hands and wrists.
   - Apply antimicrobial soap from the dispenser (Figure 7-8).
   - Keep your hands and wrists below the level of your elbows from this point on in the handwashing procedure. ☐ ☐
3. Rub your hands together vigorously to work up a lather. ☐ ☐
4. Wash vigorously for at least 15 seconds, paying particular attention to:
   - The wrists (grasp and circle with your other hand).

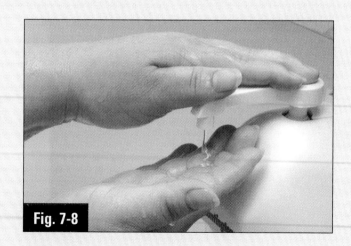

Fig. 7-8

- The palms and backs of your hands.
- The areas between the fingers.
- The nails (rub against the palms of your hands) (Figure 7-9). ☐ ☐

5. Rinse your hands and wrists under the running water (Figure 7-10), keeping your hands lower than the elbows and fingertips down. ☐ ☐

6. Using a clean, dry paper towel, dry your hands thoroughly, beginning at the fingertips and moving back toward the elbow (Figure 7-11)
- Drying your hands thoroughly keeps them from becoming chapped.
- Use a clean paper towel to turn off the faucets.
- Throw away the paper towels in a plastic trash bag or waste container. ☐ ☐

ADDITIONAL INFORMATION

For visibly soiled hands wash with soap and water.

For nonvisibly soiled hands you may use an alcohol-based rub, wash with soap and water or both. When using alcohol-based rub, use the amount of gel recommended by manufacturer. Rub it thoroughly over all surfaces of the hands including nail areas and between fingers until the product dries.

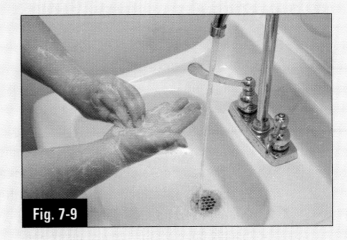
Fig. 7-9

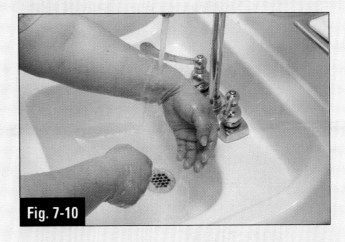
Fig. 7-10

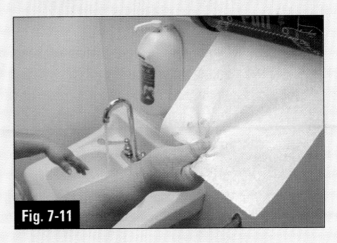
Fig. 7-11

Skill 2: Using Protective Clothing

PRECAUTIONS

- Usually, put on the protective clothing outside the person's room.
- Change the mask when it becomes moist or after you have been wearing it for 20 minutes.
- Use only gloves that are in perfect condition. If you choose gloves that are cracked, discolored, punctured or torn, discard them and choose another pair.
- Usually, take off the gloves, mask and gown in the person's room and discard them as contaminated waste.

PREPARATION

Gather supplies:
- Gown
- Mask
- Gloves
- Plastic trash bag
- Label hazardous waste bag, if needed ☐ ☐

PROCEDURE

Putting On a Gown

1. Slide your arms through armholes; keep opening of gown in back. ☐ ☐
2. Fasten ties at the back of your neck and at your waist; make sure the back is covered. ☐ ☐

Putting On a Mask

1. Put the mask over mouth and nose, and bend the nose wire. ☐ ☐

2. Tie the top strings behind your head, then tie the bottom strings or place elastic loops around the ears. ☐ ☐
3. Adjust mask for comfort. ☐ ☐

Putting On Disposable Gloves

1. Inspect both gloves carefully for tears. ☐ ☐
2. Put the gloves on carefully so that they do not tear. Pull the gloves up over the gown cuffs. ☐ ☐

Taking Off Disposable Gloves

1. Using your fingers on your gloved left hand, make a cuff on the glove on your right hand, grasp the cuff on the palm side, and pull the glove down toward the fingers of your right hand. Remove the glove only partway. ☐ ☐
2. Using your fingers on your right hand, take off the glove on your left hand by pulling it inside out and rolling it into a ball, without touching your bare left hand (Figure 7-12). ☐ ☐
3. Continue to hold the left-hand glove that you have removed in your right hand. ☐ ☐
4. With your bare left hand, grasp the glove on your right hand, touching only the clean inside of the glove (Figure 7-13). ☐ ☐
5. Remove the right-hand glove by pulling it down so that the left-hand glove you removed is now inside the right-hand glove. ☐ ☐

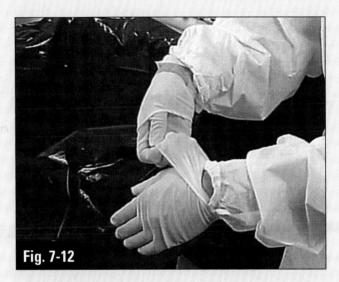

Fig. 7-12

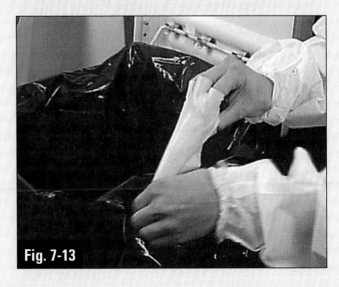

Fig. 7-13

6. Throw away the gloves in a plastic trash bag or covered trash container. ☐ ☐

7. Wash your hands now if you are not wearing any other protective gear (mask, gown). Otherwise, continue taking off your mask and then your gown and then:

8. Wash your hands. ☐ ☐

Taking Off a Mask

1. Untie the bottom strings and then the top strings, or pull the elastic loop from around one ear and then the other. ☐ ☐

2. Hold the mask by the strings and throw it away in a plastic bag or a covered trash container. ☐ ☐

Taking Off a Gown

Untie the neck and waist strings.

1. Pull off one gown sleeve by slipping your fingers under the cuff and pulling the sleeve just over your fingertips (Figure 7-14). ☐ ☐

2. Grasp the other sleeve with the covered hand and pull it off. ☐ ☐

3. Continue holding that sleeve in your covered hand. Grasp the inside of the first shoulder of the gown with your uncovered hand and pull the gown off the shoulder. Continue to bring the gown forward and turn it inside out as you pull it over your covered hand. ☐ ☐

4. Fold the outer, contaminated surface inward and roll up the gown (Figure 7-15). ☐ ☐

5. Throw the gown in the laundry hamper, plastic trash bag or covered trash container. ☐ ☐

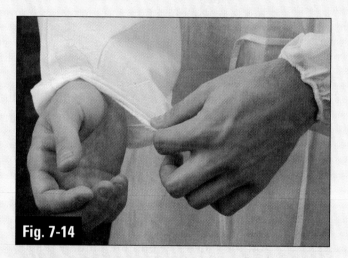

Fig. 7-14

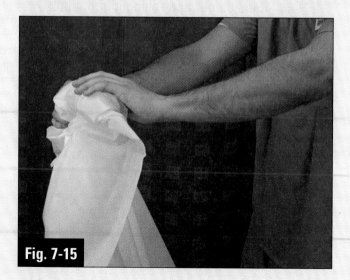

Fig. 7-15

6. Dispose of trash bag. ☐ ☐
7. Wash your hands. ☐ ☐

Note: The cuff of the gown is clean because it was covered by the clean glove.

COMPLETION

Follow Completion Standards in compliance with your facility.

ADDITIONAL INFORMATION

1. Throw the plastic trash bag in a **covered** trash container. ☐ ☐
2. Note, record, report. ☐ ☐

Skill 3: Handling a Plastic Trash Bag

PRECAUTIONS

- When closing a dirty trash bag, touch only the outside of the bag because the inside of the bag is contaminated.

PREPARATION

Gather supplies:
- Plastic trash bag(s) ☐ ☐

PROCEDURE

Opening a Plastic Trash Bag

1. Open the plastic trash bag and make a cuff around the opened edge (Figure 7-16). ☐ ☐
2. Put the opened bag on a clean surface within easy reach of your work area. ☐ ☐

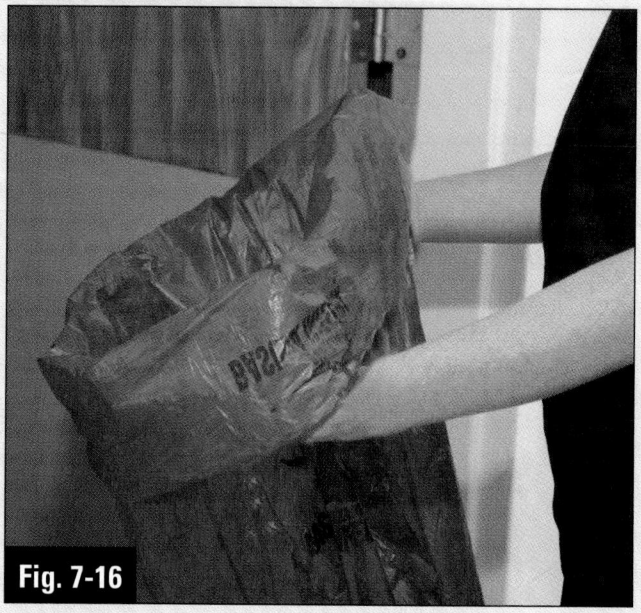

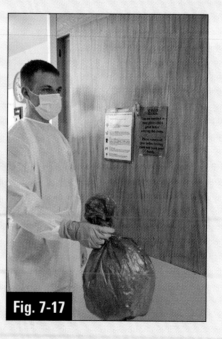

Fig. 7-16

Closing a Used Plastic Trash Bag

1. Put your fingers under the cuffed edge of the used plastic trash bag. ☐ ☐
2. Pull the cuffed edges together and close the bag. ☐ ☐

NOTE: Touch only the outside of the used bag, because the inside is contaminated.

Double-Bagging a Bag that is Contaminated with Body Fluids

1. Arrange for a co-worker to assist you at a certain time (Figure 7-17). ☐ ☐

Fig. 7-17

2. Remove the bag from the trash or laundry container inside the isolation room, close it and carry it to the door of the isolation room. ☐ ☐

3. Have your co-worker prepare a clean bag by folding down a cuff at the top of the clean bag. Have your co-worker hold the clean bag under the cuff and stand by the doorway. ☐ ☐

4. Put the bag with contaminated items into the clean bag that your co-worker is holding under the cuff (Figure 7-18). ☐ ☐

5. Have your co-worker close the outside bag by raising the cuffed area and sealing it shut. ☐ ☐

6. Put disposables in trash bag and dispose of bag. ☐ ☐

7. Wash hands. ☐ ☐

ADDITIONAL INFORMATION

Label the bag "Contaminated." Often hospitals keep a special tape in the dirty utility room for labeling contaminated trash. Take the labeled bag to the area designated for disposal or laundering of contaminated items.

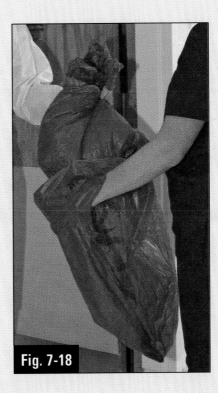
Fig. 7-18

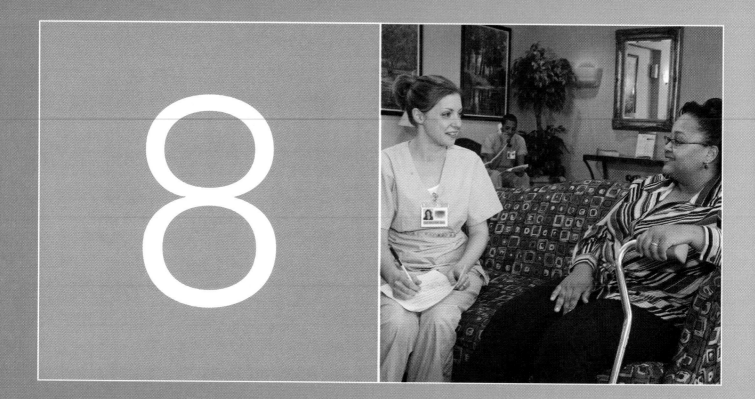

8

Keeping People Safe

GOALS

After reading this chapter, you will have the information needed to:

Explain why safety is the most important principle of care.

Use good body mechanics to help others and to protect yourself.

Maintain equipment and use it safely.

Describe restraints, what they are and why they seldom are used.

List the different types of restraints.

State how restraints affect the people in your care both physically and emotionally.

Describe a person's right to be free from restraints and how you must protect this right.

Recognize the dangers of using restraints.

Use alternative methods whenever possible to manage the behavior of the people in your care.

Meet a person's needs rather than use restraints.

Use restraints correctly, when they are ordered by a doctor.

Practice fire safety.

Help people cope with natural disasters, such as earthquakes, hurricanes and tornadoes.

After practicing the corresponding skills, you will have the information needed to:

Provide first aid for a conscious choking adult.

Provide first aid to control external bleeding.

Respond appropriately to shock, seizures, burns, falls and fainting.

The head nurse is just completing her assessment of Mrs. Clark when you enter the room. You are introduced to Mrs. Clark, who was admitted to the nursing facility to receive rehabilitation services after slipping in her home and fracturing her hip. You learn from Mrs. Clark that she slipped on a throw rug in her house. She tells you that she was in the hospital and was transferred to the nursing facility to shorten her stay at the more expensive hospital. Mrs. Clark tells you that she will be in the facility for several weeks and then will be discharged to her home. She is concerned about her safety in the facility. You tell Mrs. Clark that safety precautions are in place. There are no throw rugs, there are safety rails in the bathroom and the call signal is within easy reach. You also tell her that you will be available to assist her with care and that before she goes home, you will be happy to help her and her family identify hazards in her home.

SETTING THE STAGE FOR SAFETY

Safety is the most important principle of care because it is the foundation of everything else you do. If you are not safe, you cannot meet the needs of the people in your care. If people are not safe, they will not benefit from the care you provide them.

Practicing the other principles of care without practicing safety is like setting a table that has one short leg. No matter how clean your dishes and utensils are, or how nutritious your dinner is, you cannot eat the meal if the table tilts and your dinner falls in your lap.

The key to safety is prevention, or trying to keep things from going wrong by considering the things that *can* go wrong and taking steps to avoid them.

The first step in prevention is to check each new work site for safety hazards. Then make or request whatever changes are needed. Finally, have an emergency exit plan for you and your client, and watch for ways to use good body mechanics on the job.

Using Good Body Mechanics

As a nurse assistant, you lift and move things all day long and often rush as you carry out your responsibilities. These factors—lifting, moving and rushing—can lead to back injuries over time. Every time you twist your body quickly or in a way it is not meant to twist, you increase the chances of injuring your back. You may think that you hurt your back when you bend down to pick up a pencil, but the injury may be the result of repeated abuse from using poor **body mechanics**. The

KEY TERMS

abdominal: (ab-DOM-in-uhl) pertaining to the abdomen, the part of the body between the ribs and the groin.

alignment: (uh-LINE-ment) correct positioning to keep the spine straight and to avoid any twisting, straining, pressure or discomfort.

asphyxiation: (as-fik-see-AY-shun) suffocation caused by the lack of oxygen.

body mechanics: the way a person's body adjusts to keep its balance during movement.

chemical restraint: (KEM-e-kuhl/re-STRAYNT) any drug that is used to control behavior and is not required for medical treatment.

convenience: (con-VEE-nee-ense) something done by the caregiver or the facility to control a resident's behavior that is in the best interest of the caregiver or facility and not the resident.

disaster plan: (di-ZAHS-ter) a set of safety procedures to follow in case a fire or natural disaster occurs.

discipline: action taken by a facility to punish, penalize or otherwise control the behavior of the resident.

entrapment: (in-TRAP-ment) occurrence in which a person is caught or entangled by a nonfunctioning bed rail, often leading to injury and sometimes death.

hazard: (HAZ-erd) something that is very dangerous and could cause harm to someone.

impaired: (im-PAIRED) a condition in which something is diminished or weakened.

incident: (IN-suh-dent) anything unusual that happens and has the potential to cause harm.

medical symptom: (MED-e-kuhl/SIMP-tuhm) an indication of a physical or mental condition.

obstruction: (ob-STRUK-shun) something that blocks.

physical restraint: (FIZ-uh-kul/re-STRAYNT) any manual method that restricts freedom of movement, or any physical or mechanical device or material that is attached to or near the resident's body that restricts freedom of movement and that the resident cannot remove.

five principles of good body mechanics are:

- Use broad base of support.
- Keep object or person close to you.
- Keep upper body erect.
- Lift smoothly without jerking.
- Do not lift and twist.

Using good body mechanics is one way to prevent injuries. You practice good body mechanics if you keep your back straight when you sit or if you bend your knees when you lift. You can sit, stand and lift in certain ways that improve your body **alignment** (Figure 8-1).

If you have ever driven a car that is out of alignment, you know that it's hard to steer, the tires wear down unevenly and it's unsafe. Human bodies that are out of alignment have similar problems. Body parts get pulled out of shape, which leads to discomfort and injury.

Sitting. Sit with your knees slightly higher than your hips, your back straight, your **abdominal** muscles tightened, and your shoulders straight and centered above your hips (Figure 8-2).

Standing. Follow these tips for improving alignment when standing:

1. Relax your knees so that they are slightly bent.

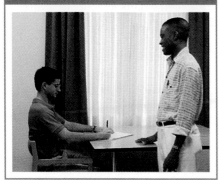

FIGURE 8-1 You may have to remind yourself several times a day to stand or sit correctly.

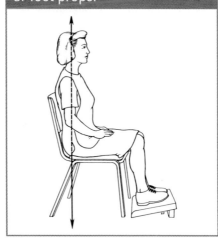

FIGURE 8-2 Sit with your shoulders and back straight and centered above your hips. If your feet do not comfortably reach the floor use firm pillows or foot props.

2. Put your weight evenly on both legs and stand with your feet shoulder width apart.
3. Stand up straight with your stomach muscles tightened and buttocks tucked under, your head up and your chin level.
4. Align your upper body by keeping your shoulders right over your hips (Figure 8-3).

Lifting. Follow these tips for improving alignment when lifting:

1. Before lifting, place your feet about 12 inches apart, with one foot slightly in front of the other. This position provides a broad base of support that makes it hard for you to lose your balance or to be knocked down.
2. Before lifting, make sure the person or object you lift is close to you so that you do not have to lean over or reach.
3. While lifting, keep the person or object close to your body.
4. While lifting, keep your upper body erect and bend only your knees.
5. Lift smoothly without jerking.

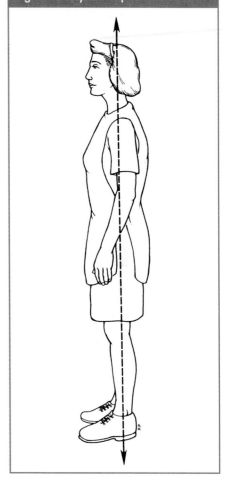

FIGURE 8-3 Align your upper body by keeping your shoulders right over your hips.

6. To turn, lift first, pivot with your feet and turn smoothly, making sure not to twist your body when your arms are loaded.

By using good body mechanics, you keep yourself safe and are better able to provide safety for others. You will also avoid injuries and be more comfortable. You can help other people maintain proper alignment when they lie in bed, sit in a chair, stand, use a walker or walk (Figure 8-4).

A person who spends most of the time in bed or in a chair may slump or lean to one side from time to time. Help the person stay comfortable and avoid injury by reminding or helping him or her to stay aligned. You can use

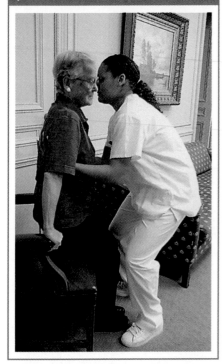

FIGURE 8-4 When helping someone sit, you must practice good body mechanics to protect the person's safety and yours.

pillows, rolled towels or other devices to support the person. You will read more about these techniques in Chapter 10, "Positioning and Transferring People."

Promoting Safety for Others

Providing a safe environment is the responsibility of all health care team members, and preventing injuries is the best safety measure. By using common sense and your knowledge of the person in your care, you can think about things that might go wrong and take steps to prevent them from happening. If a person in your care is physically weak, unfamiliar with the surroundings or confused or unsteady, you know that this person is more likely to fall or injure himself, so you take steps to prevent such a fall or injury. For example, Mr. Lightfoot's legs are unsteady when he gets up quickly

from his chair. One day he anxiously waits for a phone call. As the time of his expected call nears, you suggest that he sit by the phone.

You can use common sense and knowledge about potential **hazards** to prevent things from going wrong. To spot potential hazards, look around a room each time you enter it. If you see a safety threat, correct it right away. To help ensure the safety of the people in your care, as well as your own safety, remember these tips:

- Make sure doorways and floors are free from **obstruction.**
- Wipe up spills immediately, following infection control procedures when necessary.
- Walk. Do not run.
- Store all medicines and cleaning materials in locked cabinets and closets.
- Turn hot water on last and off first.
- Check the temperature of water coming out of faucets to be sure it is correct for performing a procedure. For general purposes, the temperature of hot tap water should be at or below 120 degrees Fahrenheit. If water seems too hot, report this concern immediately to your supervising nurse.
- Check food temperature to make sure it is not too hot. If food is steaming or a plate is too hot to touch, wait until the food stops steaming or the plate has cooled a little before serving the meal.
- Check handrails and grab bars to make sure that they are tightly fastened.
- Encourage people to use handrails and grab bars in the shower, bathroom and hallways.
- If a person wears eyeglasses, make sure they are clean.
- If a person uses a hearing aid, make sure it works and encourage the person to use it when necessary.
- Put the call signal within easy reach. Answer calls for help

promptly. Remember that there may be an emergency or that the person may be in pain, may be having trouble breathing, may need help going to the bathroom or may be frightened. Someone needing to go to the bathroom may tire of waiting for you and try to get there alone, risking a fall.

- Handle people gently, especially older adults. Their bodies may be fragile and may injure easily.
- Unless a person objects, make sure a nightlight is on at bedtime.
- Make sure people are familiar with their surroundings.
- Report any **incident** to your supervising nurse, even if no injury occurs. If an injury or incident happens, you are legally responsible for reporting it. When you report an incident, you must gather the important information and give it to your supervising nurse. The information you gather goes into an incident report, which is a written description of what happened.

Observing and reporting incidents accurately are important parts of your job. Immediately report any incident involving you or another person to your supervising nurse, because your memory of what happened is likely to be fresh and accurate right after it happens. If questions about the incident come up later, the incident report often is the only source of information. A complete incident report contains answers to the following questions:

- When did the incident happen? (time, date)
- Where did the incident happen?
- What caused the incident? (For example, was water on the floor?)
- Who was the person involved in the incident?
- Was the person injured? If so, describe the injury.
- Was the person confused before or after the incident?

- Was the person alone?
- Were there witnesses to the incident? If so, who?
- Who gave assistance or first aid?
- What kind of assistance or first aid was given?
- Did a doctor treat the person?

Include other information that would be a useful part of the record or that is required in your employer's incident report.

USING EQUIPMENT SAFELY

As a nurse assistant, you use many pieces of equipment that make your job easier and the people in your care safer. But, because most equipment has moving parts, you can cause serious injuries if you do not use it properly.

Before using any piece of equipment, be sure you understand how it works. Read the product manual and follow instructions exactly. (If no manual is available, you may find instructions on a sticker or label attached to the equipment.) Before using the equipment with the person in your care, practice the correct procedure for using it by yourself. If you are not completely confident about using the equipment, ask your supervising nurse for help rather than risking any danger to yourself or the person in your care.

Maintaining Personal Equipment

Regularly check personal equipment to make sure that it is working as it should (Figure 8-5). Anything that is broken is potentially a safety problem.

The person in your care may use a personal safety device, such as a cane or walker. To increase the safety of such devices, inspect them from time to time to make sure that the rubber tips on a cane or walker have not become worn and that the frame on a walker is tight.

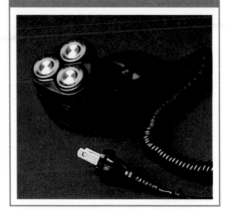

FIGURE 8-5 Small appliances can be hazardous if they do not work properly or if the cords are in bad condition.

Using Brakes

The brakes provided on equipment with wheels—beds, wheelchairs, shower chairs and carts—prevent the equipment from rolling. Imagine how unsafe and difficult it would be to help someone into a wheelchair that kept moving.

Before using a piece of equipment that has wheels, try out the brakes. Make sure you know how they work and that they work properly. If they do not work properly, do not use the equipment. Report the equipment problem to your supervising nurse. Before helping a person into or out of a wheelchair, lock the brakes and make sure the chair is secure. Also, before stepping away from a person who is in a wheelchair, make sure both wheelchair brakes are locked securely (Figure 8-6).

Following Safety Tips

Read the additional tips for using equipment safely in Table 8-1.

WHAT ARE RESTRAINTS?

A restraint is any device that inhibits a person's free physical movement or that controls her or his mood, mental status, or behavior. Until recently, most nursing homes commonly used restraints in the

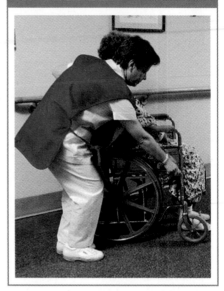

FIGURE 8-6 Remember to lock the brakes on both wheels of the wheelchair.

care of people—especially older adults—to keep them from wandering away from the nursing home, to protect others from their sometimes abusive behavior and to keep them from falling or injuring themselves. In recent years, reports of deaths and injuries related to the use of restraints have increased. Many of these incidents seem to be the result of incorrect use of these devices, including inappropriate patient selection, incorrect restraint selection, errors in correctly applying the devices and inadequate monitoring of patients when restrained. Because of these incidents, new instructions regarding restraints have been written and the reasons for using restraints better described.

When used improperly, restraints are considered a form of abuse, and a person has the right to be free from restraints. This right is protected by the Omnibus Budget Reconciliation Act (OBRA) of 1987. This law states that people receiving care in nursing homes and in their own homes have "the right to be free from any physical or chemical restraints imposed for purposes of discipline or convenience, and not required

TABLE 8-1 USING EQUIPMENT SAFELY

Always	Never	Why?
Dry your hands thoroughly before handling electrical equipment.	Pull electrical equipment out of water.	The electrical current in the water could kill you.
Plug electrical equipment into an outlet near the place where you will be using it.	Use extension cords, except in an emergency.	The cord could trip someone, or it could overload a circuit and cause a power outage or fire.
Follow the manufacturer's directions for using electrical equipment.	Use equipment—unless you have been trained to use it and feel sure of yourself.	If you use equipment incorrectly, you may injure yourself or a person in your care.
Use equipment that is clean and in good repair.	Use defective or broken equipment, and never permit the person in your care to use personal equipment that could present a hazard.	Using broken or defective equipment could cause serious injury to you or a person in your care.
Ensure that each person in your care has his own razor, toothbrush, hairbrush and other personal equipment.	Share personal equipment among people.	Keeping personal equipment personal maintains infection control.
Store equipment in closets or in other out-of-the-way areas.	Store equipment in halls or other areas where people walk.	Equipment that is improperly stored obstructs free movement.

to treat the person's medical symptoms." This law means that, with the exception of temporary use for life-threatening emergencies or medical treatments, health care workers can use restraints only under certain, specific conditions. Box 8-1 describes these conditions. Health care workers should use restraints *only* as a last resort and only when ordered by a doctor.

There are two types of restraints, **physical restraints** and **chemical restraints**. Physical restraints such as straps, special belts, or vests to hold a person down can cause bodily injury and can rob a person of his or her dignity and independence. In addition, safety is often jeopardized. Restrained people may panic and fracture or dislocate bones by struggling to get free. Some have died tragically of **asphyxiation** from restraints that squeezed their necks as they tried to escape from beds or chairs. Secluding persons—shutting them off from contact with others against their will—is also potentially harmful because it can be emotionally traumatic. The use of restraints removes dignity even when necessary to apply. Chemical restraints—drugs used to subdue a person—are just as harmful as physical restraints, because they "tie down" the person's mind instead of her or his body.

Physical Problems Caused by Using Restraints

A restraint can cause injury by keeping the restrained person in an unnatural position that violates good body mechanics. Restricting a person's ability to move can cause many other physical problems. Table 8-2 contains some examples.

Emotional Problems Caused by Using Restraints

In addition to physical problems, restrained people experience many emotional problems. Many people who are restrained experience:

- A loss of dignity.
- A loss of self-image.
- A loss of the ability to socialize with others.
- Increased dependence on health care workers and others.
- Increased agitation, confusion and combativeness.
- Withdrawal and depression.

Safety Problems Caused by Using Restraints

The use of restraints also causes safety problems. If a person is restrained, an emergency situation

TABLE 8-2 PHYSICAL PROBLEMS CAUSED BY RESTRAINTS	
Physical Problem	**Cause**
Tissue damage	Restraints applied too tightly, causing pressure and constricting blood circulation, which strains the circulatory system and decreases blood supply to certain parts of the body
Nerve damage	Restraints applied too tightly or the person fought the restraints after they were applied
Chronic constipation	Lack of exercise or lack of independent mobility
Incontinence from loss of bowel or bladder function	Lack of freedom to use the bathroom when needed
Loss of muscle tone and balance	Lack of exercise or lack of independent mobility
Pressure sores and contractures	Restraints applied too tightly or person kept in same position too long
Pneumonia	Activity restricted or lack of independent mobility
Decreased appetite	Mental depression
Injury and death	Person struggled to get free

can become deadly. Crucial lifesaving minutes would be lost by having to untie the person to provide care. Restraining people makes them helpless and puts the whole burden of their safety on you and the other health care team members.

Tips for the Use of Restraints

Physical restraints can be useful in protecting residents from falls and from wandering or straying in some states. However, restraints are not the only solution and in some cases may be more dangerous. Follow your state and local protocols when considering using any type of restraints. The following tips can make you more aware of when and how restraints might be used. Look at Table 8-3 and

ask yourself the questions provided there before applying restraints. Box 8-1 "OBRA: When Restraints Can Be Used" will show you specific examples of when to use restraints.

Side Rails

People in your care sometimes need side rails on their beds. A side rail is considered a restraint when:

- It cannot be easily lowered by the resident.
- It prevents a resident who can normally get out of bed independently from safely and easily getting out of the side of the bed.

Follow state and local protocol when using this type of restraint.

A side rail (regardless of length) is not a restraint if it does not prevent an

TABLE 8-3 GUIDELINES FOR USING RESTRAINTS CORRECTLY

Guidelines	Questions to Ask Yourself
Resident Rights	Residents have the right to be free from restraints. Restraints should not be the first choice. Why?
Facility Policy	Facility must have a written policy on use of restraints. Ask to see this document, and make sure you understand it. Why?
Prescription Only	May be used only if ordered by a doctor. The need for a restraint must be written in the chart. Why?
Resident Symptoms	An agitated or seriously confused resident may not be suited for a restraint. Why?
Right Size	Be sure that the right size restraint is selected. Why?
Good Labeling	Look at label and instructions on how to apply the restraint. Look at pictures too. Why?
Proper Use	Make sure resident is seated properly in wheelchair. In bed, tie restraint only to bed frame. Look at label for correct way to put on restraint. Why?
How Long	Resident must be free of restraint at frequent intervals. Find out the facility policy. Exercise the resident when free of restraint. Why?
Monitor Resident	Residents must be monitored on a regular basis. Why?

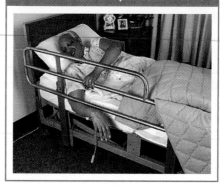

FIGURE 8-7 Entrapment in bed.

able-bodied resident from easily getting out of a side of the bed or if it is needed to protect a resident in bed who is capable of either rolling out of bed or involuntarily being "thrown" out of a bed because of his or her condition. Make sure you understand how to use side rails, because the many various types all operate a little differently. If you are unsure about how to use the type you have, ask for help. After raising or lowering side rails, test them to make sure they lock securely. If a side rail does not lock properly, stay with the person and call for help.

There have been injuries and deaths involving older adults who were entrapped by side rails. An example of one form of side rail **entrapment** is seen in Figure 8-7. When side rails are used, always check the bed frames, side rails and mattresses to find areas where a resident may become entrapped. Make sure that the side rails have been installed properly.

If there is a strong chance that the resident may fall out of bed, use a low bed or put a mattress on the floor as a last resort. When you leave the bedside of a person who is in a mechanical bed, always leave the bed in the lowest position.

Finding Alternatives to Restraints

You must have reliable information to find ways to avoid using restraints when possible, while still providing good care in a safe way. Nursing facilities must be sure that they are not putting a person in restraints because it is a **convenience** for them. Restraints cannot be used as a form of **discipline**. And finally, a resident's **medical symptom** by itself is not a reason for applying a restraint. Laws are in place to ensure restraints are only used if medically necessary.

Mental or physical illnesses may keep people from acting safely and sensibly and cause them to become agitated, confused or prone to wandering, and many common sense measures can be used instead of restraints. For example, when a resident is combative or fighting, this alone is not reason enough to put him or her in a restraint. Instead, the nurse assistant could try moving the resident to another area. Can you think of other interventions or distractions you could try that might calm the resident down? Often the best way to avoid using restraints is to help people exercise as much as they can or do other meaningful activities, such as singing, moving to music, painting or doing hobbies they have always enjoyed. These activities provide gentle physical and mental stimulation, help people feel useful and improve their self-esteem. Another alternative is having the resident wear an alarm system that will alert the staff when the resident may be in danger of harming him- or herself.

Each person in your care is an individual who has personal needs and desires. The care you provide must be special for each individual and flexible enough to meet each person's changing needs.

Many elderly and weak people cannot keep themselves in proper body alignment. Some people constantly slump forward, lean to one side or slide down in their chairs if they are not supported. Instead of using restraints, use the following techniques and devices to help the people in your care maintain proper body alignment (Figure 8-8, A and B):

- Upper-Body Positioning/Leaning Forward
  Use any of the following to support people who tend to slump forward, lean to one side or slide out of chairs: wedge cushions; positioning pillows; beanbag cushion seats; deep, inclined seats; and reclining wheelchair backrests.
- Upper-Body Positioning/Leaning to the Side
  Try a variety of chairs, such as recliners, wheelchairs with side wings, lateral stabilizer armrest boosters, lounge chairs, rocking chairs or gliders and deep-seated chairs with high backs (Figure 8-9).
- Prevention from Sliding
  Special cushions can improve positioning and reduce sliding; drop-seat bases fit most wheelchairs.

- Wheelchair Safety
  Resident-release soft belts fit over the hips to remind the resident not to leave the wheelchair without getting help. Footrest extenders prevent foot drop and allow the resident's feet to touch the floor, providing a base of support.

Review your employer's policy on restraints. Policies differ from one facility to another as changes are made to follow the OBRA laws regarding the use of restraints. Ask your supervising nurse what alternatives to restraints you may use. Remember that restraints should never be used as a substitute for nursing care.

Providing Care for a Person Who is Physically or Chemically Restrained

If a doctor orders a physical restraint for a person in your care, you must observe the person carefully and report any problems immediately to your supervising nurse. Physical restraints most commonly used are:

- Wrist restraints, which limit the movement of the arms.
- Waist restraints, which are designed to keep a person from falling out of bed or out of a chair.
- Vest restraints, which are designed to keep people from standing up or moving around.

If a person in your care is physically restrained, it is your job to help safeguard her or his well being. Follow these important rules when providing care for a person who is physically restrained:

- Remind the person and his or her family why the doctor has ordered restraints to be used.
- Understand exactly how to use the restraint, making sure to use the right size for the person's height and weight. Secure the restraint properly.

FIGURE 8-8 A. In addition to preventing a person from sliding down in the wheelchair, this cushion provides a comfortable resting place for her forearms. When the person wants to move freely, she removes the cushion. **B.** This roll bar prevents a person from slipping out of the wheelchair, but does not restrict freedom. She can release the bar and move freely whenever she chooses.

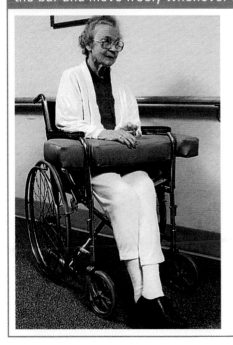
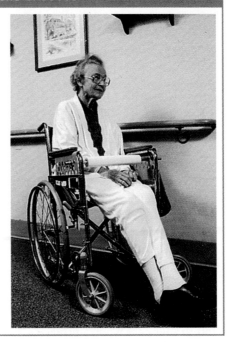

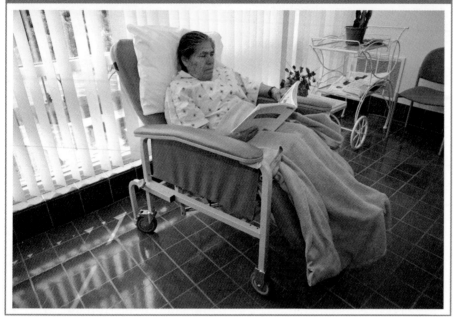

FIGURE 8-9 This resident cannot easily get out of the big chair by herself, but she has freedom to change position and move about in the chair. This is a good alternative to restraining her.

- If a person is restrained, check on her every 15 minutes. She may need to be reassured that she hasn't been abandoned. Many people injure themselves by trying to get out of restraints without assistance.
- Release the restraints every 2 hours and help the person go to the bathroom, stretch, change positions and do range-of-motion exercises. Inspect her or his skin for reddened areas and report any concerns to your supervising nurse. Release the restraints more often if the person seems to be anxious, needs to go the bathroom or is in distress.

If a doctor orders a chemical restraint for a person in your care, you must observe the person carefully and report any physical reactions or changes in behavior immediately to your supervising nurse. Such reactions might be an increase in agitation, drowsiness or decreased appetite.

COPING WITH DISASTERS

Emotional Response to Disaster

We have discussed the emotional and physical damage restraints can have on someone's health. It is just as important to recognize that a person's emotional response to disaster is part of the impact that disasters have on a person's health. How people respond to and cope with disaster depends on individual circumstances. People can and do respond differently in times of disaster. Certain characteristics make people more vulnerable to the effects of disaster than others, including the following: lack of coping skills or history of emotional problems; the experience of a recent upsetting event; recent separation from or loss of a loved one; dependency on others; or problems speaking the language. As you can see, residents in the nursing facility may show many of these characteristics.

As a nurse assistant, you will have the responsibility to assist the residents in your care when a disaster

occurs. But you need to be aware of how a disaster also affects you. While you are assisting residents in the facility, you may also be concerned about the health and safety of your own family. For example, a tornado strikes in your community while you are at work. On one hand, you are responding to the emergency at work as directed, but on the other hand, you are also afraid because you do not know whether or not your family is safe. It is normal for you to be afraid; however, pre-planning may help you to better respond. You and your family may develop a home disaster plan similar to your facility disaster plan. This plan can list the responsibilities for family members as well as direct the family on what to do if the disaster should occur while members are away from home or apart from each other. Taking the time to make and practice a disaster plan will help you to gain some control over the situation and reduce some of the stress and tension. Before a disaster make sure you and your supervisor know what plans your facility has for disasters and discuss your role and responsibilities, particularly in case of evacuation.

Fire Preparedness

Fire safety is an important concern for everyone because fires rarely affect just one person. Practicing fire safety makes sense for you, but also for the people in your care. They may be at greater risk from fire than most people because they are more likely to have limitations in mobility, hearing, vision or understanding—all of which interfere with their ability to successfully react to a fire. These limitations also make cigarette smoking especially dangerous for residents. To prevent fires, see that rules about smoking are enforced, know where fire alarms and extinguishers are located and how to use them, look for and remove fire hazards, obey all cautionary rules regarding the use of oxygen and see that emergency phone numbers are easy to find.

Help prevent fires by following these tips:

- Supervise the people in your care whenever they smoke.
- Follow your employer's rules about smoking. If you provide care for people who smoke, make sure they smoke only in appropriate places and safely extinguish their cigarettes.
- Remove smoking materials from the reach of any person who has **impaired** thinking.
- Never permit smoking around a person who is using oxygen.
- Know the location of fire doors, and keep them free from obstruction.
- Know the fire escape routes. Hospitals and nursing homes generally post fire escape routes for each room or area (Figure 8-10). Never use an elevator to escape from a fire.

Fire Safety in Nursing Facilities

Nursing facilities are protected by a system of automatic smoke detectors, water flow alarms and fire alarm pull boxes. When these systems are activated, the fire alarm will sound and all smoke barrier doors will close auto-

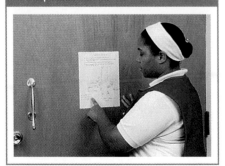

FIGURE 8-10 Know fire escape routes ahead of time so that you can proceed immediately. You may have only seconds to escape.

matically. There are special buttons to open doors in an emergency. Learn your facility's fire **disaster plan** and proceed as directed. Although the plan may designate a specific person to call the fire department, you still must know the telephone number to call. In some communities you call Emergency Medical Services (EMS), usually by dialing 9-1-1. In addition to guidelines for whom to call and how to call them, the fire disaster plan should include information about when and how to evacuate the people in the building, as well as any special measures to take to prevent a fire from spreading. These guidelines usually are practiced in periodic fire drills.

Use the following precautions and attempt to alert any other people in the building:

- Touch a door with the back of your hand before you open it (Figure 8-11). If it is hot, do not open it. Leave the room another way. If the door is cool, stand to one side and open it slowly. If you observe heavy smoke on the other side, close the door.

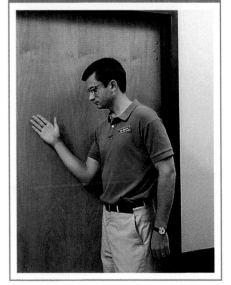

FIGURE 8-11 A door feels hot if there is a fire on the other side.

- Stay low. Smoke rises, and it is easier to breathe when you are closer to the floor.
- Use stairs, not an elevator.
- If your clothing or that of another person ignites (catches fire), *stop, drop* (to the ground), *roll* over and over (to extinguish the flames), and *cool* (use water to cool the burn site).

Natural Disasters

When a natural disaster happens, many people are injured in a short period of time. The types of natural disasters that occasionally occur where you live may differ from those that occur in other parts of the United States. For your own safety, you should know what types of disasters occur in your area.

Your employer's disaster plan or emergency plan explains your role in the event of a natural disaster (Figure 8-12). Find out what your role will be. No matter what your role, always remain calm in the event of a disaster. Because residents and their visitors may become frightened and confused, you play a critical role and can calmly explain what is happening and reassure people that you will help them move to a safe area. When helping to move a person who cannot walk, use a wheelchair or a bed. After people are moved to a safe place, make sure a staff member remains with them to keep them from wandering into dangerous areas. The presence of a staff member is especially important for people who have impaired vision or hearing or who are confused.

Earthquakes. An earthquake occurs when the earth moves, shakes or rolls. This activity in the earth may cause buildings to shake, windows to shatter and objects to shift or fall. It also can cause fires to start and can generate large ocean waves. Earthquakes can occur in most states, and they may occur at any time without warning.

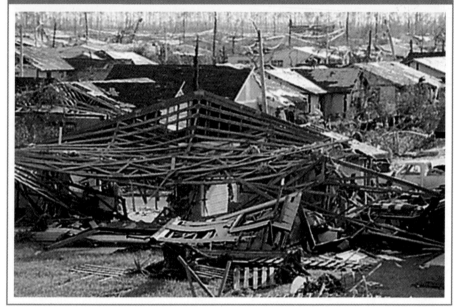

FIGURE 8-12 Because natural disasters such as hurricanes are not always predictable, you should learn ahead of time what your employer expects you to do so that you can act quickly and efficiently.

If an earthquake occurs, follow these safety tips:

- Stay calm.
- If you are inside a building, stay inside. Protect yourself and the residents, especially your head, from falling or shifting objects. Take cover under a large, heavy object, such as a desk or table.
- If you are outside, stay outside. Move away from buildings, trees and overhead wires.

After the earthquake, follow these safety tips:

- Check for injuries. Never try to move seriously injured people unless they are in danger of further injury.
- Be prepared for aftershocks (smaller quakes that occur after the first tremor).
- Use your flashlight to inspect for damage. Never use a candle. *Do not use* appliances, other electrical equipment or services requiring electricity, gas, water or sewage disposal because these systems may be damaged. If you smell gas or see a broken line, shut off the main valve or inform the person responsible. Do not try to turn utilities back on.
- Listen to the radio or television for information about the emergency.
- Watch for fallen power lines.
- Clean up spilled medicines, drugs, flammable liquids and other materials.
- Never smoke. Earthquakes can create gas leaks, and an open flame from a match or cigarette lighter can cause an explosion.
- Use the telephone only in a life-threatening emergency.

Hurricanes. A hurricane occurs when the winds of a large tropical storm increase to 74 miles per hour or more. A hurricane watch means a hurricane is possible in your area. If a hurricane watch is issued in your area, follow these safety tips:

- Listen for weather reports on the radio or television. In a hospital or nursing home, know which per-

sonnel are assigned to listen to the reports.
- Make sure you have access to a supply of fresh water.
- Have a flashlight with fresh batteries available.
- Follow your supervising nurse's instructions, which may include evacuation preparations, such as asking people to stay out of bed or moving bedridden people into chairs. Make sure a staff member stays with people after they have been moved to safety. You also may have to check outdoor areas and remove or secure loose objects and prepare to board up windows.

A hurricane warning means a hurricane is approaching your area. If a hurricane warning is issued in your area, follow these safety tips:

- If an evacuation order is issued, follow your employer's emergency procedures to safely evacuate the people in your care.
- If you are not told to evacuate, keep people away from windows.
- Move people into interior rooms.
- If some people cannot easily get out of bed, move them in their beds into the hallways or push their beds against the wall. Make sure a staff member stays with them.
- Close the doors to rooms and close fire doors (Figure 8-13).
- Make sure doorways to halls, fire doors and exits are not blocked.
- Cover people with blankets or bedspreads to protect them from flying glass in case windows break.
- Monitor weather conditions carefully.

Tornadoes. A tornado is a spinning, funnel-shaped windstorm that moves along the ground. A *tornado watch* means that weather conditions are favorable for a tornado in your area. If a tornado watch is announced, follow these safety tips:

- Listen for weather reports on the radio or television. In a nursing

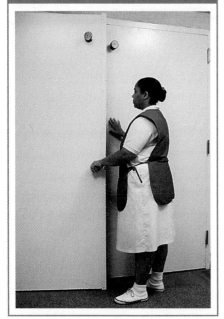

FIGURE 8-13 Closing doors during most natural disasters can help protect people from flying debris.

facility, know which personnel are assigned to listen to the report.

- Be alert to weather conditions, blowing debris and the sound of an approaching tornado. A tornado often sounds like a freight train. Inform other staff members if you see or hear anything.
- Sound alarms.
- Have a flashlight with fresh batteries available.
- Follow your supervising nurse's instructions, which may include the following:
  - Remove residents from dining rooms and sitting areas located near windows.

- Move people into interior hallways near exits or into closets or bathrooms.
- If some people cannot easily get out of bed, move them in their beds into the hallways or push their beds against the wall.
- Close the doors to rooms and close fire doors.
- Make sure doorways to halls, fire doors and exits are not blocked.
- Cover people with blankets or bedspreads to protect them from flying glass in case windows break.
- Follow evacuation procedures if necessary.

Utility Emergencies (Power Outages)

Utility emergencies may be caused by a disaster inside the facility or adjacent to it. Power outages may be the result of natural disasters such as hurricanes or tornadoes. If there is an *electrical outage,* facilities may have an emergency generator to adequately light the facility. As a precaution, have flashlights and batteries available for use. If there is a *gas outage,* depending on the season, heating may be a consideration. The facility's Food Services Department may be affected, requiring that only cold food be served. In the event that evacuation is necessary, follow your facility evacuation plan. Remember to not use elevators to evacuate residents, employees or visitors unless authorized by the local fire department.

EMERGENCY CARE AND FIRST AID

You have read about how to keep yourself safe, how to use equipment safely and how to practice fire safety. You have also looked at how you can cope with natural disasters. As a nurse assistant you also have to cope when specific emergencies occur.

When an emergency occurs, the worst thing you can do is nothing. The decision to get involved, however, can be a hard one to make. In the skills at the end of this chapter, you will read basic information about a few medical emergencies and how you can respond to them. To expand your knowledge of how to respond to emergencies, you can take an American Red Cross First Aid or CPR course. When an emergency happens, you may feel confused. However, you can train yourself to stay calm and think before you act. When responding to an emergency, remember the emergency action steps: **Check— Call—Care**.

- Check the scene and the person.
- Call 9-1-1 or the local emergency number.
- Care for the conditions you find.

These steps guide your actions in an emergency and ensure your safety and the safety of others. Turn to the skill sheets at the end of this chapter to practice how to manage emergencies such as a conscious choking adult, bleeding, shock, seizures, burns, falls and fainting.

Circle the correct answers and fill in the blanks.

1. The most important principle of care is:
   a. independence.
   b. communication.
   c. dignity.
   d. safety. *(circled)*

2. By practicing good body mechanics, you can avoid a _back_ injury.

3. Before using any equipment, you should:
   a. check to make sure it is working properly.
   b. unplug it.
   c. file an incident report.
   d. stand up straight.

4. The two categories of restraints are _physical_ and _chemical_.

5. Chemical restraints tie down a person's _mind_ instead of her or his body.

6. Before contacting the physician for an order, the nursing facility may apply a temporary restraint if:
   a. the resident is combative.
   b. other interventions were tried and were not successful. *(circled)*
   c. the staff must search for a missing person.
   d. there are not enough health care workers available.

7. What are two physical problems that can result from restraints? _____

8. Besides physical injuries, restraints also can cause_____problems for a restrained person.

9. A restrained person must be checked every _15 min_.

10. Restraints must be released at least:
    a. every shift.
    b. every hour.
    c. every 2 hours, and more often if necessary. *(circled)*
    d. whenever a relative visits.

11. Three restraint devices are _vest_, _belts_ and _wrist_.

12. What would you do if a fire alarm sounded while you were at work?
    a. Leave the building and go home.
    b. Ask another nurse assistant what was happening.
    c. Follow your employer's policies for fire alarms.
    d. Ignore the fire alarm, because it is probably only a fire drill.

13. If your clothing ignites in a fire, you should:
    a. run, cover and cool.
    b. stop, drop, roll and cool. *(circled)*
    c. call EMS.
    d. blanket, bathe and bandage.

14. One of the first things to do when a natural disaster strikes is to:
    a. unplug appliances.
    b. call the weather bureau.
    c. close all the doors. *(circled)*
    d. gather fire extinguishers.

15. In any emergency, take three basic steps: _check_ the scene and the person, _call_ 9-1-1 or your local emergency number and provide _care_ for the person.

16. Only a doctor can order _physical_ or _chemical_ restraints.

1. Mrs. Kennedy has poor vision and uses a walker. What special measures would you take to make sure her room is safe?

2. Ms. Bernstein gets into a wheelchair before you notice that the brake on the left wheel does not work. What should you do?

3. You notice that Mr. Brown's electric razor keeps shutting off by itself. Mr. Brown taps on it to get it started again. What should you do?

4. How would you feel if someone tied you down against your will?

5. What are some of the physical problems that can result from restraining a person?

6. Every time you come near Ms. Cayhill, she spits at you and tries to hit you. How can you help her with personal care without restraining her arms?

7. Why have restraints been used so much in nursing homes in the past? What is different now?

8. Think of two situations in which a person might be restrained in a nursing facility.

9. You enter Mr. Lee's room and see flames shooting out of the trash can, creating a great deal of smoke. Both Mr. Lee and his roommate are coughing and calling for help. Neither person can walk by himself. What things should you do and in what order?

10. A woman receiving care in the nursing home has been wandering into other residents' rooms. Your supervising nurse tells you to strap her into a wheelchair so that she can't wander. What should you do?

Skill 4: First Aid for Conscious Choking (Airway Obstruction)

PRECAUTIONS

NOTE:
- *If the person can cough forcefully, talk and breathe, even if it is a wheeze, do not interfere with his or her attempts to cough up the object. Encourage him or her to keep coughing.*
- *If coughing persists, call 9-1-1 (or follow facility procedure).*
- *If the person has partial airway obstruction with poor air exchange, this should be dealt with as if it were complete airway obstruction.*

PROCEDURE

1. Check the scene and the person.
   - Ask the victim if he or she is choking.
   - Identify yourself and ask the person if you can help.
   - If the person is coughing forcefully, encourage continued coughing. ☐ ☐
2. If the person cannot cough, speak or breathe:
   - Call, or have someone else call 9-1-1 (or follow facility procedure). ☐ ☐
3. Lean the person forward and give 5 back blows with the heel of your hand ☐ ☐ (Figure 8-14).

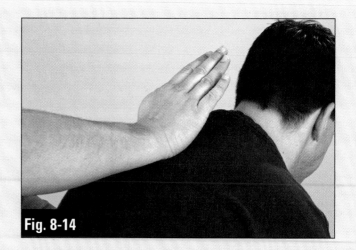

Fig. 8-14

4. Give 5 abdominal thrusts (Figure 8-15, A-C).
   - Place the thumb side of your fist just above the person's belly button.
   - Grab your fist with your other hand.
   - Give quick, upward thrusts.
   - Give chest thrusts to a choking person who is pregnant or too big for you to reach around. ☐ ☐
5. Continue giving back blows and abdominal thrusts until:
   - The object is forced out.
   - The person becomes unconscious.
   - The person can breathe or cough forcefully ☐ ☐

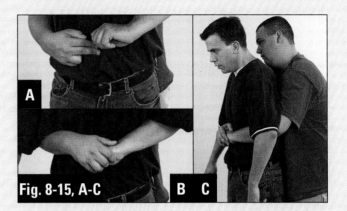

Fig. 8-15, A-C

NOTE: *If the person becomes unconscious, perform CPR. The steps to follow for an unconscious person are not part of this course. However, you may take an American Red Cross First Aid or Cardiopulmonary Resuscitation (CPR) course to learn these steps.*

Skill 5: Controlling External Bleeding

PRECAUTIONS

- Use disposable gloves and other personal protective equipment to prevent disease transmission.
- If bleeding does not stop call 9-1-1 (or follow facility procedure).
- Make sure to wash hands after providing care.

PROCEDURE

1. Check the scene and the person.
   - Identify yourself and ask the person if you can help.
   - Apply Standard Precautions to prevent disease transmission. ☐ ☐
2. Cover the wound with a sterile dressing.
   - Press firmly against the wound (direct pressure) (Figure 8-16). ☐ ☐
3. Cover the dressing with a roller bandage. (Figure 8-17).
   - Tie the knot directly over the wound. ☐ ☐
4. If bleeding does not stop:
   - Apply additional dressing and bandage. Continue to apply pressure.
   - Call, or have someone else call, 9-1-1 (or follow facility procedure).
   - Care for shock. ☐ ☐

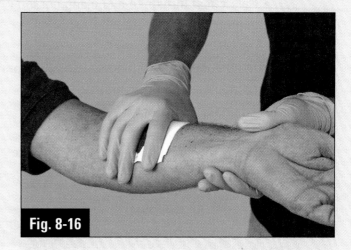

Fig. 8-16

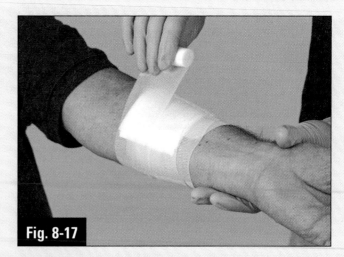

Fig. 8-17

Skill 6: Sudden Illness or Injury

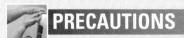 **PRECAUTIONS**

> **NOTE:** *Care for sudden illnesses follows the same general guidelines as for any emergency. Do no further harm.*

PROCEDURE: *SUDDEN ILLNESS*

- Check the scene for clues about what might be wrong, then check the person.
- Call 9-1-1 (or follow facility procedure) for life-threatening conditions.
- *Life-threatening* conditions include:
  - Unconsciousness.
  - Trouble breathing.
  - No breathing.
  - No pulse.
  - Severe bleeding.
  - Chest pain or pressure that lasts more than 3 to 5 minutes, or pain that goes away and comes back.
  - Severe (critical) burn.
  - Pressure or pain in the abdomen that does not go away.
  - Vomiting or passing blood.
  - Has a seizure that lasts more than 5 minutes or multiple seizures.
  - Has a seizure and is diabetic.
  - Has a seizure and is pregnant or fails to regain consciousness after a seizure.
  - Has a sudden severe headache or slurred speech.
  - Appears to have been poisoned.
  - Has injuries to the head, neck or back.
  - Has possible broken bones.
- If the person vomits and is unconscious and lying down, position the person on his or her side.
- Help the person rest comfortably.
- Keep the person from getting chilled or overheated.
- Reassure the person because he or she may be anxious or frightened.
- Watch for changes in consciousness and breathing.

PROCEDURE: *SHOCK*

The signals of shock are:
- Excessive thirst.
- Restlessness or irritability.
- Nausea or vomiting.
- Altered level of consciousness.
- Pale or ashen, gray, cool, moist skin.
- A blue tinge to lips and nail beds. (Called cyanosis)
- Rapid breathing and rapid pulse.

Actions

1. Check scene, and the person.
   - Identify yourself and ask the person if you can help, if possible. ☐ ☐
2. Make sure that 9-1-1 has been called (or follow facility procedure). ☐ ☐
3. Continue to monitor the person's airway, breathing and circulation (ABCs). ☐ ☐
4. Control any external bleeding (following Standard Precautions). ☐ ☐
5. Keep the person from getting chilled or overheated. ☐ ☐
6. Help the person rest comfortably. If the person is having trouble breathing you may be directed to provide oxygen to the person. If it is not suspected that the person has a head, neck or back injury or broken bones in the hips or legs, elevate the legs about 8 to 12 inches (Fig. 8-18). ☐ ☐
7. Comfort and reassure the person until medical help has arrived. ☐ ☐
8. Do not give food or drink to the person. ☐ ☐

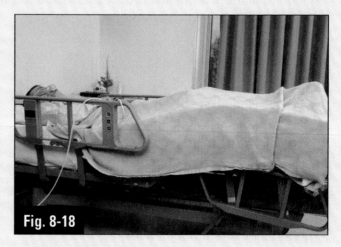

Fig. 8-18

PROCEDURE: *SEIZURE*

The signals of a seizure are:

- Confusion, dizziness or disorientation.
- Trouble breathing.
- Possible body stiffening.
- Convulsions (uncontrolled body movements).
- Fatigue and confusion.
- Headache.

Actions

1. Check scene and the person.
   - Identify yourself and ask the person if you can help, if possible. ☐ ☐
2. Call 9-1-1 (or follow facility procedure). ☐ ☐
3. Care for life-threatening conditions. ☐ ☐
4. Remove any nearby objects that may cause injury. ☐ ☐
5. Cushion the victim's head. ☐ ☐
6. After the seizure and if the person is breathing normally, place the person in recovery position (Figure 8-19). ☐ ☐
7. Do not give the victim anything to eat or drink. ☐ ☐
8. Continue to monitor airway, breathing and circulation. ☐ ☐

PROCEDURE: *BURNS*

Burns can be caused by a variety of sources. Burns can be life-threatening and can lead to shock.

You should *always* call 9-1-1 or the local emergency number if —

- Burns that cause a person to have trouble breathing, or signs of burns around the mouth and nose
- Burns covering more than one body part or a large area
- Burns on the head, neck, hands, feet or genitals
- Burns that are full thickness and the person is younger than age 5 or older than age 60
- Burns resulting from chemicals, explosions or electricity

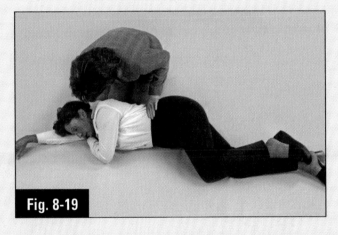
Fig. 8-19

Skill 6: Sudden Illness or Injury—cont'd

Actions

1. Check scene and the person.
   - Identify yourself and ask the person if you can help, if possible. ☐ ☐
2. Stop the burning. (Remove the person from the source.) ☐ ☐
3. Cool the burned area with cold running water until pain is relieved. (Fig. 8-20, A) ☐ ☐
4. Cover the burned area loosely (use a sterile, dry dressing, if possible). (Fig. 8-20, B) ☐ ☐
5. Provide care to minimize the effects of shock in these conditions. ☐ ☐

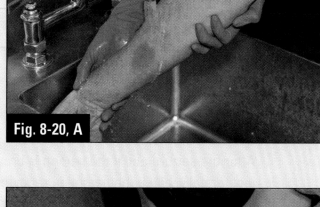
Fig. 8-20, A

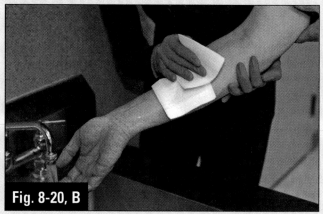
Fig. 8-20, B

PROCEDURE: *FALLS*

NOTE: *Prevention is the best safety measure. In nursing facilities, falls are an occurrence that need to be safeguarded against. Make sure the environment is free of all hazards that may cause a person to fall.*

Actions

1. If a person begins to fall, bring the person close to your body as fast as possible. ☐ ☐

2. Lower yourself and the person slowly to the floor. (Put your arms around the person's waist or underarms, keep the person close to your body, bending your knees). ☐ ☐
3. Move your leg so the person's buttocks rest on it. (Move your leg nearest the person.) ☐ ☐
4. Call for help (do not leave person alone). ☐ ☐

PROCEDURE: *FAINTING* | Syncope

Actions

1. Position the person on a flat surface on their back. ☐ ☐
2. Monitor breathing and conscious-ness. ☐ ☐
3. Call 9-1-1 (or follow facility pro-cedure). ☐ ☐
4. Loosen any restrictive clothing. ☐ ☐
5. If possible, elevate the victim's legs 8 to 12 inches. ☐ ☐
6. If person vomits, position him or her on one side. ☐ ☐
7. Do not give victim anything to eat or drink. ☐ ☐
8. Do not splash the victim with water or slap his or her face. ☐ ☐

PROCEDURE: *STROKE*

Recognize a Stroke F.A.S.T.

- **Face**—Weakness on one side of face
  Ask person to smile
- **Arm**—Weakness or numbness in one arm
  Ask person to raise both arms
- **Speech**—Slurred speech or trouble speaking
  Ask person to say a simple sentence or phrase
- **Time**—Time to CALL 9-1-1 if you see any of these signs
  If the person has difficulty with any of these tasks or shows other signals of a stroke, note the time that the signals began and CALL 9-1-1 immediately.

Other signals to look for:
- Trouble seeing in one or both eyes
- Sudden, severe headaches
- Dizziness, loss of balance
- Looking or feeling ill, abnormal behavior

Actions

1. Check scene and the person. ☐ ☐
2. Call 9-1-1 (or follow facility procedure). ☐ ☐
3. Care for the conditions you find. ☐ ☐
4. If person is drooling or has trouble swallow-ing, place him or her on one side to keep airway clear. ☐ ☐

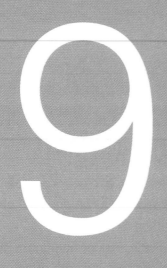

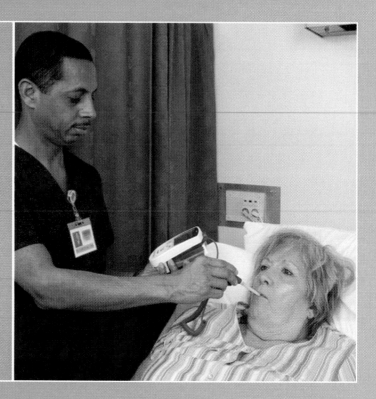

Chapter 9

Measuring Life Signs

GOALS

After reading this chapter, you will have the information needed to:

Discuss the importance of measuring vital signs.

Know when and how to measure vital signs.

Help improve a person's cardiovascular and respiratory function.

After practicing the corresponding skills, you will have the information needed to:

Take and record a person's temperature.

Count and record a person's radial and apical pulse and respirations.

Take and record a person's blood pressure.

When you arrive on duty today at Morningside Nursing Home, you learn that you will provide care for Susan Parker. You have provided care for Mrs. Parker before and know that, although she has arthritis, she is an active, interesting woman. She stays out of bed much of the day, talking with staff and other residents.

Today, however, you discover Mrs. Parker in bed, with a dry, hacking cough. When she tries to talk to you, she coughs even more. Between coughs she manages to tell you that she aches all over. Her face looks flushed, and when you touch her, she feels warm and dry.

When you report these changes in Mrs. Parker to your supervising nurse, she tells you to take her vital signs. You try to take her temperature orally, but she cannot keep the thermometer in her mouth because of the cough. Her vital signs are not normal: her temperature is 103.6 degrees Fahrenheit rectally, her pulse is 110 and thready, and her respirations are 26 and shallow. Her blood pressure is 134/94, which is higher than it usually is. You report the vital signs to your supervising nurse, who goes to Mrs. Parker's room to do a

further assessment. She says that she will phone Mrs. Parker's doctor.

Before leaving Mrs. Parker's room to call the doctor, your supervising nurse tells you to make sure that she rests in bed and drinks plenty of fluids. A short time later, while you are giving Mrs. Parker some juice, your supervising nurse returns with some medicine for the fever. Shortly after Mrs. Parker takes the medicine, her doctor arrives, examines her and orders a liquid medicine for the cough and antibiotic capsules to prevent an infection.

Later in the day, your supervising nurse commends you for being alert in your observations and taking accurate vital signs. She tells you that, because Mrs. Parker received medicine for her symptoms quickly, she will be more comfortable. In addition, she says, the antibiotic prevents pneumonia, which can be life-threatening for older people.

USING VITAL SIGNS TO MEASURE BODY FUNCTION

When you walked into Mrs. Parker's room, you knew that things were not as usual. You heard Mrs. Parker

coughing, you saw that her face was flushed as she lay in her bed, and you felt that her skin was warm to the touch. You used your senses to observe that something was wrong with Mrs. Parker.

These observations alerted you and your supervising nurse to check further. For example, you measured her body temperature to determine whether she had a fever. You also measured her pulse rate to know how fast or slow her heart was beating, her respiration rate to determine how fast or slow she was breathing and her blood pressure to see how much pressure her blood was putting on the walls of her arteries.

Temperature, pulse, respiration and blood pressure all are **vital** indicators of life. In the medical world, the measurements of a person's temperature, pulse, respiration and blood pressure are called *vital signs*. Vital signs give you information about how the person's body is functioning.

In this chapter, you will learn how to measure a person's vital signs. Health care workers use their own language for talking about vital signs. They talk about a person's TPR, which

---

KEY TERMS

abnormal: (ab-NOR-muhl) not normal or regular.

anal: (A-nuhl) of or relating to the opening at the end of the rectum, through which feces pass.

bladder: a pouch that holds air inside the cuff of a sphygmomanometer.

compression: (kum-PRESH-un) the act of pressing or squeezing together.

cuff: the inflatable band of a sphygmomanometer that wraps around the arm.

cyanosis: (si-uh-NO-sis) a condition characterized by the skin having a blue or gray color as a result of a lack of oxygen in the blood.

diaphragm: (DYE-uh-fram) the thin, usually plastic, disk of a stethoscope that is placed on the skin to magnify body sounds.

dyspnea: (disp-NEE-uh) the condition of having difficulty in breathing.

manometer: (ma-NOM-eh-ter) the gauge on a sphygmomanometer that measures systolic and diastolic blood pressure.

rectal: (REK-tuhl) of or referring to the lower portion of the large intestine just inside the anal opening.

shallow: not deep.

sphygmomanometer: (sfig-mo-ma-NOM-eh-ter) an instrument used to measure blood pressure.

stethoscope: (STETH-o-skope) an instrument used to listen to body sounds.

thready pulse: a condition in which the force of the pulse is very weak.

valve: a device that controls the flow of air in an instrument such as a sphygmomanometer or the flow of fluid in an organ such as the heart.

vital: necessary for life.

stands for *t*emperature, *p*ulse and *r*espiration, and BP, which stands for *b*lood *p*ressure. When you take someone's TPR and BP, you record the numbers as "readings." The nurse and doctor use the TPR and BP readings to decide what treatment or medication the person may need. The importance of these readings to the person's care makes it essential that you measure these signs accurately, record them correctly and report any changes in them to your supervising nurse.

When to Measure Vital Signs

The person's vital signs are always measured when (1) the person is admitted to the nursing facility and (2) when you observe a change in someone's usual condition. When a person first starts receiving care, your supervising nurse may ask you to take her vital signs frequently because it is one way to tell how her body is functioning. These frequent readings let the doctor know the usual vital sign numbers for that person. After the doctor knows a person's usual numbers, he may order the vital signs to be taken on a less frequent, but regular, basis. The frequency varies from one person to another. For example, someone who has a heart problem needs to have her vital signs measured more often than a person who has no heart problem or other major illness.

If you observe and report a change in a person's condition, your supervising nurse may ask you to take her vital signs more frequently. The changes you observe may be physical or behavioral. When you saw that Mrs. Parker was flushed and felt that she was warm to the touch, you observed a physical change (Figure 9-1). When you observed that Mrs. Parker, who is usually active and sociable, was tired and stayed in bed, you observed a behavioral change. When your supervising nurse asked you to take vital signs, your observations were verified: Mrs Parker's body temperature was

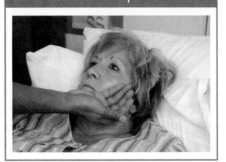

high, she had a **thready pulse,** her respirations were **shallow** and her blood pressure was high.

Responding to the Person's Needs When Taking Vital Signs

Measuring vital signs is part of providing regular care. If you work in a hospital or nursing home, you may be asked to take the vital signs of everyone who needs to have them taken at that time, or you may take just one person's vital signs. Some employers may refer to taking vital signs as "routine vital signs." The word *routine* refers to *which signs* you measure—not to *how* you measure them. You always observe the six principles of care when you take a person's vital signs. For example, you remember to provide privacy for a person while you are measuring her vital signs.

You also have to be sensitive to how a person feels about having her vital signs measured. One person may be afraid of or upset about having her temperature, pulse or blood pressure taken. Another may worry because she believes it means she is sick. Sometimes a person in your care may be tired and may not want to be bothered. Or a person may be embarrassed because you must take a **rectal** temperature through the **anal** opening.

As you take a person's vital signs, be sure to do these three things: (1) Reassure her that the procedures are important to her care; (2) ensure her dignity and privacy, especially when taking a rectal temperature; and (3) most important, perform the skills accurately.

MEASURING A PERSON'S BODY TEMPERATURE

Body temperature indicates the amount of heat in a person's body. The human body keeps its temperature fairly constant by responding to heat and cold. If the body gets hot, it sweats to get rid of some of the heat, or it breathes more air in and out of the lungs. When the body gets cold, it shivers to create heat from muscle activity.

Normal Range of Body Temperature

Body temperature can vary slightly from one person to another and among age groups (Figure 9-2). A person's normal body temperature usually changes slightly during the day. Generally, it is lower in the morning after sleeping, when body functions have slowed down, and higher in the afternoon after activity. A person's body temperature may rise when her emotions increase and may fall when she feels depressed. It also may increase

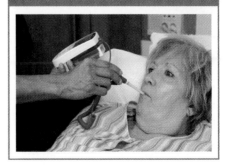

or decrease with the temperature of the air.

What is a normal body temperature? No single temperature is normal for everyone, because body temperature changes in response to many things. Instead, a range of numbers describes what is normal for most people. You have to know the normal range of body temperatures, because you must report temperatures above or below the normal range to your supervising nurse. If a person has a temperature reading above the normal range, the person is said to have a *fever*.

You will learn to measure temperature in four different ways. When you place an instrument called a *thermometer* in a person's mouth, you are taking an *oral temperature*. When you place the thermometer under a person's arm, you are taking an *axillary temperature*. (The underarm is called the *axilla*.) When you insert the thermometer in a person's rectum, you are taking a *rectal temperature*. When you place a probe in a person's ear, you are taking a *tympanic temperature*. (The eardrum is called the *tympanic membrane*.) The normal range of temperatures is different for each of the first three methods of taking body temperature, and the tympanic method can reflect either the oral or the rectal range.

A thermometer measures temperature in units called *degrees*. Degrees can be measured on two different scales: Fahrenheit or Celsius. On the Fahrenheit scale, the freezing point of water is 32 degrees, and the average, normal human body temperature is 98.6 degrees. On the Celsius scale, the freezing point of water is 0 degrees, and the average normal human body temperature is 37 degrees. In this book, temperatures are measured on the Fahrenheit scale. Fahrenheit is abbreviated as "F." Table 9-1 shows the normal range of body temperatures for each of the first three methods of measuring body temperatures.

TABLE 9-1 NORMAL RANGE OF BODY TEMPERATURES FOR THREE METHODS OF MEASUREMENT (FAHRENHEIT SCALE)

Method	Normal Range (°F)	Average (°F)
Axillary	96.6–98.6	97.6
Oral	97.6–99.6	98.6
Rectal	98.6–100.6	99.6

TABLE 9-2 NORMAL RANGE OF BODY TEMPERATURES FOR THREE METHODS OF MEASUREMENT (CELSIUS SCALE)

Method	Normal Range (°C)	Average (°C)
Axillary	35.9-37.0	36.4
Oral	36.4-37.6	37.0
Rectal	37.0-38.1	37.6

Table 9-2 shows the normal range of temperature on the Celsius scale. Some studies suggest a slightly different range of normal adult temperatures and average temperature.

At this time, however, the temperatures in Table 9-1 are still the accepted ones. The average body temperature varies quite a bit, depending on which method you use to measure it. For example, compared with the average oral temperature of 98.6 degrees Fahrenheit, the average axillary temperature is 1 degree lower and the average rectal temperature is 1 degree higher.

Types of Thermometers

To take a person's temperature, use one of three types of thermometers: glass, electronic or tympanic. See Table 9-3 for precautions, when using a thermometer.

Glass Thermometer. Glass thermometers are not often used in healthcare setting. The glass thermometer may contain mercury or nonmercury substance. When taking someone's temperature, the bulb warms from the body heat, and the nonmercury substance moves further up the shaft toward the stem.

There are two types of glass thermometers: oral and rectal. They differ in shapes of their bulbs. The oral glass thermometer, which you use for taking only oral temperatures, has a long, slender bulb. Rectal thermometers have rounder, stubbier bulbs. Once you use a thermometer to take a rectal temperature, you should never use it to take an oral or axillary temperature. To avoid confusion, the thermometer manufacturer often colors the ends of thermometers in red if they are going to be used for taking rectal temperatures.

When using a glass thermometer take the following precautions:
- Be careful not to break the glass thermometer.
- When taking a person's temperature, do not let the person bite down or break the glass thermometer.

If you should drop and break a glass mercury thermometer, do not

TABLE 9-3 PRECAUTIONS FOR USING A THERMOMETER

Situation	Problem	Solution
Person has had recent mouth surgery or has a mouth disease	Thermometer may cause injury	Take temperature using rectal, axillary or tympanic method
Confused person	May bite down on thermometer and may injure herself	Take temperature using rectal, axillary or tympanic method
Unconscious person or person paralyzed on one side of body	May not be able to keep mouth closed, resulting in inaccurate temperature reading	Take temperature using rectal, axillary or tympanic method
Person has trouble breathing or breathes through mouth, or person has tube in nose and cannot keep mouth closed	Cannot get accurate temperature reading	Take temperature using rectal, axillary or tympanic method
Person receiving oxygen experiences cooling of the body tissues around the mouth	Cannot get accurate temperature reading	Take temperature using rectal, axillary or tympanic method
Person has a blocked rectum, has hemorrhoids or has had recent rectal surgery	Rectal thermometer can cause injury	Take temperature using oral, axillary or tympanic method
Person has had a heart attack	Rectal thermometer may stimulate the urge to strain and may increase the workload of the heart	Take temperature using oral, axillary or tympanic method
Person is embarrassed about having rectal temperature taken	May be uncooperative	Explain the reason for taking rectal temperature to encourage cooperation
Person perspires under the arms	Moisture can affect the temperature reading	Dry the axilla with a tissue

touch or let anyone touch the mercury. Report it to your supervising nurse immediately. The facility will follow special procedures for cleaning up the mercury spill. Nonmercury glass thermometers are safer than mercury glass thermometers. You may read more information concerning glass thermometers in Appendix E.

Electronic Thermometer. The electronic thermometer is a small, battery-operated machine that looks something like a calculator. It is connected to a probe that resembles a thermometer, but it has no mercury. A person's body temperature is calculated electronically inside the machine. The machine beeps when the person's temperature has been registered, and the number of the temperature appears on a small digital screen.

You can use an electronic thermometer to take a temperature by any method (Figure 9-3). It measures a person's body temperature in 2 to 60 seconds. The probe of the thermometer has a disposable cover, which you

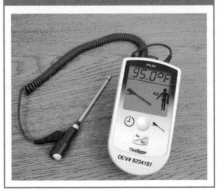

FIGURE 9-3 An electronic thermometer.

throw away after taking the person's temperature. Probes on electronic thermometers also may be colored red for the rectal method and blue for the oral and axillary methods.

Tympanic Thermometer. The tympanic thermometer, which is becoming more widely used, measures heat waves given off by the eardrum. This type of thermometer has a specially designed probe that you place in the person's ear to measure the heat waves and translate them into a temperature reading, which is displayed on a digital screen. The tympanic thermometer is a fast method for measuring a person's temperature (Figure 9-4).

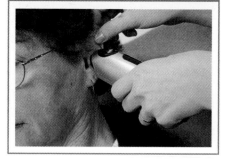

FIGURE 9-4 A tympanic thermometer is placed in the person's ear.

Taking a Person's Temperature

When taking a person's oral temperature, make sure that she has not had recent mouth surgery and does not have a mouth disease. Also make sure that she is not receiving oxygen and is not having trouble breathing, is not confused or unconscious, and is not paralyzed on one side of her body or face. Do not take an oral temperature if she is breathing through her mouth or if she has a tube in her nose. Do not take a child's oral temperature if she is under the age of 5. Also delay taking the person's temperature by 15 minutes if she has eaten, smoked or had anything to drink within the past 15 minutes.

If you take the oral temperature of an adult in your care, you usually do not have to hold the thermometer in place. You can make use of the waiting time by measuring and recording other vital signs. (If you take a rectal or axillary temperature you should hold the thermometer in place; in that case, of course, you will not be able to record other signs at the same time.) Generally, the oral method is the preferred way to measure a person's body temperature, because it is the easiest method and requires little preparation. Taken correctly, it is an accurate reflection of the body's internal temperature. Follow the specific procedure that is explained step by step in Skill 7.

The rectal method for measuring a person's body temperature also accurately reflects internal body temperature, but it requires more preparation and can be embarrassing for adults and frightening for children. Take a person's rectal temperature when an oral temperature would be inaccurate or might cause injury. Make sure that the person does not have diarrhea or a blocked rectum. Make sure that she has not recently had a heart attack or rectal surgery or injury or that she does not have hemorrhoids. Follow the specific procedure that is explained step by step in Skill 7.

The axillary method is the least accurate way to measure a person's body temperature. Take an axillary temperature only if the person cannot tolerate either an oral or a rectal thermometer. Make sure the person is sitting or lying down during the procedure and not walking around with the thermometer under her arm. Follow the specific procedure that is explained step by step in Skill 7.

Taking a Person's Temperature with an Electronic Thermometer

Electronic thermometers are quick and easy to use. You do not have to clean the electronic unit or shake it down as you provide care from one person to another. You insert the probe of the thermometer, which has a disposable cover, into the mouth, rectum or axilla of a person in your care. The unit beeps to indicate when the internal body temperature has registered and displays this number on a small digital screen. After you discard the probe cover, the thermometer is ready for reuse.

Some electronic thermometers operate on nonrechargeable batteries, and others periodically have to be plugged into recharging devices so that they are always ready to use. Because most health care facilities have a minimum number of electronic thermometers, it is important that each caregiver replaces the equipment immediately after use so that it is available for others to use.

An electronic thermometer is often used for many people, so you must practice proper infection control procedures. Remember not to put the thermometer down on dirty surfaces. If the thermometer has a cord, keep the cord in your hand and make sure that the only part that contacts the person or his or her surroundings is the probe cover.

Periodically, some electronic thermometers may have to be recalibrated or readjusted. If you suspect that a thermometer is not giving an accurate body temperature reading (for example, every person's temperature that you take is exactly the same), let your supervising nurse know so that the machine can be repaired. When taking a person's temperature with an electronic thermometer, follow the specific procedure that is explained step by step in Skill 7.

MEASURING A PERSON'S PULSE

When your supervising nurse asked you to check Mrs. Parker's vital signs, one of the signs you checked was her pulse. The pulse is one of the signs of life—breathing and movement are indicators of how the cardiovascular system is working. (See the section on the cardiovascular system in Appendix B, "Body Basics.") Each time the heart beats, it pushes blood through tiny tubes called arteries that carry blood throughout the body. The heartbeat creates a wave, which you can feel if you put your fingers over certain places on the body. Between beats, the heart rests. Then it beats again, causing another wave that you can feel. The wave that you can feel is called the *pulse*.

The pulse provides information about how a person's heart is working, and this information helps the doctor plan his or her care. Because this information is so important, you must be able to describe what the pulse feels like. You can compare a pulse that comes at regular intervals to the ticking of a clock. You can describe this pulse as having a *regular rhythm*. If the interval between pulses is uneven, describe the rhythm as being *irregular*. If the force of the pulse is easy to feel, describe it as a *full* or *strong pulse*. If the force of the pulse seems to push up against your fingertips, describe it as a *bounding pulse*. If the force of the pulse is very weak and you can barely feel it, describe it as a *thready pulse*. When you use these words to describe how the person's pulse feels, you give the doctor significant information about the person's heart.

When you count the number of times you feel a person's pulse beat in a minute, you know the rate at which the person's heart is beating. This number is called the *heart rate,* or *pulse rate*. Many things can cause the pulse rate to speed up or slow down (Figure 9-5). Think of a time when you felt like your heart was beating very fast. Perhaps you were scared or had just run up a flight of stairs. Maybe you were excited, upset or angry, which

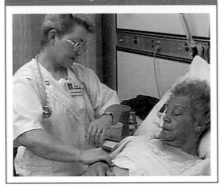

FIGURE 9-5 Even a slight amount of exercise can make a person's heart beat faster. If you know a person has been exercising, wait 5 to 10 minutes before taking his or her pulse.

caused your heart to beat faster. Other conditions that may speed up your pulse rate are pain, fever or significant blood loss. Mrs. Parker had pain and fever with the flu, and her heart rate was faster than normal. Just as some things can speed up pulse rate, other things, such as sleep, certain drugs and depression, can slow it down.

Because so many things can affect the pulse rate, it is important to count the pulse when the person is sitting quietly. The average rate for an

adult is between 60 and 100 beats per minute, although athletes have slower-than-average rates that may even fall below 60 beats per minute. The average rate for a child 1-10 years old is between 70 and 120 beats per minute, and it is even higher for infants.

You can feel the pulse in several places on a person's body. Table 9-4 describes the seven common places where you can feel the pulse. Most of the time you measure a person's radial pulse on the wrist, and except for the apical pulse at the top of the heart, you use the same procedure regardless of which pulse area you use. To measure an apical pulse, you use a **stethoscope** because you cannot feel an apical pulse with your fingers. (Read about the stethoscope later in this chapter in the section on measuring a person's blood pressure.) Because you usually take all vital signs at the same time, you can count a person's pulse while you are waiting for her oral temperature to register. You may notice that, when a person's temperature rises, her pulse rate also rises. This condition occurs because, for each degree Fahrenheit that body temperature rises, the heart beats 8 to 10 beats faster per minute.

TABLE 9-4 WHERE TO FEEL THE PULSE	
Pulse Area	Location
Apical	At the top of the heart, just under the left breast
Brachial	At the inside bend of the elbow
Carotid	On the neck on the side of the Adam's apple
Femoral	At the groin where the thigh meets the hip
Pedal	On the top of the foot
Radial	On the inside of the wrist at the base of the thumb
Temporal	At the side of the forehead above the outer corner of the eye

Counting and Recording a Person's Radial Pulse

When you are getting ready to take a person's pulse, approach her in a calm, unhurried manner so that she does not become upset or agitated and her heart rate does not increase. Make sure that she is in a comfortable, relaxed position. If she has just come back from a strenuous physical therapy session, or has just had a painful procedure done, remember that these experiences will increase her heart rate. If possible, you should come back a little later after she has had time to relax. Often a good time to do this is while taking an oral temperature (Figure 9-6).

When you are first learning to take a radial pulse, it is easy to push too hard on the wrist and flatten the artery so that you do not feel anything. Remember to press lightly against the wrist, with your fingers over the radial pulse, and count the number of beats per minute, using a watch with a second hand. Until you become comfortable with counting the pulse rate, start timing the pulse when the second hand is on the "12" so that you do not lose track of when you started counting. Never use your thumb to feel a person's pulse, because your thumb

has its own pulse and you may count *your* pulse rate instead of the person's pulse rate. Count the pulses for 1 full minute. Note the pulse rhythm and force so that you can describe them accurately. Write down the pulse rate immediately, noting any irregularities in the rhythm and any changes in the force that you feel.

Report any irregularities in rhythm and any pulse rate that is below 60 beats per minute or above 100 beats per minute to your supervising nurse. Irregular rhythms and very slow or very fast rates may indicate a medical problem. Earlier, when you measured Mrs. Parker's vital signs, her pulse was faster than usual because of her pain and fever. When taking a person's radial pulse, always keep the person's arm close to her body and not in the air. Follow the specific procedure that is explained step by step in Skill 8.

Taking an Apical Pulse

When measuring the pulse of some adults and younger children whose arteries are small and whose heart beats are fast, you must take an apical pulse. You use a stethoscope to count the apical pulse by listening to it rather than feeling it. With a stethoscope, you are listening to the heart beat, which should reflect the same beats per minute as those felt at other pulse points. Count the beats for 1 full minute, and record the number of beats as the apical pulse rate. To take an apical pulse, follow the procedure that is explained step by step in Skill 8.

Normal Values

For resting heart rate:
- newborn infants; 100 to 160 beats per minute
- children 1 to 10 years; 70 to 120 beats per minute
- children over 10 and adults; 60 to 100 beats per minute
- well-trained athletes; 40 to 60 beats per minute

COUNTING AND RECORDING A PERSON'S RESPIRATIONS

Respiration, the process of breathing, consists of two parts: inspiration and expiration. Taking breath in is called *inspiration,* and letting breath out is called *expiration.* One rise (inspiration) and fall (expiration) of the chest equals one respiration. (See the section on the respiratory system in Appendix B, "Body Basics.")

How do you know if a person's breathing is normal? A person with normal respiration breathes quietly and easily. Her breathing seems effortless and regular. If you watch her chest, you see both sides of her chest rise and fall equally.

A normal healthy adult breathes 15 to 20 times a minute. Because loud noises or pain can affect the reading, note whether either of these situations occurred while you were counting. Earlier, when you counted Mrs. Parker's respirations, they were fast and shallow because of her pain and fever.

How do you know if a person's breathing is **abnormal?** Difficult, erratic or noisy breathing is considered abnormal. Abnormal breathing indicates that the person is experiencing some medical problem. You may observe that a person is breathing abnormally if:
- She sounds like she has a rattle or wetness in her chest.
- Her breathing is uneven.
- She has **dyspnea.**
- Her lips look blue or gray and the base of her fingernails looks blue. (Either of these conditions, called **cyanosis,** develops when a person does not get enough oxygen. Oxygen-rich blood is bright red, whereas blood that is low in oxygen is darker and looks blue through the skin.)

If you observe any of these abnormal signs, report them immediately to your supervising nurse.

FIGURE 9-6 Usually you take the person's pulse along with his oral temperature.

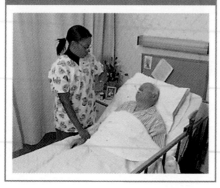

FIGURE 9-7 When someone has difficulty breathing, the head of his bed is elevated to help him breathe more easily. This resident is also receiving oxygen using a nasal cannula.

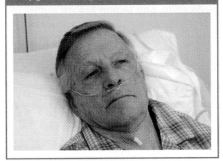

Many things affect the way a person breathes. A person who slouches may not breathe deeply, because her lungs do not have room to expand. Another person with lung or heart problems may have difficulty breathing when he is lying flat. To breathe comfortably, he may need to sit up, have his bed elevated or use several pillows (Figure 9-7).

The same things that make a person's heart beat faster also make her breathe faster, such as exercise, anger, fear, pain, excitement, fever and significant blood loss. Likewise, the same things that slow down her heart rate can also slow down her breathing, such as rest, depression and certain drugs.

Sometimes, especially after exercise, a person's body may need to take in more air. Her chest rises more to create more space for air to enter. This condition is called *deep breathing*. If the chest rises and falls very little, as it does during sleep, this type of breathing is called *shallow* (Figure 9-8).

Because a person can make herself breathe faster or slower just by deciding to do so, you must count her respirations without her being aware of what you are doing. Usually, you count a person's respirations when you take her oral temperature and

FIGURE 9-8 Respirations can be fast and shallow because of her pain and fever.

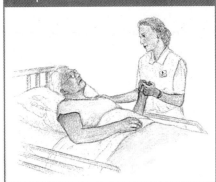

before or after taking her pulse. If you count her pulse first and continue to keep your fingers on her wrist, she may not be aware that you are counting her respirations. Count the person's respirations for 1 full minute, counting one rise and one fall of the chest for each respiration. When counting and recording a person's respirations, follow the specific procedure that is explained step by step in Skill 9.

TAKING AND RECORDING A PERSON'S BLOOD PRESSURE

Blood pressure measures the pressure of the circulating blood on the walls of the arteries. Each time the heart beats, it pumps blood through the heart and lungs and into the arteries. The pressure of the blood against the walls of the arteries when the heart pumps is called the *systolic pressure*. The pressure of the blood against the walls when the heart relaxes is called the *diastolic pressure*. A blood pressure reading consists of these two numbers, which are written like fractions. The larger systolic reading goes on the top, and the smaller diastolic reading goes on the bottom. For example, in the reading 118/78, 118 is the systolic pressure, and 78 is the diastolic pres-

sure. The systolic pressure is always higher.

To understand blood pressure, imagine the heart as a water pump and the arteries as a hose connected to the pump. When you turn on the pump, water is pushed through the hose. When you turn off the pump, water continues to go through the hose for a time, but the pressure inside the hose decreases. The water eventually stops flowing, unless the pump is turned on again. The heart is like the pump—pumping and resting, pumping and resting—as it pushes blood through the arteries.

What would happen if some sand got into the water hose? The sand would make it more difficult for the water to flow through the hose. The sand causes the pressure inside the hose to increase, because the pressure in a tube increases as the size of the opening of a tube decreases. Think about what happens when you put your finger partially over the end of a hose while the water is running through it (Figure 9-9). The opening that the water goes through gets smaller, and the water spurts out farther and harder.

FIGURE 9-9 There is more pressure in a clogged artery, just as there is more pressure in the hose when you put your thumb over the end of it.

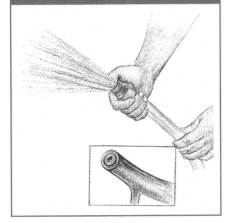

TABLE 9-5 FACTORS THAT INFLUENCE BLOOD PRESSURE

Influencing Factor	Increase(s) Blood Pressure	Decrease(s) Blood Pressure
Arteries clogged with cholesterol	X	
Eating salty foods	X	
Eating fatty foods	X	
Eating healthy foods		X
Consuming alcohol	X	
Being overweight	X	
Lack of exercise	X	
Regular exercise		X
Physical stress	X	X
Smoking	X	
Emotional stress	X	X
Some kidney diseases	X	
Medications	X	X

What is a normal blood pressure for an adult? A normal blood pressure reading is a systolic pressure that is less than 120 mm Hg and when the diastolic is less than 80 mm Hg.

A person is considered to have high blood pressure (hypertension) when either or both of the following are present:

- The top number (systolic) is consistently 140 mm Hg or higher.
- The bottom number (diastolic) is consistently 90 mm Hg or higher.

Equipment for Measuring Blood Pressure

You use two pieces of equipment when measuring a person's blood pressure. First, you place a **sphygmomanometer,** consisting of a **cuff** and a **manometer,** on the person's arm. Then you listen to the person's pulse sounds with a stethoscope (Figure 9-10).

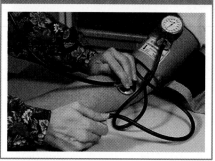

FIGURE 9-10 Properly using blood pressure equipment takes practice.

The same thing happens to the arteries in the body if they get clogged up with a fatty substance called *cholesterol*. The cholesterol buildup makes the openings of the arteries smaller. When the heart pumps blood into the arteries, the pressure inside the arteries increases because the opening is smaller. Fatty, cholesterol-rich foods can clog arteries, and people with clogged arteries may have high blood pressure.

Some other factors that influence the increase or decrease in blood pressure appear in Table 9-5. In addition, men frequently have higher blood pressure than women, and some ethnic groups tend to have higher blood pressures than others. Blood pressure in children is generally lower than in adults, and blood pressure tends to

increase with age because the arteries become narrower and more rigid.

Children whose parents had or have high blood pressure are more likely to develop high blood pressure. For all people, blood pressure varies throughout the day and is usually lowest in the morning when they first get up.

CATEGORIES FOR BLOOD PRESSURE LEVELS IN ADULTS
(in mmHg, millimeters of mercury)[a]

Category	Systolic (top number)	Diastolic (bottom number)
Normal	Less than 120	Less than 80
Prehypertension	120–139	80–89
High blood pressure		
Stage 1	140–159	90–99
Stage 2	160 or higher	100 or higher

[a]For adults 18 and older who are not on medicine for high blood pressure; are not having a short-term serious illness; and do not have other conditions, such as diabetes and kidney disease.

Note: When systolic and diastolic blood pressures fall into different categories, the higher category should be used to classify blood pressure level. For example, 160/80 mmHg would be stage 2 high blood pressure.
http://www.nhlbi.nih.gov/health/dci/Diseases/Hbp/HBP_WhatIs.html

Ranges
systolic: 90 - 140
Diastolic: 60 - 90

Using a Stethoscope. The stethoscope consists of two pieces of tubing that are connected at one end to a flat disk called a **diaphragm.** The earpieces, which are connected to the other end of the tubing, fit into your ears and allow you to hear sounds. Some stethoscopes have a bell-shaped end instead of a diaphragm. Before taking a person's blood pressure, check the tubing and diaphragm for cracks and holes that could make it difficult to hear and could cause you to make an error in the blood pressure reading. To prevent the spread of infection, use alcohol to clean the diaphragm after each contact with a person. If you use a stethoscope that is used by other caregivers and is used on a regular basis, clean the earpieces with alcohol before putting them in your ears. When using a stethoscope to measure a person's blood pressure, follow the specific procedure that is explained step by step in Skill 10.

Using a Blood Pressure Cuff. The cuff of the sphygmomanometer is placed on the person's bare arm. The cuff is made of fabric and comes in several sizes. It has a rubber **bladder** inside, which is connected at the end to a hose with a rubber ball, called a bulb. A **valve** in the bulb opens and closes to control the flow of air into the bladder. The valve is controlled by a screw. If you turn the screw to the left, it opens the valve and lets the air escape from the bladder. If you turn the screw to the right, it closes the valve so that when you pump air into the bladder with the bulb, the valve keeps the air inside the bladder, making the cuff tight. When you pump air into the cuff, the bladder pressure increases until it is strong enough to stop the blood flow through the brachial artery. At this point, you do not hear anything through the stethoscope. As you turn the valve to release pressure on the brachial artery, the cuff pressure eventually matches and

then drops below the systolic blood pressure. When the cuff pressure reaches this point, you begin to hear the pulse sounds. As the cuff pressure drops to equal the diastolic pressure in the artery, the sounds that you hear change or fade away.

Understanding the Manometer. The gauge that measures systolic and diastolic pressure is called a *manometer.* The numbers on the gauge show the pressure in millimeters. The larger the number, the greater the pressure. Three types of manometers that you may read are *mercury, aneroid,* and *electronic.*

The mercury manometer shows the pressure readings on an upright gauge with a straight column of numbers. The mercury moves up the column from zero to the higher numbers as you inflate the cuff. The numbers show the pressure in millimeters of mercury (mm Hg).

The aneroid manometer shows the pressure readings on a round dial with an arrow that points to the numbers (Figure 9-11, A). Although there is no mercury column, the numbers on the dial are equal to millimeters of mercury (mm Hg). The arrow moves from zero to the higher numbers as you inflate the cuff.

The electronic manometer (Figure 9-11, B) eliminates the need for using a stethoscope and listening for the pulse sounds, because it takes the blood pressure readings for you and displays them on a digital screen like the one on an electronic thermometer.

Taking a Person's Blood Pressure

As you use the equipment, you will learn to adjust the valve so that air is released slowly from the bladder. When you deflate the cuff slowly, it makes a quieter sound, which makes it easier to decide exactly when you hear the pulse sounds appear and disappear. Remember both numbers so that you can record the readings accurately.

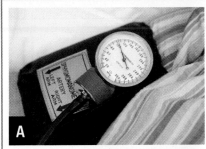

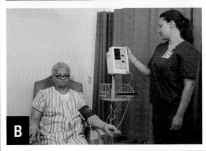

FIGURE 9-11 A, An aneroid manometer. **B,** An electronic manometer.

Sometimes you may not hear clearly or you may not be sure of what you heard. If you do not hear the pulse clearly, let all the air out of the cuff. Wait 1 minute before you try again. This pause allows time for the blood vessels to relax. Never try to take a person's blood pressure more than twice on one arm because repeated **compressions** of the arteries may give an incorrect reading.

To use the electronic manometer, place the cuff on the person's arm as you do when using the mercury and aneroid manometers. Some machines inflate the cuff automatically, while others require you to inflate the cuff manually with a bulb. When the cuff deflates automatically, the blood pressure reading and usually the pulse appear on the digital screen.

When taking a person's blood pressure, observe the precautions listed in Table 9-6 and follow the specific procedure that is explained step by step in Skill 10.

TABLE 9-6 PRECAUTIONS FOR TAKING A PERSON'S BLOOD PRESSURE

Precaution	Reason
Place the cuff on the person's bare arm.	Clothing increases the size of the arm and may give an incorrect reading. When the diaphragm is placed on clothing, it creates noises that make it difficult to hear pulse sounds.
Select the correct cuff size: adult-size for most adults, extra-large for some adults and child-size for small people.	Using the correct size results in an accurate reading.
Wrap the cuff smoothly and snugly.	A smooth wrap gives an accurate reading.
Position the cuff correctly, with the center of the bladder over the brachial artery.	Correct positioning gives an accurate reading.
Do not place the cuff on a cast.	The cuff cannot compress the cast, which results in no reading.
Do not place the cuff on an arm with an IV in place.	The pressure from the cuff could stop the flow of fluid and possibly cause the needle to clog or dislodge from the vein.
Do not place the cuff on the weak arm of a person who has had a stroke or on a person's paralyzed arm. For a woman who has had a mastectomy, do not place the cuff on the arm that is on the same side as the mastectomy.	Circulation in these conditions is impaired, resulting in an inaccurate reading. Also, an inflated cuff decreases circulation in the arm and may cause some damage.

IMPROVING CARDIOVASCULAR AND RESPIRATORY FUNCTION

When providing care to an elderly person, you can help her improve her cardiovascular and respiratory functions. In addition to observing her and monitoring her vital signs, you can remind her to do certain things and encourage her to do things in a certain way. Be patient while she does things for herself and report any concerns about her to your supervising nurse.

Helping a Person's Cardiovascular System Work Better

To help a person's cardiovascular system work better, you can:

- Provide more time for the person to complete tasks.
- Provide more time for her to rest.
- Encourage the person to exercise every day.
- Encourage her to eat healthy meals.
- Encourage her not to smoke.
- Monitor her vital signs.
- Observe any changes in her skin because poor circulation can lead to pressure sores.
- Report right away to your supervising nurse if the person has any of the following conditions:
  - Shortness of breath
  - Change in vital signs
  - Change in skin color or injury to her skin

Helping a Person's Respiratory System Work Better

To help a person's respiratory system work better, you can:

- Remind the person to take deep breaths during the day, because deep breathing fills the lungs with air and helps them stay more flexible.
- Encourage the person to rest between activities, such as between eating and bathing.
- Encourage her to take time to stop, rest and breathe deeply when walking.
- When the person is lying down, raise her upper body to make breathing easier.
- Encourage her not to smoke.
- Report right away to your supervising nurse if the person has any of the following conditions:
  - Shortness of breath
  - Difficulty breathing
  - Blue or gray color (cyanosis)
  - Unusual confusion (often the first sign of pneumonia)

Circle the correct answers and fill in the blanks.

1. Temperature, pulse, blood pressure and respirations usually are taken together and are referred to as:
   a. life measurements.
   b. **vital signs.** *(circled)*
   c. routine measurements.
   d. monitoring.

2. A person's vital signs are always measured when the person is _admitted_ to a nursing home and when you observe a _change_ in someone's usual condition.

3. The normal range for an adult's oral temperature is _97.6_ to _99.6_.

4. An elevation of body temperature is called:
   a. cyanosis.
   b. shallow.
   c. compression.
   d. **a fever.** *(circled)*

5. *Irregular* is a term used to describe the _r_ of a pulse, and *thready* is a term used to describe the _force_ of a pulse.

6. The _brachial_ pulse is located inside the bend of the elbow and is used for measuring blood pressure.

7. What instrument is used to listen to heart sounds when a blood pressure reading or an apical pulse reading is being taken?
   a. **Stethoscope** *(circled)*
   b. Diaphragm
   c. Valve
   d. Thermometer

8. Never use your _thumb_ to count another person's pulse.

9. Difficulty with breathing is called _DYSPNEA_.

10. When you count the number of times a person breathes per minute, you are counting her:
    a. pulse.
    b. temperature.
    c. **respirations.** *(circled)*
    d. emotional level.

1. *You are taking Josie's vital signs. She is complaining of being dizzy, especially when she sits up. Her BP is 90/52. What should you do?*

2. *What could you do to calm a person who is afraid of having his BP taken?*

3. *When you go into Mrs. Clement's room to take her oral temperature, you notice a cup of hot coffee on her table. What should you consider, and what should you do?*

4. *Mr. Smith is smoking when you enter his room to take his temperature. What should you do?*

5. *When you take Mr. Wilson's pulse at 8:00 a.m., the rate is 72 and the rhythm is regular. When you take it again at 9:00 a.m., it is 56 and irregular. What should you do?*

6. *Mrs. Miller breathes quietly when she is sitting up but begins to breathe noisily and faster as soon as you lower the head of her bed. What should you do?*

7. *Mr. Rivera is asleep and breathing so quietly that you have difficulty seeing his chest rise and fall. What should you do?*

8. *Josie keeps trying to carry on a conversation while you are trying to measure and record vital signs. How should you handle this situation? What should you say to her?*

Skill 7: Using an Electronic Thermometer

PRECAUTIONS
- Check to make sure equipment is working (electronically charged).

PREPARATION
1. Gather supplies:
   - Electronic thermometer
   - Probe cover
   - Lubricating jelly (for rectal)
   - Disposable gloves (for rectal)
   - Plastic trash bag
   - Pen and paper to write down the temperature
2. Check to make sure equipment is working (electrically charged).
3. Follow Preparation Standards (see Chapter 7).

PROCEDURE

NOTE: *Be sure that you have the appropriate probe. Probes are detachable and will be coded to indicate whether they are rectal or oral/axillary.*

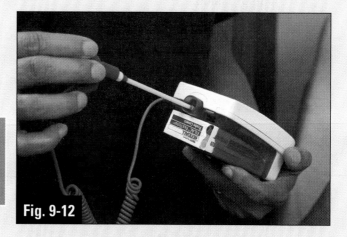

Fig. 9-12

1. Turn the thermometer "on" by removing the probe from the location in the machine where it is stored (its "home" location) (Figure 9-12). ☐ ☐
2. Insert the probe into the probe cover by pushing firmly until you feel the cover snap into place (Figure 9-13). ☐ ☐
3. Position the person appropriately.
4. Taking a Temperature
   For Oral Temperature:
   - Put the thermometer under the person's tongue and slightly to one side.

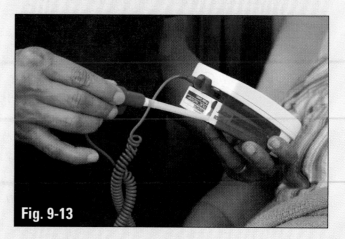

Fig. 9-13

- Ask the person to close her lips and not to bite down on the thermometer with her teeth. ☐ ☐
- Always stay with the person while you are taking an oral temperature. ☐ ☐

For Rectal Temperature:
- Lower the side rail, if used, on the side where you will be working. ☐ ☐
- Help the person lie on one side with his back toward you. Ask him to flex his top knee. Adjust his clothing and top covers so that he is covered. ☐ ☐
- Put on disposable gloves. ☐ ☐
- Put a small amount of lubricating jelly on a tissue.
- Apply lubricating jelly to the tip of the thermometer from a tissue. ☐ ☐
- Turn back the top covers and adjust or remove clothing just enough so that you can see the anal area. ☐ ☐
- Lift the person's upper buttock and gently insert the end of the thermometer into the anus, no more than 1 inch. ☐ ☐
- Wipe the person's anal area with a tissue, if necessary after taking temperature and throw away the tissue in the plastic trash bag. ☐ ☐

For Axillary Temperature:
- Uncover the person's underarm area and dry it with a tissue, if necessary. Throw the tissue in the plastic trash bag. ☐ ☐
- Put the thermometer in the middle of the person's underarm.
- Bring the person's arm across the chest to hold the thermometer in place.
- Make sure the person is sitting or lying down during the procedure and not

walking around with the thermometer
under his arm. ☐ ☐

For Tympanic Temperature:

- Ask the person to turn his head so the ear
is in front of you. ☐ ☐
- Pull up and back on the ear to straighten
the ear canal. ☐ ☐
- Gently insert the probe into the ear. ☐ ☐

5. Read the number of the temperature on the
small screen after the machine beeps. ☐ ☐

6. Eject the probe cover and throw it
into the plastic trash bag. ☐ ☐

7. Return the probe to its home. ☐ ☐

8. Take off the gloves, if you used them, throw
them into the plastic trash bag and wash
your hands. ☐ ☐

9. Write down the temperature on the paper that
you brought with you before returning the
probe to its home. If recording an oral temperature write *O* next to the number. If recording an
axillary temperature write an *A* next to the
number. If taking a rectal temperature write an
R next to the number. If taking a tympanic temperature write a *TY* next to the number. ☐ ☐

ADDITIONAL INFORMATION

If you are taking other vital signs in addition to
the temperature, do completion steps after you
take the last vital sign.

COMPLETION

Follow Completion Standards in compliance
with your facility. For a complete list of those
used in this course, see Chapter 7, "Controlling
the Spread of Germs."

Skill 8: Counting and Recording a Person's Pulse

PRECAUTIONS

- Always use your fingers to take a person's radial pulse. Never take it with your thumb.
- Do not hold the person's arm up in the air when counting the radial pulse.
- Be careful not to press too hard because this may make the radial pulse more difficult to feel.
- To take a person's apical pulse, place the person in a supine (on the back) or semi-Fowler's (sitting up with the head of the bed elevated for support) position.

PREPARATION

1. Gather supplies:
   - Stethoscope
   - Watch with a second hand
   - Alcohol wipes
   - Plastic trash bag
   - Pencil and paper for writing down the pulse rate
2. Follow Preparation Standards (see Chapter 7).

PROCEDURE

Radial Pulse

1. Make sure the person is in a comfortable, relaxed position. ☐ ☐
2. Gently press your first, second and third fingers over the person's radial pulse. ☐ ☐

Skill 8: Counting and Recording a Person's Pulse—cont'd

NOTE: *Always use your fingers to take a person's radial pulse. Never take it with your thumb.*

3. Using the second hand on your watch, count the number of beats for 1 minute. Until you are very comfortable with the skill, start counting when the second hand is at the "12" so that you do not lose track of when you started counting (Fig. 9-14). ☐ ☐

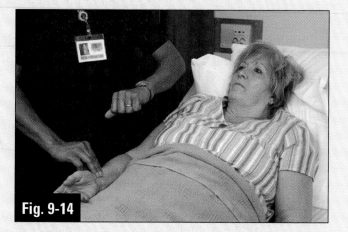
Fig. 9-14

Apical Pulse

1. Place the person in a supine or semi-Fowler's position. Make sure the person feels comfortable and relaxed. ☐ ☐

2. Clean the earpieces and diaphragm of the stethoscope with an alcohol wipe and throw away the wipe in the plastic trash bag. ☐ ☐

3. Raise the person's gown or remove the clothing from his chest/nipple area on the left side. ☐ ☐

4. Warm the diaphragm of the stethoscope by warming it in your hand. ☐ ☐

5. Locate the apical pulse. The pulse point is located 2 to 3 inches to the left of the breastbone below the left nipple. ☐ ☐

6. Put the earpieces in your ears with the tips facing forward (toward your nose). ☐ ☐

7. Place the diaphragm over the pulse point. Hold it in place with your fingers, not your thumb (because you may hear the pulse in your thumb instead of the person's apical pulse). ☐ ☐

8. Count the pulse for 1 full minute (Figure 9-15). ☐ ☐

9. Note any irregular beats, as well as the rhythm and the force, and write down the pulse rate and any irregularities on the paper that you brought with you. ☐ ☐

ADDITIONAL INFORMATION

If you are taking other vital signs in addition to the pulse, do the completion steps after you complete the last vital sign.

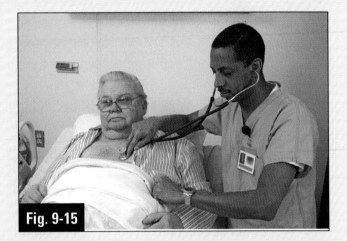
Fig. 9-15

COMPLETION

Follow Completion Standards in compliance with your facility. For a complete list of those used in this course, see Chapter 7, "Controlling the Spread of Germs."

Skill 9: Counting and Recording a Person's Respirations

PRECAUTIONS

- Always count respirations without the person being aware that you are counting them.

PREPARATION

1. Gather supplies:
   - Watch with a second hand
   - Pencil and paper for writing down the number of respirations
2. Follow Preparation Standards (see Chapter 7).

PROCEDURE

1. Hold the person's wrist as if taking a radial pulse, and count respirations by watching the rise and fall of the chest (Figure 9-16). One rise and one fall equals one respiration. Start your count when you see the chest rise. ☐ ☐

2. Observe whether the respirations are regular and whether both sides of the chest rise equally. Also notice how deep they are and whether the person seems to be having any pain or difficulty in breathing. ☐ ☐

3. Using the second hand on your watch, count respirations for 1 full minute. ☐ ☐

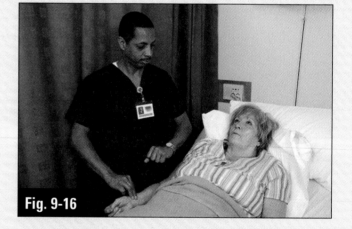

Fig. 9-16

> **NOTE:** *If you wait until the second hand gets to the "12" each time you count, it makes it easier to keep track of how many seconds have gone by.*

ADDITIONAL INFORMATION

If you are taking other vital signs in addition to the respiration, do the completion steps after you take the last vital sign.

 ## COMPLETION

Follow Completion Standards in compliance with your facility. For a complete list of those used in this course, see Chapter 7, "Controlling the Spread of Germs."

Skill 10: Taking and Recording a Person's Blood Pressure

PRECAUTIONS

- Put a cuff on a person's bare arm and never put a cuff on a person's arm that has a cast or that has an IV (intravenous infusion) in place.
- Be careful about which arm you put the cuff on. For example, you should never put a cuff on an arm on the side where a woman has had a breast surgically removed (a mastectomy). You also should avoid putting a cuff on the weak arm of a person who has had a stroke. Ask your supervising nurse for instructions if the person has had both breasts removed or has paralysis in both arms.
- Always clean the earpieces and diaphragm of the stethoscope with alcohol before and after each use.
- Check the tubing and diaphragm of the stethoscope for cracks or holes.

PREPARATION

1. Gather supplies:
   - Blood pressure machine (sphygmomanometer) with the correct size cuff
   - Stethoscope
   - Alcohol wipes
   - Plastic trash bag
   - Pencil and paper to write down the BP reading
2. Follow Preparation Standards (see Chapter 7).

PROCEDURE

1. Place the person in a comfortable position. ☐ ☐

2. Locate the person's brachial pulse. ☐ ☐

3. Before putting the cuff on the person's arm, loosen the valve. If you turn the screw to the left, it opens the valve and lets the air escape from the bladder, which makes the cuff loose. If you turn the screw to the right, it closes the valve and keeps the air inside the bladder, which makes the cuff tight. A good way to remember this is by saying, "Left equals loose. Right equals tight." Turn the screw to the left and squeeze all the air out of the cuff (Figure 9-17). ☐ ☐

4. Place the cuff on the person's upper arm, over bare skin, so that it is covering about two-thirds of the upper arm. Put the center of the cuff's bladder 1 inch above the elbow on the inside of the arm over the brachial artery (Figure 9-18). To make sure the bladder is centered over the brachial artery, fold the bladder in half and place the fold over the artery. Or, if the cuff has an arrow, make sure the arrow is directly over the brachial artery. ☐ ☐

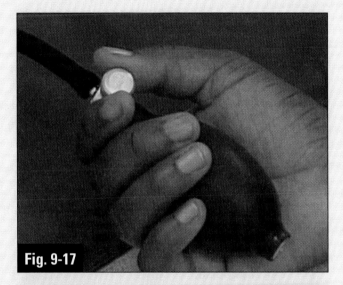
Fig. 9-17

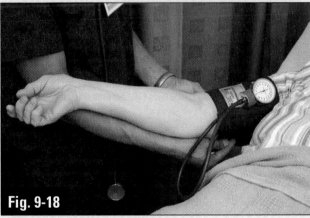
Fig. 9-18

5. Wrap the cuff around the person's arm snugly and smoothly so that the bladder presses evenly against the arm. Secure the cuff. Make sure it is snug enough to stay in place, but not uncomfortably tight. ☐ ☐

6. Find the person's brachial pulse; this is where you place the diaphragm of the stethoscope (Figure 9-19). ☐ ☐

7. Feel the wrist (radial) pulse. ☐ ☐

8. Inflate the bladder by first tightening the valve (turn the screw to the right: right equals tight) and then pumping the bulb. Look at the gauge and note the reading. The number is an estimate of systolic pressure. Let all the air out quickly by turning the valve left. Stop when you can no longer feel the pulse. ☐ ☐

9. Put the earpieces in your ears with the tips facing forward (toward your nose) (Figure 9-20). ☐ ☐

10. Place the diaphragm of the stethoscope firmly over the person's brachial pulse (Figure 9-21). ☐ ☐

11. Hold the rubber bulb in the other hand and, after tightening the valve, inflate the cuff quickly to 30 mm Hg above the estimated systolic pressure. ☐ ☐

12. Let the air out of the cuff slowly at 2 to 4 mm Hg each second. The reading when you first hear the pulse sound is the *systolic* pressure. Remember this number and continue letting the air out slowly. ☐ ☐

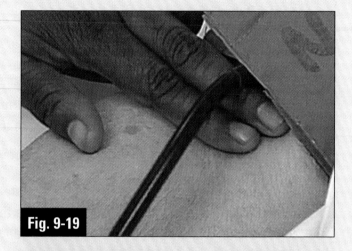

Fig. 9-19

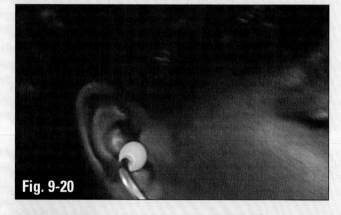

Fig. 9-20

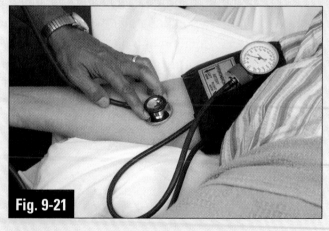

Fig. 9-21

13. The reading when the pulse sound stops or changes is the *diastolic* pressure. Remember this number and quickly let out the rest of the air. ☐ ☐

14. Immediately write down the systolic and diastolic readings on the paper that you brought with you. ☐ ☐

15. Remove the cuff from the person's arm. ☐ ☐

ADDITIONAL INFORMATION

Take the blood pressure equipment out of the room with you when you leave, and put it away after you have finished.

 ## COMPLETION

Follow Completion Standards in compliance with your facility. For a complete list of those used in this course, see Chapter 7, "Controlling the Spread of Germs."

10

Positioning and Transferring People

GOALS

After reading this chapter, you will have the information needed to:

Help prevent pressure sores on the people in your care by providing good skin care and changing their body positions.

Assess situations before positioning or transferring people.

Protect your safety and the safety of the people in your care when you position or transfer them.

Make people comfortable when you position and transfer them.

Work with another nurse assistant to position and transfer people.

After practicing the corresponding skills, you will have the information needed to:

Help move a person around in bed.

Help move a person into several different positions.

Transfer a person from a bed to a chair.

Reposition a person in a chair.

Use a mechanical lift to transfer a person from a bed to a chair.

You have been providing care for 78-year-old Victor Rivera since he was transferred from the hospital to Morningside Nursing Home several weeks ago. An earlier stroke left him paralyzed on his left side and incontinent of urine and stool. Immediately after suffering the stroke, he was unable to speak, but his speech has improved with the help of the speech therapist at the nursing home.

You are concerned that, because of his illness and poor circulation, Mr. Rivera could easily develop a bedsore if he stays in one position too long. Yet, because of his paralysis, Mr. Rivera is unable to move much by himself. So every day, according to his care plan, you help him change position at least every 2 hours. By changing his position and relieving pressure on certain parts of his body, you help provide comfort and help prevent pressure sores from developing on his dry, fragile skin. When Mr. Rivera's wife comes to visit every day, she helps by gently rubbing lotion into his skin.

This morning, when you first check on Mr. Rivera, you notice that he has been positioned on his side for sleeping. But he has moved his unaffected leg, which has caused the pillow that was between his knees to shift out of position, so his knees have been lying against each other. As you reposition him, you check the inner surfaces of his knees and notice a red spot on each knee. You report the condition of Mr. Rivera's skin to your supervising nurse.

POSITIONING

Positioning a resident in good body alignment and changing the position on a regular basis at a preset time are major tasks in the responsibilities of nurse assistants. Residents who are active will change their positions as needed; residents who are less active need to be encouraged to change their positions. Residents who are weak, frail, in pain, paralyzed or unconscious need your help in order to maintain good body alignment.

PROMOTING PROPER BODY ALIGNMENT

When you reposition Mr. Rivera, prop him up with pillows to help prevent pressure and friction and to help maintain proper body alignment. Review the sections on integumentary, muscular and skeletal systems in Appendix B, "Body Basics" to

learn more about how the body works so that you can understand the importance of promoting proper body alignment and comfort for Mr. Rivera.

Make sure Mr. Rivera's bones and joints are in a natural position that feels comfortable to him (Figure 10-1). Also, when you position him in bed, support his bones and joints to minimize the strain on them. For example, you could place a small towel under his calves to lift his heels away from the mattress and relieve pressure. Since muscles that **flex** joints are stronger than those that **extend** them, a paralyzed or inactive limb may tend to curl upward. For this reason, when positioning a person who has a weak or paralyzed arm, support the arm so that the wrist is higher than the elbow. Since the limb may curl upward, people who cannot move their wrists, hands, fingers or heels often need special devices to prevent this curling.

PREVENTING PRESSURE ULCERS

Like Mr. Rivera, someone in your care may not be able to move by himself because of illness, injury or a medical problem. A person who

KEY TERMS

bony prominence: bony part of the body that sticks out, where a pressure sore can occur.

coccyx: (COCK-siks) the "tailbone," or end of the spine.

decubitus ulcer: (duh-KYOO-bi-tuhs/UHL-ser) the medical term for a bedsore or pressure ulcer, caused by pressure or friction, which cuts off circulation. A decubitus ulcer can quickly progress into a deep, infected crater.

drawsheet: a bed sheet about 5 feet wide that is placed under a person, across the middle third of the bed.

A drawsheet is useful in positioning and transferring procedures.

extend: to straighten.

flex: to bend.

Fowler's position: a position in which a person sits up with the head of the bed elevated for support.

lateral (side-lying) position: a position in which the person lies on one side of her body.

mobility: (moe-BIL-uh-tee) the ability to move.

modified side-lying position: a position in which a person lies partially to one side with her back supported.

perception: (pur-SEP-shun) a person's awareness of his environment through his senses.

predictable: (pree-DIK-tuh-bull) can be known in advance.

pressure ulcer: another term used for bedsore or **decubitus ulcer**.

supine position: (SUE-pine) a position in which a person lies flat on his back.

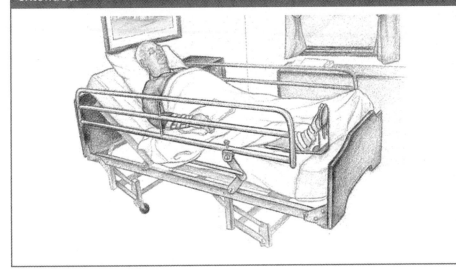

stays in one position for too long becomes stiff and uncomfortable and may develop a **pressure ulcer,** or **decubitus ulcer.** This condition is sometimes referred to as a *bedsore,* but this term is somewhat misleading because residents who sit in chairs also develop pressure ulcers. Pressure ulcers usually develop on pressure point areas, which include the ears, elbows, shoulder blades, hips, **coccyx,** knees, ankles and heels. These parts of the body are bony areas **(bony prominences)** that are protected by only a thin layer of fat and muscle under the skin (Figure 10-2). When a person stays in one position too long, pressure increases on certain points on his body. When he repeats certain activities, such as sliding down in the bed, friction affects other points on his body. Points of pressure or friction can decrease or cut off blood circulation to parts of the person's body. When he is unable to change position or repeats the same movements, pressure and friction continue and cells die, leaving a reddened, pale or darkened area that can quickly form an ulcer.

FIGURE 10-2 Bony prominences on the body are protected only by a thin layer of fat and muscle under the skin, so pressure sores can easily form.

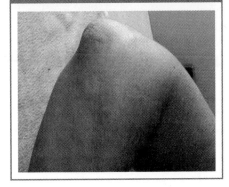

You may have experienced pressure in a minor way if your foot or arm ever "fell asleep" after being in the same position for too long. How did it feel? What did you do to relieve the discomfort? How would you feel if you could not move to stop the discomfort?

The big difference between what you experience if your foot or arm falls asleep and what some people in your care experience is that you can move to relieve pressure and restore circu-

lation and your cells can continue to function.

People who cannot move or have limited movement also have problems with friction, which causes the skin layers to tear apart. The injured skin then breaks down, which results in sores. People who are extremely overweight may develop such sores when body parts rub together in areas such as the buttocks and thighs, under folds of fat on the abdomen and under the breasts. Even the continuous rubbing of medical tubing on a person's skin can cause decubitus ulcers. Table 10-1 shows steps you can take to protect a person's skin integrity.

Several factors put Mr. Rivera at risk for developing a pressure ulcer. He:

- Has dry skin.
- Has been sick in bed for almost 6 weeks.
- Has poor circulation.
- Is unable to move himself without help, because he is paralyzed on one side.
- Has a poor appetite due to difficulty in chewing and swallowing. (Poor nutrition and poor fluid intake increase the likelihood of skin breakdown.)

When you provide care for a person who has to stay in bed, you must give frequent skin care and change his position at least every two hours. You also must be on the lookout for any clues, such as the red spot on his knees, so that you can report signs of pressure ulcers that may be developing. To know how to recognize each stage and what to do, look at Box 10-1.

Keep preventive measures in mind as you provide care for Mr. Rivera. To relieve pressure, help him roll over in bed. To make him more comfortable, help move his arms, legs and body into different positions, and help him move to different

TABLE 10-1 PROTECTING SKIN INTEGRITY

To Prevent This...	Do This...
Direct Pressure	Change the person's position at least every 2 hours.
	Observe and report immediately any reddened, pale or darkened areas of the skin.
	Make sure the person is in good body alignment. Use appropriate positioning devices when needed.
	Use special protective devices to relieve pressure and protect skin. Some examples of protective devices are air and water mattresses, special foam mattresses that look like egg cartons and heel and elbow protectors.
Friction	Get help when moving the person—be sure to lift him or her all the way off the mattress.
	Elevate the head of the bed no more than 30 degrees (except when a person is eating, requires a procedure or has difficulty breathing). This will keep the person from sliding down in bed.
	Use a drawsheet to move and turn the person.
	Keep equipment and devices such as tubes from getting caught under a part of the person's body.
Skin-to-Skin Contact	Check for skin changes under skin folds, especially under breasts, and under the folds of fat on people who are overweight.
	Position the person so that air circulates around his or her arms and legs to keep skin from touching skin.
Moisture	Wash, rinse and dry the person's skin thoroughly.
	Check people with incontinence at least every 2 hours and keep their skin clean and dry.
	Cover a vinyl chair with a pad or sheet.
	Have the person wear moisture-absorbing clothes made from natural fabrics such as cotton.
Poor Circulation	Elevate the person's arms and legs.
	Provide mild massaging, including good back and skin care.
	Observe the person's skin frequently and report any changes to your supervising nurse.
Harmful Contact from Splints and Clothing	Pad splints and check the person's circulation often.
	Check to make sure shoes and nylon stockings fit correctly.

To Improve This...	Do This...
Nutrition	Encourage the person to drink an adequate amount of fluids.
	Encourage the person to eat a well-balanced diet.
	If the person has anemia, encourage him or her to eat foods that are rich in iron.
Sleeping Conditions	Make a tight, neat, wrinkle-free bed.
	Check the bed for items such as hair pins and barrettes and remove them.
Mobility	Move the person often.
	Help with range-of-motion exercises.

BOX 10-1

SIGNS AND STAGES OF DECUBITUS ULCER DEVELOPMENT

Stage I An area is red, pale or dark and does not improve after the pressure has been removed.

What to Do...
1. **Report** this stage to your supervising nurse and discuss a plan of care.
2. Use another preventive measure to relieve pressure: Reposition the person to keep weight off areas that are red, pale or dark in color, and make sure her or his body is properly aligned.
3. Continue with other preventive measures to reduce pressure and friction, such as (a) using pillows and blankets to keep one skin surface from touching another; (b) using special protective devices, such as air and water mattresses (alternating pressure pad mattresses that fill and empty to relieve pressure and stimulate circulation), special foam mattresses that look like egg cartons, gelatin-filled pads for chairs and wheelchairs, sheepskin to protect bony areas and heel and elbow protectors with self-fasteners; and (c) keeping linens under the person as wrinkle free as possible.

4. Use additional preventive measures to reduce friction when moving the person: Get help from a co-worker, use a drawsheet and lift the person all the way off the mattress.
5. As another preventive measure to reduce friction, elevate the head of the bed no more than 30 degrees so that the person will not slide down or have pressure on the coccyx. If the bed must be elevated more than 30 degrees, such as during mealtime, slightly elevate the person's knees as well.
6. To prevent friction with people who have feeding tubes or other medical devices, keep tubes from getting caught under the person's body.

Stage II Persistent redness and blistering lead to a breakdown of the skin's surface.

What to Do...
1. **Report** this stage to your supervising nurse and discuss a plan of care.
2. Reposition the person to keep weight off this area.
3. Continue with preventive measures.

Stage III Skin breakdown has reached the inner tissue, and an ulcer now looks like a shallow crater. There may be some drainage from the wound.*

What to Do...
1. **Report** this stage to your supervising nurse and discuss a plan of care.
2. Reposition the person to keep weight off this area.
3. Continue with preventive measures.

Stage IV Skin is damaged in a deep crater that extends to the muscle or bone. Wound drainage or crust formation usually is present. The wound often becomes infected.*

What to Do...
1. **Report** this stage to, and discuss a plan of care with, your supervising nurse, who will provide treatment.
2. Reposition the person to keep weight off this area.
3. Continue to provide preventive measures so that other areas of the skin stay intact.

*Stage III and Stage IV decubitus ulcers often require surgery to remove dead skin so that healing can occur.

areas of the bed and from the bed to a chair and back. You can also use special supportive devices such as foam wedges, pillows and special mattresses; however, do *not* use donut-type devices.

Whenever you change Mr. Rivera's position, be sure to relieve the pressure points he was lying on. For example, if he is lying on his back with the head of the bed raised, reposition him on his side. When he is on his back, his shoulder blades, coccyx, heels and elbows are under pressure. If you position him on his side, his ear, shoulder, hip, knee and ankle are under pressure. It would *not* be good to change Mr. Rivera's position from lying on his back with the head of the bed raised to lying on his back with the bed flat, because the pressure points he was lying on would not be relieved.

WHEN AND HOW TO POSITION AND TRANSFER

Pressure ulcers have been around for centuries, but today more and more research has been done to find ways to improve treatment and to prevent the occurrence of pressure ulcers, and nurse assistants play a key role in their prevention. Because a person who is unable to move without help must be repositioned at least every 2 hours to avoid damage to his skin, he usually is placed on a schedule for regular turning. This rotation schedule, with 2-hour intervals for repositioning, is carried out around the clock, even while the person is sleeping. The schedule uses a sequence of positions (described later in this chapter) that allow parts of his body to be free of pressure when he is in certain positions. For example, during the first position, he may be on his back, but in the second position, he may be on his side, with no pressure on his back. A typical 12-hour rotation schedule for a person who needs regular repositioning might look like the following:

6:00 A.M.	Left-modified side-lying position*
8:00 A.M.	Semi-Fowler's position
10:00 A.M.	Right-modified side-lying position
12:00 P.M.	Supine position (raise head into semi-Fowler's position for lunch)
2:00 P.M.	Left-modified side-lying position*
4:00 P.M.	Prone position†
6:00 A.M.	Right-modified side-lying position

By paying close attention to the places where the person's body comes into contact with the bed, you ensure that he is not lying on one spot for long periods of time. You play an important role in reducing the likelihood of his developing pressure ulcers.

Whenever you move or position a person, remember two important factors: First, assess the situation and plan what to do and how to do it; and second, carry out your plan using the good body mechanics that you read about in Chapter 8, "Keeping People Safe." In addition, to successfully position and transfer someone without causing injury to him or yourself, give clear directions to the co-worker who is assisting you and to the person you are positioning. Before moving the person, check the bed for any tubes or personal items that may get in the way, and check the brakes to make sure they are locked. Finally, when you finish the procedure, make sure the person is comfortable, that his body is in proper alignment, and that he is supported by any necessary blankets and pillows.

The following sections list factors to consider and some questions to ask as you assess, communicate and complete a positioning or transferring skill for a person such as Mr. Rivera.

*If this schedule were for Mr. Rivera, you would not position him on his left side, because he is paralyzed on his left side.
†Using the prone position may require a doctor's order.

Assess

Gather information about Mr. Rivera's **mobility** and independence, as well as his environment and other risk factors, and determine a plan of how you will help him move every 2 hours.

Mobility and Independence. Find out about Mr. Rivera's mobility and level of independence by talking with your supervising nurse and checking the care plan. Find out about Mr. Rivera's weight and muscle strength and his ability to use his arms and legs so that you know how much he can help. Ask these questions:

- Can he bear all his weight on one leg or both legs?
- Is one side stronger than the other?
- Can he maintain his sense of balance?
- Does he have visual or **perception** problems?
- Do visual or language problems affect his understanding of instructions or of his surroundings?
- Does he have pain when he moves?
- Is he afraid of being moved?
- Has he ever suddenly refused to cooperate?
- Are his movements **predictable?**

Environment. Ask yourself these questions about the room and equipment:

- How much room do you need to complete the move?
- Is there a co-worker available to assist?
- What obstacles, such as tubes or personal items, are in the way?
- Where do you get a **drawsheet?** (In a home setting, make a drawsheet by folding a top sheet in half, widthwise.)
- What equipment do you need? (Check to see what equipment is available, and be sure you know how to use it.)
- What height should the bed be?
- How will you position yourself to avoid injury?

- Do the bed and wheelchair have brakes? (Be sure to lock them when necessary.)

Sometimes you may have to use special equipment, such as a mechanical lift or a metal trapeze above the bed (Figure 10-3). This equipment is designed to help with positioning and transferring when the person being moved cannot assist you with the move. You also can use it if the person is too heavy or if there is any risk to you or the person being moved. Lack of this specialized equipment, however, is not an excuse for improper positioning. Have you been trained on the proper use of this equipment? If special equipment is not available and you believe it is necessary, discuss this concern with your supervising nurse.

Other Risk Factors. As you have learned, each person that you care for is different and needs to be considered on an individual basis. This is also true in assessing your resident for the risk of developing pressure ulcers. There may be factors or conditions that will put him at risk. These factors may include incontinence, poor nutritional status and obesity. The person you are caring for may be unconscious or paralyzed. You can observe each

person in your care to identify factors that may put him at risk for developing pressure sores.

Determining a Plan. After you have the necessary information about the person and his environment, determine whether you need any help to move him. To prevent injury to yourself and Mr. Rivera, you need another nurse assistant to help you with most positioning techniques. Two people can lift or move someone more easily than one person can. You must arrange for a co-worker to help you and then remember to return the favor when he or she asks you for help.

Communicate

After you decide what to tell Mr. Rivera and the co-worker assisting you, explain each step of your plan to them.

What to Communicate. Emphasize good body mechanics to both Mr. Rivera and your co-worker as you explain each step of the plan to them. Tell Mr. Rivera what he can do to help make the move easier. Encourage him to help as much as possible and make sure he understands and agrees with your plan. Tell your co-worker exactly what his or her responsibilities are and make sure he or she understands the

plan. For example, you could tell Mr. Rivera to use his unaffected arm to lock arms with you so that you can support his head while your co-worker moves his pillow or ties his nightgown.

When to Communicate. Explain the procedure before you begin. Then, as you move through the steps, explain each step as you come to it. For example, you might say to Mr. Rivera, "Now, we are going to help you roll over onto your right side." And you might say to your co-worker, "When I count to 3, lift the drawsheet."

Complete

Finish the procedure and make sure Mr. Rivera is comfortable and safe. Ask yourself:

- Did I protect all the pressure points of his body?
- Does this new position put pressure on different bony parts of his body than the last position did?
- Did I support his back, arms and legs with pillows?
- Did I smooth out the sheets under him to prevent his lying on uncomfortable wrinkles?
- Does Mr. Rivera look comfortable?

Ask Mr. Rivera whether he is comfortable. Complete the procedure by checking to see whether his spine is straight and his body is in proper alignment by putting up the side rails, if necessary, and by making sure the call signal is within reach of his strong hand. If a person in your care is unable to speak at all, it is important to watch his facial expressions. If he grimaces or frowns, he may be uncomfortable. If he is unable to communicate at all, you must look at his position to make sure his body is in proper alignment.

TYPES OF POSITIONS AND TRANSFERS

You can position people in many ways to provide safety and comfort. For example, you go to Mr. Rivera's room to prepare him for breakfast. He is lying on his right

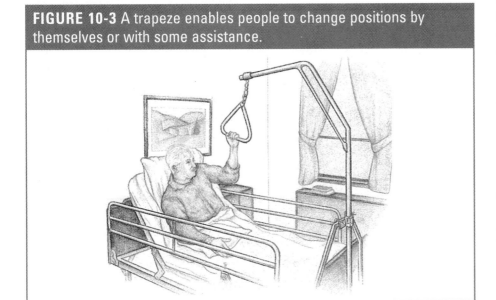

FIGURE 10-3 A trapeze enables people to change positions by themselves or with some assistance.

side in a **modified side-lying position,** with a rolled blanket supporting his back. He has a pillow between his knees to reduce strain on his upper hip and to prevent pressure on his knees and ankles. His paralyzed arm rests on a pillow (Figure 10-4). You ask a co-worker to help you position Mr. Rivera in a high **Fowler's position** for eating. You roll him onto his back, move him up in bed, and elevate the head of his bed so that he can sit up and eat (Figure 10-5). After breakfast, you collect Mr. Rivera's food tray and tell him it will soon be time for his personal care. He shakes his head and, with effort, tells you that he wants to rest. Although you had planned to start your day by providing personal care for Mr. Rivera, you observe that he seems tired, and you adjust your schedule to meet his needs. Because he has just eaten, you encourage him to rest in the semi-upright position called the *semi-Fowler's position*. You lower his head and make him comfortable.

Later you return to Mr. Rivera's room to help him with his bath. To per-

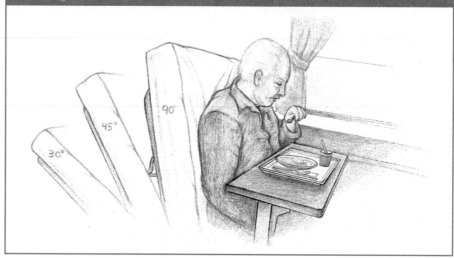

FIGURE 10-5 Three types of Fowler's positions are:
- High Fowler's position with the head of the bed elevated almost 90 degrees.
- Fowler's position with the head of the bed elevated about 45 degrees.
- Semi-Fowler's position with the head of the bed elevated about 30 degrees.

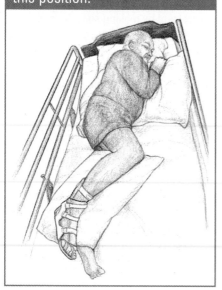

FIGURE 10-4 Use the modified side-lying position when you reposition a person in bed to prevent pressure ulcers. Many people prefer to rest or sleep in this position.

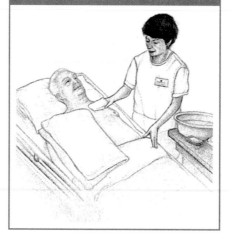

FIGURE 10-6 Help a person into the supine position when he needs to lie flat on his back to rest or sleep. This position is also useful when helping someone with a bed bath.

form this personal care procedure, you lower the head of the bed and put him in a **supine position** (Figure 10-6). During the bath you have to turn him onto his side in the **lateral (side-lying) position** to wash his back and give him a

backrub (Figure 10-7). Because of his paralysis, he finds it difficult to position himself but is able to help turn with his unaffected side. After his bath, Mr. Rivera agrees that he would like to get out of bed and sit in his wheelchair. His mobility is limited because of his left-sided paralysis, but he can balance himself with assistance and can support his own weight. You ask a co-worker to help you transfer Mr. Rivera into the wheelchair using a transfer belt. Later, when you check on him, you notice that he has slumped over and slipped down in the wheelchair. You and a co-worker reposition him (Figure 10-8).

Throughout the day and night, you and other nurse assistants reposition Mr. Rivera every 2 hours. Even though it may seem inconsiderate to awaken someone to move him, it is better to interrupt his sleep than to let him sleep in the same position for more than 2 hours, which could cause pressure ulcers. If you are gentle and quiet, you can move him without bringing him to a full waking state.

FIGURE 10-7 Use the lateral or side-lying position to complete a bed bath, a backrub or to assist with getting onto a bedpan.

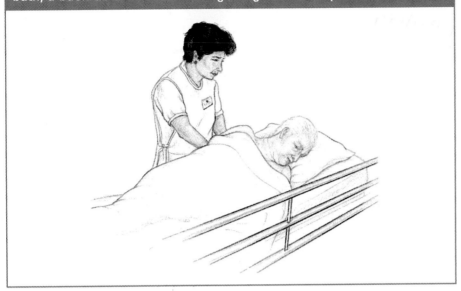

FIGURE 10-8 Help a person reposition in a chair when he has slouched down and cannot move back up without assistance.

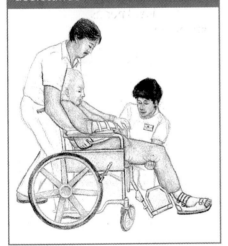

Occasionally you assist a person into the prone position when you help him lie on his stomach. This position is useful for relieving pressure on other areas of the body, but it is not used often because many people find it uncomfortable. In many health care settings, the prone position requires a doctor's order.

When positioning or transferring someone, follow the specific procedures that are explained step by step in Skills 11 through 19 at the end of this chapter. You must perform these skills well, because, as a nurse assistant you have the important job of positioning and transferring people in your care. You provide for their safety and comfort by understanding the importance of using good body mechanics to protect yourself and others and by putting people in proper body alignment to prevent pressure ulcers and injury. You apply your skills to the people in your care in a personalized manner, taking into consideration their needs and their ability to help you. You also recognize the importance of teamwork when you ask a co-worker for help or when you help another co-worker in positioning and transferring people.

TRANSPORTING A PERSON IN A WHEELCHAIR

If you work in a hospital or nursing home, you may have to transport people from one part of the facility to another. Sometimes you will transport the person on a stretcher. The other way to safely transport a person is in a wheelchair. Follow these important tips:

- Always walk on the right side of the hall.
- When going down wheelchair ramps, turn the chair around and walk down backwards, with the person facing uphill. This backward positioning decreases the risk of tipping the chair and injuring the person.
- To avoid bumping into other people, use caution when walking past doorways and around corners or when entering hallway intersections.
- To enter an elevator, turn the chair around and enter the elevator backwards. Once inside, turn the chair around again and exit the elevator backwards. This backward positioning prevents the small wheels on the front of the chair from jamming in the space between the elevator and the floor.
- Always lock the brakes when the wheelchair is stopped and when the person remains in the wheelchair for a period of time.
- Always check with your supervising nurse before leaving a person unattended in a wheelchair.

Circle the correct answers and fill in the blanks.

1. Decubitus ulcers, or _pressure ulcer_, can easily develop on pressure points of the body, because these areas are protected only by thin layers of _fat_ and _muscle_ under the skin.

2. On which areas can pressure sores develop?
   a. Eyes, ears, nose and throat
   b. Ears, elbows and ankles _(circled)_
   c. Heels and wrists
   d. Coccyx and buttocks

3. What is the *first* sign of a decubitus ulcer?
   a. A reddened area on the skin _(circled)_
   b. A fever
   c. An open sore
   d. Bleeding

4. To avoid damaging the skin of a person who is unable to move without help, you should reposition him:
   a. when you can fit him into your schedule.
   b. every 4 hours.
   c. at least every 2 hours. _(circled)_
   d. when you come to work and before you go home.

5. When planning to move a person, your first action is to assess. Some of the things you must know are:
   a. the person's height.
   b. how much time you have to move the person.
   c. how recently the person ate.
   d. the person's mobility, level of independence and ability to help. _(circled)_

6. A _draw sheet_ is placed under a person to help with positioning and turning him.

7. It is important that you _explain_ your plan to the person so that he understands what you are going to do and how he can _help_.

8. When you help a person sit up in bed with the head of the bed raised, that person is in a _High-Flowers_ position. (Fowler's)

9. Supine position means the person is flat on his _back_.

10. Always lock the ~~brea~~ _brakes._ on a wheelchair when the chair is stopped and the person is remaining in the chair for a period of time.

1. Mr. Rivera has been sitting in a Fowler's position and watching television for the past 2 hours. When you come to help him change position, he wants to lie on his back and sleep. What should you do?

2. Why is it important to change Mr. Rivera's position so often? How often should his position be changed?

3. Why could Mr. Rivera easily develop pressure sores or decubitus ulcers? Give three reasons.

4. What do you consider before getting Mr. Rivera out of bed and into the wheelchair? Which type of transfer method should you use?

5. What important things should you think about to protect yourself from injury when positioning and transferring Mr. Rivera?

6. You are wheeling Mrs. Paulson down the hallway in a wheelchair. Because she has a cast on her right leg, you have raised the leg supports of the wheelchair so that her leg is supported out in front of her. You are approaching an intersecting hallway. What would you do to ensure her safety as you enter the intersection?

7. Mr. Eller, who is paralyzed on his right side, is sitting in a chair next to his bed. Every time you look into his room, he has slumped over to his weaker side. What could you do to position him properly and maintain his alignment?

8. Mrs. Hillman, who weighs 200 pounds, begins to stand up from the chair where she is sitting. Knowing that she often gets dizzy without warning, you offer to help her, but she insists that she is able to stand up by herself. What safety precautions should you take to prevent potential injury? How many people are needed to move her safely?

9. Mrs. Romano is sitting in the chair in her room while her niece is visiting. When Mrs. Romano says she wants to get back into her bed, her niece says that she will help her. You offer to help, but the niece says she can do it by herself. What should you do?

Skill 11: Moving a Person Around in Bed

PRECAUTIONS

- Assess the person and the room environment to determine your plan for moving him or her safely. Talk with your supervising nurse and check the care plan.
- Use proper body mechanics to prevent injury. To keep from injuring your back, always tighten your abdominal and buttocks muscles while positioning or transferring someone.
- Make sure bed brakes are locked (Figure 10-9).
- Ask a co-worker to help, if needed.

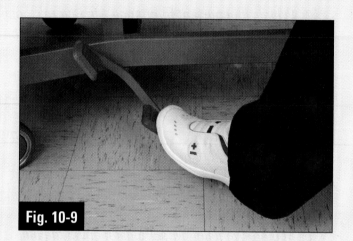

Fig. 10-9

PREPARATION

1. Gather supplies: Moving a person around in bed is most frequently done during the performance of another procedure. Think about the supplies you will need for that procedure and bring those. Be sure to bring the bed protectors.
2. Follow Preparation Standards (see Chapter 7).

ADDITIONAL INFORMATION

1. Introduce your co-worker, if one is helping you.
2. Explain your moving plan to the person and the co-worker. Tell them what they can do to help. Encourage the person to help as much as possible.
3. Check for the placement of drainage tubes; move them as necessary to prevent their being pulled out.

Option 1: Moving Up in Bed Using a Drawsheet (One Nurse Assistant)

This procedure is used in home health situations where you may not have anyone to help you. To accomplish this procedure, you must be able to stand comfortably at the head of the bed. The bed must be pulled away from the wall and must *not* have a headboard. You cannot use proper body mechanics if you have to lean over a headboard.

1. Raise the height of the bed, if possible. ☐ ☐

NOTE: *This decreases the amount you have to bend over.*

2. Lower the side rail, if used, and loosen the drawsheet on one side of the bed. Raise the side rail and repeat this step on the other side of the bed. ☐ ☐

3. Make sure the person is lying as flat as possible. Ask the person to lift her head, or if she is unable, gently lift her head and remove the pillow. Place it alongside her or in a chair. ☐ ☐

NOTE: *Lower the head of the bed as low as the person can tolerate.*

4. Stand at the head of the bed with your feet 12 inches apart and one foot slightly behind the other (Figure 10-10). ☐ ☐

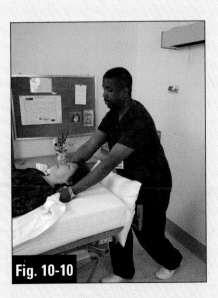
Fig. 10-10

Skill 11: Moving a Person Around in Bed—cont'd

NOTE: *Do not reach over a headboard.*

5. Roll the top of the drawsheet close to the person's head and shoulders. Ask her to bend her knees if she is able and place her feet flat against the mattress so that she can help push up. □ □

6. With your palms up, grasp the rolled drawsheet with both hands, on either side of her head. This will enable you to lift better and avoid injury to your wrists. □ □

7. Bend your hips and knees so that your upper back remains straight. □ □

8. Tell the person to get ready to move on the count of 3. On the count of 3, rock backward, pulling the drawsheet and the person up toward the head of the bed. □ □

9. Retuck the drawsheet (Figure 10-11). □ □

10. Help the person lift her head and replace the pillow for comfort (Figure 10-12). □ □

11. Raise the side rail, if used. □ □

12. Lower the height of the bed. □ □

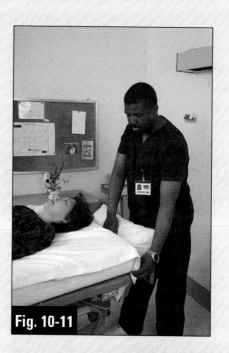
Fig. 10-11

Option 2: Moving Up in Bed When the Person Can Help (One Nurse Assistant)

1. Raise the height of the bed, if possible. □ □

2. Lower the side rail, if used. □ □

3. Make sure the person is lying as flat as possible. Ask the person to lift her head, or if she is unable, gently lift her head and remove the pillow. Place the pillow against the headboard. □ □

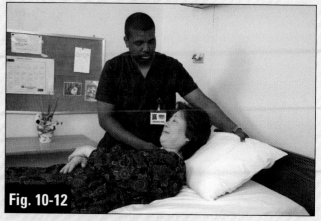
Fig. 10-12

4. Stand with your feet about 12 inches apart. Point the toe of the foot nearest the headboard toward the headboard (Figure 10-13). ☐ ☐

5. Ask the person to bend her knees and place her feet firmly on the bed. Then ask her to place her hands palm side down on the bed. Place one arm under her shoulders and one hand under her buttocks. Ask her to help by pushing up with hands and feet on the count of 3. Or, if the person is able, ask her to reach back and hold on to the headboard with both hands. Ask her to assist you by pulling herself up on the count of 3 (Figure 10-14). ☐ ☐

6. Count to 3 and, by shifting your weight onto the foot nearest the headboard, move the person toward the head of the bed. ☐ ☐

7. Repeat as necessary until the person is appropriately positioned. ☐ ☐

NOTE: *Move the person only in short distances at one time so that you do not twist your back.*

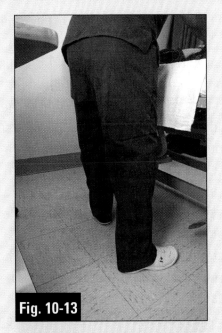
Fig. 10-13

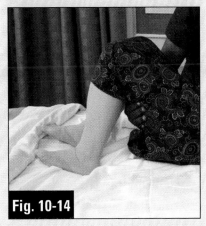
Fig. 10-14

8. Gently lift the person's head and replace the pillow for comfort. ☐ ☐

9. Raise the side rail, if used. ☐ ☐

10. Lower the height of the bed. ☐ ☐

Option 3: Moving Up in Bed (Two Nurse Assistants)

1. Tell your co-worker to stand on one side of the bed while you stand on the other side. Explain to your co-worker what to do. ☐ ☐

2. Lower both side rails, if used. ☐ ☐

Skill 11: Moving a Person Around in Bed—cont'd

3. Help the person lift her head and remove the pillow. Place it against the headboard. ☐ ☐

4. Make sure the person is lying as flat as possible in the *center* of the bed. ☐ ☐

5. Loosen the drawsheet on each side of the bed and roll it toward the side of the person until your hands are close to her body. Place a bed protector (a cloth or disposable absorbent pad) on the bed along each side of the person to avoid contaminating your uniform. ☐ ☐

6. You and your co-worker stand as close to the bed as possible. Each of you lifts your knee that is facing the direction of the move (the one closest to the head of the bed) and places it on the bed on top of the bed protector (Figure 10-15). ☐ ☐

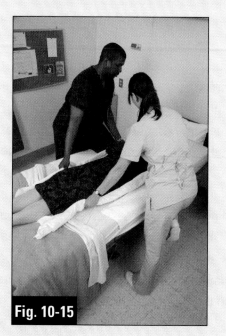

Fig. 10-15

NOTE: *Be sure the bed is in a lower-than-working-height position so that you can keep one foot firmly on the floor while your knee is on the bed.*

7. Grasp the rolled-up drawsheet. ☐ ☐

8. Tell the person that, if she is able to help, she should bend her knees and push up with her feet at the count of 3. Tell your co-worker that on the count of 3 together you will move the person to the top of the bed by moving the drawsheet toward the head of the bed. ☐ ☐

9. On the count of 3, gently lift the person to the top of the bed using the drawsheet to support most of her body. Lift her smoothly, without jerking, and lift her high enough off the bed so that she does not slide along the bottom sheet. Otherwise, the friction of rubbing against the sheet can injure her skin. Keep your elbows as close to your body as you can to avoid straining your back. Shift your weight onto the knee that is on the bed as you lift. Repeat step 9 until the person is correctly positioned at the top of the bed. ☐ ☐

> **NOTE:** *Move the person a little at a time rather than all the way up in one attempt so that you do not twist your back.*

10. Gently lift the person's head and replace the pillow for comfort. ☐ ☐
11. Retuck the drawsheet. ☐ ☐
12. Raise the side rails, if used. ☐ ☐

Option 4: Moving to the Side of the Bed (One Nurse Assistant)

> **NOTE:** *Do not use this procedure if the person has a spinal cord injury or has had spinal surgery or spinal anesthesia.*

1. Make sure the person is lying as flat as possible. ☐ ☐
2. If side rails are used, lower the one closer to you. ☐ ☐

Skill 11: Moving a Person Around in Bed—cont'd

3. Ask the person to lift her head, or if she is unable, gently lift her head and take away the pillow. Place it against the headboard. ☐ ☐

4. Stand with your feet 12 inches apart and one foot slightly behind the other. Bend your knees and keep your upper back as straight as possible (Figure 10-16). ☐ ☐

5. Ask the person to cross her arms over her chest. ☐ ☐

6. Place one arm under her neck and shoulders and the other arm under her upper back (Figure 10-17). ☐ ☐

7. On the count of 3, rock backwards and pull her upper body toward you. ☐ ☐

8. Reposition your hands, placing one hand under the person's waist and the other under her thighs (Figure 10-18). Using the same motion, count to 3 and rock backwards, pulling her lower body toward you. ☐ ☐

9. Finally, reposition your hands under her lower legs and feet and, on the count of 3, move her legs and feet toward you (Figure 10-19). Be careful to move legs just enough to keep proper body alignment. (You can check body alignment of the resident, by standing at the foot of the bed and looking at the person for straight alignment.) ☐ ☐

10. Help the person lift her head and replace the pillow for comfort. ☐ ☐

11. Raise the side rail, if used. ☐ ☐

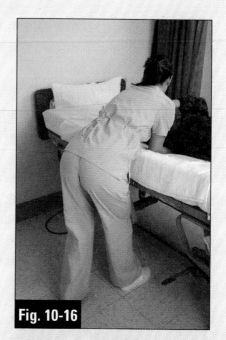

Fig. 10-16

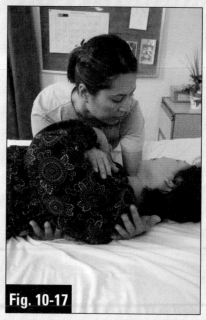

Fig. 10-17

Option 5: Moving to the Side of the Bed (Two Nurse Assistants)

1. Make sure the person is lying as flat as possible. □ □
2. Tell your co-worker to stand on one side of the bed while you stand on the other side. □ □
3. Lower both side rails, if used. □ □
4. Ask the person to lift her head, or if she is unable, gently lift the person's head and take away the pillow. Place it against the headboard. □ □
5. You will move the person away from yourself and toward your co-worker. Loosen the drawsheet on each side of the bed and roll it toward the side of the person until your hands are close to her body. Put a bed protector on the bed alongside the person in front of you. □ □
6. Have your co-worker position his or her feet about 12 inches apart, with one foot slightly behind the other and the knees slightly bent.
7. Stand as close to the bed as possible, lift one knee, and place it on the bed on top of the bed protector, while keeping the other foot firmly on the floor (Figure 10-20). □ □

NOTE: *Be sure the bed is in a lower-than-working-height position so that you can keep one foot firmly on the floor while your other knee is on the bed.*

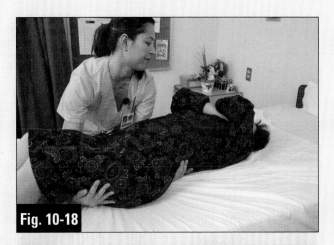

Fig. 10-18

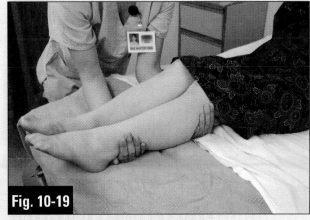

Fig. 10-19

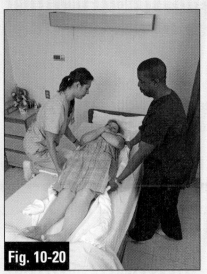

Fig. 10-20

Skill 11: Moving a Person Around in Bed—cont'd

8. Both you and your co-worker grasp the rolled-up drawsheet. ☐ ☐

9. Tell your co-worker that on the count of 3 both of you together will move the person toward your co-worker's side of the bed by lifting the drawsheet. ☐ ☐

10. Tighten your abdominal and buttocks muscles and straighten your back. On the count of 3, gently lift the person and move her to the side of the bed, using the drawsheet to support most of her body. Lift her smoothly, without jerking, and lift her high enough off the bed so that she does not slide along the bottom sheet. ☐ ☐

NOTE: *Shift your weight from the foot on the floor to the knee on the bed as you lift.*

NOTE: *Your co-worker shifts his or her weight from the forward foot to the back foot as he or she lifts.*

11. Help the person lift her head and replace the pillow for comfort. ☐ ☐

12. Retuck the drawsheet. ☐ ☐

13. Raise the side rails, if used. ☐ ☐

Option 6: Turning a Person (One or Two Nurse Assistants)

1. Tell your co-worker to stand on one side of the bed while you stand on the other side. ☐ ☐

2. Lower both side rails (or one side rail if you are turning the person by yourself). ☐ ☐

3. Ask the person to lift her head, or if she is unable, gently lift the person's head and remove the pillow. Place it against the headboard. ☐ ☐

4. Make sure the person is lying as flat as possible on one side of the bed, not in the center of the bed. If she is lying in the center of the bed, move her to the side following the steps in Option 4 or Option 5. ☐ ☐

5. Tell the person that she can help you by crossing her arms over her chest and crossing her ankles toward the direction that you are turning her. For example, if the person is turning onto her right side, have her put her left ankle on top of her right ankle. Assist her if necessary (Figure 10-21). ☐ ☐

6. Stand on the side toward which the person is turning. Put a bed protector on the bed alongside the person. Stand as close to the bed as possible, lift one knee and place it on the bed on top of the bed protector, while keeping the other foot firmly on the floor. Place one hand on the person's far shoulder and the other hand on her upper thigh (Figure 10-22). For example, if the person is turning onto her right side toward you, put your left hand on the person's left shoulder and your right hand on the person's left thigh. ☐ ☐

7. Your co-worker loosens the drawsheet and rolls it close to the side of the person's body. Grabbing the rolled-up drawsheet with palms up and using a broad

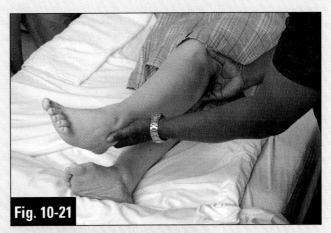

Fig. 10-21

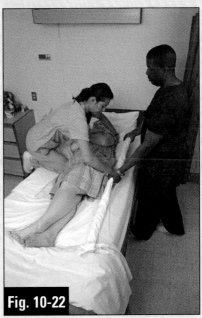

Fig. 10-22

base of support, your co-worker counts to 3, lifts the drawsheet, and rolls the person onto her side (Figure 10-23). You help to roll her toward you by transferring your weight to your foot on the floor. ☐ ☐

8. Help the person lift her head and replace the pillow for comfort. ☐ ☐

9. Raise the side rails, if used. ☐ ☐

NOTE: If you are turning the person by yourself, without the assistance of a co-worker, follow steps 2 through 9, omitting step 7, and then roll her on her side toward you.

NOTE: Stand as close to the bed as possible. Be sure the bed is in a lower-than-working-height position so that you can keep one foot firmly on the floor.

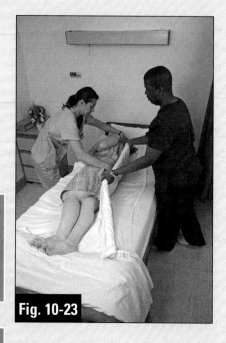
Fig. 10-23

Option 7: Lifting a Person's Head and Shoulders off the Bed (One Nurse Assistant)

You may have to adjust a pillow or help someone sit up to readjust her clothing. To do this, you must raise the head and shoulders of the person off the bed.

1. Lower the side rail, if used. ☐ ☐

2. Stand on one side of the bed facing the head of the bed. Position your feet about 12 inches apart. ☐ ☐

3. If the person can help, ask her to place her arm that is nearer to you under your arm and to hold on behind your shoulder. ☐ ☐

4. Place your arm that is nearer to the person under her arm and behind her shoulder and your arm that is farther from the person under her upper back and shoulders (Figure 10-24). ☐ ☐

5. Raise the person's head and shoulders off the bed by shifting your weight toward the foot of the bed. Remember not to twist when you lift. Ask the person to assist you as much as she can by helping to support herself with her free hand (Figure 10-25). Use your hand that is under her shoulders to readjust the pillow. ☐ ☐

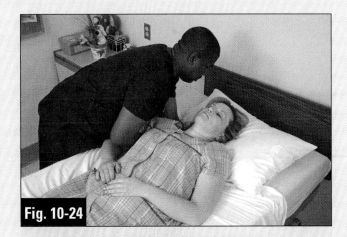

Fig. 10-24

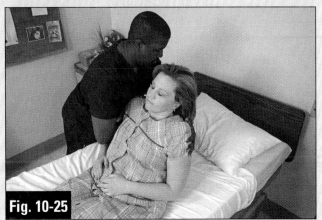

Fig. 10-25

 COMPLETION

1. Follow Completion Standards in compliance with your facility. For a complete list of those used in this course, see Chapter 7, "Controlling the Spread of Germs."

2. Report:
   • Dizziness on movement
   • Pain
   • Red or swollen areas

Skill 12: Positioning a Person in a Supine Position

PRECAUTIONS

- Assess the person and the room environment to determine your plan for moving her safely. Talk with your supervising nurse and check the care plan.
- Use proper body mechanics. To avoid injuring your back, always tighten your abdominal and buttocks muscles while positioning or transferring someone.
- Make sure bed brakes are locked.
- Ask a co-worker to help, if needed.

PREPARATION

1. Gather supplies:
   - Pillows
   - Rolled blanket or towels
   - Foot support
2. Follow Preparation Standards (see Chapter 7).

PROCEDURE

1. If necessary, lower the head and foot of the bed to make it flat. ☐ ☐
2. Lower the side rail, if used, on the side where you are working. ☐ ☐
3. If drainage tubes are used, move them, as necessary. ☐ ☐
4. Position the person so that she is lying on her back in the center of the bed. ☐ ☐
5. Place her in proper body alignment. In the supine position, her body is in proper alignment when:
   - Her head is supported with a pillow (Figure 10-26).

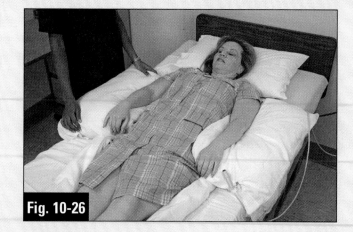

Fig. 10-26

- Her arms are extended and, if there is paralysis or weakness, they are supported by small pillows. This position improves blood return to the heart. If a person is unable to move her hands, position her palms so that they face down.
- Her thighs are in a straight line from her hips. ☐ ☐

NOTE: *Use a small cushion or rolled towel to support the small of her back.*

NOTE: *If the person's foot tends to roll outward, place a rolled towel or pillow against her outer thighs.*

NOTE: *Use a splint or foot board to keep her toes pointing upward. To keep pressure off her heels, use a small pad under her calves and ankles.*

6. Raise the side rail, if used. ☐ ☐

COMPLETION

1. Follow Completion Standards in compliance with your facility. For a complete list of those used in this course, see Chapter 7, "Controlling the Spread of Germs."
2. Report:
   - Dizziness on movement
   - Pain
   - Red or swollen areas

Skill 13: Positioning a Person in a Fowler's Position

PRECAUTIONS

- Assess the person and the room environment to determine your plan for moving her safely. Talk with your supervising nurse and check the care plan.
- Use proper body mechanics. To keep from injuring your back, always tighten your abdominal and buttocks muscles while positioning or transferring someone.
- Make sure bed brakes are locked.
- Ask a co-worker for help, if needed.

PREPARATION

1. Gather the following supplies and bring these to the person's room:
   - Pillows
   - Rolled blanket or towel
   - Foot support
2. Follow Preparation Standards (see Chapter 7). Check for the placement of drainage tubes; move them as necessary.

PROCEDURE

1. Lower the side rails, if used, on the side where you are working. ☐ ☐
2. Make sure the person is supine, in the center of the bed, and remove all pillows. Raise the head of the bed 90 degrees for high Fowler's position, 45 degrees for Fowler's position (Figure 10-27), and 30 degrees for semi-Fowler's or low Fowler's position. Replace the pillows. ☐ ☐

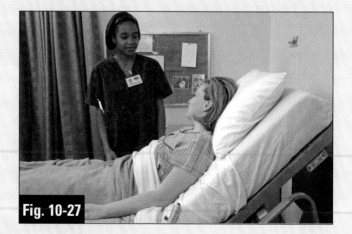

Fig. 10-27

NOTE: *A person sitting up in bed is in Fowler's position.*

3. Raise the foot of the bed very slightly, just enough to prevent the person from sliding down in the bed (or place a pillow or folded blanket under her legs). Make sure the person is in proper body alignment. ☐ ☐

4. If the person has a weak forearm and wrist, support these with a pillow, keeping the wrist higher than the elbow. If the person is unable to move her hands, position them so that her palms face down: the forearm and wrist must be elevated when the person's arm is weak or paralyzed to aid the return of blood to her heart and to prevent swelling of her hand. ☐ ☐

5. Place a foot support, if needed. Maintaining proper position of the person's feet prevents "foot drop." Foot drop causes the toes to drop downward; then the person is unable to bring her foot up into a normal walking position.

☐ ☐

NOTE: *Some people may have forearm, wrist, hand or foot splints to keep their bodies in proper alignment. If a person uses splints, check to see that they are properly applied and that they are clean and dry.*

6. Raise the side rail, if used. ☐ ☐

 ## COMPLETION

1. Follow Completion Standards in compliance with your facility. For a complete list of those used in this course, see Chapter 7, "Controlling the Spread of Germs."

2. Report:
   • Dizziness on movement
   • Pain
   • Red or swollen areas

Skill 14: Positioning a Person in a Modified Side-Lying Position (One or Two Nurse Assistants)

PRECAUTIONS

- Assess the person and the room environment to determine your plan for moving her safely. Talk with your supervising nurse and check the care plan.
- Use proper body mechanics. To keep from injuring your back, always tighten your abdominal and buttocks muscles while positioning or transferring someone.
- Make sure bed brakes are locked.
- Ask a co-worker for help, if needed.
- Check for the placement of drainage tubes; move them as necessary.

PREPARATION

1. Gather supplies:
   - Pillows
   - Rolled blanket or towel
   - Bed protector
2. Follow Preparation Standards (see Chapter 7).

PROCEDURE

1. Lower the side rail, if used, on the side where you are working. ☐ ☐
2. Make sure the bed is as flat as possible. ☐ ☐
3. Ask the person to help with the move by crossing her arms on her chest and ankles toward the direction you are turning her. ☐ ☐
4. *Follow the procedure in Skill Sheet 11 for moving a person to the side of the bed. If working alone follow the procedure in Option 4. If working with a co-worker follow the pro-*

cedure in Option 5. Move the person to the far side of the bed, away from the direction she will be facing. ☐ ☐

5. Turn the person onto her side so that she is off her coccyx (tail bone), but not directly on her hip, by doing the following:
   If working with a co-worker and you are on the side toward which the person is turning, put one knee on the mattress or, if available, on a bed protector placed on top of the mattress. Keep your other foot firmly on the floor.
   If working alone, stand with your feet 12 inches apart and bend your knees and keep your back straight as possible.

6. Place one hand on her shoulder and the other hand on her upper thigh. For example, if the person is turning onto her right side toward you, put your left hand on her left shoulder and your right hand on her left thigh. ☐ ☐

7. *If working alone,* slowly roll the person away from you onto her side.
   If you are working with a co-worker, your co-worker loosens the drawsheet and rolls it up close to the person's body. She grabs the drawsheet. Using a broad base of support, she counts to 3, lifts the drawsheet and rolls the person onto her side, while you help to roll her toward you (Figure 10-28). ☐ ☐

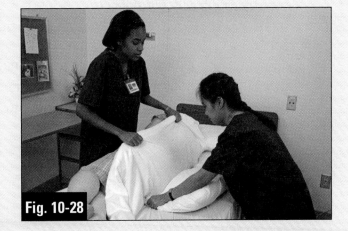
Fig. 10-28

NOTE: *Your co-worker keeps her body close to the bed and her knees slightly flexed.*

8. Position the person in proper body alignment:
   - Support her head with a pillow.
   - Adjust her shoulder so that she is not lying on her arm.
   - Support her back with a rolled blanket or towel to keep her in proper position.
   - Support her top arm with a pillow (Figure 10-29).
   - Flex her top knee.
   - Place her top leg forward and support the knee and ankle with pillows so that they do not rest on top of her lower leg and do not pull on the hip joint.
   - If the person is wearing alignment splints, check to make sure they are properly applied and that they are clean and dry.

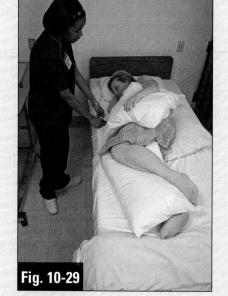
Fig. 10-29

☐ ☐

9. Retuck the drawsheet. ☐ ☐
10. Raise the side rail, if used. ☐ ☐

COMPLETION

1. Follow Completion Standards in compliance with your facility. For a complete list of those used in this course, see Chapter 7, "Controlling the Spread of Germs."
2. Report:
   - Dizziness on movement
   - Pain
   - Red or swollen areas

Skill 15: Positioning a Person in a Prone Position

PRECAUTIONS

> **NOTE:** *When you help someone lie on her stomach, you help her into the prone position. This position is not often used, because many people find it uncomfortable and it often requires a physician's order.*

- Assess the person and the room environment to determine your plan for moving her safely. Talk with your supervising nurse and check the care plan.
- Use proper body mechanics. To avoid injuring your back, always tighten your abdominal and buttocks muscles while positioning or transferring someone.
- Make sure the bed brakes are locked.
- Ask a co-worker to help, if needed.
- Check for the placement of drainage tubes; move them as necessary.

PREPARATION

1. Gather supplies:
   - Bed protector
   - Rolled blanket or towel
2. Follow Preparation Standards (see Chapter 7).
3. Check for the placement of drainage tubes; move them as necessary.

PROCEDURE

1. Lower the side rail, if used, on the side of the bed where you are working. ☐ ☐
2. Make sure the person is lying as flat as possible. ☐ ☐
3. Gently lift the person's head and remove her pillow. ☐ ☐

4. Tell the person that she can help to roll over, if she is able. ☐ ☐

5. With the help of your co-worker, follow the procedure for moving a person to the side of the bed (Skill 11 Option 5). ☐ ☐

6. Put one hand on her far shoulder and one hand on her far hip and your knee on top of a bed protector on the bed. ☐ ☐

> **NOTE:** *Be sure the arm close to you is tucked close to the person or extended up alongside her head so that it will not be trapped or caught under her body when she rolls over. Tuck a folded blanket or small pillow alongside her upper abdomen.*

7. Your co-worker loosens the drawsheet, grabs it with her palms up, and rolls it close to the person's body. Using a broad base of support, she counts to 3, lifts the drawsheet and rolls the person, while you gently turn her toward you and onto her stomach with her head turned to the side. ☐ ☐

8. Position the person in proper body alignment:

   • Help her move down slightly so that her feet are over the end of the mattress or place a pillow under her shins to raise her toes off the bed (Figure 10-30). Use the drawsheet, if necessary, to move her down in the bed.

   • Place a small pillow or folded blanket under her head, and adjust the one under her upper abdomen.

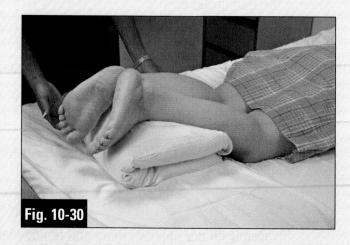

Fig. 10-30

- Place the arm the person is facing with the elbow bent at a 90-degree angle at her side and her other arm straight along the other side (Figure 10-31). ☐ ☐
9. Retuck the drawsheet. ☐ ☐
10. Raise the side rail, if used. ☐ ☐

COMPLETION

1. Follow Completion Standards in compliance with your facility. For a complete list of those used in this course, see Chapter 7, "Controlling the Spread of Germs."
2. Report:
   - Dizziness on movement
   - Pain
   - Red or swollen areas

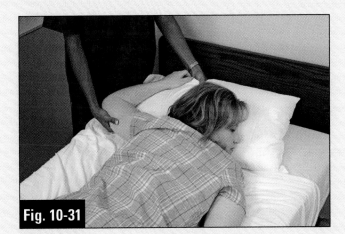

Fig. 10-31

Skill 16: Transferring a Person from the Bed to a Chair

PRECAUTIONS

- Assess the person and room environment to determine your plan for transferring her safely. Talk with your supervising nurse or check the care plan.
- Use proper body mechanics. To keep from injuring your back, always tighten your abdominal and buttocks muscles while positioning or transferring someone.
- Make sure bed brakes are locked.
- If a wheelchair is used, fold back footrests and lock the brake.
- Ask a co-worker to help, if needed.
- Do not use a safety belt if the person has the following:
  - Recent abdominal, chest or back surgery
  - Severe respiratory problems
  - Severe cardiac problems

PREPARATION

1. Gather supplies:
   - Safety belt (transfer belt or walking belt with handles), if you are using one
2. Gather the person's own:
   - Robe
   - Slippers
   - Wheelchair or straight chair
3. Check for the placement of drainage tubes; move them as necessary.
4. Adjust the bed to the same height as the chair.

NOTE: *The person's feet should touch the floor when she is sitting on the edge of the bed.*

5. Follow all other Preparation Standards (see Chapter 7).

PROCEDURE

1. Place the wheelchair or stationary chair at a slight angle against the bed on the person's stronger side. ☐ ☐
2. Lock the bed brakes. If a wheelchair is used, remove or fold back the wheelchair footrests, and lock the brakes (Figure 10-32). ☐ ☐
3. Raise the head of the bed so that the person is almost in a sitting position. ☐ ☐
4. Lower the side rail, if used, that is nearer to the wheelchair. ☐ ☐
5. With your knees bent and back straight, put one of your arms under the person's shoulders and the other arm under her thighs. Do not twist your back at the waist. If a co-worker is helping, one nurse assistant holds the person with one hand under the person's arm and around her shoulder and the other nurse assistant uses both hands to support her legs. ☐ ☐
6. Turn the person toward you into a sitting position, bringing her legs to a dangling position over the side of the bed, making sure her feet are flat on the floor. ☐ ☐

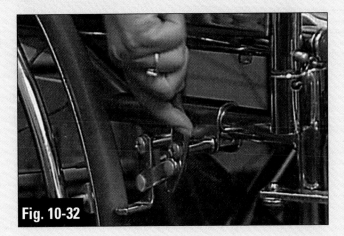

Fig. 10-32

Skill 16: Transferring a Person from the Bed to a Chair—cont'd

NOTE: Stay with her and encourage her to sit on the side of the bed for 2 minutes before going on with the procedure. Some dizziness is common when a person sits up after being in bed for a while. See if the dizziness passes in 2 minutes. If it does not pass, if it gets worse, if she becomes sweaty or short of breath, or if she is in any pain, lay her back down and raise the side rail, if used. Report the situation to your supervising nurse.

7. Help the person put on her clothing, including footwear. ☐ ☐

Option 1: One Nurse Assistant, Without a Safety Belt, When the Person Can Help

To safely transfer a person by yourself without a safety belt, the person must need only steadying and minimal support. She must be able to stand with support, must be able to pivot and must be predictable.

1. Tell the person you are going to put your arms under her arms and that she should place her hands on the bed to push herself up, if she is able (Figure 10-33). ☐ ☐

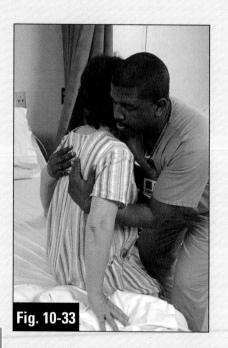

Fig. 10-33

NOTE: When she gets ready to move, her buttocks should be at the edge of the bed so that she can keep her balance when you shift her weight forward. Her feet should be flat on the floor about 12 inches apart, giving her a broad base of support. One foot, closest to the chair, should be a few inches in front of the other foot.

2. Block the person's lower extremities to prevent her from slipping. To do this, face the person, placing your feet almost "toe-to-toe," but toes turned slightly outward to create a supportive base. The foot closest to the chair should be farther back than the other foot. When you stand up, you will be shifting some of your weight onto the foot that is farther back. Bend your knees, deeply, so that they rest against, or near, the person's knees. Keep your knees bent and tighten your abdominal and buttocks muscles, and keep your back straight. (Figure 10-34)   ☐   ☐

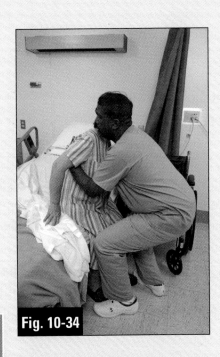
Fig. 10-34

NOTE: Get as close as possible with the person's leaning forward toward you. Remember to use proper body mechanics—use a good base of support, keep the person close, keep your back straight, lift smoothly, do not jerk and do not twist.

NOTE: Do not put pressure under the person's arms.

3. Tell the person that on the count of 3 you are going to assist her to a standing position. On the count of 3, raise her to a standing position (Figure 10-35). Tell her to place her arms on your upper arms or shoulders to steady herself during the move, but not around the neck.

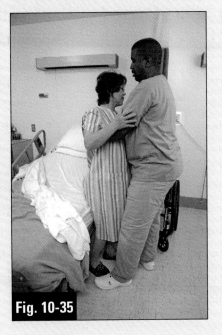
Fig. 10-35

NOTE: Placing arms around a caregiver's neck can injure the caregiver.

Skill 16: Transferring a Person from the Bed to a Chair—cont'd

Take small steps together. Move around until she is right in front of the wheelchair. Ask her to tell you when she can feel the chair against the back of her legs. ☐ ☐

4. Lower her into the chair by bending your knees and keeping your back straight (Figure 10-36). She can help by placing her hands on the chair arms and helping to lower herself into the chair. Help her to feel for the arms of the chair, one arm at a time, while keeping your other arm around her waist for support.

5. Assist her to position herself in the chair so that her back is against the back of the chair. Place her feet on the footrests, if used. ☐ ☐

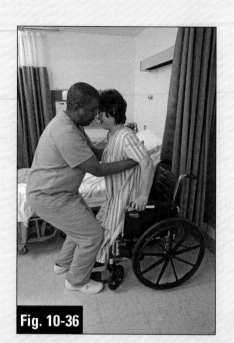
Fig. 10-36

Option 2: One Nurse Assistant, with a Safety Belt, When the Person Can Help

Transferring a person by yourself with a safety belt can be safely accomplished only under the following conditions: the person must be able to stand with support, take a few steps with support and must be predictable.

1. Stand in front of the person, facing her, and put the safety belt around her waist. The belt should be snug but not tight (Figure 10-37). She should be sitting with her buttocks on the edge of the bed, her feet flat on the floor. ☐ ☐

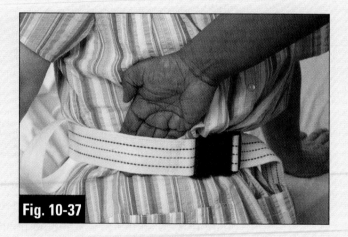
Fig. 10-37

2. Tell the person that when you grasp the safety belt on the back side or by the handles, she must hold you around your shoulders. Grasp the safety belt on the back side of the person's waist, or by the handles, and have her hold you around your shoulders. Block the person's lower extremities to prevent her from slipping. To do this, face the person, placing your feet "toe-to-toe," but toes should be turned slightly outward to create a supportive base. The foot closest to the chair should be farther back than the other foot. Bend your knees, deeply, so that they rest against, or near, the person's knees. When you stand up, you will be shifting some of your weight onto this foot. Keep your knees bent, tighten your abdominal and buttocks muscles and keep your back straight. ☐ ☐

3. Tell the person that on the count of 3 you are going to assist her to a standing position. On the count of 3, raise her to a standing position. Tell her to place her arms on your upper arms or shoulders to steady

Skill 16: Transferring a Person from the Bed to a Chair—cont'd

herself during the move, but not around the neck. Placing arms around a caregiver's neck can injure the caregiver. Taking small steps, together, move around until she is right in front of the wheelchair. Ask her to tell you when she can feel the chair against the back of her legs. □ □

4. Lower her into the chair by bending your knees and keeping your back straight. She can help by placing her hands on the chair arms and helping to lower herself into the chair. Help her to feel for the arms of the chair, one arm at a time, while keeping your other around her waist for support. □ □

5. Assist her to position herself in the chair so that her back is against the back of the chair. Place her feet on the footrests, if used. □ □

6. Place one foot facing the person with your knee (the one farther from the chair) between the person's knees and your other foot in the direction of the move. Flex your knees, tighten your abdominal and buttocks muscles and keep your back straight. Put your head to the person's side closest to the chair so that you can keep the chair in sight during the move. □ □

7. Lower the person into the wheelchair by bending your knees and keeping your back straight. The person can help by placing her hands on the chair arms and helping to lower herself into the chair. □ □

8. Remove the safety belt.

Option 3: Two Nurse Assistants Using a Safety Belt

Use this option if the person is usually predictable but may not be consistent about helping to bear his own weight. If the person weighs over 125 lbs and cannot support her weight, use a mechanical lift. The caregiver must be able to get close enough to the person to avoid reaching.

1. Stand in front of the person, facing her, and put the safety belt around her waist. The belt should be snug but not tight. The person should be sitting with her buttocks on the edge of the bed and her feet flat on the floor and her heels pointed slightly toward the direction of the move. ☐ ☐

> **NOTE**: *If possible, use a safety belt that has handles on the sides, because it is more comfortable for the person and provides less stress for you.*

2. Tell the person that you and your co-worker will grasp the safety belt on the back sides or on each handle and put an arm under each of her arms to move her into a standing position. ☐ ☐
3. You and your co-worker should stand on each side of the person, facing each other. You and your co-worker block the lower extremities to prevent slipping by each placing one foot in front of the person's feet. Flex your knees and keep your back straight. ☐ ☐

Skill 16: Transferring a Person from the Bed to a Chair—cont'd

4. You and your co-worker grasp the safety belt on the back side or by the handles, with one hand, and you each put your free arm under one of her arms and hold on to her back. If you are using a walking belt, grasp the handles of the belt at her sides (Figure 10-38). ☐ ☐

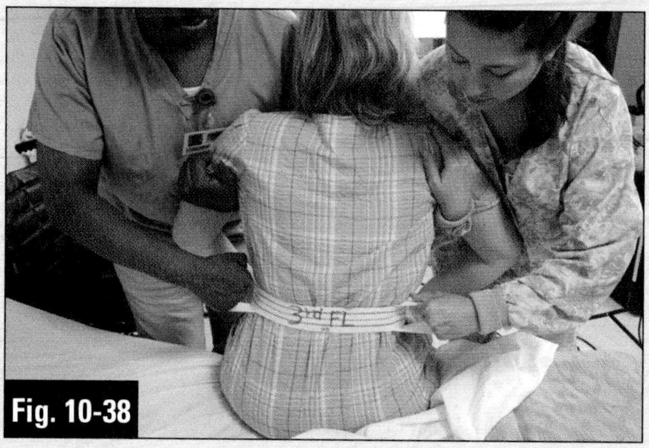

> **NOTE:** *Do not put pressure under the person's arms.*

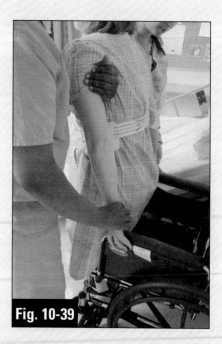

Fig. 10-38

5. Tighten your abdominal and buttocks muscles, flex your knees and keep your back straight. ☐ ☐

6. Tell the person and your co-worker that on the count of 3 you are going to assist the person to a standing position. Ask the person to place her hands on the bed to help push herself up, if she is able. On the count of 3, pull the person toward you into a standing position by straightening your knees. ☐ ☐

7. Taking small steps together, move around until she is in front of the wheelchair. Ask her to tell you when she can feel the wheelchair against the back of her legs. ☐ ☐

8. You and your co-worker each move to one side of the wheelchair and lower the person into the wheelchair, by bending your knees and keeping your back straight. The person can help by reaching back to hold on to the arm rests of the chair (Figure 10-39). ☐ ☐

9. Remove the safety belt. ☐ ☐

Fig. 10-39

COMPLETION

1. Follow Completion Standards in compliance with your facility. For a complete list of those used in this course, see Chapter 7, "Controlling the Spread of Germs."

2. Before you leave, check:
   • Wheelchair footrests replaced or readjusted

3. Report:
   • Dizziness on movement
   • Pain
   • Red or swollen areas

Skill 17: Repositioning a Person in a Chair (Two Nurse Assistants)

PRECAUTIONS

- Use proper body mechanics. To avoid injuring your back, always tighten your abdominal and buttocks muscles when positioning someone.
- Make sure the wheelchair brakes are locked.
- Ask a co-worker to help you.
- Do not use a safety belt if the person has the following:
  - Recent abdominal, chest or back surgery
  - Severe respiratory problems
  - Severe cardiac problems

PREPARATION

1. Gather supplies:
   - Safety belt (if person is not already wearing one)
2. Follow Preparation Standards (see Chapter 7).

PROCEDURE

1. Lock the brakes of the person's wheelchair and put a safety belt on her, if she is not already wearing one. ☐ ☐
2. Stand as close as possible to the back of the wheelchair, facing the person's back. ☐ ☐
3. To give yourself a broad base of support, place one leg against the back of the wheelchair and put the foot of your other leg slightly behind and shoulder-width apart from the first leg. Bend your knees. ☐ ☐
4. Ask your co-worker to assist by kneeling on one knee close to the person's legs and placing an arm under her knees. ☐ ☐

5. Support the person's head against your chest or one shoulder, and grip the safety belt firmly with your palms up. Tighten your abdominal and buttocks muscles; keep your back straight. ☐ ☐

6. Tell the person and your co-worker that on the count of 3 you are going to move her back. ☐ ☐

7. On the count of 3, your co-worker slightly lifts the person's legs and guides them toward the back of the chair, while you lift her by slowly straightening your legs (Figure 10-40). ☐ ☐

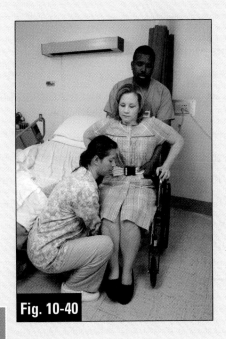
Fig. 10-40

NOTE: *Slide the person's legs and hips by transferring her weight toward the back of the chair at the same time you lift. Your co-worker must be careful not to twist her back.*

 COMPLETION

1. Follow Completion Standards in compliance with your facility. For a complete list of those used in this course, see Chapter 7, "Controlling the Spread of Germs."

2. Report:
   • Dizziness on movement
   • Pain
   • Reddened areas on skin

Skill 18: Using a Mechanical Lift to Transfer a Person from the Bed to a Chair (Two Nurse Assistants)

PRECAUTIONS

- Do not use a mechanical lift:
  - Until you have been properly instructed on how to use it and have practiced using it (Figure 10-41).
  - If parts are missing or broken.
- Assess the person and the room environment to determine your plan for moving him safely. Talk with your supervising nurse and check the care plan.
- Use proper body mechanics. To avoid injuring your back, always tighten your abdominal and buttocks muscles when positioning or transferring someone.
- Make sure bed brakes are locked.
- Ask a co-worker to help.

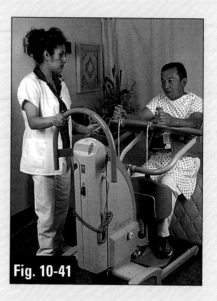

Fig. 10-41

NOTE: *For safety, two nurse assistants should always perform this transfer together. However, sometimes in a home setting you may have no choice except to operate the lift by yourself. Do not do this until you have the skill to do it safely and properly.*

PREPARATION

1. Gather supplies:
   - Mechanical lift, which has the following parts:
     - Base, or frame
     - Sling—a canvas or plastic seat that extends from the back of the knees to the shoulder blades to provide support to the person being lifted

- Chains or straps—used to attach the sling and suspend it from the base. On newer models, the sling may attach directly to hooks on the lift frame
  - Crank, handle or electronic buttons— used to raise or lower the sling (Figure 10-42)
2. Gather the person's own:
   - Robe
   - Slippers
   - Wheelchair or straight chair
3. Check for the placement of drainage tubes; move them as necessary. Adjust the bed to a height that allows you to get the sling under the person and still maintain proper body mechanics.
4. Follow Preparation Standards (see Chapter 7).

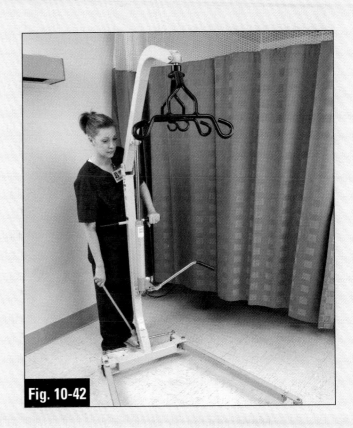

Fig. 10-42

PROCEDURE

1. Detach the sling from the lift and fanfold half of it. ☐ ☐
2. Roll the person toward you and place the fanfolded part of the sling along her back, making sure it is smooth for comfort. Make sure the top of the sling is under her shoulders and the bottom end is at her knees. Roll her over the fanfolds, toward your co-worker, and onto the flat part of the sling. Straighten out the fanfolds. Help her lie flat. ☐ ☐

NOTE: *You can help the person put on her bathrobe while she is turning from side to side. Make sure her clothing is wrinkle-free. Put her slippers on at this time too.*

3. Wheel the lift into place over the person with the base beneath the bed. Make sure the bottom frame of the lift is in its widest position to provide a wide base of support during the move (Figure 10-43). Set the brakes on the lift. Also set the brakes on the wheelchair. ☐ ☐

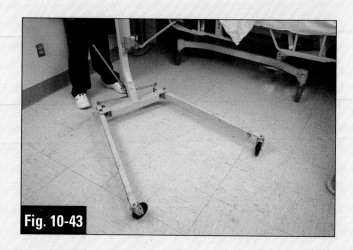

Fig. 10-43

4. Attach the sling to the mechanical lift according to the manufacturer's instructions. If using metal hooks, make sure the open ends of the S-shaped hooks face away from the person. Otherwise, the hooks can catch clothing or scrape skin if they are not facing the correct way. ☐ ☐

5. Slowly lift the person from the bed, release the brakes and guide the lift away from the bed to the chair. Your co-worker guides the person's legs and watches carefully so the person's head and feet do not have contact with the lift. Make sure the person is properly aligned and securely suspended. She may feel more secure if her arms are placed across her chest or if she can grasp the straps or chains. ☐ ☐

6. Set the brakes on the lift, and slowly lower the person into the chair and position her comfortably. Your co-worker should gently push on the person's knees while lowering her into the chair so that she moves into a sitting position in the chair. Your co-worker guides and steadies the person. ☐ ☐

7. Remove the sling from the lift. Keep the sling under the person, since you will later move her back to the bed. Make sure the fabric of the sling is wrinkle-free. ☐ ☐

COMPLETION

1. Follow Completion Standards in compliance with your facility. For a complete list of those used in this course, see Chapter 7, "Controlling the Spread of Germs."
2. Report:
   - Dizziness on movement
   - Pain
   - Red or swollen areas

Skill 19: Turning a Person Using a Log-Rolling Technique

PRECAUTIONS

- Arrange for help from a co-worker.

PREPARATION

1. Gather supplies:
   - Towels, pillows or blankets to be used for support and positioning
   - Bed protectors
2. Follow Preparation Standards.

PROCEDURE

1. With you and a co-worker standing on the same side of the bed, place your hands under the person's head and shoulders (Figure 10-44). The co-worker places her hands under the person's hips and legs. ☐ ☐

2. Stand with one foot slightly behind the other. On the count of 3, rock backwards, transferring weight to the back foot, and together, move the person toward the side of the bed (Figure 10-45). ☐ ☐

3. Lower the bed. Go to the opposite side of the bed. Place a pillow between the person's knees. Cross the person's arms over her chest. ☐ ☐

4. Place your hands on the person's shoulders and hips. ☐ ☐

5. Have your co-worker place her hands on the person's far thigh and lower leg (Figure 10-46). ☐ ☐

6. On the count of 3, turn the person on her side, keeping the head, back and legs in a straight line. ☐ ☐

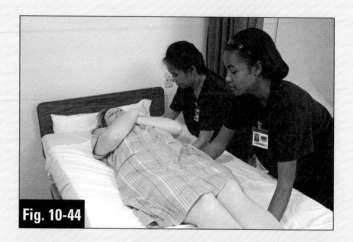

Fig. 10-44

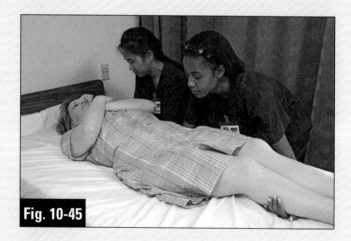

Fig. 10-45

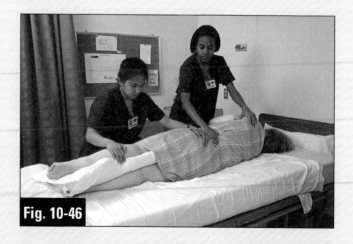

Fig. 10-46

7. Position a pillow behind the person's spine to maintain the position. Support the top arm with pillow or folded blankets. Place a small pillow or folded blanket under the person's head, if allowed (Figure 10-47). ☐ ☐

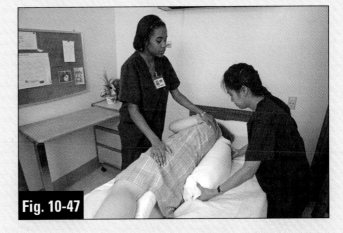
Fig. 10-47

COMPLETION

1. Follow Completion Standards in compliance with your facility. For a complete list of those used in this course, see Chapter 7, "Controlling the Spread of Germs."

2. Report:
   - Dizziness on movement
   - Pain
   - Red or swollen areas

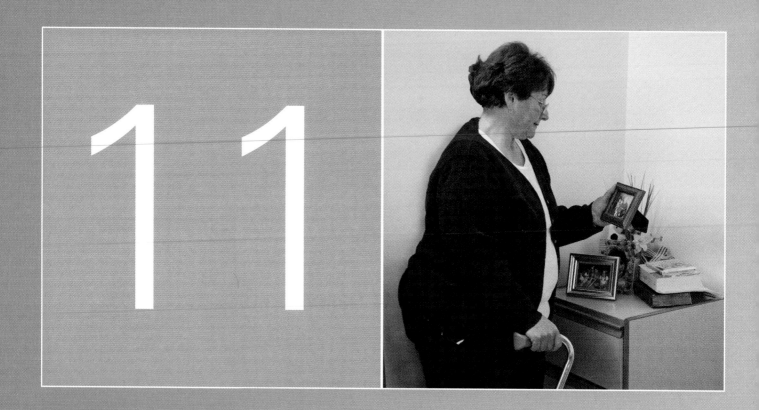

11

Providing Care for the Person's Surroundings

GOALS

After reading this chapter, you will have the information needed to:

Respect a person's belongings while maintaining his or her place.

Operate and maintain different types of beds.

Use and maintain different types of equipment for a bed.

After practicing the corresponding skills, you will have the information needed to:

Make an unoccupied and an occupied bed.

Agnes Ryan shares a room with Louise Wang at Morningside Nursing Home. Mrs. Ryan's part of the room has become home to her. A quilted wall hanging, which she made many years ago, hangs on the wall next to her bed. Every day she straightens one of her quilts, which is folded at the foot of her bed. She keeps a little stack of books, a pad of paper and pen and an arrangement of silk flowers. She likes to keep these things arranged in a particular way so that she knows just where they are.

Mrs. Ryan also enjoys the family photos that are arranged on her nightstand as well. She likes to keep the pictures in a certain order so that she can tell visitors her favorite stories about her loved ones without having to search for the pictures.

One day, a new nurse assistant, who had never assisted with Mrs. Ryan's care, moved things around as she was providing morning care. Mrs. Ryan became very upset when she discovered all her things had been moved from her nightstand. She yelled at the new nurse assistant and told her not to touch her things again. She then told her to leave the room and not to come back. She wanted someone else to provide care for her—someone who would respect her home. The new nurse assistant was surprised at how upset Mrs. Ryan became. "It's not like I took anything," she said to her supervising nurse. Then her supervising nurse talked with her to help her

understand the importance of respecting each resident's home space and personal belongings.

WHAT IS A PERSON'S PLACE?

Think about the word *home*. What do you picture in your mind when you think of home? Do you think of a favorite, comfortable chair where you sit down after a long, hard day? Do you picture a special gift that someone gave to you? Does *home* trigger thoughts about family pictures on the wall?

What do you feel when you hear the word *home?* Do you feel that home should be a place where you feel safe and where you belong? A place where you would want to find comfort, love and security?

Home is your personal space. It is where you reside. As a nurse assistant, one way that you help with a person's care is by maintaining her **environment,** or her place. One person's place may be the hospital, where her "home space" is usually part of a room. Another person's place may be a nursing home, where she receives care in her room and in shared areas, such as a dayroom. Still another person's place may be her own home, where she receives home health care.

Has someone ever come into your home and picked up or moved your things so that you could not find them? How did you feel? Did you feel as if

that person came into your space where he or she did not belong?

All your personal belongings are special. They say something about who you are. They often hold special meaning and may remind you of a certain place, person or time.

A person in your care is sensitive about who touches her belongings or comes into her personal space. You must be sensitive to that person's needs by showing that you care and that you respect her belongings and her immediate surroundings. You show your sensitivity by always:

- Asking the person if there is something special that she would like, such as two pillows instead of one.
- Telling the person you would like to move something and asking where to place it (Figure 11-1).
- Telling the person you would like to make or change her bed.

As a home health aide, you work in different kinds of homes. Many older people and people with disabilities may live in small apartments, or sometimes in one room. You may work with families in a poor area of a city or in a rural area. Space and materials may be limited. In some areas, you may find outdoor toilets. It is important for you to be able to "make do" with the materials that are available in the home.

Whether home is a person's own home, a nursing home or a hospital, you help maintain that place so that it is special and personal. You help each person by maintaining a place that is safe, loving and secure. In addition, you provide care for each person's place by keeping belongings tidy, making and changing beds and practicing infection control so that the home space is clean and odor-free.

Types of Beds

People in your care may be in different types of beds, depending on where they are receiving care and what their particular needs are. You should not

---

KEY TERMS

bed linens: (LIN-ens) sheets, pillow cases, mattress covers, blankets and bedspreads.

environment: (en-VY-run-ment) the surroundings in which a person lives.

incontinent: (in-KON-ti-nent) unable to control the release of urine or feces.

miter: (MY-ter) to square off the corners of bed linens by neatly tucking them under each other.

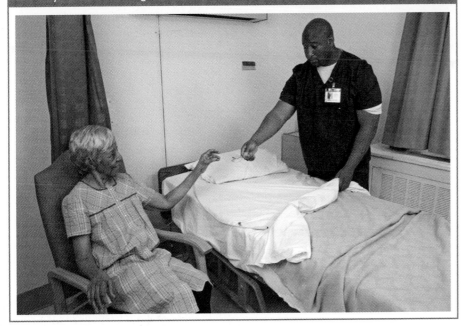

FIGURE 11-1 If you find glasses or other personal items in the bed while you are making it, ask the owner where you should put them.

operate any special bed unless you have:

- Received instructions on how to operate the bed properly.
- Practiced operating the bed.

Gatch-Frame Bed. A gatch-frame bed has joints at places that allow the head and/or foot of the bed to be raised. A simple gatch-frame bed operates manually. You raise either the head piece or the foot piece and then adjust a horizontal bar (which lies across the bed), securing the bar into notches on the frame of the bed. You can adjust the bed to several different heights, depending on which notches you use.

Other manual gatch-frame beds have cranks that you turn to raise the head or foot portion of the bed. With some gatch-frame beds, you can raise or lower the entire bed, while others are stationary.

Electric Bed. An electric bed has head and foot sections that you can raise and lower electrically. Because the control panel normally is located within the person's reach, she or he

usually can operate the bed without your assistance.

Specialty Beds. Some facilities have the following specialty beds that licensed nurses generally operate:

- **Stryker frame.** This special bed is used when it is necessary to change a person's position from prone to supine or supine to prone without moving her or him in the bed. To accomplish this repositioning, the person is secured into the bed, sandwiched between two frames, and gently "flipped" over.
- **Clinitron.** This bed has a mattress filled with a sandy material that supports and conforms to the shape of the person's body. Warm air circulates through the mattress to provide an even temperature. It is used for people who have severe bedsores or burns.
- **Low bed.** This may be any hospital bed that is placed in its lowest position. In some instances mattresses are placed on the floor for the safety of the resident.

- **Air bed.** This bed has a mattress filled with air which circulates to reduce pressure against the body.

Special Equipment for Beds

People who need increased comfort in a standard bed can use special equipment, such as a pressure reduction mattress or polycore mattress (Figure 11-2), foam mattress pads, alternating pressure pads and foot boards.

Foam Mattress Pad. A foam mattress pad increases comfort and reduces the risk of developing pressure sores. Often it is contoured, resembles an egg carton and is called an EGGCRATE mattress. It is placed on top of the standard mattress, and the bottom sheet is tucked in loosely around it. A person may need more than one foam pad on the mattress to aid in the treatment of pressure sores. To put a foam mattress pad on a bed:

- Transfer the person from the bed to a chair, if possible. If the person is unable to be placed in a chair, use the procedure for making an occupied bed to position the pad. When making an occupied bed, follow the procedure that is explained step by step in Skill 21.
- Strip the linens from the bed.

FIGURE 11-2 A pressure-reduction or polycore mattress is used for persons who have pressure sores or have the potential to develop them.

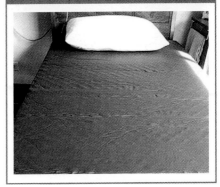

- Place the foam mattress pad on the bed with the wavy side up.
- Place the bottom sheet over the foam mattress pad.
- **Miter** the corners by following the procedure for making an unoccupied bed that is explained step by step in Skill 20. Tuck the sheet in loosely, so that it does not reduce the cushioning effect of the pad. If one sheet is not large enough to cover both the mattress and the pad, use two sheets. Use one to cover and tuck in around the mattress, and then lay the foam mattress pad over the sheet. Use the other sheet to cover and tuck in around the foam mattress pad.
- Put on a drawsheet and tuck it in loosely (Figure 11-3). Also use the drawsheet to move and position the person. Do not use the foam mattress pad as a lifting sheet: it is not strong enough to support the weight of a person and may tear.

Alternating Pressure Pad (Air Mattress). An alternating pressure pad, which is placed on top of the standard mattress, has channels that are connected to a pump that alternately fills and empties the channels with air. The

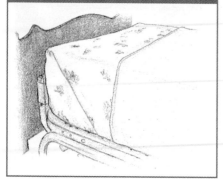

FIGURE 11-3 The sheet and drawsheet are loosely tucked so that the EGGCRATE mattress does not flatten, and the corners of the sheet are mitered so that they will not come untucked.

pad is useful in preventing pressure sores and stimulating circulation.

Before using the pad, read the manufacturer's instructions for operation and safety practices. Follow these instructions, as well as general rules of electrical safety. To use the pad:
- Transfer the person from the bed to a chair, if possible. If the person is unable to be placed in a chair, use the procedure for making an occupied bed (Skill 21) to position the pad.
- Strip the linens from the bed.
- Unfold the alternating pressure pad on the bed with the inlet tubes facing up at the foot of the bed.
- Hang the air pump on the bedframe, or place it on the floor on a clean surface.
- Check the tubing to make sure it has no kinks, holes or cracks.
- Attach the tubing to the air pump connectors.
- After following the instructions on the pump to determine the proper start-up pressure setting, plug the pump into an electrical outlet and turn on the motor. Make sure the cord is out of the way so that no one trips over it.
- After several minutes, check the filling and emptying of the channels.
- Cover the alternating pressure pad with a large sheet tucked loosely under the mattress, rather than mitered, to avoid pinching the tubing. Also, limit the layering of linens, because the thickness reduces the effectiveness of the pad. You may use a drawsheet to help with positioning and transferring.
- Check the effectiveness of the pad by placing your hand under the person's thigh. If you can feel the bottom of the pad when the channel is inflated, increase the pressure of the pump. Check periodically to make sure the mattress is functioning.
- To avoid puncturing the pad, do not use pins to attach anything to it.

- When changing linens, check to see that the alternating pressure pad is clean and dry. If it is not, clean it, using the manufacturer's method of cleaning.

Foot Board. A board placed at the foot of the bed keeps the resident's foot at a right angle to the leg and the toes pointed straight.

Bed Cradle. A bed cradle is a framework that keeps the top **bed linens** from rubbing against and putting pressure on various parts of a person's body, especially the toes. The top linens are placed on the bed over the bed cradle to prevent direct contact.

BEDMAKING

Bedmaking may seem like a very routine task. At home, you may make your bed every day. Or you may hardly ever make your bed. You may change your sheets once a week. Or you may change your sheets every few days. No matter what routine you follow for bedmaking in your own home, the *way* you do it and *when* you do it are important to you. A clean, fresh bed is important to almost everyone. It is especially important to people who spend most of their time in bed.

As a nurse assistant, you provide care for many people who spend much of the day out of bed. However, you also provide care for some people who are unable to get out of bed. The frequency with which you change bed linens depends on how much time the person spends in bed, and it also depends on your employer's policies. One universal rule to follow: Change all linens immediately if they are wet or contaminated, because they can cause skin irritation that can lead to sores.

In a hospital or nursing home, change the bed linens according to the policies of your employer. For people who are able to get out of bed, you may change the linens every day, or only on days when people shower. For those people who cannot get out of bed, change the linens every day.

Generally, most facilities change beds in the morning after bathing, grooming and dressing are completed. But the time of day for changing beds also varies according to the needs of the person in your care.

How to Make a Bed

Bedmaking in a health care setting is probably different from the way you perform this task at home. First, you probably make many more beds at work than you do at home, which places extra strain on your back muscles. For this reason, you must protect your back by conserving your energy and using good body mechanics. Second, you must take special infection control measures when making beds in a health care setting.

When making beds in a health care setting, save time and energy by stacking bed linens in the order in which you use them, so that the bottom sheet or the mattress pad is on the top. Also, save time by folding reusable linens, such as blankets and spreads, and putting them over a clean place, such as the back of a chair, until you are ready to put them back on the bed.

Save more time and energy by making one side of the bed at a time. When you work from one side of the bed, you also use better body mechanics because you do not reach across the bed. Keep from twisting your upper body by standing in front of the section of linen that you are tucking under the mattress. When making an unoccupied bed, work with the bed in a flat position and at a comfortable height so that you do not injure your back. When making an occupied bed, put the bed only as flat as the person can tolerate, because some conditions and diseases make it hard for a person to tolerate lying flat. In a home setting, the bed may be low, and you may not be able to raise it. In such situations, you may have to squat or kneel, keeping your upper body erect, to make the bed.

When you gather supplies for bedmaking, take only the linens you need into the person's room. In a hospital or nursing home, once linens have been taken into a person's room, they cannot be used for another person, and they have to be laundered, even if they were not used. This practice maintains infection control.

In a facility, you will be asked to make an unoccupied bed (the person is not in bed) or occupied bed (the person is in the bed when you make it). You may use a fitted or a flat sheet on the bottom of the bed. Bed linens may also include mattress pads or covers.

Whether you are making an occupied or unoccupied bed, be sure to follow these precautions:

- Before removing dirty linens, check the linens for personal items such as eyeglasses and dentures.

- Keep the side rail up on the side where you are not working.
- Help the person roll onto their side.
- Keep clean linens on a clean surface.
- Keep clean and dirty linens from touching the floor.
- Remove and replace linens carefully, without shaking them. Shaking linens causes air currents that may spread dust and germs around the room.
- Keep dirty, contaminated linens away from your uniform.
- Never leave the person alone.

Put the person first when you are making her bed, and after you have finished making her bed, make sure that she is comfortable and safe before you leave her room.

Bedmaking is an opportunity for you to spend some time in conversation with the person in your care. In addition to providing a clean, comfortable bed for her, you can use this time to show her that you think she is an important and special person.

When making an occupied bed or unoccupied bed, follow the specific procedure explained step by step in Skills 21 and 20.

- Remember when making beds that side rails can sometimes be considered a restraint. Also, beds that are pushed against a wall may be a type of restraint. Therefore, always explain to the person what you are doing and get her permission.

Circle the correct answers and fill in the blanks.

1. To show respect for a person when you make her bed:
   a. make the bed when it is convenient for you to do so, no matter what the person is doing.
   b. tell the person you would like to move something and ask her where to place it.
   c. throw away any personal items left in the bed without asking the person first.
   d. rearrange items on the overbed table and nightstand as you would like them.

2. Foam mattress pads are:
   a. placed between the drawsheet and the bottom sheet.
   b. used to lift and turn a person in the bed.
   c. used to prevent bedsores.
   d. tightly covered with a sheet.

3. When making a bed in a home health care setting, you should do all of the following except:
   a. make one side of the bed at a time.
   b. store many linens in the person's room so that you do not have to go back and forth to get them.

   c. wash your hands before handling clean linens.
   d. hold dirty linens away from your uniform.

4. When you make an unoccupied bed:
   a. the person sits in a chair outside the room.
   b. do not talk, so you can finish the task quickly.
   c. use this time to talk and listen to the person.
   d. the person sits on the side of the bed where you are not working.

5. A(n) _____ has channels that are connected to an air pump; it is useful in preventing pressure sores and stimulating circulation.

1. *Mrs. McDay keeps a large, framed picture of her daughter on her nightstand. While making her bed, you find it necessary to move the picture to avoid knocking it over. What must you remember to do before leaving the room?*

2. *Mrs. Ross cannot get out of bed, and you have to change her bed linens. You know that her delicate skin is particularly vulnerable to irritation and bedsores. What can you do to protect her skin and maintain her comfort?*

3. *While Mr. Gilbert showers, you change his bed linens. As you lift a pillow, his reading glasses slip from the pillowcase and fall to the floor, unharmed. What should you do to retrieve them?*

4. *In the clean utility room, you pick up a supply of bed linens to change Tamara Frazier's bed and stack them in the order that you will use them. In Ms. Frazier's room, you begin to remove the top sheet and realize that she has been* **incontinent** *of feces and her nightgown and bed are soiled. What should you do?*

Skill 20: Making an Unoccupied Bed

PRECAUTIONS

- Keep clean linens on a clean surface.
- Keep clean and dirty linens from touching the floor.
- Remove and replace linens carefully, without shaking them. Shaking linens causes air currents that may spread dust and germs around the room.
- Keep dirty, contaminated linens away from your uniform.
- Use proper body mechanics.

PREPARATION

1. Gather supplies:
   - Pillowcase
   - Top sheet
   - Drawsheet
   - Bottom sheet
   - Laundry bag (or plastic bag for wet or soiled linens)
   - Disposable gloves
2. Follow Preparation Standards (see Chapter 7).

PROCEDURE

Task 1: Removing Dirty Linens

1. Check the dirty linens for personal items the person may have left in bed. ☐ ☐
2. Move personal items found to a safe place. ☐ ☐
3. Loosen all sheets while moving around the bed. ☐ ☐
4. Remove dirty pillowcase off the pillow. Place the pillow on a clean surface. ☐ ☐

Skill 20: Making an Unoccupied Bed—cont'd

5. Remove reusable linens, such as the unsoiled blanket and spread. Place them in clean place (Figure 11-4). ☐ ☐

6. With disposable gloves, roll all dirty linens tightly and put them in the laundry bag (Figure 11-5).

7. Dispose of gloves and wash hands before touching clean linens. ☐ ☐

Task 2: Placing Clean and Reusable Linens on the First Side of the Bed (Unoccupied Bed)

1. Put the clean bottom sheet on the bed. ☐ ☐

2. If using a flat sheet:
   • Tuck in the sheet at the head of the mattress. ☐ ☐

3. Prepare a tight-fitting corner by mitering the corner, using the following steps:
   • Face the head of the bed with your side next to the bed. With the hand that is next to the bed, lift the edge of the sheet at the side of the bed about 12 inches from the top of the mattress, making a triangle.
   • Lay the triangle on top of the bed, holding the top of the triangle firmly.
   • Tuck the hanging portion of the sheet under the mattress (Figure 11-6).
   • Bring the triangle down and tuck it in. With your palms facing up, continue tucking in the sheet on the side, all the way to the foot of the mattress. The sheet should be even at the foot of the mattress.

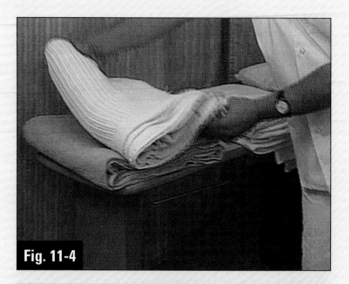
Fig. 11-4

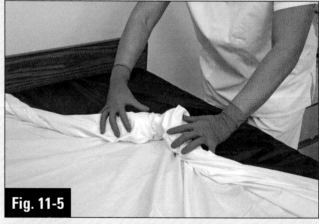
Fig. 11-5

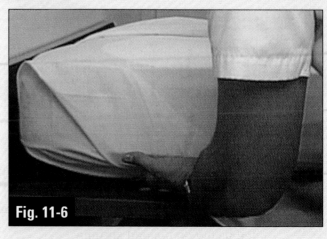
Fig. 11-6

If using a fitted sheet:

- Tuck in sheet smoothly and firmly. ☐ ☐

4. Place the drawsheet across the middle of the mattress with the centerfold in the center of the bed. Unfold the drawsheet. With your palms facing up, tuck the drawsheet under the side of the mattress, tucking in the middle third first, then the top third and then the bottom third. ☐ ☐

5. Put the clean top sheet on the bed with the centerfold in the center. Place the wide hem even with the head of the mattress, with the seam on the outside. ☐ ☐

6. Place the blanket over the top sheet about 6 inches down from the top edge. Center blanket on the bed so that the sides hang evenly. ☐ ☐

7. Place the spread over the blanket. Center spread on bed so that the sides hang evenly. ☐ ☐

8. Tuck in the top sheet, blanket and spread together under the foot of the mattress. Miter the corners together. Do not tuck in the sides as you did with the bottom sheet. ☐ ☐

9. Fold the top of the spread down far enough to allow room to cover the pillow. ☐ ☐

Task 3: Placing Clean and Reusable Linens on the Second Side of the Bed (Unoccupied Bed)

1. Move to the opposite side of the bed. ☐ ☐
2. Tuck in the bottom sheet at the head of the mattress. ☐ ☐

Skill 20: Making an Unoccupied Bed—cont'd

3. Miter the corner of the sheet, if using a flat sheet. ☐ ☐

4. Tuck the sheet in all the way to the foot of the bed. ☐ ☐

5. Tighten the drawsheet by tucking in the middle third first, then the top third and then the bottom third. ☐ ☐

6. Straighten the top sheet. Tuck in the top sheet, blanket and spread together under the foot of the mattress. Miter the corners together. Do not tuck in the sides, as you did with the bottom sheet. ☐ ☐

7. Fold the top of the spread down far enough to allow room to cover the pillow. ☐ ☐

8. Fold the top sheet down 6 inches over the blanket's edge on each side of the bed. ☐ ☐

Task 4: Placing Clean Linens on the Pillow (Unoccupied Bed)

1. Hold the pillowcase at the center of the end seam. ☐ ☐

2. With your hand on the outside of the pillowcase, turn the pillowcase back over your hand. ☐ ☐

3. Hold the pillow through the pillowcase at the center of one end of the pillow (Figure 11-7). ☐ ☐

4. Bring the pillowcase down over the pillow. ☐ ☐

5. Fit the corners of the pillow into the corners of the pillowcase. ☐ ☐

6. Put the pillow on the bed. ☐ ☐

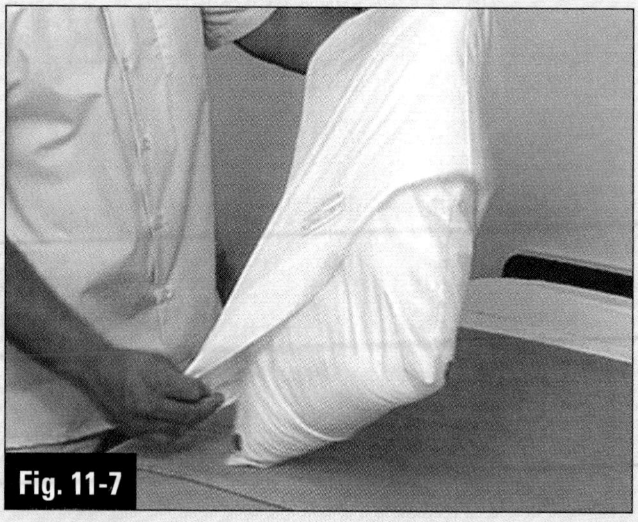

Fig. 11-7

7. Cover the pillow with the bedspread (Figure 11-8). ☐ ☐

8. If the person is going back to bed, open the bed by fanfolding the linens to the foot of the bed and lowering the bed to its lowest position. Help the person into the bed. ☐ ☐

ADDITIONAL INFORMATION

Some nursing homes, hospitals and private homes use fitted bottom sheets instead of flat sheets.

 ## COMPLETION

Follow Completion Standards in compliance with your facility. For a complete list of those used in this course, see Chapter 7, "Controlling the Spread of Germs."

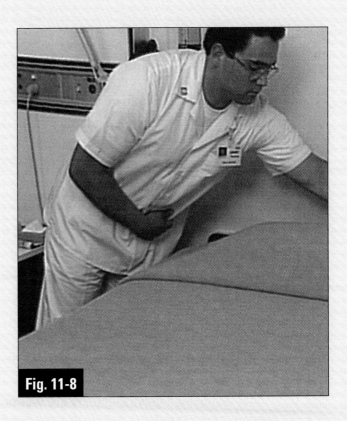

Fig. 11-8

Skill 21: Making an Occupied Bed

PRECAUTIONS

- Keep the side rail up on the side where you are not working.
- Roll the person toward you, never away from you. There is less risk of injury to you and the person when you roll him or her toward you.
- Always stay with the person; never leave him or her alone.
- Keep clean linens on a clean surface.
- Keep clean and dirty linens from touching the floor.
- Remove and replace linens carefully, without shaking them. Shaking linens causes air currents that may spread dust and germs around the room.
- Keep dirty, contaminated linens away from your uniform.
- Wear disposable gloves if linens are wet or soiled. After discarding gloves, wash hands before touching clean linen.

PREPARATION

1. Gather supplies:
   - Disposable gloves (if linens are wet or soiled)
   - Pillowcase
   - Top sheet
   - Drawsheet
   - Bottom sheet
   - Bath blanket (optional)
   - Extra sheet or bed protector (optional—use if you know the sheets are wet or soiled)
   - Laundry bag (or plastic bag for wet or soiled linens)
2. Follow Preparation Standards (see Chapter 7).

PROCEDURE

Task 1: Removing and Replacing Linens on the First Side of the Bed (Occupied Bed)

1. While moving around the bed, take off reusable linens, such as the unsoiled blanket and spread. Fold and put them in a clean place. ☐ ☐

2. Keep the top sheet on the person for privacy and warmth or cover the person with a bath blanket and then remove soiled top sheet. ☐ ☐

3. Check the side of the bed opposite to the one you are going to make first for personal items, such as dentures, eyeglasses or hearing aids. Move found items to a safe place after asking the person where he or she would like you to put them. ☐ ☐

4. Raise bed to working height. ☐ ☐

5. Lower the side rail, if used. Help the person roll on their side. Raise side rail. ☐ ☐

6. Return to the opposite side of the bed, where you are working. Lower the side rail, if used. ☐ ☐

7. Adjust the pillow under the person's head for comfort and for proper body alignment. ☐ ☐

8. Check that side of the bed for personal items. If you find any, move them to a safe place of the person's preference. ☐ ☐

Skill 21: Making an Occupied Bed—cont'd

9. Loosen the dirty bottom sheet and draw-sheet. Roll them toward the person and tuck them against her back (Figure 11-9). If sheets are soiled with body fluids, place bed protector down so that the clean bottom sheet will not become contaminated. ☐ ☐

10. Put the clean bottom sheet on the bed. ☐ ☐

11. Tuck in the sheet at the head of the mattress (or use fitted sheets). ☐ ☐

12. Miter the corner. ☐ ☐

13. Tuck in the sheet all the way to the foot of the mattress. ☐ ☐

14. Place the centerfold of the drawsheet on the middle of the mattress. Fanfold the top of the drawsheet next to the rolled dirty sheet (Figure 11-10). Tuck the remaining part under the side of the mattress. ☐ ☐

15. Flatten the rolled dirty sheets as much as possible. Help the person roll over the dirty linens toward you. Adjust the pillow under the person's head. Check for proper body alignment. ☐ ☐

16. Raise the side rail, if used, on the side of the bed where you have been working. Go to the opposite side of the bed. ☐ ☐

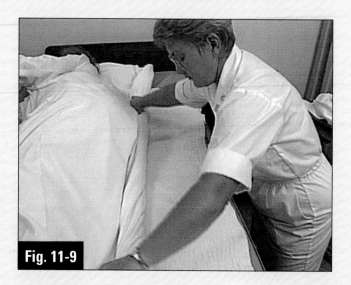
Fig. 11-9

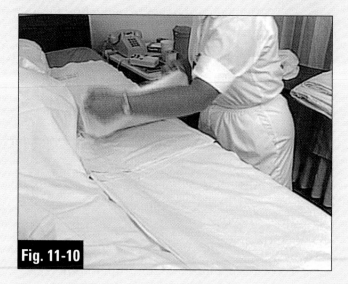
Fig. 11-10

Task 2: Removing and Replacing Linens on the Second Side of the Bed (Occupied Bed)

1. Lower the side rail, if used, on the side where you are working. ☐ ☐

2. With gloves, roll up the dirty bottom sheets and put them in the laundry bag (Figure 11-11). After removing your gloves, wash your hands. ☐ ☐
3. Pull the clean, fanfolded bottom sheet toward you until it is completely unfolded. ☐ ☐
4. Tuck in the bottom sheet at the head of the mattress and miter the corner. ☐ ☐
5. Tuck in the sheet all the way to the foot of the mattress (Figure 11-12). ☐ ☐
6. Pull the drawsheet out from under the person. Tighten it by tucking in the middle third first, then the top third and then the bottom third. ☐ ☐
7. Help the person roll onto his back in the center of the bed. Adjust the pillow under his head. ☐ ☐
8. Put the clean top sheet over the dirty top sheet or bath blanket. ☐ ☐
9. Place the wide hem of the sheet at the head with the smooth side of the hem next to the person. Center the sheet so that the sides hang evenly and the top of the sheet is even with the top of the mattress. ☐ ☐
10. Raise the side rail, if used. ☐ ☐
11. Have the person hold the clean top sheet in place while you remove the dirty sheet or bath blanket if used from underneath. ☐ ☐

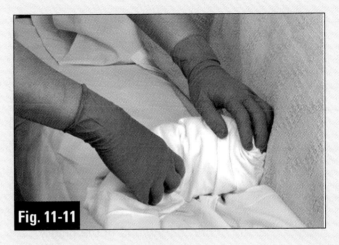
Fig. 11-11

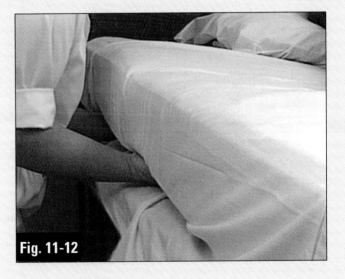
Fig. 11-12

Task 3: Removing and Replacing Linens on the Pillow (Occupied Bed)

1. Lower the side rail, if used, on the side where you are working. ☐ ☐

Skill 21: Making an Occupied Bed—cont'd

2. Remove the pillow from under the person's head. ☐ ☐
3. Remove the dirty pillowcase from the pillow. ☐ ☐
4. Hold the clean pillowcase at the center of the end seam. ☐ ☐
5. With your hand on the outside of the pillow-case, turn the pillowcase back over your hand. ☐ ☐
6. Hold the pillow through the pillowcase at the center of one end of the pillow. ☐ ☐
7. Bring the pillowcase down over the pillow. ☐ ☐
8. Fit the corners of the pillow into the corners of the pillowcase. ☐ ☐
9. Replace the pillow under the person's head. ☐ ☐
10. Raise the side rail, if used. ☐ ☐

Task 4: Replacing Reusable Linens (Occupied Bed)

1. Lower the side rail, if used, on the side where you will be working. Put the blanket over the top sheet about 6 inches down from the top of the mattress. Center the blanket on the bed so that it hangs evenly. ☐ ☐
2. Center the spread over the blanket so that it hangs evenly and the top hem is even with the head of the mattress. ☐ ☐
3. Tuck in the top sheet, blanket and spread together under the foot of the mattress. Miter the corners together. Do not tuck in the sides (Figure 11-13). ☐ ☐

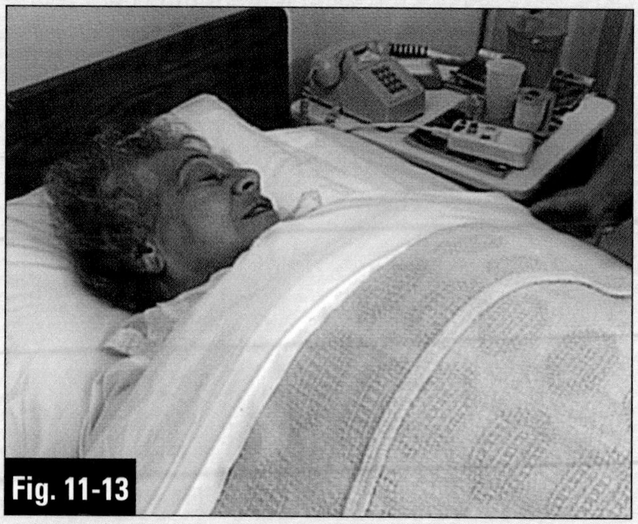

Fig. 11-13

4. Fold the hem of the top sheet down over the blanket and spread. Fold the top sheet down 6 inches over the blanket and spread. Raise the side rail, if used. ☐ ☐

5. Complete the other side. ☐ ☐

Task 5: Making a Toe Pleat

1. Standing at the foot of the bed, grasp both sides of the top covers about 18 inches from the foot of the bed. Pull the top covers toward the foot of the bed (Figure 11-14). ☐ ☐

2. Make a 3- to 4-inch fold across the foot of the bed to make a toe pleat. ☐ ☐

3. Lower bed (if raised) to lowest position, then lower side rails unless ordered. ☐ ☐

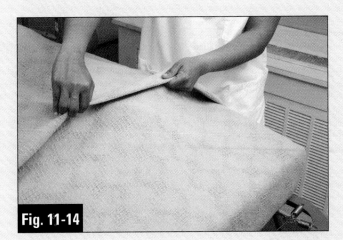

Fig. 11-14

ADDITIONAL INFORMATION

Some nursing homes, hospitals and private homes use fitted bottom sheets instead of flat sheets.

COMPLETION

Follow Completion Standards in compliance with your facility. For a complete list of those used in this course, see Chapter 7, "Controlling the Spread of Germs."

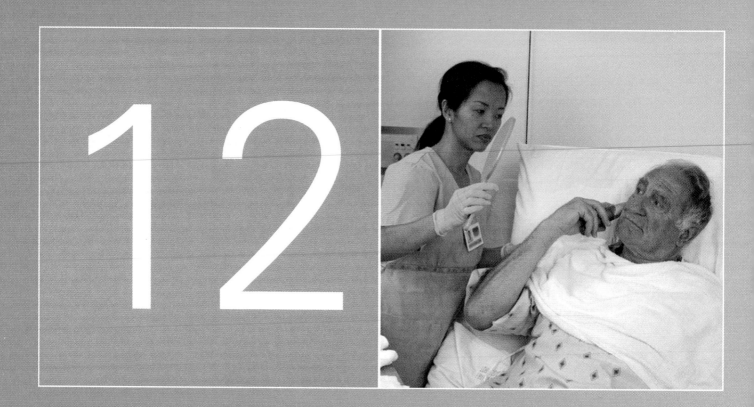

12

Assisting People with Personal Care

GOALS

After reading this chapter, you will have the information needed to:

Be better prepared to provide each person with thoughtful, individualized care that respects the private nature of personal care.

Know how to incorporate the six principles of care when assisting adults with personal care.

After practicing the corresponding skills, you will have the information needed to:

Assist with good mouth care, including mouth care for someone who has dentures, as well as for someone who is unconscious.

Assist with good grooming care by helping people brush and comb their hair, shave, clean and trim their fingernails and clean their feet and toenails.

Help a person with dressing and undressing.

Help people bathe and shampoo in bed, in the shower and in the tub.

Every other day you are assigned to give Mr. Rivera a complete bed bath. On the days when you do not give him a complete bed bath, he receives a partial bed bath.

As you enter his room, you see Mr. Rivera lying in his bed. You tell him that you are here to help him with his bath and to shampoo his hair. He looks your way, smiles, and lifts his hand in a weak wave. "G'morning," he says.

You ask Mr. Rivera's permission and you explain to him how you will be helping him with his personal care. You gather supplies and close the door to his room. First you help him brush and floss his teeth. Mr. Rivera is able to shave his face, using an electric razor, so you wash his face and then stand by to help if he needs assistance. You help him undress for his bath, take care to keep him warm during the bath and pay special attention to his skin. During the bath, you have him soak his hands so that you can clean and trim his fingernails. You also have him soak his feet in a basin of water so that you can clean his toenails. After the bath, you shampoo, condition and towel dry his hair.

Now that Mr. Rivera is bathed, you help him into the bedroom chair so that he can get dressed and rest for a few minutes while you comb his hair and make his bed.

FOCUSING ON PERSONAL CARE

Personal care includes positioning and transferring people, which you will read about in Chapter 10; healthful eating, which you will read about in Chapter 14; and elimination, which you will read about in Chapter 15. It also includes mouth care, bathing, shampooing, grooming and dressing and undressing, which you will read about in this chapter.

ASSISTING WITH PERSONAL CARE

To assist with personal care in a sensitive manner, put yourself in the place of the people in your care. Imagine what it would feel like to have a stranger brush your teeth, bathe you, comb your hair and dress you.

Every day you make choices about what to wear, when to get up, how to style your hair and many other personal decisions. These actions and decisions say something about you and your personal needs, self-image and independence. The people in your care need to make these same decisions for themselves, but they may need your help to carry out the actions. You must respect the way people want their personal care done because they each must maintain their own personal needs, self-image and independence.

Remember to think about what the people in your care need to feel good, how much they can do for themselves and how you can help them feel good about themselves. For example, even though Mr. Rivera is very weak, he still wants to brush his teeth, shave and help dress himself. It takes him longer to do each of these tasks than it would take you to do them for him. But your patience in encouraging him to do these tasks independently helps him feel better about himself.

Because it is so important to respect a person's needs and promote a good self-image and independence, assisting with personal care involves making many decisions.

When to Help with Personal Care

As nurse assistants, you and your co-workers make sure the people in your care are clean, safe and comfortable throughout the day and night. In the morning, you help a person prepare for breakfast by helping him go to the bathroom or using another method to eliminate. You also help him wash his face and hands and brush his teeth. You offer him fresh drinking water and assist with any other care that makes him comfort-

---

KEY TERMS

abrasion: (uh-BRAY-zhun) a tiny cut or scrape.

antiseptic: (an-tuh-SEP-tik) a substance that stops the growth of germs.

aspirate: (AS-puh-rate) to breathe in. The breathing of fluid or an object into the lung.

dandruff: (DAN-druff) flaking skin from the scalp.

depilatory cream: (duh-PILL-uh-tor-ee) a lotion that dissolves hair and removes it from the surface of the skin.

fluoride: (FLOOR-ride) a chemical that helps decrease tooth decay. Toothpaste and drinking water often contain fluoride.

perineal care: (per-uh-NEE-uhl) a nursing procedure in which a person's body is cleaned from the genitals to the anus.

plaque: (PLAK) a sticky, colorless layer of bacteria that forms constantly on the teeth.

unconscious: (un-KON-shus) a state of mind in which a person does not respond to the world around him or her.

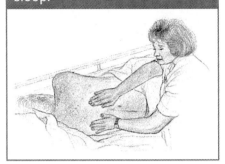

FIGURE 12-1 A backrub is relaxing and helps promote sleep.

able. After breakfast, you usually help the person bathe and dress. During the day, you take care of any other personal care needs that arise.

At night, you help a person prepare for bed by helping him undress, use the bathroom, wash his face and hands and brush his teeth. You also make sure his bed linens are smooth and wrinkle-free, offer him fresh drinking water and assist with any other care that makes him comfortable (Figure 12-1).

ASSISTING WITH MOUTH CARE

When you get up in the morning, how does your mouth feel? What do your teeth feel like after you eat a meal? Part of your responsibility in assisting with personal care is to help provide dental care, also called *oral hygiene*. This important part of daily care includes care of the mouth, teeth, gums, tongue, lips and soft parts of the inside of the mouth, such as the cheeks and the roof. A person in your care may want to take care of his own mouth, as Mr. Rivera did.

Encourage the people in your care to be independent, but make sure they all receive proper mouth care. Assist them as much as necessary, which may involve helping some people brush and floss their teeth, helping others clean their dentures or provid-

ing special mouth care for **unconscious** people. Remember to use Standard Precautions, especially wearing disposable gloves, when you assist with mouth care.

Why Help with Mouth Care?

A clean mouth and clean teeth help prevent mouth odors and infection. An unclean mouth and unbrushed teeth can cause discomfort, loss of appetite and a reduced desire for water. In addition to making a person unhealthy, it may also keep him or her from wanting to talk or be with other people.

If a person does not brush his or her teeth, **plaque** builds up on the gums and teeth. Eating sugars and starches causes the bacteria in plaque to grow. These bacteria, in turn, produce acids, which destroy the outer surface of the tooth, leading to tooth

decay. If plaque is not removed by brushing the teeth, it hardens into tartar, which only a dentist can remove. If tartar is not removed, it can cause gum irritation, infection and possibly tooth loss.

Good mouth care is important for people of all ages, but it is especially important for older adults. Table 12-1 contains examples of dental conditions that affect the elderly.

How to Help with Mouth Care

When assisting with mouth care, always wear disposable gloves. Use a toothbrush that has soft bristles with rounded ends to remove plaque and food particles from the teeth and to stimulate circulation in the gums, which helps keep them healthy. Generally, you should use toothpaste that contains **fluoride** when you clean a

TABLE 12-1 DENTAL CONDITIONS AFFECTING OLDER ADULTS

Sign of Change	Reason
Plaque builds up faster.	Decreased saliva production
Teeth appear slightly darker.	Changes in bonelike tissue under tooth enamel
Mouth is drier.	Decreased saliva production; medications, especially for high blood pressure
Teeth are more susceptible to decay.	Drier mouth; other conditions or diseases that may decrease the ability to brush and floss the teeth effectively
Dentures become uncomfortable.	Drier mouth
Gums may bleed easily.	Gum disease
Pus forms between gums and teeth.	Gum disease
Denture fit changes.	Gum disease
Bad breath persists.	Insufficient or improper brushing or flossing; gum disease

person's teeth. Fluoride is important for keeping teeth strong and healthy, but too much fluoride can cause teeth to discolor. In a few areas of the United States, the water supply contains a high percentage of fluoride, and dentists recommend using toothpaste that does not contain fluoride.

To finish cleaning the teeth, use dental floss to remove plaque and food particles from between the teeth. Waxed dental floss slides between the teeth more easily than unwaxed dental floss does, and it makes the procedure more comfortable for a person who has sensitive gums. Flossing, like brushing, also stimulates the gums (Figure 12-2).

Use mouth sponges to remove mucus and secretions from the gums, tongue, and palate of people who are unconscious or who wear dentures. Mouth sponges are soft enough to clean the tender tissues of the mouth without injuring them.

Brushing and Flossing. When brushing and flossing teeth, be sure to follow these precautions:

- Use a toothbrush with soft bristles.

- Brush the upper teeth first and then the lower teeth to control the amount of saliva produced.
- Slide (do not snap) the floss carefully between the teeth without pressing against the gums.
- Replace the person's toothbrush every 3 to 6 months or when it begins to fray or show wear.
- Bring a mask and protective eyewear if there is a likelihood that you may be splashed with bloody saliva, or if the person is HIV- or HBV-positive.

Before flossing a person's teeth, check with your supervising nurse or the person's care plan to see whether there are any restrictions or special precautions to be considered. For example, some people taking certain medications may bleed excessively if their teeth are flossed. To keep a person's gums from bleeding when you floss, insert floss without pressing against the gums. Whenever you brush or floss, observe changes in the person's mouth and report any swollen, red or tender gums, as well as bleeding, white patches or pain.

Denture Care. You may also provide mouth care to residents who wear dentures or false teeth. People in your care may wear complete (full-mouth) dentures, which replace all of their teeth, or partial dentures, which replace only a portion of their teeth. Wearing dentures decreases gum shrinkage after teeth have been removed and maintains the shape of the mouth. It also improves a person's speech and makes it easier to eat. In addition, wearing dentures improves a person's self-image. You should observe the following precautions when caring for a person's dentures.

- Remind the person to remove the devices for at least 8 hours each day to rest his or her gums (usually at bedtime).
- Handle dentures carefully so that they do not chip or break.
- Always mix mouthwash with water to help protect the person's gums.
- Be sure to label each person's dentures and denture cup to keep them from being misplaced or lost. Read the information in Box 12-1 on labeling dentures to learn how to do this.

Observe changes in the person's mouth and report any swollen, red or tender gums; bleeding, white patches, sores or pus between gums and natural teeth; and ill-fitting or broken dentures.

Providing Mouth Care for an Unconscious Person

You may be responsible for providing care to a person such as 25-year-old Tamara Frazier, who is unconscious as the result of a car crash.

An unconscious person cannot swallow adequately and does not have normal mouth movements to keep the mouth clean and moist. Mucus and other mouth secretions, which tend to coat the teeth of a person who is unconscious, must be removed regu-

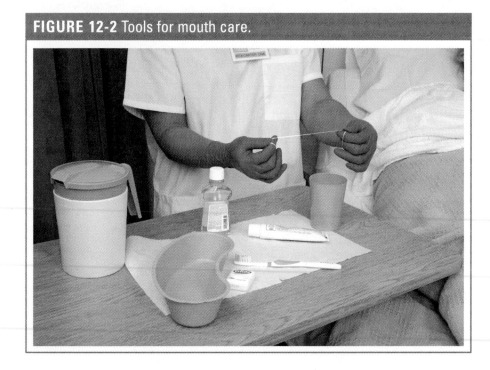

FIGURE 12-2 Tools for mouth care.

BOX 12-1

HOW TO LABEL DENTURES

Professional dentists and dental employees can mark dentures permanently. If dentists or dental employees are not available, you can mark them with surface-marking techniques that are not as durable as permanent denture labeling but that help to avoid losing or misplacing dentures. Often hospitals and nursing homes have denture-labeling kits that contain all necessary supplies. If a kit is not available, use the following method:
1. Thoroughly clean and dry the dentures.
2. Use an abrasive pad to roughen the area on the lingual (tongue) side of the denture.
3. Use an extrafine felt-tip pen* to print the wearer's name or initials in the roughened area of the dentures.
4. Allow markings to dry and then coat them with two layers of clear, acrylic resin.† Ask a local dentist for the product available in your area. (From *Techniques for Denture Identification,* Chicago, 1984, The American Dental Association Council on Prosthetic Services and Dental Laboratory Relations.)

*Sharpie pens by Sanford Corporation have been tested for toxicity and, according to research reports, are not toxic when used in small quantities inside the mouth.
†Clear fingernail polish should *not* be used as a coating, because it has not been tested for toxicity or durability.

larly. You must provide mouth care for an unconscious person every 2 hours throughout the day and night because her or his mouth can become very dry (Figure 12-3). For more information see Skill 24 on page 249.

An unconscious person may not respond to you, but he or she may be able to hear you. People who regain consciousness sometimes remember and talk about the frustration of hearing what was going on but not being able to move or talk while they were unconscious. Therefore, as you provide care, always talk to an unconscious person and tell him or her what you are doing.

To prevent aspiration, elevate the head of the bed or turn him on his side so that fluids will run out of his mouth instead of going down his throat, which could cause him to choke. Observe changes in the person's mouth and report any swollen, red or tender gums, as well as bleeding, white patches or sores.

Remember to follow these precautions when providing mouth care to an unconscious person:
- Open the mouth gently, without using force.
- Always position the person's head to the side so that he will not **aspirate,** or breathe fluids into the lungs.

- Always mix mouthwash with water.
- Always use a soft bristle brush.

When to Help with Mouth Care

As a nurse assistant, help the person with mouth care:
- Every morning
- Every evening
- After the person eats a meal (as often as possible)
- Every 2 hours, if the person is unconscious
- After the person vomits, if the person is unconscious, on oxygen therapy or is a mouth breather.

ASSISTING WITH GROOMING

Why is grooming important to you? What does your hairstyle say about you? What does your beard or mustache say about who you are? How are your fingernails an expression of

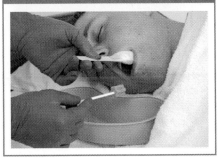

FIGURE 12-3 Reposition an unconscious person and provide mouth care for him every 2 hours during the day and night.

who you are? Does the way you look affect how you feel about yourself? A clean, well-groomed appearance improves your sense of well-being and makes you feel better about yourself.

Part of your responsibility in assisting with personal care is to help people with grooming. This important part of personal care includes brushing and combing the hair, shaving or grooming the beard, cleaning and trimming the fingernails and cleaning the feet and toes. Some people in your care may want to do their own grooming, as Mr. Rivera did when he used his electric shaver. Team up with the person by helping him with the tasks he cannot do and encouraging him to do the ones that he is capable of doing. For example, Mr. Rivera could shave but was not able to clean his nails, so you helped him with that task. If someone in your care is unable to groom himself, you must provide the care for him.

You must know what kind of grooming each person in your care needs. Think about how you would feel if a stranger had to do your grooming. What if someone styled your hair in pigtails? Or what if someone shaved off your mustache? Or how would you feel if someone hastily applied the wrong color of lipstick to your mouth? How would you feel if your parent or grandparent was treated in this way?

If you can relate personally to these situations, you understand why each person must be treated as an individual. If you can imagine what it would feel like to depend on someone else to help you with your grooming, these feelings will help you provide better care to others.

Why Help with Grooming?

In addition to improving the person's self-esteem, grooming can help prevent painful tangles in the hair and possible injuries from jagged or long nails. Good foot care is an essential part of grooming because the feet

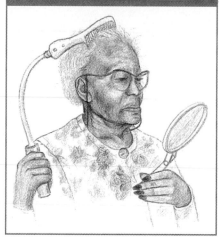

have a large number of sweat glands that remove wastes from the body. Foot care is especially important for anyone who has poor circulation in the legs and feet and for older adults who may not be mobile enough to care for their own feet.

How to Help with Grooming

Generally, people like to groom themselves. If physical limitations prevent this, you may have to help with grooming or encourage the use of adaptive devices (Figure 12-4).

To make good use of personal care time, combine tasks. For example, while a person in your care soaks his hands for nail care, use this time to brush and comb his hair. If a man in your care wears a beard or mustache, periodically wash it during bath time to remove accumulated oil and food residue. Follow the person's desire for grooming. For example, he may want to use a special soap on his beard or mustache.

Brushing and Combing Hair. The way a person wears her hair generally reflects how she feels about herself. The amount of time she spends on her hairstyle on a given day may reflect

how she feels that day. You must consider the person's feelings along with variations in hair types and styles when you help brush, comb and style someone's hair (Figure 12-5).

Remember to brush hair gently so that you do not pull it out. Some medications and medical treatments cause hair to be brittle or fall out. To prevent hair from breaking and to detangle the ends, start brushing from the ends of the hair, working toward the scalp, and work in small sections.

If a person's hair is tangled, use a comb with widely spaced, blunt teeth so that you do not hurt the person's scalp. Work slowly and in small sections so that you do not break the hair. In extreme cases, wet the hair and apply conditioner before combing and then wash and rinse the hair after you have removed all the tangles.

People of African descent may have very curly hair and dry scalps. If the person prefers, use oils, creams or lotions when assisting with hair care to make the hair easier to comb and to moisturize the scalp. Generally, apply

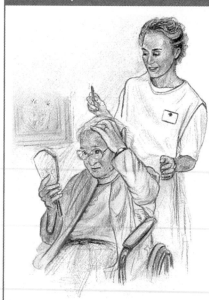

these creams to the scalp after shampooing and massage them into the scalp and hair. For people who have coarse hair, it may be easier to comb the hair when it is wet, after shampooing. Some people with very curly hair may find it easier to keep their hair tangle-free if it is braided. Check with the person to make sure that she wants her hair braided. If she does, be careful not to braid the hair too tightly, because hair tends to draw tighter as it dries and may pull too tightly on her scalp.

As you groom a person's hair, encourage him or her to look in the mirror. Report to your supervising nurse any unusual conditions, such as sores on the person's scalp, unusual flaking or **dandruff,** excessive hair loss or tangles that cannot be removed.

Shaving with a Safety Razor. Many men prefer to shave with a safety razor instead of an electric razor. Safety razors may either be disposable or have standard handles that hold replaceable blades. Whenever you handle a razor blade, you must take special precautions to avoid nicking or cutting yourself and the person in your care.

Because certain medical disorders and some medications can cause excessive bleeding if a person is cut, *always ask your supervising nurse whether a person should be shaved with a safety razor.* Before helping a man shave, inspect his skin for moles, birthmarks or sores. Shave carefully around these areas to avoid scraping or cutting, which could cause bleeding. Encourage the person to use shaving cream, because it softens the skin and helps the razor glide over the skin. Also encourage him to use aftershave lotion, because the alcohol in aftershave helps keep germs from growing and acts as an **antiseptic** on **abrasions.** Men who have very curly beards may prefer not to shave, but to use **depilatory cream** or powder to remove facial hair.

After helping a man shave, report any red areas, sores, nicks or cuts on his skin to your supervising nurse. To avoid cutting yourself or the person in your care, place the used razor in a sharps container or, if it is reusable, place the blade end down in a container, but do not recap it. *Make sure each razor is used by only one person,* because blood particles may be left on the blade, which could spread infection from one person to another.

Shaving with an Electric Razor. Some people use electric razors for convenience. Other people may have to use them for medical reasons. Before shaving a person, always ask your supervising nurse whether the person is allowed to be shaved. Use electric razors instead of safety razors on all people with blood-clotting disorders and on people taking medication that changes how fast the blood clots. For safety, check the condition of the razor to make sure that the screen has no holes and the cord is not frayed. Use an electric razor only in a room where no one receives oxygen because the combination of the electric razor and the oxygen could set off a spark and start a fire. A battery-operated or rechargeable razor may be safe to use in a room with oxygen, but you must first clear such use with your supervising nurse.

To keep the razor in good working order, take it apart and clean it when finished. As when shaving with the safety razor, report any red areas, sores, nicks or cuts on the person's face to your supervising nurse.

Cleaning and Trimming Fingernails. Helping to wash someone's hands is part of daily personal care, and assisting with care for the fingernails is done as needed. Keeping a person's fingernails trimmed and smooth will help prevent injury to his or her skin.

Note: *Use caution when trimming the nails of a person who has diabetes, poor circulation, paralysis (on*

the paralyzed side) or decreased sensation in the hand. Check with your supervising nurse before trimming a person's nails.

Report to your supervising nurse any changes in the person's hands, such as reddened or discolored areas, sores, hangnails or badly torn nails.

Helping with Foot Care and Cleaning Toenails. Although you may assist a person with general foot and toenail care, it is generally a doctor or nurse who cuts a person's toenails because of the chance of injury that may come from cutting nails too short or cutting the skin around the nails. Remember that using orange sticks to clean under the toenails may also cause injury. Do not use them if the person has diabetes, poor circulation in the feet, paralysis of the legs or decreased sensation in the feet.

After assisting with foot care, report to your supervising nurse any changes in the person's feet, such as reddened or discolored areas, sores, breaks in the skin between the toes, injuries to the feet, toenails that need trimming and ill-fitting shoes and socks.

When to Help with Grooming

Help a person with grooming:
- As part of regular care
- When the person asks
- When your supervising nurse asks

ASSISTING WITH UNDRESSING AND DRESSING

How important are clothes to you? What does it feel like when you wear your favorite clothes or when you wear something you do not like? Deciding what to wear is part of who you are. It is part of your self-image. Getting dressed every day helps you maintain your sense of identity. Making choices about what to wear encourages you to maintain control over your independence.

Every day when you get up and decide what to wear, you consider the weather, where you are going, who you will be with and how you feel that day. Can you imagine if someone else made the decision for you? Suppose he or she selected clothing that was wrinkled, too big or small or mismatched? What would that do to your self-image?

The person in your care also likes to decide what to wear. Even though you may think it is easier to pick out clothes for her, she needs to decide what outfit to wear each day. How can you help someone decide what to wear? Even if the person has difficulty making decisions, you can help by offering two selections from which she can choose (Figure 12-6).

When helping someone select clothing, consider:

- The person's preferences
- The person's physical capabilities

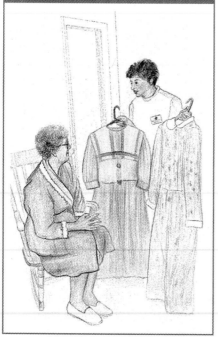

FIGURE 12-6 For someone like Mrs. McDay, who has a hard time making decisions and selecting clothing, you can offer two appropriate choices and ask, "Which one would you like to wear today?"

- Changing conditions, such as the time of day, scheduled activities, and the weather

Why Help with Undressing and Dressing?

Dressing properly is important to help people maintain dignity, stay warm and prevent their bodies from being exposed. Wearing shoes also helps to protect the feet from possible injury.

Undressing is also important. Over a period of time, a person's clothing absorbs perspiration, a waste product from the body, which needs to be washed out of the clothes.

How to Help with Undressing and Dressing

Today, you encourage Mr. Rivera to wear a nice, warm sweat suit. He sits in the bedroom chair to get dressed while you make his bed. Mr. Rivera takes a long time to fasten his sweat suit jacket, but you make the bed and talk with him as he completes the task. Taking the time to talk with Mr. Rivera provides you with an opportunity to learn more about him and helps him to feel more comfortable with you. By providing time for Mr. Rivera to finish snapping his jacket, you encourage his independence.

When helping someone get dressed, provide safety by making sure he or she sits down when putting on or taking off clothing. Sitting down eliminates the risk of the person standing on one foot, possibly losing balance, and falling. Make sure the person is dressed appropriately for the weather and situation. Provide privacy and warmth by keeping the person covered as much as possible while undressing and dressing.

When to Help with Undressing and Dressing

Help a person undress and dress:

- Every morning
- Every evening

- Before and after the person takes a shower or bath
- Whenever the person's clothes are soiled

ASSISTING WITH BATHING AND SHAMPOOING

Have you ever had to be bathed by another person? If so, how did you feel? Was the person who bathed you sensitive to your feelings? Have you ever bathed another person? Do you have any fears about bathing another person?

Part of your responsibility in assisting with personal care is to help people with bathing. Helping a person with bathing is important because it gives you an opportunity to observe physical and emotional changes in the person. When you help someone bathe, observe his or her skin for redness, open sores or bruises (see Appendix B, "Body Basics," the integumentary system), as well as any signs of physical abuse. During bathing, you may notice changes in the person's mood, which may be a clue that something is wrong.

What does it feel like to have someone else wash your hair? What does it feel like to have someone gently rub or massage your head or scalp? How do you feel after your clean hair is dried and styled? Many people enjoy having someone else wash their hair.

Helping a person shampoo his or her hair also is an important part of your responsibility in assisting with personal care. Shampooing helps clean the scalp, stimulate circulation and improve the person's self-image. The ideal way to shampoo someone's hair is in the shower or tub, although the same procedures can be used for shampooing at the sink.

Many people like to have their hair washed in a beauty shop. You can encourage a nursing home resident to arrange for an appointment with the hairdresser. Oftentimes, the facility may have a hairdresser on the premises.

When you help a person with bathing or shampooing, you often have to consider whether he bathes and shampoos in the bed, the shower or the tub. If he bathes in the bed, will you shampoo his hair while he is in the bed, or will you transfer him to a stretcher and wash his hair over a sink? If the person bathes in the shower or tub, can he get there by walking, or will you need to push him in the wheelchair? If the person bathes in the tub, will you have to use a mechanical lift?

The person in your care also has needs and preferences that influence your decision making. Does he prefer the tub or the shower? Does he like to use soap on his face? When he is not shampooing in the shower, does he like to wear a shower cap? How often does he like to shampoo? Does he like to use conditioner after shampooing?

Why Help Bathe and Shampoo?

Bathing does a lot for a person: It refreshes and relaxes, eliminates body odor, removes dirt and dead skin cells and stimulates movement and blood flow, or circulation, through the body (Figure 12-7). In addition, washing with soap and water reduces oily secretions, which provide a place for odor-producing bacteria to grow. Shampooing removes dirt, oil and bacteria from the hair and also prevents dandruff.

How to Help with Bathing and Shampooing

When you help a person bathe and shampoo his or her hair, you must observe the principles of care. As always, safety is the most important principle. Because bathrooms, showers and tubs can be dangerous places, make sure that showers and tubs have nonskid mats and surfaces and that grab bars are tightly fastened to the wall. To prevent burns, check the temperature of shower or bath water by using a bath thermometer or by touching the inside of your wrist to the water if a thermometer is not available. Your fingers are less sensitive than the inside of your wrist, and by using them you could underestimate the water temperature. Always follow these precautions when giving a person a complete bed bath or shampoo.

- Keep the person well covered to provide privacy and warmth (Figure 12-8).

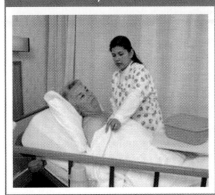

FIGURE 12-8 When helping someone bathe, be sure that you know and respect her personal and cultural feelings about modesty.

- Check the water temperature; it should be at 105 degrees F. It should not be warmer than 105 degrees F.
- Use proper body mechanics as you wash the person and move him from side to side.
- Inspect the person's skin for injuries, changes in condition and color (reddened areas or sores).
- When giving a shampoo, cover the person's eyes with a washcloth.
- Check for placement of drainage tubes and unhook or move them as necessary.

Note: *Get your supervisor's permission to unhook tubes.*

- Ask a coworker to help, if needed.
- Wash the perineal area of a female from front to back.

Practice proper infection control measures by wearing disposable gloves when providing **perineal care.** When assisting a woman with perineal care, bathe her from front to back (the genitals to the anus). Cleaning in this direction avoids contaminating the urethral opening with bacteria from the anal area. (Review Appendix B, "Body Basics," the reproductive system.)

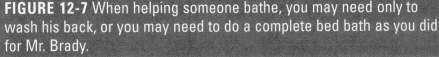

FIGURE 12-7 When helping someone bathe, you may need only to wash his back, or you may need to do a complete bed bath as you did for Mr. Brady.

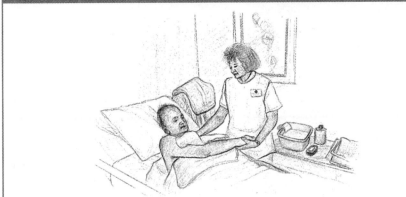

Bathing and Shampooing a Person in Bed. A complete bed bath involves bathing all parts of a person's body while she is in bed, as well as giving a backrub. A partial bed bath involves bathing only these parts of the body: face, hands, axillae, perineal area, back and buttocks. When assisting with a complete bed bath, help the person maintain her independence by discussing with her how she can help. A person may be able to help only by washing her face, but any amount of self-care is good. If the person has more ability, you may suggest that she do her own perineal care. In this case, hand her the washcloth and provide privacy for her, after making sure she is safe.

When shampooing the hair of someone who is in bed, place a waterproof sheet under the person's head to keep the bottom sheet from getting wet. Or position the person on a stretcher with side rails and wash her hair at the sink (Figure 12-9).

Many people enjoy a backrub after a bath. After washing and drying a person's back, put lotion on your hands and rub them together to warm the lotion. Rub the lotion into the person's skin, using circular motions, to relax her and stimulate circulation.

Showering and Shampooing. Many people enjoy bathing and shampooing in the shower. Before helping someone shower, reserve the shower, if necessary, and determine whether you need any special equipment. Assess the person to decide whether he is steady on his feet or needs to use a shower chair or shower seat (Figures 12-10 and 12-11).

Determine the best way to get the person to the shower room or bathroom: by walking or by riding in a wheelchair or shower chair. Accompany him to the shower room or bathroom to ensure his safety.

Tub Bathing and Shampooing. Today at the nursing home, you help Mr. Wilson with a tub bath after his evening meal. He always enjoys a bath before he goes to bed. He says he sleeps better after a nice, warm bath.

Before helping someone with a tub bath, reserve the tub room, if necessary. Assess the person to determine whether he can get into and out of the tub by himself or whether you have to help him with a mechanical lift (Figure 12-12). The information in Box 12-2 helps you make this decision.

Determine the best way to get the person to the tub room or bathroom: by walking or by riding in a wheelchair or shower chair. Accompany him to the tub room or bathroom so that you can prevent a possible fall. When you fill the bathtub, check the water temperature with a bath thermometer to make sure that the temperature is not over 105 degrees F. Shut off the hot water first to prevent hot water in the faucet from dripping on the person's skin.

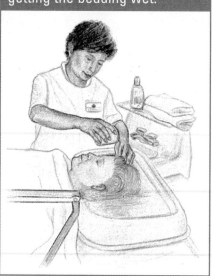

FIGURE 12-9 When you use this method for shampooing, water from the shampoo tray flows directly into the sink, avoiding any possibility of getting the bedding wet.

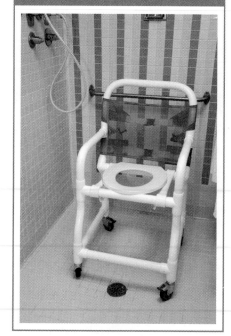

FIGURE 12-10 A shower chair is a waterproof chair on wheels. It is used to move a person into and out of the shower.

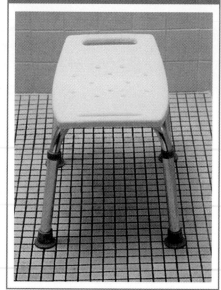

FIGURE 12-11 A shower seat is a removable chair or bench that enables a person to sit while showering.

FIGURE 12-12 This mechanical lift is used to help a person from a bed or chair into a shower chair.

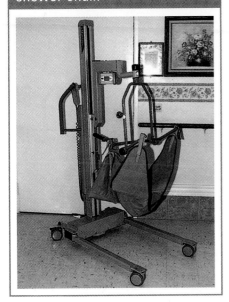

WHEN CAN A PERSON SAFELY GET IN AND OUT OF THE TUB WITHOUT A LIFT?

To help a person into the bathtub without the use of a lift, the person should be:

- Predictable.
- Able to reliably bear all or most of his or her own weight.
- Able to stand on one foot and lift the other foot over the edge of the tub with a minimum of assistance.
- Able to lower his or her body onto the tub seat or into the tub.

When to Help with Bathing and Shampooing

Set up regular bathing times based on the person's independence level, his preference for when to bathe, and your employer's policy on bathing. Assist him with shampooing as part of his personal care, following whatever schedule he would like, although it is recommended that a person wash his hair at least once or twice each week.

To practice the skills described in this chapter, follow the specific procedures that are explained step by step in Skills 22 through 35.

INFORMATION REVIEW

Circle the correct answers and fill in the blanks.

1. When you provide care, you must respect each person's need to maintain his own:
   a. toothbrush, razor and wardrobe.
   b. personal needs, self-image and independence.
   c. grooming.
   d. toenails.

2. When you help a person with mouth care:
   a. use a stiff toothbrush to clean his or her teeth thoroughly.
   b. first rinse the person's mouth with plain water.
   c. rinse the person's mouth with full-strength mouthwash after brushing.
   d. rinse the person's mouth with diluted mouthwash before and after mouth care.

3. When providing mouth care for an unconscious person, you should:
   a. position the person in a supine position.
   b. use a lot of water to clean the person's mouth thoroughly.
   c. turn the person on his side so that he does not aspirate.
   d. remain silent, because the person cannot hear you talk.

4. When assisting a woman with perineal care, always wipe from _____ to _____, using a clean part of the washcloth for each stroke.

Continued

5. When giving a person a complete bed bath and shampoo, do all of the following except:
   a. inspect the person's skin for injuries or changes in condition.
   b. ensure that water is at 140 degrees F.
   c. keep the person well covered.
   d. cover the person's eyes with a washcloth while shampooing.

6. What should you do when you finish using a disposable safety razor to shave someone?
   a. Recap the razor. Put it in the person's drawer.
   b. Do not recap the razor. Put it in the person's drawer.
   c. Do not recap the razor. Put it in the "sharps" container.
   d. Do not recap the razor. Put it in a plastic bag and put the bag in a trash can.

QUESTIONS TO ASK YOURSELF

1. Mrs. Jaskowitz is right-handed, but because of her stroke, she is not able to use her right hand to grip the toothbrush. How should you help Mrs. Jaskowitz brush her teeth?

2. Mr. Randal is unconscious. What should you talk about while you provide mouth care for him?

3. What should you look for on a person's skin during bath time? What should you report to your supervising nurse?

4. You are bathing Mrs. Feld when Mr. Lloyd, a confused gentleman from down the hall, walks into the room. He tries to enter the privacy curtain, but cannot seem to find the opening immediately. What should you do?

5. You walk by Mrs. Kitzmiller's room while a new nurse assistant is styling her hair. You have assisted Mrs. Kitzmiller before and you know she likes to wear her hair in a bun. The new nurse assistant is putting it in pigtails. What should you do?

6. Because of a problem with his leg, Mr. Wingard has been having bed baths without a shampoo for 11 days. He likes to wash his hair only in the shower. Today your supervising nurse has asked you to make sure his hair is washed. How should you do this?

7. Mrs. Lanver wants to help dress herself, but she is very slow. What can you do to increase her independence and maintain her dignity?

Skill 22: Brushing and Flossing a Person's Teeth

PRECAUTIONS

- Slide (do not snap) the floss carefully between the teeth without pressing against the gums. Gums are soft, and dental floss can easily cut them.
- Always mix mouthwash with water. Gums are sensitive, and full-strength mouthwash may hurt them.
- Replace the person's toothbrush every 3 to 4 months or when it begins to fray or show wear. A worn toothbrush cannot properly clean the teeth and may injure the gums.
- Use a toothbrush with soft bristles. Also, use just enough pressure so that you get good contact with the tooth surface without flattening the bristles.

PREPARATION

1. Gather supplies:
   - One towel
   - Two pairs of disposable gloves
   - Lip cream or petroleum jelly and cotton-tipped applicator
   - Toothbrush, toothpaste and emesis basin
   - Plastic trash bag
   - Laundry bag (or plastic bag for wet or soiled linens)
2. Follow Preparation Standards (see Chapter 7).

PROCEDURE

1. In a drinking cup, prepare a solution of half water and half mouthwash (Figure 12-13). ☐ ☐

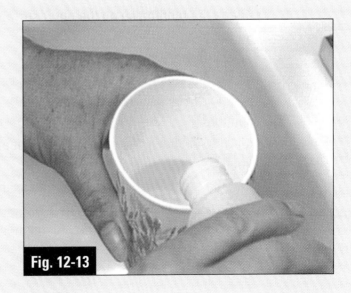

Fig. 12-13

2. Help the person turn her head toward you and raise the head of the bed. ☐ ☐

3. Unfold the towel. Place it across the person's chest. ☐ ☐

4. Put on disposable gloves and any other necessary protective gear, such as protective eyewear and disposable gown, as needed. ☐ ☐

5. Place the emesis basin on the towel under the person's chin. ☐ ☐

6. Give the person a mouthful of the mouth-wash mixture to rinse her mouth. Hold the emesis basin under her chin to catch the liquid. ☐ ☐

7. Wet the toothbrush by pouring mouthwash solution over it. ☐ ☐

8. Put toothpaste on the wet brush (Figure 12-14). ☐ ☐

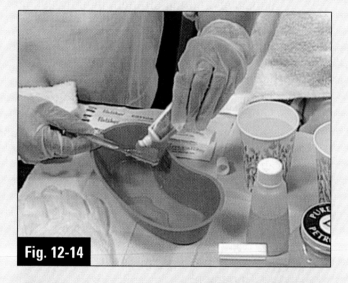

Fig. 12-14

9. Clean the person's mouth by first brushing the upper teeth and gums:

   • Place the toothbrush on the outer surface of the upper teeth at about a 45-degree angle (Figure 12-15).

   • Move the brush back and forth, using very short strokes and a gentle scrubbing motion.

   • Scrub the chewing surfaces of the upper teeth.

   • Put the brush vertically against the inside surfaces of the front upper teeth and brush with a gentle up-and-down motion.

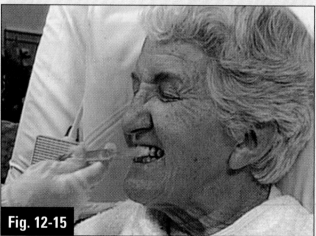

Fig. 12-15

- Brush the lower teeth and gums in the same way, and brush the tongue very gently (Figure 12-16). ☐ ☐

10. Help the person rinse her mouth with the mouthwash mixture. Hold the emesis basin under her chin to catch the liquid. ☐ ☐

11. Break off about 18 inches of floss from the dispenser. Wrap most of the floss around the middle fingers of both hands, leaving 1 inch of floss between your hands (Figure 12-17). Stretch it tightly between your thumbs and index fingers. ☐ ☐

12. Gently insert the floss between each of the person's teeth without pressing against her gums. Use a gentle sawing motion to guide the floss between the teeth, never "snapping" it into the gums.

- Hold the floss against the tooth and scrape the side of the tooth, moving the floss away from the gum. After you floss each tooth, unwrap a clean 1-inch section of floss from your finger and wrap the soiled floss around the other finger.

- Floss the teeth in this order: Start between the two front teeth, then do the first half of the upper teeth, the second half of upper teeth, the first half of lower teeth, the second half of the lower teeth. ☐ ☐

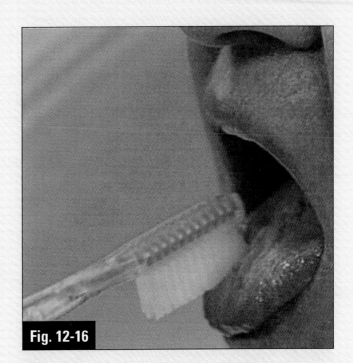

Fig. 12-16

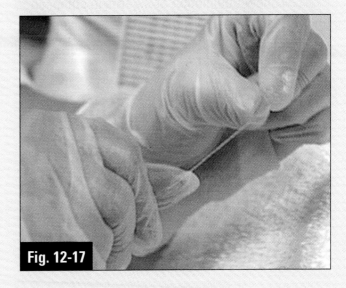

Fig. 12-17

Skill 22: Brushing and Flossing a Person's Teeth—cont'd

13. Help the person rinse her mouth with the mouthwash mixture (Figure 12-18). Hold the emesis basin under her chin to catch the liquid. ☐ ☐
14. Wipe resident's mouth and remove towel.
15. Clean and dry supplies.
16. Remove disposable gloves and wash your hands. ☐ ☐

ADDITIONAL INFORMATION

Encourage the person to apply lip cream or petroleum jelly to her lips, or use a cotton-tipped applicator to apply the lip cream or petroleum jelly to the person's lips.

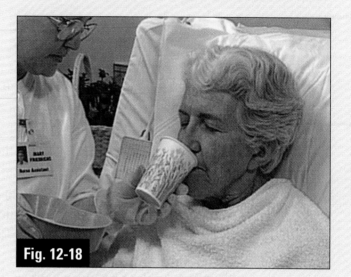

Fig. 12-18

 ## COMPLETION

Follow Completion Standards in compliance with your facility. For a complete list of those used in this course, see Chapter 7, "Controlling the Spread of Germs."

Skill 23: Providing Denture Care

PRECAUTIONS

- Dentures, or false teeth, are very expensive. You must handle them very carefully so that they do not get damaged. Dentures are very slippery when coated with mucus or saliva.
- Always mix mouthwash with water. Gums are sensitive, and full-strength mouthwash may hurt them.
- The person should remove his or her dentures for a least 8 hours every day to rest the gums, usually at night.

PREPARATION

1. Gather supplies:
   - One washcloth
   - One towel
   - Two pairs of disposable gloves
   - Tissues
   - Disposable mouth sponges
   - Lip cream or petroleum jelly and cotton-tipped applicator or gauze squares
   - Plastic trash bag
   - Laundry bag (or plastic bag for wet or soiled linens)
2. Follow Preparation Standards (see Chapter 7).

PROCEDURE

Task 1: Removing Dentures

1. In a drinking cup, prepare a solution of half water and half mouthwash. ☐ ☐
2. Ask the person to turn her head toward you and raise the head of the bed. ☐ ☐
3. Put on disposable gloves. ☐ ☐

4. Unfold the towel. Place it across the person's chest. ☐ ☐
5. Place the emesis basin on the towel under the person's chin. ☐ ☐
6. Have the person rinse her mouth with the mouthwash mixture. ☐ ☐
7. Have the person remove her dentures and put them in the denture cup. ☐ ☐
8. If the person needs assistance, use a tissue to hold her teeth firmly with your thumb and index finger (Figure 12-19). Use a rocking motion to gently remove the teeth and put them in the denture cup. ☐ ☐
9. Place the denture cup in the proper storage place. ☐ ☐
10. Remove disposable gloves and wash your hands. ☐ ☐

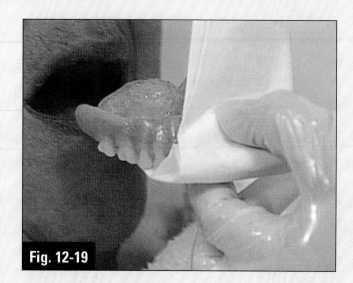
Fig. 12-19

Task 2: Providing Care for the Person's Mouth

1. Put on disposable gloves and have the person rinse her mouth with the mouthwash mixture. ☐ ☐
2. Help the person clean her mouth with mouth sponges dipped in the mouthwash mixture (Figure 12-20). If she has any of her natural teeth, help her clean and floss them, using the toothbrush and flouridated toothpaste. Help her clean her entire mouth. ☐ ☐
3. Have the person rinse her mouth with the mouthwash mixture. ☐ ☐

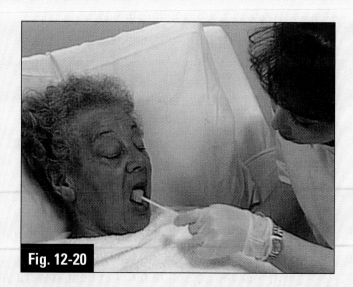
Fig. 12-20

Task 3: Cleaning and Replacing Dentures

1. Line the sink with the washcloth or several paper towels. ☐ ☐
2. Turn on the faucet with a fresh paper towel. Adjust the water temperature so that it is cool. ☐ ☐
3. Put on disposable gloves. ☐ ☐
4. Wet the toothbrush and apply toothpaste. ☐ ☐
5. Fill the sink half full with cool water. ☐ ☐
6. Turn off faucet with paper towel. ☐ ☐
7. Rinse denture cup and lid. ☐ ☐
8. Rinse dentures and place on clean paper towel. ☐ ☐
9. Hold dentures over the sink. Use the toothbrush to clean them. Brush all surfaces (Figure 12-21). ☐ ☐
10. Rinse the dentures under cool, running water. ☐ ☐
11. Put the clean dentures back in the denture cup. Turn off the faucet with a paper towel. ☐ ☐
12. Help the person put the dentures back in his or her mouth, if needed. If the dentures are not to be worn, place them in the denture cup and add enough water to cover them (Figure 12-22). ☐ ☐
13. Remove your disposable gloves and wash your hands. ☐ ☐

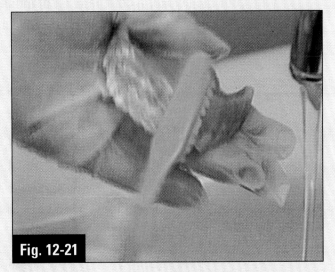

Fig. 12-21

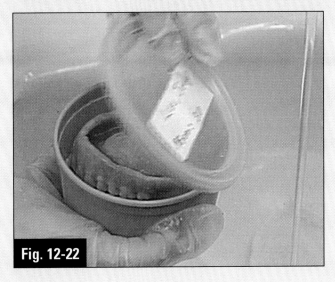

Fig. 12-22

Skill 23: Providing Denture Care—cont'd

 COMPLETION

Follow Completion Standards in compliance with your facility. For a complete list of those used in this course, see Chapter 7, "Controlling the Spread of Germs."

Skill 24: Providing Mouth Care for an Unconscious Person

PRECAUTIONS

- When working on an unconscious person, open the mouth gently, without using force.
- Always position the person's head to the side so that he will not aspirate, or breathe in, any fluids into the lungs. An unconscious person cannot swallow fluids.
- Always mix mouthwash with water. Gums are sensitive, and full-strength mouthwash may hurt them.
- Use a toothbrush with soft bristles. Us just enough pressure to give you good contact with the tooth surface without flattening the bristles.

PREPARATION

1. Gather supplies:
   - Two towels
   - Two pairs of disposable gloves
   - Gauze
   - Disposable mouth sponges
   - Petroleum jelly and gauze squares or cotton-tipped swabs
   - Plastic trash bag
   - Laundry bag (or plastic bag for wet or soiled linens)
   - Wooden tongue depressor and tape (optional)
2. Follow Preparation Standards (see Chapter 7).

PROCEDURE

1. Make a padded tongue depressor if needed. ☐ ☐

2. Prepare a solution of half water and half mouthwash in a cup. ☐ ☐

3. To prevent aspiration, elevate the head of the bed. ☐ ☐

4. Turn his head toward you. ☐ ☐

5. Place a towel under the person's head and across his chest. ☐ ☐

6. Put on disposable gloves. ☐ ☐

7. Place the emesis basin on the towel near the person's cheek. ☐ ☐

8. Without using force, gently separate the person's upper and lower teeth. To do this, cross the middle finger and thumb of one hand. Put the thumb against the person's top teeth and the middle finger against his lower teeth and gently push the finger and thumb apart (Figure 12-23). This causes the jaw to open. ☐ ☐

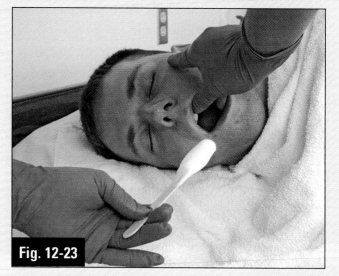

Fig. 12-23

9. You may need to use a padded tongue depressor as a prop to hold the person's mouth open. Check with your supervising nurse before using it. Padded tongue depressors may or may not be used in your facility. ☐ ☐

10. Clean the soft tissues of the person's mouth with a mouth sponge dipped in diluted mouthwash. Use just enough fluid to moisten the sponge. Clean the entire mouth:
   • Roof
   • Inside of cheeks
   • Teeth
   • Gums
   • Under tongue
   • Lips ☐ ☐

11. Wrap gauze squares or use a mouth sponge around your finger to remove thick mucus or secretions. ☐ ☐

12. Use a soft toothbrush moistened with diluted mouthwash to clean the person's teeth. ☐ ☐

13. Apply a small amount of petroleum jelly to the person's lips, using a cotton swab or gauze square. ☐ ☐

14. Remove disposable gloves and wash your hands. ☐ ☐

COMPLETION

Follow Completion Standards in compliance with your facility. For a complete list of those used in this course, see Chapter 7, "Controlling the Spread of Germs."

Skill 25: Brushing and Combing a Person's Hair

PRECAUTIONS

- Brush and comb hair gently so that you do not pull out the person's hair.
- Use a brush or a comb with blunt teeth so that you will not hurt the person's scalp.

PREPARATION

1. Gather supplies:
   - Towel
   - Laundry bag
2. Follow Preparation Standards (see Chapter 7).

PROCEDURE

1. Place the towel over the person's shoulders (or under the shoulders if the person is lying in bed). ☐ ☐
2. Remove the person's eyeglasses and hairpins from hair. ☐ ☐
3. Brush the hair gently, beginning at the ends, and work up in sections to the scalp (Figure 12-24). ☐ ☐
4. Style the person's hair the way she likes it. ☐ ☐
5. Provide a mirror during styling. ☐ ☐

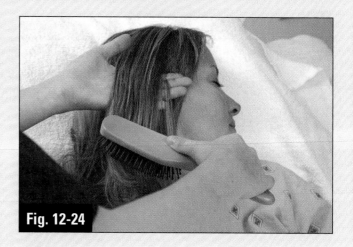

Fig. 12-24

ADDITIONAL INFORMATION

It is easier to comb a person's hair when she is sitting, but you also can comb a person's hair when she is lying in bed. To do this, turn her head first to one side and then to the other.

COMPLETION

Follow Completion Standards in compliance with your facility. For a complete list of those used in this course, see Chapter 7, "Controlling the Spread of Germs."

Skill 26: Helping a Man Shave with a Safety Razor

PRECAUTIONS

- Always ask your supervising nurse if a person should be shaved. Some medicines can cause excessive bleeding if a person is cut.
- Make sure each razor is used by only one person. Because blood particles may be left on the blade, sharing a razor may spread blood-borne infections.

PREPARATION

1. Gather supplies:
   - Towel
   - Washcloth
   - Disposable gloves
   - Disposable razor
   - Shaving cream
   - Plastic trash bag
   - Laundry bag (or plastic bag for wet or soiled linen)
2. Follow Preparation Standards (see Chapter 7).

PROCEDURE

1. Fill the washbasin with warm water and place the basin on a clean surface. ☐ ☐
2. Help the person into a sitting position. ☐ ☐
3. Place the towel over his chest. ☐ ☐
4. Put on disposable gloves. ☐ ☐
5. Inspect his skin for moles, birthmarks or sores. ☐ ☐
6. Assist the person in washing his face with soap (optional) and warm water. Remove soap, if used, with wet washcloth. ☐ ☐

7. Assist the person in applying shaving cream to his face. ☐ ☐
8. Assist the person with shaving, if needed. ☐ ☐
9. With the fingers of one hand, hold the person's skin tight as you use the razor to shave downward. By shaving downward, you are shaving in the direction that his hair grows (Figure 12-25). ☐ ☐
10. Rinse the razor often in the washbasin of water to remove hair. ☐ ☐
11. Use shorter strokes around the person's chin and lips. Work downward toward his neck under his chin. Shave one side of the face first and then the other. ☐ ☐
12. Use the wet washcloth to remove the remaining shaving cream. ☐ ☐
13. Dry the person's face with the towel that is covering his chest. ☐ ☐
14. Give the person a hand mirror so that he can inspect the shaved area. ☐ ☐
15. Assist the person to apply aftershave lotion (optional). ☐ ☐
16. Remove disposable gloves and wash your hands. ☐ ☐

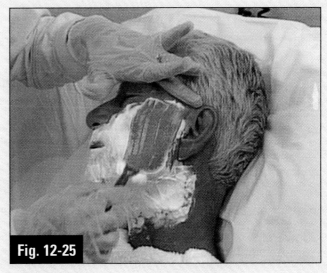
Fig. 12-25

COMPLETION

Follow Completion Standards in compliance with your facility. For a complete list of those used in this course, see Chapter 7, "Controlling the Spread of Germs."

Skill 27: Helping a Man Shave with an Electric Razor

PRECAUTIONS

- Use electric razors instead of safety razors on all people with blood-clotting disorders or on people undergoing special drugs that change how fast the blood clots.
- Always ask the supervising nurse if a person should be shaved.
- Check to see if the razor is in good shape (the screen has no holes, the cord is not frayed.)
- Use an electric razor only in a room where no one is receiving oxygen. If oxygen is present, you could set off a spark and start a fire.

PREPARATION

1. Gather supplies:
   - Towel
   - Washcloth
   - Electric razor
   - Preshave lotion
   - Laundry bag (or plastic bag for wet or soiled linens)
   - Aftershave lotion
2. Follow Preparation Standards (see Chapter 7).

PROCEDURE

1. Fill the washbasin with warm water and place it on a clean surface. ☐ ☐
2. Help the person into a sitting position. ☐ ☐
3. Place the towel over his chest. ☐ ☐
4. Put on disposable gloves. ☐ ☐
5. Inspect the person's skin for moles, birth-marks or sores. ☐ ☐

6. Have the person wash his face with soap (optional) and warm water, if he is able. Remove the soap, if used, with the wet washcloth. ☐ ☐

7. Assist the person in applying preshave lotion to his face. ☐ ☐

8. With the fingers of one hand, hold the person's skin tight as you use the razor to shave as the manufacturer suggests—usually in a circular motion (Figure 12-26). ☐ ☐

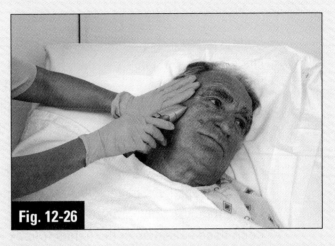
Fig. 12-26

9. Work downward toward the person's neck under his chin. ☐ ☐

10. Use the wet washcloth to rinse the person's face. ☐ ☐

11. Dry the person's face with the towel that is covering his chest. ☐ ☐

12. Give the person a hand mirror so that he can inspect the shaved area. ☐ ☐

13. Apply aftershave lotion (optional). ☐ ☐

14. Remove disposable gloves and wash your hands. ☐ ☐

COMPLETION

Follow Completion Standards in compliance with your facility. For a complete list of those used in this course, see Chapter 7, "Controlling the Spread of Germs."

Skill 28: Cleaning and Trimming a Person's Fingernails

PRECAUTIONS

- Keep a person's fingernails trimmed and smooth to prevent injury to his or her skin.
- When trimming a person's fingernails, make sure his or her nails extend slightly beyond the tip of the fingers so that you do not injure the skin on the fingers.
- Use extra caution when you cut the fingernails of people who have diabetes, poor circulation, paralysis (on paralyzed side) or decreased sensation in the hands. *Check with your supervising nurse before trimming a person's nails.*

PREPARATION

1. Gather supplies:
   - Washcloth
   - Disposable gloves
   - Nail clippers
   - Orange stick (wooden stick with an angled edge used in manicuring)
   - Emery board or nail file
   - Towel
   - Plastic trash bag
   - Laundry bag (or plastic bag for wet or soiled linens)
   - Bed protector (if the basin will be placed on the bed)
2. Follow Preparation Standards (see Chapter 7).

PROCEDURE

1. Fill the washbasin with warm water and place it on a clean surface. Check the temperature of the water. ☐ ☐

2. Help the person to a sitting position, if possible. ☐ ☐

3. Place the basin of water within the person's reach. ☐ ☐

4. Put on disposable gloves. ☐ ☐

5. Help the person soak her or his hands in warm water for 5 minutes (Figure 12-27). ☐ ☐

6. Apply soap to a wet wash cloth. ☐ ☐

7. Lift the person's hands from the water, one at a time, and hold each over the washbasin as you wash the hand, push the skin at the base of the nails, or cuticles, back gently with a washcloth (Figure 12-28). Place wash cloth in laundry bag when finished. ☐ ☐

8. Rinse the person's hands. ☐ ☐

9. Clean under the fingernails with the orange stick (Figure 12-29). Wipe the orange stick on the towel after cleaning under each fingernail. ☐ ☐

10. Unfold a towel and rest the person's wet hands on it. ☐ ☐

11. Dry the person's hands thoroughly. Make sure the skin is dry between her fingers. ☐ ☐

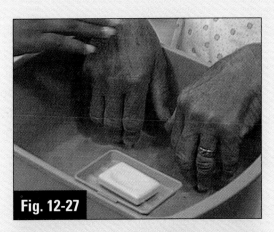

Fig. 12-27

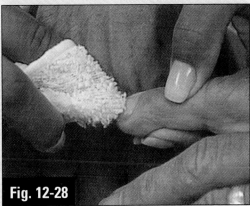

Fig. 12-28

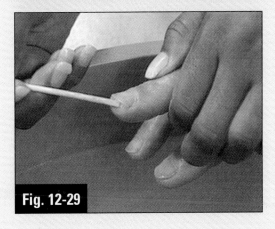

Fig. 12-29

12. Use nail clippers to cut the person's fingernails straight across, if safe to do so (Figure 12-30). ☐ ☐

13. Use a nail file or an emery board to shape, trim, smooth and remove sharp edges from her fingernails. ☐ ☐

14. Put lotion on the person's hands. Gently massage each hand from the fingertips toward the wrist. ☐ ☐

15. Remove your gloves and wash your hands. ☐ ☐

16. Raise the side rail, if used. ☐ ☐

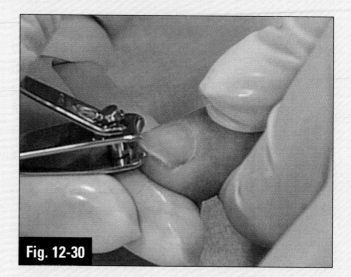

Fig. 12-30

COMPLETION

Follow Completion Standards in compliance with your facility. For a complete list of those used in this course, see Chapter 7, "Controlling the Spread of Germs."

Skill 29: Providing Foot Care and Cleaning a Person's Toenails

PRECAUTIONS

- Although you provide a person with general foot and toenail care, only a doctor or a nurse should cut a person's toenails because of the chance of injury from cutting nails too short or cutting the skin around the nail.

PREPARATION

1. Gather supplies:
   - Disposable bed protector
   - Disposable gloves (optional)
   - Towel
   - Washcloth
   - Plastic trash bag
   - Laundry bag (or plastic bag for wet or soiled linens)
2. Follow Preparation Standards (see Chapter 7).

PROCEDURE

1. Fill the washbasin with warm water, check temperature and place it on a clean surface. ☐ ☐
2. Help the person out of bed and into a chair, if possible. ☐ ☐
3. Place a disposable bed protector on the floor in front of the person. ☐ ☐
4. Place the washbasin on the bed protector. ☐ ☐
5. Help the person soak her feet for at least 5 minutes. ☐ ☐
6. Put on disposable gloves (optional) and help the person wash her feet with a soapy washcloth (Figure 12-31). ☐ ☐

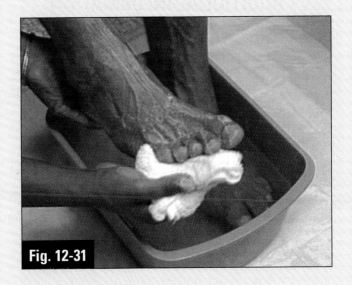

Fig. 12-31

Skill 29: Providing Foot Care and Cleaning a Person's Toenails—cont'd

7. Empty the washbasin into the sink and rinse it out. Refill it with warm water and check the temperature. ☐ ☐
8. Rinse the person's feet in the fresh, warm water. ☐ ☐
9. Dry the person's feet thoroughly, especially between the toes, pushing back the cuticles with a towel (Figure 12-32). ☐ ☐
10. Inspect the condition of the skin on the person's feet, including between all toes. ☐ ☐
11. Massage the person's feet with lotion. Begin with the toes and move upward toward the legs, but massage only the feet, *not* the legs (Figure 12-33). ☐ ☐
12. Remove disposable gloves if worn. ☐ ☐
13. Help the person put on clean socks and shoes. ☐ ☐
14. Wash your hands. ☐ ☐

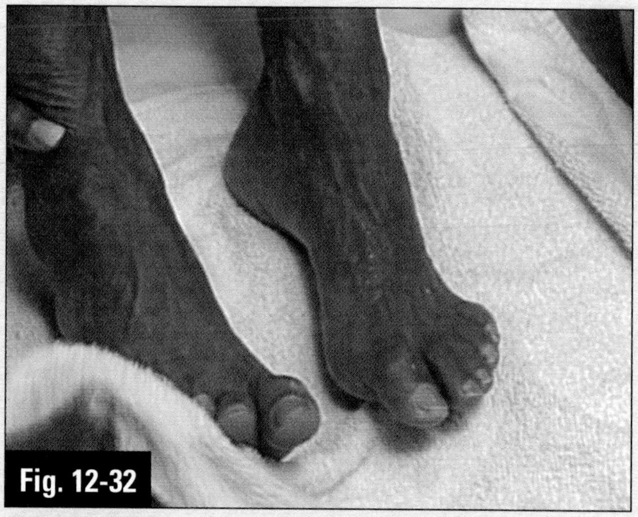

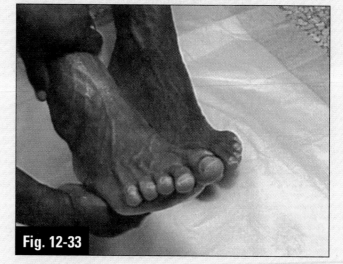

Fig. 12-32

Fig. 12-33

ADDITIONAL INFORMATION

If the person cannot get out of bed, help her lie flat or in a semi-Fowler's position. Place the washbasin on a bed protector near her feet. Flex the person's knee and place her feet into the basin.

COMPLETION

Follow Completion Standards in compliance with your facility. For a complete list of those used in this course, see Chapter 7, "Controlling the Spread of Germs."

Skill 30: Helping a Person Undress

PRECAUTIONS

- To avoid the possibility of the person falling, make sure he or she sits down when taking off his or her clothing.
- To provide privacy and warmth, keep the person covered as much as possible while he or she undresses.

PREPARATION

1. Gather supplies:
   - Bath blanket
   - Laundry bag (or plastic bag for wet or soiled laundry)
2. Follow Preparation Standards (see Chapter 7).

PROCEDURE

1. Help the person sit on the side of the bed. ☐ ☐

2. Help him take off his shirt (or her dress). If the person has a weak or paralyzed side, remove the clothing from the strong or unaffected side first (Figure 12-34). ☐ ☐

   If the person has an IV:
   - Carefully gather the clothing material, starting at the shoulder of the sleeve that has the IV. Glide the sleeve over the needle site and tubing.
   - Holding the gathered sleeve, carefully unhook the IV bottle from the IV pole and slide the tubing, the bag and your hand through the gathered sleeve.
   - Hook the IV bottle back on the IV pole. ☐ ☐

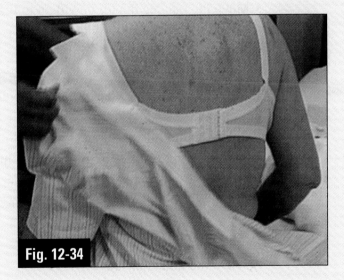

Fig. 12-34

3. Cover the person, as necessary, with the bath blanket. ☐ ☐

4. Help the person take off his undershirt (or her bra and slip). ☐ ☐

5. Help the person put on his pajama top (or her nightgown). ☐ ☐

   If the person has an IV:

   • Gather the sleeve of the pajama top (or gown) that will be going on the arm with the IV.

   • Carefully unhook the IV bottle from the pole.

   • Slide the bottle, the tubing and the person's arm through the sleeve.

   • Move the pajama top (or gown) up to the person's shoulder. ☐ ☐

6. Help the person take off shoes and socks. ☐ ☐

7. Help the person lie down in bed, and cover him with the bath blanket. ☐ ☐

8. Help the person remove underpants and pants. Ask the person to raise his or her hips (Figure 12-35) so that you can reach under the bath blanket to help slip the pants down over the hips. ☐ ☐

9. Help the person put on pajama bottoms. Remove the bath blanket. ☐ ☐

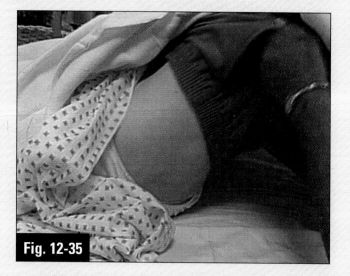

Fig. 12-35

ADDITIONAL INFORMATION

If a person cannot raise the hips to wiggle out of his or her underpants and pants while lying down in a supine position:

- Unfasten the zipper, buttons or ties and turn the person on his or her side and pull the pants over the buttocks and hip on that side.
- Repeat the process on the other side.
- Turn the person back into a supine position.
    Use the same process in reverse to assist in putting on pajama bottoms.

COMPLETION

Follow Completion Standards in compliance with your facility. For a complete list of those used in this course, see Chapter 7, "Controlling the Spread of Germs."

Skill 31: Helping a Person Dress

PRECAUTIONS

- To avoid the possibility of the person falling, make sure he or she sits down when taking off his or her clothing.
- Make sure the person is dressed appropriately for the weather and situation.
- To provide privacy and warmth, keep the person covered as much as possible while he or she undresses.
- If the person has a weak or paralyzed side, dress the affected side first.

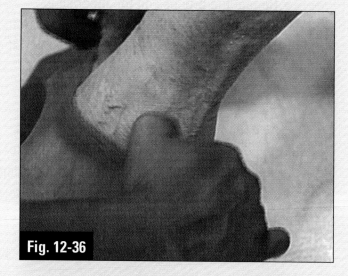

Fig. 12-36

PREPARATION

1. Gather supplies:
   - Bath blanket
   - Laundry bag (or plastic bag for wet or soiled laundry)
2. Follow Preparation Standards (see Chapter 7).

PROCEDURE

1. Help the person lie flat and cover with a bath blanket. ☐ ☐
2. Remove the person's pajama bottoms (or underwear). ☐ ☐
3. Sit the person on the side of the bed, and help put on socks (or stockings) (Figure 12-36). ☐ ☐
4. Help the person put on underwear and pants partway (Figure 12-37). ☐ ☐
5. Help the person put on shoes. Check for proper shoe fit. ☐ ☐
6. Assist the person to stand and pull up both underwear and pants. ☐ ☐

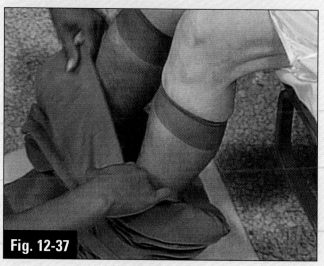

Fig. 12-37

7. Help the person sit back down. ☐ ☐

8. If the person is female, adjust the bath blanket so that it covers her shoulders and upper body. Remove her gown from underneath the bath blanket to avoid exposing her. If the gown must come off over her head, pull it off one arm at a time while she uses the other arm to hold the bath blanket over herself. Help her hook her bra in front and turn it around so the hooks are in the back. Assist her to pull up her bra straps. ☐ ☐

9. Help with putting arms into the armholes of undershirts (or slips). ☐ ☐

10. Help with putting arms into the sleeves of shirts (or dresses). Smooth out the back of the shirt (or dress) and fasten it. ☐ ☐

11. Help the person to stand to tuck in the shirt and fasten or zip the pants. ☐ ☐

12. Help the person with accessories, if he or she asks you. ☐ ☐

ADDITIONAL INFORMATION

If a person cannot sit up for dressing, help him lie in a supine position and:

- Put both his legs into the legs of the underpants and pants.
- Turn him on his side and pull his pants over his buttocks and hip on that side.
- Repeat the process on the other side by turning him onto his other hip.
- Turn him back into a supine position.
- Fasten the zipper, buttons or ties as needed.

Skill 31: Helping a Person Dress—cont'd

COMPLETION

Follow Completion Standards in compliance with your facility. For a complete list of those used in this course, see Chapter 7, "Controlling the Spread of Germs."

Skill 32: Helping a Person with a Complete Bed Bath and Shampoo

PRECAUTIONS

- Keep the person well covered to provide privacy and warmth.
- Check the water temperature. It should be warm to the touch on the inside of your wrist. If the water is too hot, it can injure the person's skin. If the water is too cold, it can chill the person.
- Use proper body mechanics as you wash the person and move him or her from back to side.
- Inspect the person's skin for injuries, changes in condition and color (such as reddened areas or bruises) and sores.
- Wash the perineal area of a female from front to back. This decreases the chance of infection.
- When giving a shampoo, cover the person's eyes with a washcloth to prevent shampoo from getting in the eyes.
- Check for placement of drainage tubes, and unhook or move them as necessary.
- Ask a co-worker to help if needed.

PREPARATION

1. Gather supplies:
   - For the bath:
     - Bath blanket (a flannel sheet used to keep the person warm during bathing)
     - Two towels
     - Two washcloths
     - Disposable bed protector
     - Disposable gloves
     - Plastic trash bag
     - Laundry bag (or plastic bag for wet or soiled linens)

- For the shampoo:
  - Two towels
  - Two washcloths
  - Waterproof chair
  - Waterproof sheet
  - Shampoo tray, plastic sheet or large plastic trash bag
  - Cup or pitcher (for rinsing the hair)
  - Empty washbasin
2. Follow Preparation Standards (see Chapter 7).

PROCEDURE

Task 1: Bathing the Person

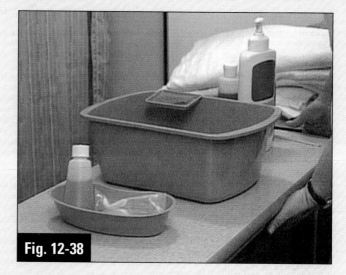

Fig. 12-38

1. Fill the washbasin with warm water, check temperature with your wrist, and place it on the over-bed table (Figure 12-38). ☐ ☐
2. Adjust the angle of the head of the bed to a flat position. ☐ ☐
3. Help the person move closer to the side of the bed where you are working. ☐ ☐
4. Put on disposable gloves. ☐ ☐
5. Remove and fold the bedspread and blanket for reuse. Put the bath blanket over the person. ☐ ☐
6. Have the person hold the bath blanket under his chin or tuck the edges of the bath blanket under his shoulders or pillow while you roll the top sheet down to the bottom of the bed. ☐ ☐
7. Take off the person's gown by slipping it off each arm and pulling it from under the bath blanket on the side closest to you. ☐ ☐

8. Place a towel across the person's chest. □ □

9. Wet the washcloth and make a mitt with it by:
   - Holding a corner of the washcloth between your thumb and fingers.
   - Wrapping the rest of the cloth around your hand and holding it with your thumb.
   - Folding the cloth over your fingers and tucking it under the fold in your palm. □ □

10. Without using soap, use the washcloth to bathe the eye farther from you. Always begin at the inner corner of the eye, near the nose. Then move the washcloth across the eye to the outer corner. Use the towel to dry the eye. Use the opposite end of the mitt and towel to bathe and dry the other eye. □ □

11. Using soap sparingly; wash, rinse and dry the person's face, neck and ears (Figure 12-39). □ □

12. Fold back the bath blanket on the person's arm that is farther from you. Place the towel lengthwise under the arm. □ □

13. Wash, rinse and dry the shoulder, arm and underarm, or axilla. Use the towel that was under the arm to dry it (Figure 12-40). □ □

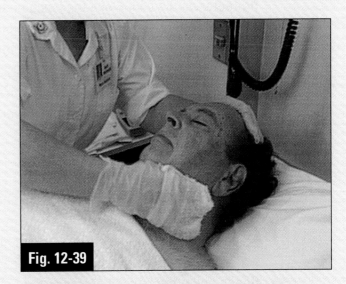
Fig. 12-39

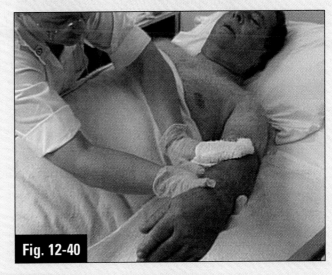
Fig. 12-40

14. Wash, rinse and dry the person's hand. When possible, place his hand in the washbasin (Figure 12-41). To do this, place a bed protector on the bed. Place the basin on top of the bed protector, and place the person's hand in the basin or place the basin on the over-bed table. ☐ ☐

15. Fold back the bath blanket on the person's arm that is nearer to you. Place the towel lengthwise under the arm. ☐ ☐

16. Wash, rinse and dry the shoulder, arm, axilla and wash hand as in Step 14. ☐ ☐

17. Remove the towel from under the arm, and cover it with the bath blanket. ☐ ☐

18. Place the towel over the person's chest and abdomen on top of the bath blanket. ☐ ☐

19. Reach under the towel that is over the bath blanket and fold the bath blanket down to the person's pubic area without exposing it. Leave the towel in place so that the person is not completely exposed. ☐ ☐

20. Fold back the towel to expose the side of the person's chest that is farther from you. Wash, rinse and dry the person's chest. Inspect under the person's breast and skin folds as you work. ☐ ☐

21. Dry the person's skin completely. Recover the chest with the towel. ☐ ☐

22. Fold back the towel to expose the side of the person's chest that is nearer to you (Figure 12-42) as in Step 20. ☐ ☐

23. Wash, rinse and dry the chest. ☐ ☐

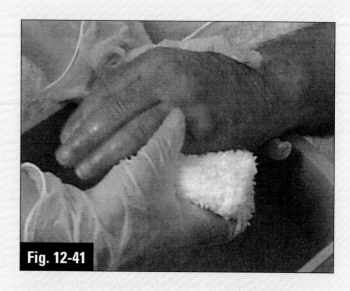

Fig. 12-41

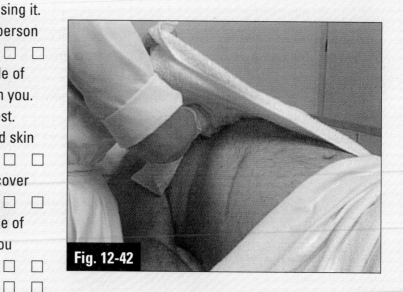

Fig. 12-42

24. Wash, rinse and dry the person's stomach, or abdomen, in the same manner as the chest, doing the farther side first, and then the nearer side. ☐ ☐

25. Pull the bath blanket back up to cover the chest and abdomen, and remove the towel from underneath. ☐ ☐

26. Change the water if it becomes too soapy or cool. ☐ ☐

27. Fold the bath blanket away from the person's leg that is farther from you. Place the towel lengthwise under the leg (Figure 12-43). ☐ ☐

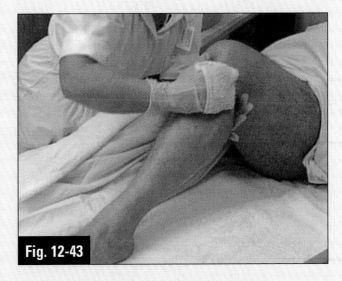

Fig. 12-43

28. Wash the leg and foot. When possible, place the foot in the washbasin. To do this, move the towel down under the foot. Move the washbasin onto the towel. Help the person bend the knee and place the foot into the washbasin (Figure 12-44). ☐ ☐

29. Use the mitt to wash the person's foot. ☐ ☐

30. Rinse the leg and foot. Help the person to move the leg out of the washbasin and onto the towel. Move the washbasin back to the over-bed table or nightstand. ☐ ☐
Use the towel to dry the person's legs and feet, making sure the skin between the toes is dry. ☐ ☐

31. Recover the leg with the bath blanket. Remove the towel from under the leg. ☐ ☐

32. Fold the bath blanket away from the person's leg that is nearer to you. Place the towel under the leg. ☐ ☐

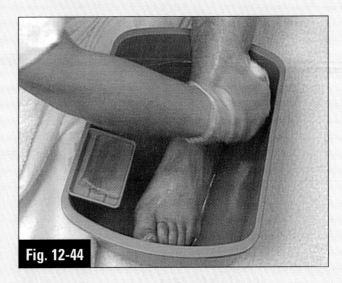

Fig. 12-44

33. Wash, rinse and dry the leg and foot as in Steps 28-30. ☐ ☐

34. Recover the leg with the bath blanket. Remove the towel from under the leg. ☐ ☐

35. Change the water. ☐ ☐

36. Help the person turn onto one side so that his or her back is facing you. ☐ ☐

37. Place the towel on the sheet behind the person's neck, back and buttocks. Drape the bath sheet over the person's chest, shoulders, abdomen and legs. ☐ ☐

38. Wash, rinse and dry the person's neck, back and buttocks. Inspect the skin as you work. ☐ ☐

Task 2: Rubbing the Person's Back

The person may want a back massage after the bath.

1. Squeeze some lotion onto the palm of your hand. Warm it by rubbing your hands together (Figure 12-45). ☐ ☐

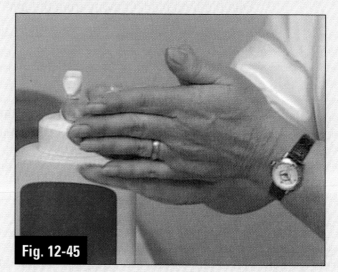

Fig. 12-45

2. Gently rub the person's back. Use big circular motions. Start at the base of the back and move upward toward the shoulders. Without stopping the motion or taking your hands away, rub the back, moving downward toward the buttocks. Continue the backrub for 3 to 5 minutes. ☐ ☐

3. If you are doing the backrub as part of the person's bed bath and will be going on to bathe the perineal area, place a bed protector on the bed under the buttocks and roll the person onto his or her back. If you are doing the backrub separately from the bed bath, roll the person onto the back and go on to the completion steps. ☐ ☐

Task 3: Cleaning the Person's Perineal Area

1. Fill the washbasin with warm water and check the temperature. ☐ ☐
2. Place a bed protector under the person's hips. ☐ ☐
3. If the person is able to do his or her own perineal care, offer a fresh washcloth, soap and clean water. Give the person a few minutes alone to bathe. ☐ ☐

Perineal Care for Females

1. Drape the woman's perineal area by doing the following:
   - Place the bath blanket over her like a diamond. Put one corner at her neck, a corner at each side, and one corner between her legs (Figure 12-46).
   - Help her bend her knees and spread her legs.
   - Wrap each side corner around her feet. ☐ ☐
2. Elevate her pelvis by placing either a bedpan or a folded towel (or bath blanket) under her buttocks. ☐ ☐

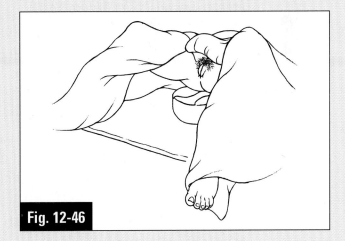

Fig. 12-46

3. Put on disposable gloves. ☐ ☐

4. Make the washcloth into a mitt. ☐ ☐

5. Lift the corner of the bath blanket between her legs, and fold it back onto her abdomen to expose her perineal area. ☐ ☐

6. Put soap on the mitt and wash her perineal area with the soapy washcloth by the following steps:

   • Wash the pubic hair on her lower abdomen.

   • Separate her labia with one hand.

   • Wash one side of her labia in one gentle, even stroke; then, using a different part of the wash cloth, wash the other side. Move in the direction from her hair, or pubic area, to her anal area (Figure 12-47).

   • Using a different part of the washcloth, wash gently down the middle. Move in the direction from her pubic area to her anal area. ☐ ☐

7. Rinse the soap out of the washcloth. Rinse her perineal area by using the same steps as you did when washing. Always use a different part of the washcloth for each stroke when rinsing. ☐ ☐

8. Dry her perineal area with a clean towel, using the same steps as you did when washing and rinsing. ☐ ☐

9. Remove the bedpan or the folded towel or blanket. ☐ ☐

10. Assist the person as she rolls onto her side. ☐ ☐

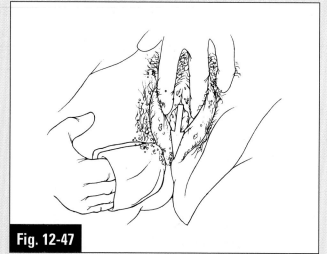

Fig. 12-47

7. Place a waterproof sheet under the person's head so that it covers the bottom sheet. ☐ ☐

8. Place the shampoo tray under the person's head so that the drainage through it is directed toward the empty washbasin on the chair. ☐ ☐

9. If you are using a plastic sheet or large trash bag, place a rolled towel inside the bag. Twist it into a C shape. Place the person's head in the center of the C. Drape the sheet or bag toward the side of the bed so that water drains into the washbasin on the chair. ☐ ☐

10. Place a clean washcloth over the person's eyes (Figure 12-50). ☐ ☐

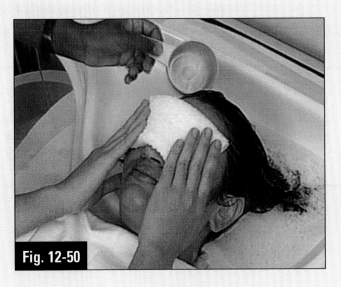
Fig. 12-50

11. Wet the hair with cups of (clean) water from the washbasin until it is fully wet. ☐ ☐

12. Apply a small amount of shampoo to the hair and massage the scalp with your fingertips, starting at the hairline working toward the back of head, until completely lathered. ☐ ☐

13. Rinse the person's hair with cups of water from the washbasin until all shampoo is removed. ☐ ☐

14. Wash and rinse the hair again (optional). ☐ ☐

15. Apply conditioner to the hair (optional). Work it through with your fingertips. ☐ ☐

16. Fill the cup with water and rinse the hair until the conditioner is removed. ☐ ☐

17. Unfold a clean, dry towel and dry the hair. Wrap the person's head in the towel (Fig. 12-51). ☐ ☐

18. Remove shampoo tray and waterproof pad.

19. Raise head of bed and style hair to the person's preference.

COMPLETION

Follow Completion Standards in compliance with your facility. For a complete list of those used in this course, see Chapter 7, "Controlling the Spread of Germs."

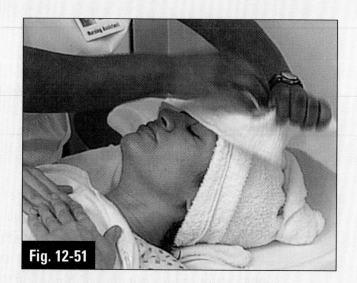

Fig. 12-51

Skill 33: Helping a Person with Showering and Shampooing

PRECAUTIONS

- Make sure the person is well covered with a bathrobe and wears slippers when you take him or her to the shower room.
- Check the water temperature. It should feel warm to the touch on the inside of your wrist. If the water is too hot, it can injure the person's skin. If the water is too cold, it can chill the person.
- Inspect the person's skin for injuries, changes in conditions and color (such as reddened areas or bruises) and sores.
- When giving a shampoo, cover the person's eyes with a washcloth to prevent shampoo from getting into them.
- To prevent injury, always stay with the person.

PREPARATION

1. Gather supplies:
   - Bath blanket (a flannel sheet used to keep the person warm after bathing or showering)
   - Two towels (three towels if the person is going to shampoo)
   - One washcloth
   - Shower cap (if not shampooing)
   - Disposable gloves (if you need to help the person with perineal care)
   - Plastic trash bag
   - Laundry bag (or plastic bag for wet or soiled linens)
   - Wheelchair (if person does not have his or her own) or shower chair, if needed
   - Plastic apron (optional)
2. Follow Preparation Standards (see Chapter 7).

Skill 33: Helping a Person with Showering and Shampooing—cont'd

PROCEDURE

1. Accompany the person to the shower room or bathroom. If using a wheelchair or shower chair, have the person hold the supplies in his or her lap. ☐ ☐

2. Turn the water faucet on, and adjust the temperature of the water so that it is warm to the touch. ☐ ☐

3. Help the person undress. ☐ ☐

4. If no shampoo is needed, offer a shower cap. ☐ ☐

5. Help the person into the shower. If a shower chair is used, lock the brakes or place the chair against the shower wall. ☐ ☐

6. If the person is going to wash his or her own hair, give assistance as needed. ☐ ☐

7. If you are shampooing the person's hair:
   - Put on a plastic apron, if desired.
   - Give the person a clean washcloth to hold over his or her eyes.
   - Wet the hair thoroughly.
   - Apply a small amount of shampoo to the person's hair. Massage the scalp until the hair is completely lathered.
   - Rinse the shampoo out of the person's hair.
   - Shampoo and rinse again (optional).
   - Apply conditioner (optional). Work it through with your fingertips.
   - Rinse the conditioner out of the person's hair. ☐ ☐

8. Give the person the soap and encourage him or her to wash as much of him- or herself as possible (Figure 12-52). ☐ ☐

9. Assist with washing the perineal area, if needed. ☐ ☐

10. Make sure all soap is rinsed off the skin. ☐ ☐

11. Help the person get out of the shower and have him or her sit on the towel-covered chair. ☐ ☐

12. Shut off the water. ☐ ☐

13. Use the second towel to dry the person's hair and wrap the head. ☐ ☐

14. Use the third towel to help the person dry off. ☐ ☐

15. Help the person put on slippers and bathrobe. ☐ ☐

16. Assist the person, if needed, to his or her room. ☐ ☐

17. Apply deodorant or antiperspirant. Apply lotion and powder, if tolerated. ☐ ☐

18. Assist the person with getting dressed and combing hair, if needed. ☐ ☐

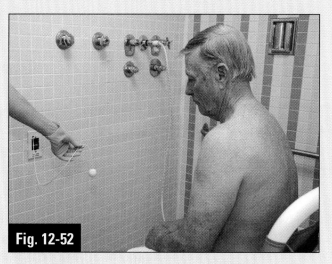
Fig. 12-52

ADDITIONAL INFORMATION

1. Determine the need for a shower chair or shower seat.
2. Reserve the shower room.

COMPLETION

Follow Completion Standards in compliance with your facility. For a complete list of those used in this course, see Chapter 7, "Controlling the Spread of Germs."

Skill 34: Helping a Person with Bathing and Shampooing in the Tub

PRECAUTIONS

- Make sure the person is well covered with a bathrobe and wears slippers when you take him or her to the tub to provide privacy and warmth.
- Check the water temperature with a bath thermometer. It should not be higher than 105° Fahrenheit. If the water is too hot, it can injure the person's skin. If the water is too cold, it can make the person chilled. If possible, ask the person if the water feels okay. Sometimes even water at 105° Fahrenheit will feel too warm for a person.
- Shut off the hot water faucet first. This prevents hot water from dripping from the faucet, which could scald the person.
- Be sure to use proper body mechanics when you help the person into and out of the tub.
- Inspect the person's skin for injuries, changes in conditions and color (such as discoloration or bruises) and sores.
- Check with supervising nurse and care plan for special instructions before shampooing the person's hair.

PREPARATION

1. Gather supplies:
   - Bath blanket
   - Bath thermometer
   - Two towels (three towels if the person is going to shampoo)
   - Pitcher
   - Disposable gloves

- One washcloth (two washcloths if the person is going to shampoo their hair)
- Laundry bag (or plastic bag for wet or soiled linens)

2. Follow Preparation Standards (see Chapter 7).

PROCEDURE

1. Help the person undress and put on bathrobe and slippers with nonskid soles. ☐ ☐

2. Accompany the person to the tub room or bathroom. If a wheelchair is used, have the person hold the supplies on her lap. ☐ ☐

3. Have the person sit in a chair next to the tub until you run the bath water. ☐ ☐

4. Fill the tub half way. Check the water temperature, using a bath thermometer, to make sure water is 105° F (Figure 12-53). ☐ ☐

5. Help the person into a sitting position in the tub (Figure 12-54). ☐ ☐

6. Place a folded towel on the chair (Figure 12-55). ☐ ☐

7. If the person seems chilled, offer her a towel to throw over her shoulders as she bathes. ☐ ☐

8. Encourage her to wash herself as much as possible. ☐ ☐

9. Assist with cleaning the perineal area, if needed. ☐ ☐

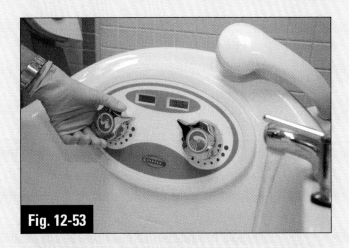
Fig. 12-53

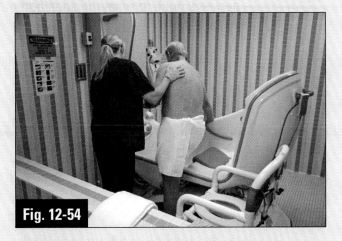
Fig. 12-54

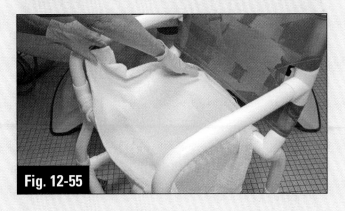
Fig. 12-55

10. Make sure all the soap is rinsed off the skin (Figure 12-56). ☐ ☐
11. Wash the person's hair.
    • Offer a washcloth for the person to hold over their eyes.
    • Wet the hair thoroughly.
    • Apply a small amount of shampoo to the hair and massage the scalp gently with your fingertips until the hair is completely lathered.
    • Use the pitcher to pour water over the person's head to rinse the shampoo out of the hair.
    • Shampoo and rinse again (optional).
    • Apply conditioner to the hair (optional).
    • Rinse the conditioner out of the hair. ☐ ☐
12. Towel-dry the person's hair. Wrap her head in a towel. ☐ ☐
13. Assist the person out of the tub and into the towel-covered chair. Wrap the bath blanket around her. ☐ ☐
14. Help the person dry off her body. Make sure the areas between the toes are completely dry. ☐ ☐
15. Assist the person with putting on slippers and bathrobe. ☐ ☐
16. Escort the person to her room. ☐ ☐
17. Apply lotion to the person's dry skin areas. Offer the person deodorant. ☐ ☐
18. Assist with dressing and hair grooming, if needed. ☐ ☐

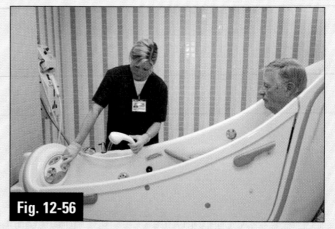
Fig. 12-56

ADDITIONAL INFORMATION

Make sure the person's hair is dry before she goes to bed or goes outside.

 COMPLETION

Follow Completion Standards in compliance with your facility. For a complete list of those used in this course, see Chapter 7, "Controlling the Spread of Germs."

Skill 35: Assisting with a Whirlpool Bath

PRECAUTIONS

- During a whirlpool bath, the increased blood flow to some parts of a person's body might cause him or her to become dizzy or faint. Observe the person often for signs of faintness, dizziness, fatigue or weakness.
- Make sure the water temperature is between 95 and 110° Fahrenheit to prevent burns or injury (Figure 12-57).
- Never leave the person alone in the tub.

PREPARATION

1. Gather supplies:
   - One towel
   - Laundry bag (or plastic bag for wet or soiled linens)
   - Bath thermometer
2. Follow Preparation Standards (see Chapter 7).

PROCEDURE

1. Place a chair near the whirlpool. ☐ ☐
2. Check the water temperature with a bath thermometer. ☐ ☐
3. Help the person remove his clothing and help him into the tub. ☐ ☐
4. Press the whirlpool turbine control button (agitation or mixing) and adjust for desired turbulence (motion). ☐ ☐
5. Remain with the person until the bath is finished. ☐ ☐
6. Help the person out of the tub and, as needed, with toweling dry and dressing. ☐ ☐

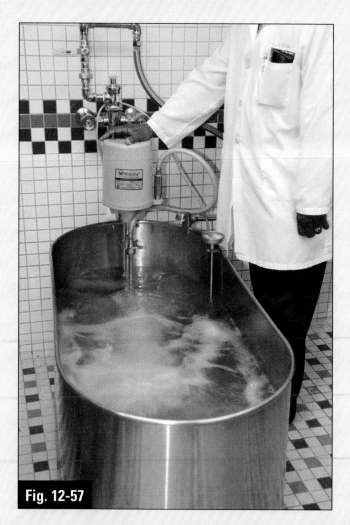

Fig. 12-57

ADDITIONAL INFORMATION

Check with the nurse or physical therapist for the length of time the person should remain in the tub.

COMPLETION

Follow Completion Standards in compliance with your facility. For a complete list of those used in this course, see Chapter 7, "Controlling the Spread of Germs."

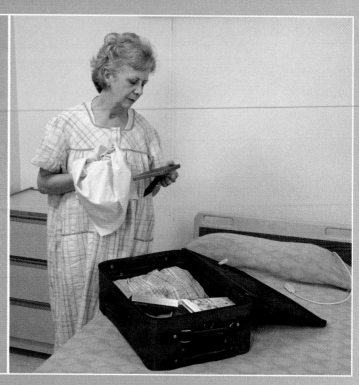

13

Admitting, Transferring and Discharging

GOALS

After reading this chapter, you will have the information needed to:

Help people when they are admitted to a nursing home.

Help people when they are transferred within a nursing home.

Help people when they are discharged from a nursing home to a hospital or home health care agency.

Weigh and measure people correctly.

After practicing the corresponding skill, you will have the information needed to:

Measure a person's height and weight.

One day in the lunch room, you talk with another nurse assistant about a resident that you helped discharge that morning. You talk about how difficult it was to say good-bye to someone that you had helped for several months.

"I always have mixed feelings about admitting and discharging residents," says your co-worker, Kathy Barnes. "When a resident first arrives, I feel a little nervous. I really want the person to be as comfortable and relaxed as possible. I know how important my role is in making the person feel that way.

"I remember when I first started working, a woman, Mrs. McDay was admitted. One of the other nurse assistants was out sick, so the rest of us split up her work load. I was rushing around trying to get everything done. I even rushed through Mrs. McDay's admission. Just before I was getting ready to leave at the end of my shift, I checked on her one more time and saw that she was crying. When I asked her how I could help her, she snapped back at me, 'Well, I certainly wouldn't want to bother you. You obviously have too many other things to do without having to worry about me.' I felt terrible. She was right. I hadn't even taken the time to make her feel welcome because I had so much to do. Now, I always think about Mrs. McDay whenever I help with someone's admission. I learned how important it is to slow down, work in an unhurried manner, and treat each person as if she's the most important person at that moment.

"When the time comes to discharge residents whom I've gotten to know fairly well, I often have mixed feelings. I'm glad that they are well enough to go home, but at the same time, I'm sad to see them go. I know I'll miss them."

ADMITTING, TRANSFERRING AND DISCHARGING A PERSON

Have you ever had to spend time away from home in a strange place? What do you remember as being important? Were you made to feel comfortable, or did you feel unwelcome or ill at ease? Did you plan to stay for a short or long time? Were things ready for you when you arrived, or did you have to wait for arrangements to be made? Thinking about your own answers to these questions may help you understand what people feel when they are admitted to health care. In addition to emotional uncertainties, people may experience physical pain or discomfort at the time they are admitted.

As a nurse assistant, how you perform your role in admitting a person to health care may influence her attitude about the care she receives. One of your tasks is to make the admission process as smooth as possible. Another is to help a person transfer from one part of a hospital or nursing home to another part of the facility as easily as possible, ensuring that the person and her possessions are moved safely and completely. The care that you provide in helping to discharge a person when she leaves a health care situation may leave a lasting impression about the care that she received.

Each employer and each health care facility has its own procedures for admitting, transferring and discharging people. Some procedures, such as taking vital signs, are basic to all situations. And in most situations, the role of the nurse assistant is basi-

cally the same: to look after and help ensure the safety of the person and her possessions as she is admitted, transferred and discharged.

Admitting a Resident to the Nursing Home

Today, you prepare for the arrival of 72-year-old Alma Garcia, who is recovering from surgery and who will be transported from the hospital to the Morningside Nursing Home by ambulance. To get ready for Mrs. Garcia's arrival, follow the admission sheet and instructions from your supervising nurse. Gather and bring to her room the equipment and materials you need for admission: blood pressure cuff and stethoscope, thermometer and any other items listed by your supervising nurse. Put a pitcher of water and a cup on the nightstand. Put a gown, washcloth and towel in the nightstand, and be prepared to put a washbasin, bedpan, emesis basin, soap and soap dish in the nightstand if she doesn't bring these items from the hospital. Also bring a laundry marker, personal belongings sheet, pen and paper to her room. Prepare Mrs. Garcia's bed. In some nursing homes, the nurse assistant fanfolds the top linens down to the bottom of the bed so that the bed is ready for the new resident when she arrives.

Your supervising nurse has already told you a little about Mrs. Garcia and her physical condition, so you know that she broke her hip and will be receiving physical therapy. You think about other things to explore when she arrives, such as how she feels about being in a nursing home. Entering a nursing home can be a very emotional experience, and people may react in many different ways. They may be sad, frightened, anxious, relieved or withdrawn. It is important for you to recognize and support new residents' feelings and to report any extreme behaviors that you observe to your supervising nurse.

When a new resident is admitted to the nursing home, you and other members of the nursing home staff follow a planned series of events. Sometimes an admissions clerk or social worker manages the admissions and introduces the new resident to the nurse assistant. However, if you are the one admitting the new resident, knock on the door, smile at her and greet her with a friendly "hello." Make the person feel welcome by introducing yourself. To help lessen feelings of anxiety about the health care experience, explain what is happening and what is going to happen.

Check her name band; remove the hospital name band and replace it with one that your unit secretary or administrative assistant has prepared. Explain that you are the nurse assistant who will be providing care for her. Ask her what she would like to be called, and be sure not to use her first name unless she gives you permission. Introduce her to her roommate. Ask her if she needs to use the bathroom before continuing with the admissions process.

One way to help ensure the safety of a person in your care is to interview her. In addition to asking the questions on the admission form, encourage the person to tell you anything that would make her stay more comfortable. Ask about special preferences, habits or problems. One way to organize the interview is to ask questions, working your way from head to toe. The admission form often prompts you to work this way. For example, you might ask the person: "Do you wear glasses? Is there anything special I should know about them? Do you have a hearing aid? Is there anything special I should know about it or about your hearing in general? Do you wear dentures? Do you have trouble sleeping at night?" Continue asking similar questions about diet, mobility and elimination. Record the answers and report important information to your supervising nurse.

It also is important to remember the person's needs and feelings when you transfer her from one room of a nursing home or hospital to another and when you discharge a person to a nursing home or hospital, or to her own home. Even in the home health care setting, it is important to think about how the person may feel about having you in her own home, doing the things that she once did for herself.

Looking after the Person's Possessions

An important part of looking after a person's possessions in a nursing home or hospital is filling out the admission checklist, which also may include an envelope for valuables and a personal belongings list. Following your employer's guidelines, fill out the admission checklist, noting valuables and personal belongings. When describing possessions such as jewelry, use words that do not assign value to the object. For example, describe a ring as "a yellow metal ring with one clear stone," being careful not to use words such as *gold, silver,* or *diamond.* When describing a watch, write down the brand name found on the watch face. Encourage the person

to send as many valuables home as possible. If necessary, you can arrange for valuable items to be locked in the facility's safe. After completing the checklist, give it to your supervising nurse.

When you help a person transfer within a nursing home or hospital, you must take special care of his possessions to make sure that they arrive safely in his new room.

After helping the new resident fill out a personal belongings list, help her label her clothes with the laundry marker. Be sure to mark the clothes in an area where the ink will not show through to the outside (the label is often a good place). Encourage her to send any valuables home. If she decides not to send them home, list them and lock them in the safe. Help her put her things away.

Once you have finished both the interview and the checklist of the resident's belongings, explain nursing home policies, schedules and visiting hours to the new resident and her family. Show her how the call signal works and ask her to demonstrate her understanding of its use (Figure 13-1). Demonstrate how to raise and lower the bed and over-bed table.

FIGURE 13-1 Explain to a new patient how the call signal works and the location of anything else she might need.

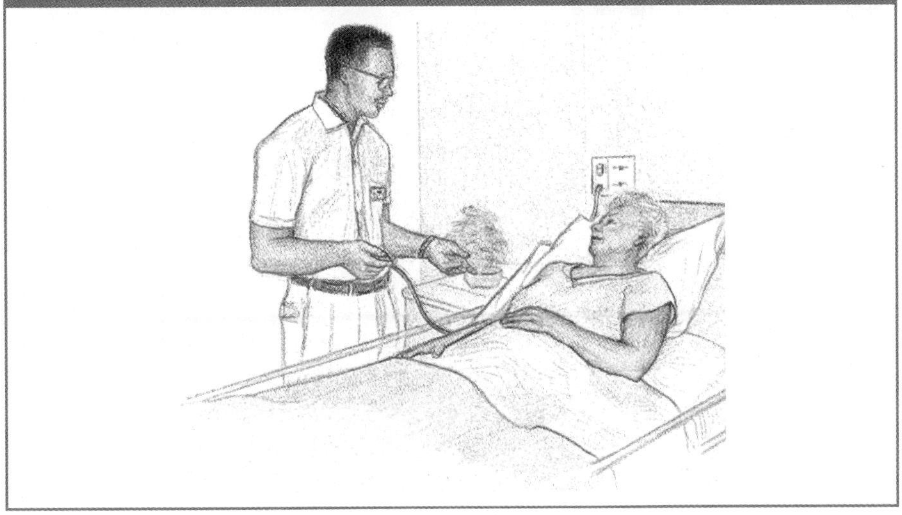

Measuring and Recording Weight and Height

When a person is first admitted to health care, you will take and record his or her vital signs. (Review the information in Chapter 9, "Measuring Life Signs.") It is important to keep an accurate record of a person's weight, because weight gain or loss could be related to a person's medical condition. These measurements at admission are important for other health care workers to use as a **baseline** reference point when vital signs are taken at other times. Perform your tasks in a warm, unhurried manner to help the person relax and feel better about being in a health care situation (Figure 13-2).

Some people may have to be weighed every day, whereas others may need to be weighed only occasionally. In addition to weighing a person in your care, you must measure her height so that the doctor can evaluate the person's weight based on the normal weight range for someone of her particular height.

Because scales can vary, always weigh the person on the same scale. Also, whenever possible, weigh her at the same time of day. Have her wear as few clothes as possible, and follow your employer's guidelines about having her use the toilet before weighing.

You can use several types of scales, depending on the person's condition. When you weigh a person who can stand, use a balance scale (upright scale) or bathroom scale. If the person cannot stand, use a scale that enables you to weigh her in her wheelchair, in bed or in a chair that resembles a mechanical lift (Figure 13-3).

When you bring a person to a balance scale to be weighed, first make sure the balance is set at zero to ensure accurate weighing. If the balance is not set at zero, ask your supervising nurse to help you change it. Observe this precaution: use good body mechanics when measuring or weighing a person. To learn how to use a balance scale and a bathroom scale, as well as how to measure someone's height, follow the specific procedure that is explained step by step in Skill 36.

After explaining the surroundings to the new resident and her family and recording her vital signs, height and weight, offer to take her and her family on a tour of the facility. If she wishes to go, introduce her to other members of the staff and to other residents.

After the tour, help the new resident get comfortable in her room and put the call signal within her reach. Ask her whether she needs anything. If not, wash your hands, tell her when you will return and report your completion of the admission checklist, as well as any observations about the new resident's physical condition and emotional status, to your supervising nurse.

HELPING A RESIDENT FEEL AT HOME

Once you have helped a new person's admission to a nursing home, it is important to continue to help her feel welcome and become as comfortable as possible, knowing she may stay for a few months or perhaps for the rest of her life. Because of the long stay and because she may never go home again, it is important to be sensitive to her feelings.

As one of the first people to have contact with a new resident, you can help her feel comfortable and trusting in her new environment. Because her first impression of the nursing home may influence how she feels about being there, your approach and consideration can help make her experience pleasant and give her confidence in the care she is about to receive. To ensure a good first impression, take some of the following steps:

- Each time you greet a new resident, smile, call her by name and be attentive to her feelings. Find out her needs. Does she need to use the bathroom, be repositioned or have a drink of water?

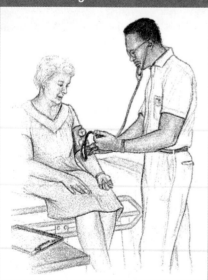

FIGURE 13-2 Take vital signs in an efficient and competent manner to reassure a person who is being admitted.

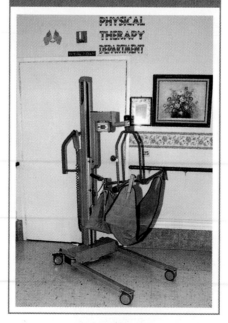

FIGURE 13-3 You can use this type of mechanical-lift device to weigh a person who cannot stand on an upright scale or a bathroom scale.

- When family members visit, respect their privacy but be willing to answer questions about mealtime, activities, using free time and making positive use of visiting time.
- Always include the resident in conversations that concern her.

Transferring a Resident Within the Nursing Home

Two weeks ago, a resident, Mrs. Eastman, broke two vertebrae in her back and was admitted to Morningside Nursing Home to receive physical therapy. From the first day that she arrived, she refused to cooperate with the physical therapist, and eventually, she refused to leave her room to go to physical therapy. Today, when she tells the doctor that she won't go to physical therapy, he reports this situation to the nursing home administrators. Because the unit where she now resides is specified for residents who receive physical therapy and nursing care, they arrange for Mrs. Eastman to be transferred to a unit where she will receive only basic nursing care.

When you help transfer a resident to a different unit in the nursing home, go to her room, greet her and wash your hands. Explain to her that you are going to help her get ready for her transfer. As you help her pack her belongings, check the closets, drawers and nightstand for personal items. Pack all of her equipment, such as the washbasin and bedpan, to take to the new room. As you help gather her things, talk with her about the transfer. Ask her whether she wants to share her feelings about what is going to happen, and answer any questions she may have (Figure 13-4). Give her time to say good-bye to her roommate.

Ask your supervising nurse for the records and charts that must go with the resident, and ask the unit secretary to inform the staff on the new unit that you are bringing the resident from your unit. It may be necessary to

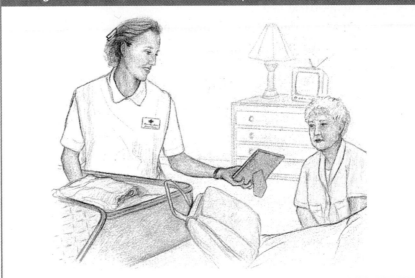

FIGURE 13-4 Any move may have an emotional impact on a resident. Whether the resident moves down the hall or to another floor, tell her why she is being transferred, encourage her to talk about her feelings and reassure her, if necessary.

adjust the time of her arrival in the new unit so that the nurse assigned to her is available to receive her.

Help the resident into a wheelchair. (Some facilities prefer that you move the resident in her bed from one room to another.) Ask a co-worker to help you, if necessary. Move the resident and her possessions to her new room, and introduce her to her new nurse and nurse assistant. Report important information, as necessary.

To help the resident make a comfortable transition from one nursing home unit to another, and as a courtesy to her new nurse assistant, you may stay and assist her new nurse assistant with some of the tasks to help get her settled in her new room. Then spend a few minutes talking with her about how you enjoyed helping her. Wish her well in her new room and say good-bye to her.

Return to your own unit. Remove any equipment that the resident did not take from her old room. If she wasn't moved in her bed, strip it of dirty linens. Follow your employer's policy for preparing the room for use by another resident.

After finishing these tasks, wash your hands. Report to your supervising nurse that the resident's transfer has been completed. Provide important information, such as the time of the transfer, her mode of transportation, how she responded and any important observations.

Discharging a Resident from the Nursing Home

A resident may be discharged from the nursing home to a hospital or to her own home. In either situation, you must help her make the transition as smoothly and safely as possible.

Discharging a Resident to a Hospital. Mr. Wilson has been doing very well at Morningside Nursing Home. Suddenly his temperature goes up, he complains of pain in his chest and he develops a cough. His doctor writes orders to send him by ambulance to the hospital, and your supervising nurse notifies his family of the decision to hospitalize him. As his nurse assistant, you help him get ready to be transferred.

Pack only the clothing and belongings that he needs for the hospital stay (robe, slippers and personal care items such as a comb, brush, toothbrush, toothpaste, eyeglasses and dentures). Help him dress appropriately. In this case, pajamas, a robe and slippers are appropriate, because the ambulance crew will make sure that he is covered and warm.

Check with your supervising nurse to make sure that the proper forms are filled out and are ready to go with the resident. (It is helpful to send a detailed description of his physical needs and personal habits, as well as medications and usual vital signs, to the hospital.) Stay with him and comfort him until he is in the ambulance, because he may be very frightened.

Check the resident's name band and introduce him to the ambulance crew. If they need assistance, help the ambulance attendants transfer the resident to the stretcher. Make sure that his belongings and forms are in the ambulance with him. Follow your employer's policy for listing and storing his personal belongings that he didn't take to the hospital, and make sure that his room is clean.

Report to your supervising nurse that the resident's discharge has been completed. Provide important information, such as the time of the discharge, his mode of transportation, how he responded and any important observations.

Discharging a Resident to Her Home. For several weeks, Mrs. Garcia has been receiving physical therapy at the nursing home to help strengthen her hip. You have helped her with bathing, dressing and walking, as well as with special exercises that she learned from the physical therapist. Over time, Mrs. Garcia has become strong and independent enough to walk with a walker. Today, her doctor explains to her that she is well enough to go home but says that she will need help at home for a while. He refers her to a home health care agency.

On the day that a resident is ready to go home, help her gather all her belongings and pack her suitcase. Check items against the personal belongings sheet to make sure that she has everything she brought with her. After your supervising nurse gives verbal and written instructions to the resident and her family members, help the resident into a wheelchair and transport her to the nursing home exit where her family's car is waiting (Figure 13-5). Tell her how much you have

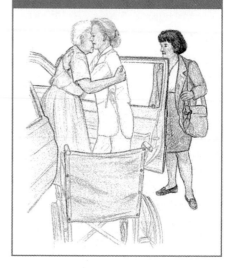

FIGURE 13-5 When discharging a resident, provide for her safety by transporting her out of the building in a wheelchair and carefully helping her into the waiting vehicle.

enjoyed helping her. Wish her well in her recovery and say good-bye.

Return the wheelchair to your unit, clean it and return it to the proper place. Then strip the discharged resident's bed, pick up discarded items and report important observations to your supervising nurse.

Circle the correct answers and fill in the blanks.

1. When a person first enters a health care setting, you help with a procedure called

    _____.

2. When a person moves from one unit in a nursing home or hospital to another unit, you help with a procedure called _____.

3. When a person leaves a health care situation, you help with a procedure called

    _____.

4. When a person moves into and out of health care situations, the nurse assistant looks after the person and the person's:
    a. family.
    b. pets.
    c. doctor.
    d. possessions.

5. One of the basic tasks performed in all admitting procedures is measuring _____

    _____.

6. In a nursing home and hospital, it is important to keep records of a person's personal:
    a. belongings.
    b. thoughts.
    c. desires.
    d. remarks.

7. You can help a resident or patient feel more comfortable in her new health care setting by introducing her to her _____.

8. When you admit a new resident to a nursing home, one of your tasks is to use a laundry marker to help label:
    a. her new bed.
    b. her clothing.
    c. the back of her hand.
    d. her bed linens.

1. *Mrs. Marker insists on wearing her opal and diamond ring in the nursing home. One day, after Mrs. Marker has become very ill and is slipping in and out of consciousness, the ring slips off her finger onto the bed. What would you do?*

2. *Mr. Yoder, a patient with diabetes, has been admitted to the nursing facility. As you help him unpack his suitcase, you notice that he brought along a stash of cookies and cupcakes. What would you do?*

3. *After Mrs. Garcia has been discharged home from the nursing home, as you are changing the bed linens, you find a picture of a small boy just under the bed. What would you do?*

Skill 36: Measuring a Person's Height and Weight

PRECAUTIONS
- Use proper body mechanics.

PREPARATION
1. Gather supplies:
- Appropriate scales to weigh the person
- Tape measure, if needed
- Paper towel
- Towel (optional)
- Chair (optional)
- Paper and pen to record measurements
2. Follow Preparation Standards (see Chapter 7).

PROCEDURE

Option 1: Measuring a Person's Height in Bed
1. Have the person lie as flat and straight as possible. ☐ ☐
2. Using a tape measure, measure the person from the top of her head to the soles of her feet (Figure 13-6). ☐ ☐
3. Record her height in feet and inches. ☐ ☐

Option 2: Measuring a Person's Weight Using a Bathroom Scale
1. Make sure the scale is balanced before directing the person to stand on the scale. ☐ ☐
2. Place a paper towel on the scale. ☐ ☐
3. Help the person to stand alone safely on the scale without shoes. ☐ ☐

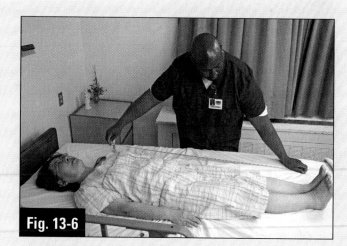
Fig. 13-6

4. Record the weight shown on the scale dial. ☐ ☐
5. Help the person off the scale. ☐ ☐
6. Help the person with clothing and shoes, as needed. ☐ ☐

Option 3: Measuring a Person's Height and Weight Using an Upright Scale

1. Check the balance of the scale by moving the weight all the way to the left (zero). The pointer should swing evenly between the top and bottom of the metal square. If the scale is not balanced, notify your nurse supervisor. ☐ ☐
2. Put a paper towel on the scale (Figure 13-7). ☐ ☐
3. Help the person remove his or her robe and slippers. ☐ ☐
4. Assist the person onto the scale platform. ☐ ☐
5. Measure the person's height. ☐ ☐
6. Measure the person's weight. ☐ ☐
7. Record the height and the weight of the person. ☐ ☐
8. Help the person of the scale. ☐ ☐

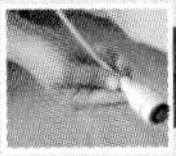

COMPLETION

Follow Completion Standards in compliance with your facility. For a complete list of those used in this course, see Chapter 7, "Controlling the Spread of Germs."

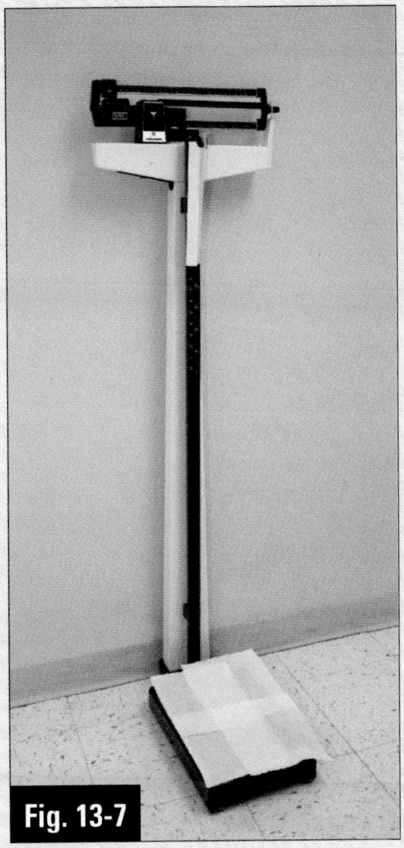

Fig. 13-7

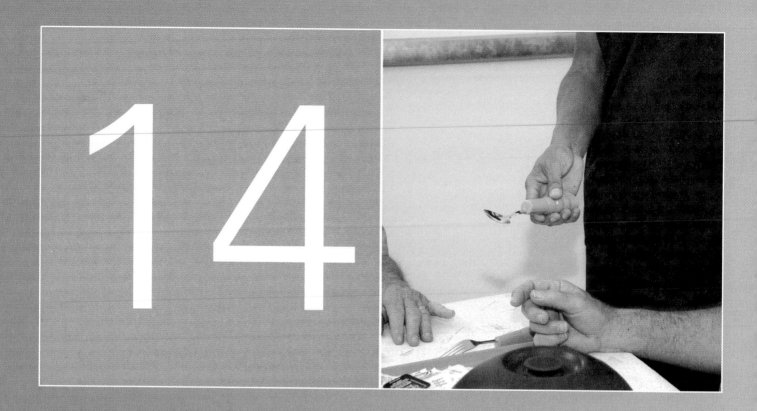

14

Chapter 14

Healthful Eating

GOALS

After reading this chapter, you will have the information needed to:

Explain how social customs, religious practices, economic factors and family
   background shape attitudes about food.

Describe the nutrients in food.

Describe the five food groups.

Explain how seven kinds of special diets help people who have special dietary needs.

Explain why it is important to make mealtime pleasant.

Explain why and how to measure the amount people eat and drink.

After practicing the corresponding skill, you will have the information needed to:

Help people eat.

Victor Rivera's wife comes to the nursing home every day around 2:00 P.M. and stays until after Mr. Rivera has finished eating his dinner. When Mr. Rivera first came to Morningside Nursing Home from the hospital, where he had received treatment for a stroke that left his left side paralyzed, Mrs. Rivera asked how she might help with her husband's care. You taught Mrs. Rivera how to help her husband at mealtimes, and now she comes every day to make dinner time a special part of the day.

During the day, you help Mr. Rivera eat his breakfast and lunch. In the nursing home's dining room, filled with light and fresh flowers, he sits at a table with Mr. O'Reilly, who also has had a stroke. Mr. O'Reilly receives help from family members who are frequent guests in the dining room. During lunch, the two men talk about the day, the weather and local news. They have become good friends, and they look forward to having mealtimes together.

Mr. Rivera is trying to learn to eat with his left hand and finds mealtime a major challenge. His shaky left arm has been getting stronger, but he often becomes tired after feeding himself the first few bites. Today at lunch you encourage him to eat all of his mashed potatoes by himself, using the new large-handled spoon the occupational therapist taught him how to use. When he finishes, he sighs heavily and slouches back in his wheelchair. "I knew you could do it, Mr. Rivera," you say, and help him with the rest of his meal.

ATTITUDES ABOUT FOOD

As a nurse assistant, it is important for you to know about food and nutrition. If you eat the recommended foods, you may be healthier and better able to enjoy your life and work. The same is true for the people in your care. The right foods can help people stay healthy. They also can play a big part in helping people who are sick or injured get better.

Yet people differ in what they eat, when they eat and how they prepare food. Each person has certain likes and dislikes. One person may not like green beans, while another may not like chocolate. What you like to eat may seem strange to someone who grew up in a different place or who has a different religion.

Your food choices, likes and dislikes have been influenced by where you come from and who you are. Social customs, religious practices, economic factors and the availability of ingredients all play a part in what you choose to eat. They shape your attitudes about food—attitudes that may last a lifetime. For example, one person who grew up in a Southeast Asian culture may eat rice every day with a variety of cooked vegetables, fish, eggs and meat. He may season his foods with strong flavors such as garlic, chilies, ginger and fresh coriander. These foods may remain part of his **diet** even if he moves far from his native country. But another person who grew up in the same culture may learn to enjoy other kinds of foods, such as pizza and tacos.

Do not depend on what you know about the person's culture or religious

---

KEY TERMS

appetite: (AH-puh-tite) the desire to eat and drink.

arteriosclerosis: (ar-teer-ee-oh-skluh-ROW-sis) hardening and thickening of the arteries.

calorie: (KAL-uh-ree) a unit of heat or energy produced when the body uses food.

cholesterol: (ko-LES-ter-all) a white, fatty substance that occurs naturally in the blood and tissues of the human body and that also is found in meat, egg yolks, liver, most dairy products and animal fat.

dehydrated: (de-HI-dray-ted) not having enough water in the body.

diabetes: (dye-uh-BEE-tez) a disease in which the pancreas does not secrete

enough insulin and the body is not able to use all the carbohydrates, resulting in a high concentration of glucose in the blood.

diet: (DYE-it) the foods and liquids that a person usually consumes.

incision: (in-SIZH-un) a cut made during surgery.

malnutrition: failure to obtain enough calories and essential nutrients.

nauseated: (NAW-zee-ay-ted) a feeling of sickness in the stomach.

nutrient: (NEW-tre-ent) a substance that the body needs to grow, maintain itself and stay healthy.

obesity: (oh-BEE-suh-tee) having too much body fat.

saturated fat: (SAH-tyur-ay-ted) a form of fat found in meats, cheese, dairy products and certain vegetable oils, such as palm and coconut oil.

suture: (SUE-tyur) the stitch used to join the edges of a cut or wound.

therapeutic diet: (ther-uh-PEW-tik) a special diet that helps a person regain his or her health.

turgor: (TER-jer) the ability of the skin to return to its normal shape when it is squeezed or gently pinched

preferences to give you clues about what he may like to eat, because individual preferences differ. The best way to find out what someone likes to eat is to ask the person.

THE BASICS OF NUTRITION

You may have heard an old saying, "You are what you eat," meaning that what you eat is reflected in your health. This saying is only partly true. Heredity, environment and lifestyle also play a part in how healthy you are. Eating properly helps maintain overall good health, and following good nutritional habits can improve poor health.

Diet is What You Eat

You may hear someone who is trying to lose weight say he or she is on a "diet." In this book, the word *diet* means all the food and liquid a person consumes. A person may choose to eat an unbalanced diet of ice cream, cookies, cake, fudge and broccoli. Another person may choose meat, potatoes, vegetables and fruit. Someone who is ill may need just liquids, such as broth, gelatin and fruit juice. All these selections of food are diets.

Selecting the Major Nutrients

It is important to know what foods are in a person's diet and what **nutrients** are in those foods. Foods contain some or all of the following major nutrients:

- Carbohydrates
- Protein
- Fat
- Minerals
- Vitamins
- Water

To get all the necessary nutrients, a person needs to eat a variety of foods. No single food or group of foods supplies all the nutrients you need. Carbohydrates, protein and fat supply

energy for the body. The amount of energy that a food has is measured in **calories.** Have you ever looked at the label on a package of food to check the number of calories? If you eat more calories than your body uses for energy, the leftover calories are stored in your body as fat. In addition to identifying the number of calories, many food labels also identify the amounts of carbohydrate, protein and fat that are in a serving of that food item (Box 14-1). Look at Table 14-1 to learn what each nutrient does and in which foods each nutrient is found.

A Healthy Diet

One Size Does Not Fit All. USDA's new MyPyramid (Figure 14-1) symbolizes a personalized approach to healthy eating and physical activity. The MyPyramid symbol has been designed to be simple. It has been developed to remind consumers to make healthy food choices and to be active every day. The different parts of the symbol are described below.

The nutritional needs of an ill or injured person vary, depending on what type of illness or injury he has.

TABLE 14-1 MAJOR NUTRIENTS

Nutrient	What It Does	Where It Is Found
Carbohydrate	Supplies energy that is easy for the body to use; adds bulk (fiber) to the diet that helps eliminate waste material	Grains such as wheat and rice Vegetables such as potatoes, sweet potatoes, lima beans, corn and carrots Fruit such as apples, bananas and oranges Sugars such as honey and syrup
Protein	Builds body tissue, regulates water balance and fights disease	Milk, cheese, yogurt, meat, poultry, fish and eggs Dried beans and nuts, seeds, grains and peanut butter*
Fat	Provides a concentrated source of energy for the body to store	Nuts, seeds, peanut butter, whole milk, yogurt, cheese, meat, fatty fish (such as tuna), poultry with skin, eggs, olives and avocados Vegetable cooking oils, margarine, butter, mayonnaise and salad dressing
Minerals	Regulate many body functions; build and renew bones, teeth, blood and tissue	In all foods, but types of minerals and their amounts vary
Vitamins	Break down other nutrients into smaller parts so that the body can use them	In all foods, but types of vitamins and their amounts vary
Water	Keeps substances in solution in body tissue and regulates body temperature, circulation and excretion	A major component of vegetables and fruits

*Incomplete proteins—must be eaten in combination with certain other foods to provide complete proteins when the person does not eat animal products.

For example, when a person has **diabetes,** his diet often limits the number of calories he should consume, as well as the amount of carbohydrate and fat. Or when a person has a burn or open sore and the body needs to repair tissue, his diet contains more protein and total calories for healing.

Because very active people need more calories for energy, they need to eat more food, especially carbohydrates, which provide energy that is easy for the body to use. Men tend to need more calories than women do.

To help people know how much from each food group to eat, doctors and dietitians/nutritionists make recommendations for the average person. Some guidelines for the recommended amount from each food group appear in the following paragraphs and in Figure 14-1. The suggested amounts are for those individuals on about a 2,000 calorie diet.

What is the Right Amount of Grain?
You read that carbohydrates supply the body with easy energy, which is what the body needs to do its work. The body's work occurs even when people are sleeping or unconscious. A healthy person needs more carbohydrates than anything else in his or her diet. Because grains supply the type of carbohydrate that is used most efficiently by the body, a healthy person should eat more foods from the grain group than from any other food group.

Bread, rice, pasta and cereal are examples of foods in the grain group (Figure 14-2).

Depending on how active he is, a healthy adult should eat about 6 oz of grain every day. The size of a serving depends on what kind of grain the person is eating. For example, one slice of bread is 1 oz as is ½ cup of cooked cereal, rice or pasta. When he eats a sandwich made with two slices of bread for lunch, he is having two servings of grain. What else could he eat at breakfast and dinner to get the rest of the grain he needs for 1 day?

What is the Right Amount of Vegetables?
Vegetables also contain large amounts of carbohydrates, as well as

FIGURE 14-1 MyPyramid

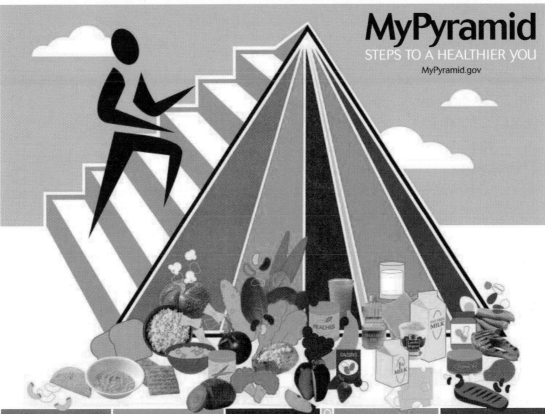

MyPyramid
STEPS TO A HEALTHIER YOU
MyPyramid.gov

GRAINS	VEGETABLES	FRUITS	OILS	MILK	MEAT & BEANS
Make half your grains whole	Vary your veggies	Focus on fruits		Get your calcium-rich foods	Go lean with protein
Eat at least 3 oz. of whole-grain cereals, breads, crackers, rice, or pasta every day 1 oz. is about 1 slice of bread, about 1 cup of breakfast cereal, or ½ cup of cooked rice, cereal, or pasta	Eat more dark-green veggies like broccoli, spinach, and other dark leafy greens Eat more orange vegetables like carrots and sweetpotatoes Eat more dry beans and peas like pinto beans, kidney beans, and lentils	Eat a variety of fruit Choose fresh, frozen, canned, or dried fruit Go easy on fruit juices		Go low-fat or fat-free when you choose milk, yogurt, and other milk products If you don't or can't consume milk, choose lactose-free products or other calcium sources such as fortified foods and beverages	Choose low-fat or lean meats and poultry Bake it, broil it, or grill it Vary your protein routine -- choose more fish, beans, peas, nuts, and seeds

For a 2,000-calorie diet, you need the amounts below from each food group. To find the amounts that are right for you, go to MyPyramid.gov.

Eat 6 oz. every day	Eat 2½ cups every day	Eat 2 cups every day	Get 3 cups every day; for kids aged 2 to 8, it's 2	Eat 5½ oz. every day

Find your balance between food and physical activity
- Be sure to stay within your daily calorie needs.
- Be physically active for at least 30 minutes most days of the week.
- About 60 minutes a day of physical activity may be needed to prevent weight gain.
- For sustaining weight loss, at least 60 to 90 minutes a day of physical activity may be required.
- Children and teenagers should be physically active for 60 minutes every day, or most days.

Know the limits on fats, sugars, and salt (sodium)
- Make most of your fat sources from fish, nuts, and vegetable oils.
- Limit solid fats like butter, margarine, shortening, and lard, as well as foods that contain these.
- Check the Nutrition Facts label to keep saturated fats, *trans* fats, and sodium low.
- Choose food and beverages low in added sugars. Added sugars contribute calories with few, if any, nutrients.

MyPyramid.gov
STEPS TO A HEALTHIER YOU

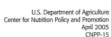

U.S. Department of Agriculture
Center for Nutrition Policy and Promotion
April 2005
CNPP-15

USDA is an equal opportunity provider and employer.

FIGURE 14-2 Grains

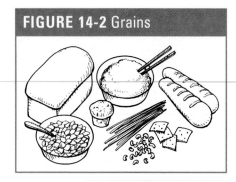

vitamins (Figure 14-3). A healthy adult should eat about 2½ cups of vegetables each day. The person should vary the kinds of vegetables eaten; dark green, orange and dry peas and beans subgroup.

What is the Right Amount of Fruit?
Like vegetables, fruits contain high levels of carbohydrates and vitamins. A healthy adult should eat about 2 cups of fruit each day. Any fruit or 100% fruit juice counts as part of the fruit group.

What is the Right Amount of Meat?
The body needs protein to build muscle and other body tissue. High levels of protein are found in foods in the meat group (Figure 14-4). This group includes:
- Eggs
- Red meat, such as beef, lamb and pork
- Poultry, such as chicken and turkey
- Fish and shellfish, such as shrimp, crab, lobster, scallops and oysters

FIGURE 14-3 Vegetables and Fruit

A healthy adult should have up to about 5½ ounces of meat each day.

When choosing foods from the meat group, keep in mind that these foods contain varying amounts of fat. Dietitians/nutritionists recommend cutting down on the amount of fat consumed. Red meat usually contains more fat than poultry, and fish is generally lower in fat than meat. If you eat red meat, it is better to choose lean red meat and trim off all the visible fat before cooking. It also is better to take the skin off chicken and turkey before cooking, because most of the fat in poultry is in the skin.

Some people do not eat meat or milk for religious, personal, medical or cultural reasons. These people can get the protein they need by eating other high-protein foods, such as whole grains, beans and nuts, as well as extra servings of leafy green vegetables. Beans and whole grains at the same meal provide a high-quality protein.

What is the Right Amount of Milk?
Like the meat group, foods in the milk group contain high levels of protein (Figure 14-4). An average adult should have about 3 cups from the milk group each day.

Foods in the milk group also can contain large amounts of fat. One way to reduce the amount of fat is to drink milk that contains 2 percent or 1 percent of milk fat instead of whole milk. Nonfat milk is even lower in fat than 1 percent milk. Another way to reduce fat in dairy foods is to choose low-fat cheese and reduced and nonfat yogurt.

What about Oils? Oils are fats in liquid form. Because people naturally get fats from other sources, such as meats and milk products, they should limit how much they choose to eat from this other group. Fats and oils should be the smallest part of any diet because they are high in calories. It is better to use very little fat when cooking and to bake, roast or boil meat instead of fry-

FIGURE 14-4 Meat and Dairy

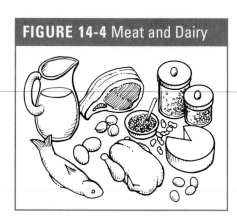

ing it. It also is better to use only a small amount of salad dressing and spreads, such as butter, margarine and mayonnaise. An average adult is allowed about 5-6 teaspoons of oils a day. In addition to limiting the amount of fat in their diets, people should limit their consumption of alcohol and sweets, such as candy.

A person needs to find balance between eating the recommended foods and participating in physical activity. MyPyramid further explains those requirements.

Activity
Activity is represented by the steps and the person climbing them, as a reminder of the importance of daily physical activity. To reduce the risk of chronic disease, engage in at least 30 minutes of moderate- to vigorous-intensity physical activity above usual activity at work or home on most days of the week.

Moderation
Moderation is represented by the narrowing of each food group from bottom to top. The wider base stands for foods with little or no solid fats or added sugars. These should be selected more often. The narrower top area stands for foods containing more added sugars and solid fats. The more active you are, the more of these foods can fit into your diet.

Personalization

Personalization is shown by the person on the steps; the slogan and the URL. Find the kinds and amounts of food to eat each day at MyPyramid.gov.

Proportionality

Proportionality is shown by the different widths of the food group bands. The widths suggest how much food a person should choose from each group. The widths are just a general guide, not exact proportions. Check the Web site for how much is right for you.

Variety

Variety is symbolized by the 6 color bands representing the 5 food groups of the Pyramid and oils. This illustrates that foods from all groups are needed each day for good health.

Gradual Improvement

Gradual improvement is encouraged by the slogan. It suggests that individuals can benefit from taking small steps to improve their diet and lifestyle each day.

EATING FOR HEALTH AND PLEASURE

Proper nutrition and long-term good health are closely linked. Proper nutrition means eating a wide variety of foods and choosing those that are low in fat, salt and sugar. Eating too much of these substances can cause health problems. For example, people who eat too much **cholesterol** and **saturated fat** may develop high cholesterol levels in the blood, which can cause problems with the heart and circulatory system. Eating too much fat also has been linked to certain types of cancer. Eating too much salt can cause problems for people who have high blood pressure. Eating large amounts of sugar adds calories without adding other nutrients and contributes to tooth decay.

Building good nutritional habits early in life helps keep the digestive system healthy, helps prevent **obesity** and helps avoid the risk of long-term diseases such as cancer, heart disease, high blood pressure, **arteriosclerosis** and diabetes in later years. When people develop health problems, they may have to change their diets.

Monitoring Special Dietary Needs

Many people require special diets because of physical disabilities or diseases. Doctors and dietitians help decide what a person should eat. For example, Mr. Rivera once enjoyed eating fried foods, but because he had a stroke and has high blood pressure and high cholesterol, his doctor has ordered a low-fat diet that eliminates all fried foods. As a nurse assistant, you have to know what foods are in such special diets and why they are ordered. In many cases you are responsible for serving these diets, and sometimes you also must monitor how much of the food the person in your care eats. Commonly ordered **therapeutic diets** are described in the following paragraphs.

Soft, Mechanical or Pureed Diet. Food can be prepared in special ways to make it easier for a person to chew, swallow and digest than food in a regular diet (Figure 14-5). In a soft diet, food such as hot breakfast cereal and mashed potatoes is prepared soft or mashed. In a mechanical diet, food such as ground meat is ground with a mechanical device. Pureed food, such as pureed vegetables and meat, is boiled to a pulp and rubbed through a sieve. Any of these three diets can meet a person's daily nutritional needs.

Liquid Diet. A liquid diet may be ordered for a person who has digestive problems, has had recent surgery, or cannot swallow solid food. Depending on the person's condition, the doctor may order a clear liquid diet or a full liquid diet.

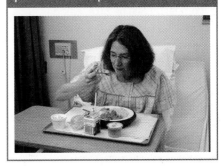

FIGURE 14-5 The soft foods in a mechanical diet are ordered for someone who cannot chew because of a stroke or other problem. This diet is chosen over a liquid diet because it provides complete nutrition.

A clear liquid diet includes liquids you can see through, such as broth, gelatin, sport or electrolyte drinks, carbonated beverages, tea, as well as clear juices such as apple, grape and cranberry. A person with a short-term illness such as flu, diarrhea or vomiting may be on a liquid diet for only 1 or 2 days to give his digestive system a rest. Because this diet is lacking in protein, fiber and certain vitamins and minerals, it cannot provide adequate nutrition; therefore, a doctor must reorder this diet every 48 hours.

A full liquid diet includes fruit juices such as orange and grapefruit juice, strained soups, ice cream, milk, diluted (thinned) cooked cereal and eggnog. A doctor orders this diet for 1 or 2 days for a person with an illness that causes digestive problems. It provides more nutrients than the clear liquid diet but still does not provide adequate nutrition. It also must be reordered by the doctor every 48 hours.

No-Added-Salt (NAS) or Sodium-Controlled Diet. Sodium may be limited for people with high blood pressure or kidney or circulatory diseases. Foods in this diet must be prepared with no added salt. The person on this diet may not use table salt, but may use a salt substitute with the doctor's approval. This diet provides adequate nutrition but limits foods that are high in salt or sodium, such as ham, bacon, cheese, regular canned soups, potato chips, lunch meat, pickles, olives and many packaged or canned foods (Figure 14-6).

Calorie-Restricted Diet. A diet with 1,200, 1,500, 1,800 or 2,000 calories per day may be ordered for a person who needs to control his weight. A well-planned diet contains all the proteins, carbohydrates and fats the person needs. The doctor or dietitian may recommend multivitamin and mineral supplements for a daily diet of 1,200 calories or fewer. For minor calorie restriction, the doctor or dietitian may order a regular no-concentrated-sweets (NCS) diet that eliminates only cookies.

High-Protein Diet. A doctor prescribes this diet for people who do not eat enough protein or who need additional protein to build skin or organ tissues. A person who has been burned or has developed decubitus ulcers may be put on a high-protein diet.

Diabetic Diet. Two types of diets are available for people who have diabetes. The older, traditional diabetes diet carefully defines the number of calories, as well as the amount and type of carbohydrates, protein and fat a person may eat. A newer and more convenient approach is to simply allow the patient a specific number of carbohydrates, protein and fats per day (Figure 14-7).

Low-Fat Diet. A doctor may order a low-fat diet for people with heart, gallbladder or liver disease. This diet calls for increased protein and carbohydrates and restricted amounts of fat.

Thickened Liquids. For people who have problems swallowing liquids such as orange juice, milk, tea, etc., the doctor will sometimes order a special liquid thickener such as Pro Mod™. These thickeners are added to the liquid and cause the drink to thicken to a pudding-type consistency. Always follow the directions on the container when using a thickening product.

Food Supplements. When a person has not been eating well or is losing weight because of an illness, the doctor usually orders a food supplement that is given with each meal. These supplements usually have a higher caloric, fat and protein content. Some examples of food supplements are Ensure™, Jevity™, Glucerna™ and Boost™. Remember to check with your supervising nurse regarding how often a person should receive food supplements.

People may need to limit the number of calories. Others require a limited amount of fluid. For example, a person with severe congestive heart disease or kidney disease may be allowed to receive only the amount of fluid ordered by the doctor. He may not be allowed to drink or eat at all for a certain amount of time. A person who undergoes certain blood tests or procedures may be forbidden to eat or drink after midnight or for a specific number of hours before the test or procedure.

If a doctor orders a therapeutic diet for someone in your care, make sure the person gets only the food permitted in that diet. Eating other foods or more food than is recommended can cause health problems.

To remind everyone that the person may not eat or drink, post a sign on their room door saying "NPO." If you have a resident or client that is on a special diet, it should be communicated during shift report.

Making Mealtime Enjoyable

Malnutrition can be a serious problem for nursing home residents. This condition is largely due to a loss of appetite, but a person who enjoys mealtime may eat more. You can play a big part in encouraging residents to eat by making mealtime pleasant for the people in your care. The following general rules will help you achieve that purpose:

- Keep the atmosphere as cheerful and comfortable as possible and provide adequate lighting.
- For people who eat in their rooms, keep the rooms neat, clean and free of odors.
- Allow adequate time for a person to prepare for his meal. Encourage him to go to the bathroom and wash his hands before eating.
- If needed, help the person into a comfortable, upright, sitting position, with his head up and his hips

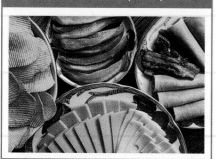

FIGURE 14-6 A person who eats a lot of these foods consumes a large amount of sodium. These foods are inappropriate for a low sodium or a no-added-salt (NAS) diet.

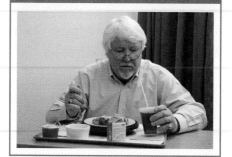

FIGURE 14-7 The people in your care may have medical reasons for avoiding certain foods or eating special foods. Because this resident is diabetic, the dietary department plans special meals for him that are low in carbohydrates and fat.

at a 90-degree angle. This position makes it easier for him to chew and swallow, as well as to manage his eating utensils.

- Serve meals promptly to make sure hot food stays hot and cold food stays cold. Some foods spoil quickly if you allow them to stand at room temperature.
- If a person is on a therapeutic diet, make sure that he gets the proper food. If sugar, salt or butter is not included with his meal, do not serve it without checking first with your supervising nurse.
- Identify a person's food allergies and dislikes so that these foods will not be served to him. If any of these foods are present, report this problem to your supervising nurse before serving the meal.
- Serve pureed food separately. Add seasoning, such as salt (if permitted) and pepper, to pureed food. A pureed meal does not have the appealing look of a regular diet, but a positive attitude toward the food can help a person accept it. Pureed food should have the consistency of pudding and should maintain a distinct identity from other pureed food. If you think the food needs to be thinned, check with the dietitian to determine the liquid to use. Also, check with your supervising nurse before thinning food if the person you are feeding has had a stroke or is paralyzed on one side. Some people who have difficulty swallowing may not be able to swallow thinned, pureed food or liquid.
- Report any uneaten food to your supervising nurse so that a substitute may be offered. Substituting food is especially important to prevent an insulin reaction in people with diabetes who must have a specific number of calories in their diets. Ask the person why he did not eat or whether he would like something else to eat.

- Observe people during mealtime to determine whether they need help with eating. Sometimes people leave part of a meal uneaten because they get too tired to finish. If the person does tire, you may have to help him eat more or give him a snack later.

In a nursing home, encourage residents to eat in the dining room, if possible (Figure 14-8). Assure them that they will receive as much help and direction as needed. For example, help or direct a resident to the dining room, and help him sit down. Provide protective covering for his clothing if he needs and wants it.

Helping People Eat

Some of the people in your care need assistance when they are eating, and this task may make them feel helpless. It is important for you to encourage a person to do as much as possible on his own. You may have to open a milk carton for someone whose hands are unsteady or weak. You may have to cut up meat for someone who is paralyzed on one side. You may have to steady or support the elbow of a person whose arm is weak while he feeds himself. At each meal, talk with the person about the amount of help he needs, because he may have different needs at different meals. The amount of help he needs depends in part on the kind of

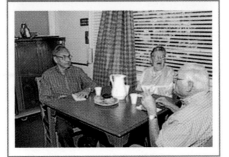

FIGURE 14-8 Being in the company of others and socializing are positive aspects of eating.

food served. For example, a person may be able to hold a sandwich but may not be able to cut up meat.

If you are helping someone eat, follow the specific procedure that is explained step by step in Skill 37 at the end of this chapter. Also follow these suggestions for helping people eat:

- When serving a person's meal, remove the dishes from the tray and place them on the table to create a more homelike environment. Some nursing homes may serve food directly on trays with compartments for different parts of the meal.
- Make sure the person is positioned correctly for eating. If possible, use a dining room or kitchen chair that pulls close to the table. Make sure the person's feet are flat on the floor, and have him rest his elbows or forearms on the table if he needs support. If the person wishes, provide protection for his clothing by spreading a towel or napkin over his chest.
- Encourage him to hold finger foods.
- If you must help feed the person, ask whether he has a preferred order for eating foods and ask about preferred seasonings.
- If the person is going to drink hot liquids such as coffee or tea, test the temperature before serving by placing several drops on your wrist. If the liquid feels too hot on your wrist, allow it to cool slightly before serving it. Serving liquid at the correct temperature is especially important if the person drinks hot liquid through a straw, because the liquid bypasses the lips as the straw delivers liquid far back in the mouth, where it could cause serious burns to the mouth and throat.
- To offer a hot liquid by straw, first stir the liquid with the straw to distribute the heat evenly. Place the straw in the person's mouth. He can suck and swallow the liquid as he desires. If the person sucks

too much liquid, you may have to pinch off the straw and pull it away so that he can swallow.

- To offer fluids by cup to a person who is not sitting up, use one hand to raise and support the person's head. Use the other hand to hold the cup while the person drinks.
- Offer liquids to a person only when he has no food in his mouth.
- Feed the person slowly. Offer a liquid first to moisten his mouth and make it easier to swallow. Then begin offering solids by filling a spoon two-thirds full. Touch the spoon to the person's bottom lip so that he opens his mouth. Then touch the spoon to his tongue (Figure 14-9). This touch to the lips and tongue lets him know where the spoon is in his mouth. Allow time between bites for the person to chew and swallow. Offer liquids after several swallows of solid food, making sure the liquids are not too hot. End the meal with water to rinse the mouth.
- Name each food as you offer it.
- Wipe the person's mouth with a napkin, as needed.

When the person in your care has finished with a meal, remove the dishes and tidy up the table. If needed, help the person wash his hands and brush his teeth or rinse his mouth as desired.

Good nutrition is more than just eating the correct food. When helping someone eat, you can help his body work more efficiently by following the general principles related to digestion that appear in Box 14-2.

Helping a Person Who is Blind with Mealtime. If you provide care for a person with a visual impairment, remember that he can probably eat by himself if he has no other disabilities. Unless he has a special condition, you probably need to do only the following:

- Identify the foods on the table and on the plate. Describe their locations as if the plate were the face of a clock (Figure 14-10). For example, if peas are on the dinner plate at the place closest to the person, you could say, "Peas are at 6 o'clock." If potatoes are directly across from the peas, you could say, "Potatoes are at 12 o'clock." If a glass of water is on the table near the upper right portion of the plate, you could say, "A glass of water is at 2 o'clock."
- Cut up meats or anything else that needs cutting.
- Open containers.
- Describe the location of the dining utensils.
- During the meal, occasionally check on the person to see whether he has overlooked some of the food and, if so, to offer assistance.

Helping Someone Who has Difficulty Swallowing. A person who has had a stroke that has resulted in speech difficulties may also have trouble swallow-

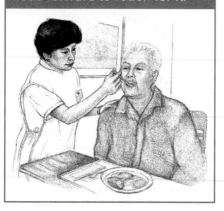

FIGURE 14-9 When helping someone eat, put the spoon into the person's mouth so that he will not have to move his head forward to reach for it.

BOX 14-2

WHAT CAN YOU DO TO HELP THE DIGESTIVE SYSTEM WORK AS WELL AS POSSIBLE?

1. Encourage people to drink liquids.
2. Encourage people to eat high-fiber foods, such as cereal, whole-grain bread, vegetables and fruit.
3. Allow enough time for eating and completely chewing food before swallowing.
4. Be sensitive to a person's eating patterns. Many older people cope better with frequent small meals than with a few larger ones.
5. Remember that mealtime also serves a social need.
6. Encourage the person to remain in an upright position for 60-90 minutes to aid digestion (gastric reflux).
7. Encourage regular bowel functioning by the following:
   • Provide privacy and time for using the toilet.
   • Encourage exercise to stimulate bowel activity.
8. Provide good mouth care.
9. Report any of the following occurrences to your supervising nurse:
   • A person's appetite changes.
   • A person's bowel habits change.
   • A person has signs of nausea and vomiting.

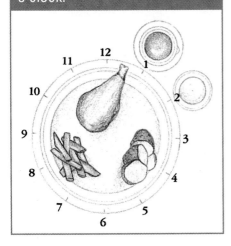

ing food. The doctor and speech therapist will make an initial assessment of the person's ability to swallow and, if the person is able to swallow, will order the appropriate diet. Generally, soft foods are easier for the person to swallow than liquids, which run down the throat. When you help feed him, observe the following guidelines:

- Remain with the person while he is eating.
- Place food toward the back of his mouth and on the unaffected side, because he cannot feel the food on the affected side and it may accumulate in his cheek.
- Encourage him to chew slowly and thoroughly.
- Eliminate distractions, such as television or many visitors, from the room so that the person can concentrate on eating.
- Encourage him to tilt his chin down as he swallows.

- Keep his head elevated during eating and for at least 30 minutes after eating.

Some people will be able to feed themselves with the help of special utensils or feeding aids, described in the next section.

Helping Someone Use Adaptive Feeding Devices. A variety of adaptive feeding devices help a person with disabilities to gain as much independence as possible when eating. Before serving a meal, check to see whether the person uses any adaptive feeding equipment.

The most common problems people have with feeding themselves are using utensils while trying to cope with conditions such as weak or paralyzed limbs and poor eyesight. Information about adaptive feeding devices and methods used to solve problems with feeding appears in Table 14-2.

Providing Care for Someone Who is Fed through a Gastrostomy Tube. If a person cannot swallow, has trouble swallowing or cannot take foods by mouth, a doctor may order a gastrostomy tube so that the person can receive food. A doctor inserts the gastrostomy tube directly into the person's stomach through a surgical **incision.** The tube is clamped and held in place by **sutures** and covered with a dressing.

A nurse puts commercially prepared formula and water into the tube, which gives the person a nutritionally adequate diet even though he cannot swallow. When you provide care to a person who has a gastrostomy tube, you must observe the following important rules:

- Never feed the person any food or fluid by mouth. Only a nurse may feed him through the tube or give him food or fluid by mouth.
- When the nurse inserts food into a gastrostomy tube, she elevates the head of the bed at least 45 degrees (semi-Fowlers) to prevent aspiration. Keep the head of the bed elevated for at least 30 minutes after a gastrostomy tube feeding.
- Follow the instructions of your supervising nurse for cleaning the area around a person's gastrostomy tube. Be careful not to wet the dressing when giving the person a bath. Notify your supervising nurse if the person complains of pain or discomfort in the abdomen, nausea or gas problems, or if you see any redness, irritation or drainage around the tube insertion site.
- When providing care for a person with a gastrostomy tube, always position him so that he is not lying on the tube. Occasionally a person may attempt to pull out his tube. Talk with your supervising nurse about methods to use to prevent this action from happening. To maintain proper gastric suctioning, follow the procedure that is explained step by step in Skill 38.

Helping Someone in Isolation with Mealtime. Before bringing a meal tray to a person who is in isolation, first put on protective clothing as described in Chapter 7, "Controlling the Spread of Germs." Once you are in the person's room, help him into a comfortable position for eating and assist him with his meal as needed. Since a person in isolation cannot socialize with others, it is important to give him companionship if he wants it and allow him enough time to finish his meal. When the person has finished eating, dispose of any leftover food or liquid in the toilet or sink. Double-bag any reusable utensils, as well as any garbage. To avoid the spread of infection, your employer may serve meals on disposable plates, with disposable cups and utensils, to people in isolation.

Monitoring the Amount a Person Eats and Drinks

A person's **appetite** is affected by many things. For example, he may not have a very good appetite if he is ill or

TABLE 14-2 ADAPTIVE FEEDING DEVICES

If Someone is Having Trouble With . . .	Use This Device	How to Use the Device/How the Device Helps	How to Improvise When the Device Is Not Available
1. Trying to get food on the utensil	Plate guard	Keeps food from falling off the plate as the person tries to scoop it onto the fork or spoon.	Ask the person to use his weak hand or arm to hold a piece of bread on the plate to block the food and then use his unaffected hand to push the food onto the fork or spoon.
	Scoop dish	This plate with a rounded side keeps food from falling off the plate.	
	Spork	This spoon-fork combination allows the person to either spear or scoop food onto the utensil.	
2. The plate slipping around or moving	Suction base	Place the suction base underneath the plate to hold it more securely in place.	Place a wet washcloth under the plate to increase suction and stability.
3. Grasping and holding onto utensils	Built-up utensils: Vertical or horizontal palm self-handle utensils	Slip the handle over the palm of the person's hand.	Use foam rubber or leather to build up the handles of a standard utensil or put the utensil into a bicycle handle or tennis ball.
	Utensil holder	Place the holder over the person's palm. Put the utensil inside the holder.	
	Universal cuff	Fasten the strap to the person's hand. Put the utensil handle inside the strap.	
4. Food falling off a utensil because of an arm tremor or weakness	Swivel utensil (fork or spoon)	The bowl of the fork or spoon can remain horizontal even if the person's hand shakes. It may have a built-up handle. Guide the person's hand as necessary.	Rest the person's elbow on a piece of sponge rubber on the table to lessen tremors. Guide the person's hand as necessary.
5. Using both hands and a knife to cut food	Rocker knife	A person can use one hand to cut by rocking the sharp edge over the food to cut it.	
6. Spilling liquids as he attempts to drink from a cup	Modified drinking cup	The cover and spout keep liquid from spilling.	Secure plastic wrap over the top of a cup with a rubber band and put a straw through a small opening in the top.
	Commercial straw holder	The holder keeps the straw in place.	
7. Reaching his mouth with a utensil because of limited arm movement	Extension utensil	The utensil handle is longer.	

nauseated. He may feel either very hungry or not very hungry because of medication he is taking. His appetite may change if he is worried, afraid or sad. He may eat even when he is not hungry because he is happy, excited, bored or lonely.

A person's appetite may be affected by the smell of food. The smell may make one person hungry, yet make another person feel nauseated. Smell also affects how food tastes. When a person cannot smell food, he cannot taste much. A person whose nose is stuffed up may not be hungry because he cannot smell or taste the food. The next time you eat, try holding your nose to see whether it makes a difference.

If the person in your care does not have much of an appetite or if his appetite changes suddenly, report these situations to your supervising nurse.

It is often important to measure and record how much the person in your care eats and drinks (intake). It is also important to measure and record how much fluid passes through his system (output). The medical abbreviation for measuring intake and output is I&O. You will learn about measuring output in Chapter 15, "Elimination."

Recording the Amount of Food Eaten

It is important to record the amount of food each person eats. If someone on a special diet does not eat all his food, he may need a snack or food supplement between meals. To judge how much extra food he needs, you may be asked to record the amount of food he eats at each meal. You also may be asked to record the amount of the snack or supplement the person eats. Between-meal snacks are offered to people who have special conditions, including diabetes, poor appetite, weight loss and pressure ulcers. These foods may be liquid, such as milk-shakes or liquid supplements, or solid, such as a sandwich.

When determining how much a person has eaten, you will find that most facilities ask that you determine the amount of food eaten and then record it on a food acceptance record (Figure 14-11). The food acceptance record lists foods that are usually served at the facility for each meal, as well as snacks. After a meal or snack, you must check off the foods eaten. If the person is on a special diet that requires them to eat a certain amount of food and they refuse or they only eat ¾, or 75%, of the required food, the resident is offered a food substitute.

Try this: Look at Figure 14-12. Using the food acceptance record in Figure 14-11, what would you check off, and how much food would you estimate that the person ate? Would you offer a food replacement?

Following are examples of different ways to estimate how much food a person eats. Try completing the food acceptance record, and think about whether or not you would offer a food replacement substitute and, if so, what type of food substitute should be offered.

- At lunch, you serve Mrs. Wang a cheese sandwich, tomato soup, a bowl of cherries, milk and coffee. She eats only a few bites of the sandwich. You would record *R* (refused) for the few bites of the sandwich and *R* for the rest of the food. Mrs. Wang should be offered a menu substitute.
- For dinner, you serve Josie Miller a small breast of chicken, potatoes, broccoli, fruit cocktail, milk and cookies. She eats all of the meat on her plate, but none of the other foods. In this case, you would record *A* (all) for all of her meat and *R* for the rest of her food. Ms. Miller should be offered substitutes for the food she did not eat.
- At dinner, Mrs. McDay sits down to a meal of mixed vegetables, potatoes, a pork chop, an apple,

pudding and coffee. She eats half of the vegetables and all of the potatoes from her plate, but none of the other foods. What would you record on her food acceptance record?
- At breakfast, you serve Mrs. Ryan one egg, two pieces of toast, orange juice and coffee. She eats the egg and one piece of toast and drinks her coffee. Would you offer Mrs. Ryan a food substitute?
- Mr. Lightfoot eats all of the food that you serve him for lunch (a piece of baked chicken, a serving of broccoli, a serving of rice, a piece of apple pie and a cup of coffee). How would you fill out his food acceptance record?

If you are uncertain how to complete the food acceptance record, check with your supervising nurse. Recording guidelines vary among health care facilities.

The Importance of Fluid Intake

With certain illnesses, it is important to know how much fluid someone drinks and how much passes through her body. Most people must drink 6 to 8 cups (or about 1,500 to 2,000 cc or ml) of fluid each day to stay healthy or become well. A person can take fluid in liquid form, such as water, coffee, juice, milk, soup and tea, or in solid form, such as ice cream, sherbet or gelatin. She must consume enough fluid to replace the fluid lost each day in the form of urine, perspiration, bowel movements and breath vapor. (When you breathe on a cold glass or mirror and it fogs up, you can see that this is fluid that you are losing from your body.)

A person must take in the same amount of fluid as her body puts out to maintain fluid balance. If a person consumes a large amount of fluid and does not lose much fluid, it could be a sign of disease. Likewise, if a person loses more fluid than she takes in, this also could be a sign of

FIGURE 14-11 Food Acceptance Record

FOOD ACCEPTANCE RECORD

Name: _____ Room # _____ Month/Year _____ Reason: _____

Food	1	2	3	4	5	6	7	8	9	10	11	12	13	14	15	16	17	18	19	20	21	22	23	24	25	26	27	28	29	30	31
BREAKFAST																															
Total Meal Eaten																															
Fruit/Juice cc's																															
Milk cc's																															
Other Beverages cc's																															
Bread/Margarine																															
Meat/Egg																															
Cereal																															
Substitute																															
Supplement cc's																															
Initials																															
AM SNACK																															
Initials																															
LUNCH																															
Total Meal Eaten																															
Fruit/Juice cc's																															
Milk cc's																															
Other Beverages cc's																															
Meat/Main Dish																															
Bread/Margarine																															
Starch/Potato																															
Vegetable																															
Dessert																															
Substitute																															
Supplement cc's																															
Initials																															
AFTERNOON SNACK																															
Initials																															
SUPPER																															
Total Meal Eaten																															
Fruit/Juice cc's																															
Milk cc's																															
Other Beverages cc's																															
Meat/Main Dish																															
Bread/Margarine																															
Starch/Potato																															
Vegetable																															
Dessert																															
Substitute																															
Supplement cc's																															
Initials																															
HS SNACK																															
Initials																															

Substitutes offered (same food category) when <u>less than 3/4</u> of tray is eaten or if <u>food is refused.</u>   © Mercy Continuing Care, 2000

- Fruit/Juice includes fruited Jello and fruit as dessert
- Meat/Main Dish includes egg, casserole or entrée
- Starch/Potato includes pasta, rice
- Dessert includes cake, cookie, ice cream, sherbet or other
- Supplement = canned or house liquid

Recording of eating each item:
R = Refused
— = Not on tray

Amount of Item Eaten
A = All Food Eaten
3/4 = 75% of Item Eaten
1/2 = 50% of Item Eaten
1/4 = 25% of Item Eaten

Amount of liquids taken in cc's:
Milk carton 8oz = 240cc's
Juice glass 4oz = 120cc's
Cup – tea/coffee 6oz = 180cc's
Supplement 8oz = 240cc's

Glass 6oz = 180cc's
Tall Glass 8oz = 240cc's

---

disease. When a person perspires heavily (as with a fever), vomits (as with a stomach virus) or has diarrhea, she must replace lost fluids quickly.

Sometimes a person's fluid balance may be off because she does not drink enough. If someone in your care is losing a lot of fluid in one of these ways or is **dehydrated,** you must tell your supervising nurse. The symptoms of dehydration include the following:

- Confusion
- Constipation
- Drowsiness
- Very dry skin or chapped lips
- Poor skin **turgor**
- Decreased urination or scanty, dark-colored urine
- Elevated temperature

Dehydration is a serious condition. If you suspect that someone in your care is dehydrated, tell your supervising nurse immediately.

A person in your care may become dehydrated because she does not consume enough fluid. She may be afraid she will not get to the bathroom in time. She may be sick or have a disability—such as arthritis—that makes

FIGURE 14-12 How would you report how much food the person ate?

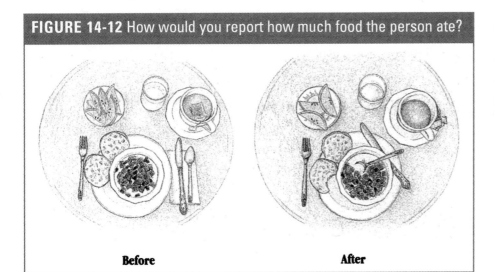

Before   After

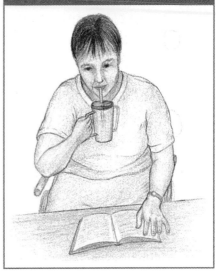

it difficult to get up to get a drink or to hold a glass. She may be afraid that she might spill the liquid and get her bed or clothing wet. Or she may simply forget to drink fluids. You can encourage her to drink the fluid she needs by following these guidelines:

- Offer fluids that the person likes at the temperature she prefers. (Be sure to ask what these fluids and temperatures are.)
- Encourage her to drink plenty of fluids with her meal. (Drinking with a meal may not be her usual habit.)
- Frequently provide her with a pitcher of clean, fresh water. Encourage her to drink each time you enter the room. (Follow your employer's policy for cleaning and refilling pitchers.)
- Be sure the person has a clean drinking glass or cup within easy reach. Refill the glass if she cannot do it. Supply a drinking straw if she needs it or a plastic container with a screw-on lid and a plastic straw if she has trouble with a

glass or is afraid of spilling fluids (Figure 14-13).

The doctor may give an order to "force fluids" for a person who is dehydrated. Forcing fluids means that the person should be urged to drink as much fluid as possible. You do not actually force the person to drink, but you encourage her to drink each time you enter the room and again on your way out. Keep a record of the amount of fluid the person does drink.

Record the amount of fluid intake and output on the specified sheet of paper. One side of the sheet is for recording intake measurements, and the other side is for output. Each time a person finishes drinking a container of liquid, record the amount in that container on the sheet. Sometimes printed information on the container indicates how much it holds. For example, a small prepackaged milk container contains 8 ounces. In other cases, you may have to determine how much a container holds. Some facilities have lists of the amount each of

their serving containers holds. If you are measuring a client's intake at home, you may have to measure how much each serving container holds. If the person does not finish the full amount in the container, estimate how much she drank and write that amount, usually in cubic centimeters (cc), on the sheet. At the end of your shift, add up the amount of fluid the person drank and record the total amount on the sheet.

Apply the information in this chapter to yourself, your family and the people in your care. Make what you serve and what you eat reflect the very best you can offer. Providing proper nutrition is more than a science. It is also an art. Eating for health and pleasure is one area in which you can be both scientist and artist.

INFORMATION REVIEW

Circle the correct answers and fill in the blanks.

1. In this book, *diet* means:
   a. a way to lose weight.
   b. a list of dos and don'ts about eating.
   c. all the food and liquid a person consumes.
   d. therapeutic.

2. A person needs more of which nutrient than all the others?
   a. Carbohydrates
   b. Protein
   c. Vitamins
   d. Fat

3. _____Fat_____ should be the smallest part of any diet.

4. Which therapeutic diet does not provide enough nutrients to maintain good nutrition?
   a. NAS
   b. Diabetic
   c. Full liquid
   d. Pureed

5. A clear liquid diet has to be reordered by the physician every _____ 24 8 _____ hours.

6. A high-protein diet is often prescribed for people who have decubitus ulcers or burns.

7. When a person has difficulty swallowing, it is easier for him or her to swallow _____ pureed _____ foods than liquids.

8. If a person in your care is fed through a gastrostomy tube, you should:
   a. keep the person lying flat for 30 minutes after a tube feeding.
   b. give the person water by mouth.
   c. use cotton balls moistened with alcohol to clean around the person's mouth and nose.
   d. keep the head of the bed elevated for 30 minutes following a tube feeding.

9. Which of these symptoms is *not* a sign of dehydration?
   a. Dark urine
   b. Dry skin
   c. Frequent urination
   d. Confusion

10. To promote healthy eating habits, you would:
    a. be patient, positive and consistent.
    b. force the person to eat everything on her plate.
    c. reward the person's good behavior with special treats.
    d. tell the person not to do what you do, but to do what you say.

QUESTIONS TO ASK YOURSELF

1. You notice that Mr. Rivera did not eat much of his breakfast or lunch. He says he feels okay and asks you not to worry. What would you do?

2. Mrs. Morgan tells you that her diabetic roommate has been stealing her cookies at lunch. You know that Mrs. Morgan's roommate cannot have cookies. What would you do?

3. Mrs. Garcia eats very little. She says she is not hungry. You suspect that she may tire easily and find it difficult to feed herself. You offer to help her eat, but she says she is too old to be fed like a baby. What would you do?

Skill 37: Helping a Person Eat

PRECAUTIONS
- When offering hot fluid through a straw, use caution so that the person does not burn his or her throat.
- Offer food slowly and in small amounts to prevent the person from choking.
- To avoid possible aspiration, make sure the person is awake and alert before offering food or drink.
- Check the person's diet before offering food.

PREPARATION
1. Gather supplies:
   - Towel
   - Washcloth
   - Special eating utensils, if needed
   - Special cups or drinking straws, if needed
2. Follow Preparation Standards (see Chapter 7).

PROCEDURE

Task 1: Preparing a Person for Mealtime
1. Help the person prepare for mealtime by assisting with toileting, appropriate dress, oral care, glasses and hair care. ☐ ☐
2. Assist the person in the dining room with table seating or wheelchair placement. ☐ ☐
3. Assist the person dining in his or her room with good lighting and comfortable seating at bedside. ☐ ☐
4. If you are using a geriatric feeding chair, make sure that the wheels are locked, that

the person's feet are on the footrest and that the adjustable tray is locked securely in the tray notches.

- Position a tray table in front of the person.
- Place a clothing protector on the person's chest and lap to protect against spills (Figure 14-14).
- Place fresh drinking water and the call signal within the person's reach. ☐ ☐

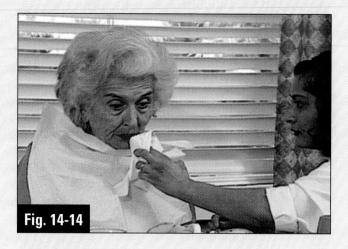

Fig. 14-14

For the person staying in bed for mealtime:

- Change any soiled bed linens.
- Position the person in Fowler's position with the tray table across the bed.
- Place a clothing protector under the person's chin to protect against spills.
- Place fresh drinking water and the call signal within the person's reach. ☐ ☐

Task 2: Serving a Meal Tray

1. Bring the tray to the person. Make sure the name on the tray matches the name of the person and that the tray of food matches the type of diet that the person is following. ☐ ☐
2. Check for any missing items. Correct any problems with the tray. ☐ ☐
3. Hand the napkin to the person or tuck it under his or her chin.
4. Open any containers or packages, butter bread, cut up meats or other food if the person needs help. ☐ ☐
5. Position the overbed table so that the person can easily reach the food. ☐ ☐
6. Assist the person to sit in an upright position. ☐ ☐

Task 3: Feeding a Person

1. Ensure the person is sitting in an upright position. ☐ ☐

2. Describe what is on the tray if the person cannot see, and ask in which order she prefers to eat things. ☐ ☐

3. Encourage the person to hold any finger foods. ☐ ☐

4. To offer liquids by cup to a person who cannot sit upright, raise and support her head with one hand while holding the cup with the other and allowing the person to drink. ☐ ☐

5. To offer liquids by straw, stir the liquid with the straw to distribute the heat evenly. Place the straw in the person's mouth so that she can suck and swallow the liquid as desired. (If the person sucks too much liquid, you may need to pinch off the straw and pull it away so that she can swallow.) Try to avoid having the person finish all the liquid first so that she is not too full to eat the solids. ☐ ☐

6. Feed the person slowly, naming each food as you offer it. ☐ ☐

7. Fill a spoon only two-thirds full. Touch the spoon to the person's lower lip and then to the tongue to let her know where the food is and when to open her mouth. Allow time between bites for the person to chew and swallow. Offer a liquid and then a few bites of food, followed by liquid again. ☐ ☐

8. Remove the tray when the person has finished eating. ☐ ☐

9. Provide mouth care after the meal. ☐ ☐

COMPLETION

Follow Completion Standards in compliance with your facility. For a complete list of those used in this course, see Chapter 7, "Controlling the Spread of Germs."

Skill 38: Maintaining Gastric Suctioning

PRECAUTIONS

- Follow universal precautions and use infection control techniques when handling stomach contents.

PREPARATION

1. Gather supplies:
   - One or two pairs of disposable gloves
   - Lip cream or petroleum jelly and cotton-tipped applicator
   - Plastic trash bag
   - Laundry bag (or plastic bag for wet or soiled linens)
   - Replacement suction container, if needed
2. Follow Preparation Standards.

PROCEDURE

1. Provide oral hygiene every 2 hours. ☐ ☐
2. Keep the person's nose clean and apply recommended lubricants to the nasal membranes. ☐ ☐
3. Check to make sure the suction is working and that fluid is collecting in the suctioning equipment (Figure 14-15). ☐ ☐

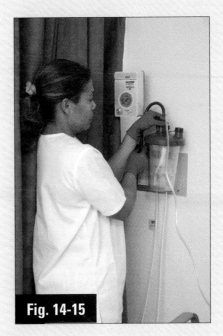

Fig. 14-15

ADDITIONAL INFORMATION

To provide oral hygiene to a person who has dentures, see Skill 23. If the person is unconscious, see Skill 24.

COMPLETION

Follow Completion Standards in compliance with your facility. For a complete list of those used in this course, see Chapter 7, "Controlling the Spread of Germs."

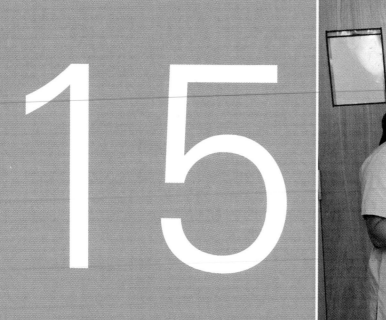

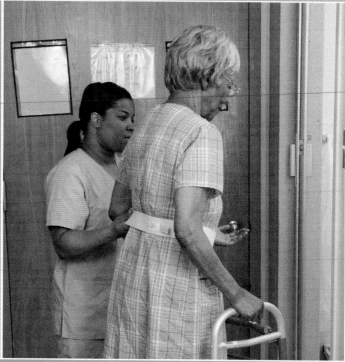

Chapter 15

Elimination

GOALS

After reading this chapter, you will have the information needed to:

Discuss daily elimination patterns and needs.

Explain special urinary needs.

Explain special bowel elimination needs.

After practicing the corresponding skills, you will have the information needed to:

Help a person use the bathroom toilet, portable commode, bedpan or urinal.

Provide perineal care for a person with a urinary catheter.

Empty a urinary drainage bag.

Apply an external catheter to a male resident.

Collect urine and stool specimens.

Strain urine.

Test urine for glucose and acetone.

Give a tap water, soap solution, commercial cleansing or oil-retention enema.

This morning, just as you are about to help Mr. Wilson with his bath, Josie Miller presses her call signal. You make sure that Mr. Wilson is safe and comfortable and tell him that you must answer a call signal and will return as soon as possible. You then go to Josie's room, where she is trying to get to the edge of her bed. She says she needs to have a bowel movement. You think this is a bit unusual, because she already had a bowel movement just after breakfast as she normally does.

You move the portable commode to the side of her bed, put on the brake and begin to prepare a basin of warm water when Josie says, "I don't want to use that thing today. I want to go to the bathroom and use a real toilet." You ask her whether she feels well enough to walk to the bathroom or if she wants to ride to the bathroom in her wheelchair. "I'll walk," says Josie.

Although you know that she usually uses the portable commode and that you must get back to Mr. Wilson's room to help him with his bath, you tell her that you understand. You help Josie put on her bathrobe and slippers before helping her use her walker to walk to the bathroom where she can use the "real toilet." You help her onto the toilet, rearrange her bathrobe and gown and

then step outside the bathroom door, where you wait for her to finish.

After 5 minutes, you knock on the door and ask Josie whether she needs help. She says she's taking care of things herself. You wait another few minutes and ask her again if she needs help. This time, you hear the frustration in her voice, and she agrees to let you come in to help her.

When you go into the bathroom, you discover that Josie has diarrhea and that she needs some assistance. You ask her permission to help her, and when she agrees, you put on gloves and clean her carefully, washing from front to back, and reassuring her.

Later, after you get Josie settled back in her bed and put away the portable commode and supplies, you stop at the nurses' station to report to your supervising nurse that Josie has diarrhea. Then you return to Mr. Wilson's room, where he begins to complain about your being gone for such a long time.

ELIMINATING BODY WASTE

Every living thing eats to provide nutrients to its body. The valuable parts of the food are absorbed into the body.

The wastes that are not used are **eliminated** from the body in several forms. Two of these forms of waste are **urine** and **feces,** or **stool.** Another form is **perspiration.**

For most people, going to the bathroom to eliminate body wastes is a regular occurrence. It is a natural and normal process that everyone does, although the words people use to describe the process may differ. As a nurse assistant, you must use the terms that people in health care use for elimination. Two correct terms for the elimination of urine are **urinate** and **void.** The correct term for the elimination of feces is **defecate** (you may also use the phrase "move the bowels"). It is important for you to use these words, but in some situations it is okay to use the term preferred by the person in your care. For example, on days when Mrs. McDay is extremely confused, the only way you can get her to cooperate in using the bathroom is to use her words, "number 1" and "number 2."

Most people in our society think elimination is a personal, private matter and may be embarrassed to talk about it. Some people are brought up to think that the parts of the body used for elimination are unclean or "dis-

KEY TERMS

concentrated: (KON-sen-tray-ted) containing a small percentage of water, less diluted.

constipation: (kon-stuh-PAY-shun) difficult elimination of a dry, hard stool.

defecate: (DEF-uh-kate) to eliminate solid waste from the body.

dehydration: (dee-hi-DRAY-shun) serious fluid loss.

diarrhea: (dye-uh-REE-uh) the frequent passage of liquid feces.

diluted: (di-LOO-ted) containing a large percentage of water.

eliminate: (uh-LIM-uh-nate) to get rid of.

enema: (EN-uh-muh) a solution introduced into the rectum and lower colon to relieve fecal impaction or constipation.

feces: (FEE-seez) solid body waste.

incontinence: (in-KON-ti-nense) the inability to control the release of urine or feces.

perspiration: (pur-spi-RAY-shun) body waste eliminated through the skin.

stool: solid body waste, or feces.

urinary catheter: (YUR-uh-nair-ee/KATH-uh-ter) a small tube (ordered by a doctor) that is inserted (usually by a nurse or doctor) through the urethra into the bladder. A small balloon at the end of the tube on the bladder end is blown up, or inflated, to hold the tube in place. On the other end, the tube connects to a bag that collects the urine.

urinate: (YUR-uh-nate) to eliminate liquid waste from the body.

urine: (YUR-in) liquid body waste.

void: to urinate.

gusting." They are taught not to touch those parts of the body on themselves or on other people.

As a nurse assistant, one of your responsibilities is helping the people in your care with elimination. You will learn how to provide this care with respect for their privacy and dignity. How do you feel about helping someone with her elimination needs? Feeling uncomfortable when you help a person who needs to urinate or move her bowels is normal.

How do you think people in your care feel about needing your help when they urinate or have a bowel movement? Do you think they might feel embarrassed, helpless or angry? It's extremely important for you to be sensitive to people's feelings about needing help with a very personal function. It's also important that you always act in a positive, professional way when you help them.

DAILY ELIMINATION

A person normally eliminates 1 to 1 ½ quarts of urine each day. Normal urine is clear and golden yellow to amber in color and has a slight odor. In the morning, the color of urine is darker, and as the day goes on, it gets lighter. Urine changes color because a person usually takes in less fluid at night than during the day. Decreased fluid intake causes urine to be more **concentrated,** which makes the color darker. During the day, when a person drinks more fluids, the urine becomes more **diluted,** which makes the color lighter. Drinking fluids frequently helps keep urine diluted and light yellow. If urine remains concentrated for too long, it irritates the bladder and can cause an infection.

Feces are normally brown in color, soft in texture and formed. Because feces are about three-fourths water and one-fourth solid waste products, it is important for people to drink water to maintain regular bowel movements.

The frequency with which a person has bowel movements is called her or his *pattern of bowel elimination.* This pattern varies from person to person. Some people have bowel movements every day, others every 2 to 3 days. A change in routine can disrupt a person's bowel elimination pattern.

PATTERNS OF ELIMINATION

An elimination pattern indicates the number of times each day a person uses the bathroom, how much time passes between voiding, and what time and how often a person usually has a bowel movement. Every person has her or his own normal pattern of elimination. You must learn the elimination pattern of each person in your care so that you can help maintain the pattern and recognize changes in it.

Think about your own elimination pattern. How would you feel if you had to rely on another person to take you to the bathroom at those times? How would you feel if someone tried to change your elimination pattern? For example, let's say that every day, all your life, you have moved your bowels after breakfast. It would be important for the person providing care for you to know this pattern. What would happen if that person decided it was more convenient for you to have your bowel movement after lunch?

Maintaining Normal Elimination Patterns

You can help maintain a person's normal elimination pattern in the following ways: (1) learn about her elimination pattern, (2) answer her call signal promptly, (3) provide her privacy during elimination, (4) give her as much time as she needs to eliminate, (5) be sensitive to her feelings about having to ask for assistance, (6) have a professional attitude about elimination, and (7) help her urinary and digestive systems work more efficiently.

Learn About the Person's Elimination Pattern. To learn about the person's elimination pattern, ask her these questions:

- How often do you urinate?
- Is there anything special about your urinating habits that I should know?
- How often do you have a bowel movement?
- What time of day do you usually have a bowel movement?
- Is there anything special about your bowel movement habits that I should know?

If the person cannot provide the information, ask her family members or check her chart to determine a pattern.

Answer the Person's Call Signal Right Away. Because of illness, a person may not always be able to control the urge to urinate or defecate, so it is important to answer her call signal right away. As people age, muscle tone may decrease, making it difficult to control the flow of urine.

Even for the person who has control over her elimination, it is important to answer the call signal right away, because she may need help getting out of bed or getting to the bathroom. If she cannot get out of bed, she may need help using a bedpan. When a person cannot control the release of urine or feces, this condition is called **incontinence.** The person may be truly incontinent, or she may simply have been unable to find the bathroom or get there on her own. Another possibility is that the person needed help, but a staff member did not answer her call signal right away (Figure 15-1). Think about Josie and how she was trying to get out of bed when you answered her call signal. What might have happened if you had decided to ignore her call signal and give Mr. Wilson his bath first?

Provide Privacy for the Person During Elimination. To provide privacy, pull the curtain around the bed or

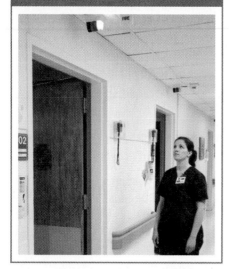

close the door. Encourage the person to eliminate in private, but let her know that you are nearby to help if she needs you. Make sure the call signal is easy for her to reach.

Give the Person as Much Time as She Needs to Eliminate. Give the person plenty of time to take care of her elimination needs, but check on her regularly so that you do not leave her stranded on the bedpan or alone in the bathroom for too long. Encourage her to remain on the toilet a few minutes after voiding to make sure her bladder is empty.

Be Sensitive to a Person's Feelings About Having to Ask for Assistance. Often a person may be too embarrassed to ask for help using the bathroom. She may feel ashamed or not in control if she cannot get to the bathroom by herself. She may be embarrassed if she needs help with perineal care.

Have a Professional Attitude About Elimination. In response to the feelings of a person in your care,

approach the elimination task positively, show her respect and make sure that your facial expressions and gestures do not show displeasure.

Help the Person's Urinary and Digestive Systems Work More Efficiently. Offer the person fluids frequently during the day and encourage her to drink six to eight glasses of liquid each day to help her urinary and digestive systems work more efficiently (Figure 15-2). Also, encourage her to exercise and to eat high-fiber foods, such as whole grains and fresh fruits and vegetables.

Helping a Person Use a Bathroom Toilet

Often when you answer a person's call signal, she needs you to help her use the bathroom toilet. If she is in bed, help her put on her bathrobe and slippers before going to the bathroom. When assisting someone to use the bathroom toilet, please observe these precautions:

- Make sure the person in your care is safe before leaving him alone in the bathroom.

FIGURE 15-2 Extra fluid intake is essential to maintaining healthy urinary and digestive systems. Because Josie has diarrhea, she needs to drink fluid to help avoid dehydration.

- Stay just outside the bathroom door.
- Check on him at least every 5 minutes to make sure he is okay and to see whether he needs assistance.

To learn the step-by-step procedure for helping someone use the toilet, see Skill 39 at the end of this chapter.

Always report any significant changes or difficulty with urination or defecation.

Maintaining a Normal Environment with an Alternative Toilet

Not everyone can use a bathroom toilet. Some people have to use an alternative toilet, such as:

- A portable commode, which the person sits on by the side of the bed.
- A bedpan, which the person sits on while in the bed.
- A urinal, which a man uses while in the bed or standing beside the bed.

A person who must use an alternative toilet may see elimination as a more difficult, or even distasteful, task. You can make this experience more comfortable if you make it as similar as possible to using a bathroom toilet.

Helping a Person Use a Portable Commode. A portable commode looks like a chair with a toilet seat (Figure 15-3). Under the seat is a collection container, bedpan or bucket (with or without a lid) that can be removed for emptying and cleaning. Some portable commodes have wheels, and some do not. Sometimes they remain at the person's bedside. In other situations, you may have to bring one to the person's room for a short period of time. When assisting someone to use a commode, observe these precautions:

- Check with your supervising nurse before moving the person from the bed to the commode.

FIGURE 15-3 A portable commode is a good solution for a person who does not use a bedpan and cannot get to the bathroom. To use a commode, a person must be able to sit up with little assistance.

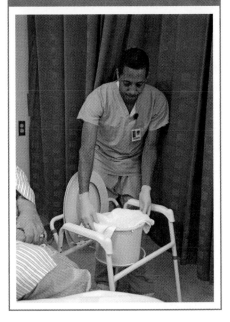

FIGURE 15-4 A regular bedpan is less likely to spill and is used most often. If a person cannot move enough to get on a regular bedpan (on the left), have him use a fracture pan (on the right).

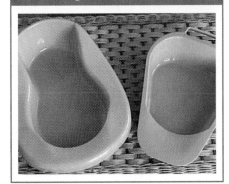

or using a urinal at least every 5 minutes to make sure he is okay and to see whether he needs assistance. If the person is on the bedpan or has a urinal in place for longer than 5 minutes, he can develop pressure ulcers. To learn the procedure for helping

someone use a bedpan or urinal, see Skill 41.

Measuring Fluid Output

You will occasionally need to measure a person's fluid output for two reasons: to compare it with the normal range of output and to compare it with her fluid intake (see the discussion on measuring fluid intake in Chapter 14) to determine the balance of fluids in her body.

To measure a person's output of fluid, use a graduate (a pitcher with measurement marks on its side). When the person finishes using a portable commode, bedpan or urinal, pour the contents of the container into the graduate. Look at the fluid level to determine the amount to record on the intake and output (I&O) sheet. Each time a person is incontinent of stool (with **diarrhea**) or urine, make a check mark in the right place on the I&O sheet. Ask a nurse to measure or estimate the fluid output from vomit, blood or diarrhea, if necessary. In hospitals

- Make sure the collection container is under the seat.
- If the commode has wheels, lock the wheels before moving the person from the bed to the commode.
- Check on the person at least every 5 minutes to make sure he is okay and to see whether he needs any assistance.
- Ask a co-worker to help, if needed.

To learn the step-by-step procedure for helping someone use a portable commode, see Skill 40.

Helping a Person Use a Bedpan or Urinal. When a person cannot get out of bed to urinate or defecate, he must use a bedpan (Figure 15-4). A man may use a urinal to urinate (Figure 15-5). Using a bedpan is not very comfortable and may feel unnatural. Check on a person who is sitting on the bedpan

FIGURE 15-5 If a man cannot stand at the side of the bed to use a urinal, he may prefer to sit on the side of the bed. Both of these positions are preferable to lying in bed.

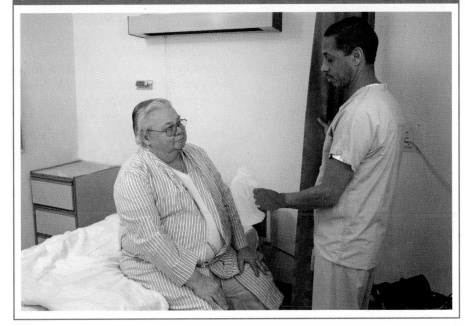

and nursing homes, I&O sheets are totaled at the end of each shift.

SPECIAL URINARY ELIMINATION NEEDS

As a nurse assistant, you play a key role in identifying potential urinary elimination problems by observing and reporting changes in a person's urinary elimination pattern. For example, if someone in your care usually voids every 2 to 3 hours and suddenly starts asking to void every ½ to 1 hour, you would report the change to your supervising nurse.

You might identify another potential problem when you observe and report that a person is not taking in enough fluid. You would suspect this problem if the amount of the person's urine decreased and the color and smell became darker and stronger.

Some people develop urinary problems as a result of physical conditions, changes in diet or poor personal hygiene. Also, as people grow older, they often develop urinary problems because of changes that occur in the urinary system. Common urinary problems include urinary incontinence and urinary tract infection. Urinary incontinence is loss of control of the release of urine from the bladder, and it is not a normal process of aging. Several factors can lead to urinary incontinence:

- Damage to the brain that prevents the individual from feeling the urge to urinate
- Weakness of the muscles surrounding the opening of the bladder
- Medications (diuretics)
- Confusion about where to go to the bathroom
- Difficulty in moving, making it hard to get to the bathroom
- Not having a call signal answered in a timely manner
- Urinary tract infection

A urinary tract infection can occur in any part of the urinary system (or urinary tract)—kidney, bladder, ureter or urethra—and it can be painful. Several of the following symptoms may indicate such an infection:

- Pain or burning sensation when urinating
- Frequent or urgent need to urinate but with only a little urine released at a time
- Cloudy, concentrated (dark yellow) and possibly foul-smelling urine
- Milky mucus discharge or blood in the urine
- Fever

If someone in your care has any of these symptoms, you should report this information to your supervising nurse. However, keep in mind that older adults may not show these symptoms yet still have infection.

Causes of a urinary tract infection include any of the following:

- Inadequate fluid intake
- Incomplete emptying of the bladder
- Poor perineal care
- Poor urinary catheter care

When you respond to people who have special urinary elimination needs, you must remember that the people in your care cannot meet their own needs. They rely on you to help them and to offer support and encouragement. Give the best care possible when you provide care for a person who is incontinent, when you help someone who has a urinary tract infection, when you assist a person with a urinary catheter and when you collect and test urine specimens.

Preventing Urinary Tract Infections

The stroke that left Mr. Rivera paralyzed on his left side also left him incontinent of urine. As part of his training program to help him regain control of his bladder, you encourage him to be patient and to take the time

he needs to completely empty his bladder. But Mr. Rivera becomes irritated and impatient about this part of the training program. You think he may be embarrassed about all the attention he is getting about urinating. So he always insists that you take away the urinal immediately. As a result of his failure to empty his bladder completely, Mr. Rivera develops a urinary tract infection.

To help a person prevent the development of a urinary tract infection, do all the things you normally do for any person in your care. In addition:

- Offer the person fluids frequently.
- Provide time for the person to empty the bladder completely when eliminating urine.
- Encourage female residents to wipe from front to back.
- If the person is incontinent, change adult briefs often.

Assisting People with Special Urinary Elimination Needs

Because she has Alzheimer's disease, Shirley McDay is often confused about where she has been and what she has done. She often forgets whether she has used the toilet and even forgets where the bathroom is. As a result, she often doesn't get to the bathroom in time to void. She has episodes of incontinence. To help Mrs. McDay, do all the things you normally do for any person in your care. In addition:

- Offer her fluids frequently throughout the day. Increasing fluid intake dilutes the urine so that it is less irritating to the bladder, which results in a decrease in the problems of incontinence, urinary dribbling and urinary tract infection.
- Help her if she has trouble rising or walking to get to the bathroom.
- Offer her frequent opportunities to go to the bathroom, particularly if she is confused. Give her sufficient time and provide privacy.

- Learn about her voiding pattern and offer her assistance just prior to the time she usually voids.
- Be sensitive to the embarrassment she may feel about being incontinent. Be aware that she may be concerned about the need to wear adult briefs to protect her clothing. It is important to call the protective underwear *briefs,* not *diapers.* Adult briefs should be used only when absolutely necessary and not as a convenience for the health care team.
- Offer her emotional support and encouragement.
- Help her with a bladder training program.

A doctor or nurse may sometimes recommend that a person participate in a bladder training program to help her regain urinary control. The training schedule is written on the person's care plan. Support the person in her bladder training program by taking her to the toilet on a regular schedule or at least every 2 hours, allowing her sufficient time to urinate, and following the training schedule 24 hours a day. Supporting a bladder training program means following the schedule during the night as well, although the intervals between using the toilet may be longer during the night.

Providing Perineal Care for a Person with a Urinary Catheter

Sometimes when a person has a urinary problem, he needs a **urinary catheter** to help eliminate urine from his body (Figure 15-6). A person also may need a urinary catheter if he has nerve damage following a stroke or spinal cord injury and has no control over elimination, he may need one if he is incontinent (and is prone to developing pressure sores on the skin), or if he is undergoing or has undergone certain kinds of surgery. (You may hear health care professionals refer to the catheter by other

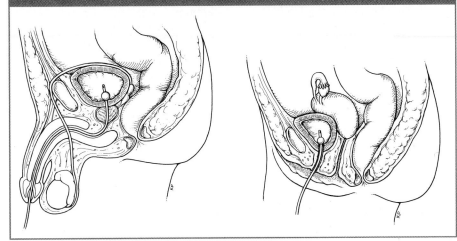

FIGURE 15-6 An indwelling urinary catheter is inserted through the urethra and into the bladder. It is held in place by a small balloon inflated in the bladder. The catheter drains into a plastic bag.

names, such as a *Foley catheter* or an *indwelling catheter.*)

To show special concern and provide special care for someone who has a urinary catheter:

- Offer fluids frequently to help dilute urine, which decreases the chance of developing a urinary tract infection.
- Provide perineal care on a regular schedule and whenever the person is soiled with secretions or feces. Use Standard Precautions and Isolation Precaution standards, if necessary, when providing perineal care for a person who has a catheter, which includes wearing disposable gloves. Make sure the perineal area is kept clean, dry and free from skin irritation. Clean the perineum from the front to the back. Report any blood, redness or swelling.
- Keep in mind that a catheter can be uncomfortable, and without proper care a person can develop an infection.

To learn the procedure for providing perineal care to someone with a urinary catheter, see Skill 42. To clean around tubes and catheters, follow the procedure in Skill 43. To change on ostomy appliance, see Skill 44.

FIGURE 15-7 When positioning a urinary drainage bag, make sure the bag is always placed lower than the person's bladder so urine can flow into it. Also, make sure the tubing is not kinked or hanging below the bag.

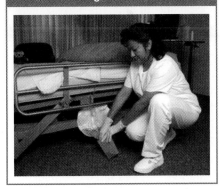

Urinary Catheter Care. In addition to providing care for the person who has a urinary catheter, remember to observe the following precautions:

- Maintain the urinary drainage flow by keeping the drainage bag below the person's bladder (urine flows downward by the force of gravity) (Figure 15-7).

- Make sure the catheter tubing is not kinked, bent or creased. If the tubing kinks, urine backs up into the bladder. An infection or serious damage to the bladder could occur if the tubing kinks for a long period of time. Also make sure that extra tubing does not loop down below the bag.
- For security, make sure the catheter tubing is taped or secured by a fastener to the top part of the person's thigh. Securing the tubing prevents it from rubbing and pulling at the entrance to the urethra.
- Keep the tubing or drainage bag from touching the floor, because the floor is dirty.
- When transferring a person to a chair, move the drainage bag before moving the person. If you do not move the bag first, the catheter could be pulled, causing injury and pain to the person.
- Notify your supervising nurse if you learn that the catheter has come out.
- Empty the drainage bag and note the color and volume of the urine.

Emptying a Urinary Drainage Bag. To measure output from a urinary drainage bag, release the clamp on the drainage bag and let the urine flow from the tube into the graduate (Figure 15-8). Never let the tip of the tube touch anything. When all the urine has emptied out of the bag, secure the clamp. Record the time of the collection and the amount collected in the graduate on the intake and output sheet. Also note any important observations, such as cloudy or foul-smelling urine, a change in the amount of urine, a change in the color of the urine and any complaints of pain by the person. When emptying a urinary drainage bag, follow the specific procedure explained step by step in Skill 45.

Applying an External Urinary Catheter to a Male. An external urinary catheter is used for many of the same reasons as an indwelling catheter. Used only for males, it consists of a condom-like device, tubing and a drainage bag (Figure 15-9). The condom fits over the man's penis and is attached to tubing, which is connected to the drainage bag. The bag may be the same type as the indwelling catheter drainage bag, or it may be designed to be strapped to his calf or thigh. This smaller leg bag is useful to wear under pants. Because it is smaller, it must be emptied every 2 hours. Remove the catheter once each day for bathing and then apply a new catheter. After bathing or perineal care, make sure the person's penis is dry so that the tape will stick during application. When applying an external urinary catheter, make sure the condom is completely unrolled so that it does not interfere with the person's circulation. Check the person frequently to make sure the condom is not too tight and that circulation is good. If you notice any swelling or color change in his penis, remove the condom and report your observations to your supervising nurse. When applying an external urinary

catheter, follow the procedure explained in Skill 46.

Collecting Urine Specimens
In addition to measuring and recording urinary output, you may collect urine when a doctor orders other laboratory tests. These tests, to be performed on a person's urine, help the doctor make decisions about his or her medical treatment. When you collect urine, you use one of three methods, and for people who have diabetes, you may actually perform one of the tests on the urine.

Three methods of collecting urine specimens are routine urine collection, clean catch or midstream collection and 24-hour collection. Each method is ordered by the doctor for a particular purpose, so use only the method ordered. Follow your supervising nurse's instructions for specimen collection. Remember to observe the prin-

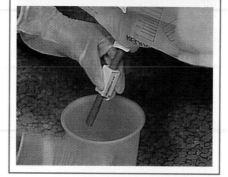

FIGURE 15-8 When emptying a urinary drainage bag, never let the tip of the tube touch anything.

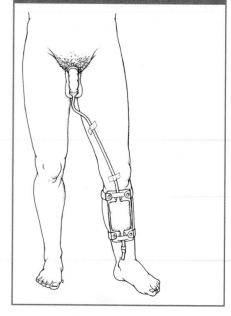

FIGURE 15-9 An external urinary catheter is less likely to interfere with body function or to cause a urinary tract infection than an indwelling catheter.

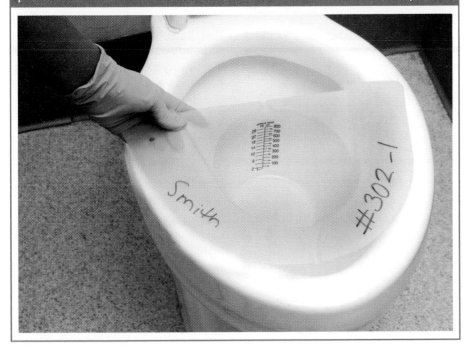

FIGURE 15-10 A urinary collection device, often called a "hat," is placed in a toilet or commode to collect and measure urine output.

ciples of Standard Precautions when collecting any specimen.

Routine Urine Specimen Collection. A routine urine specimen is collected for lab tests or to test for sugar and acetone in the urine of a person with diabetes. This specimen can be collected while the person is using the bathroom toilet, portable commode (Figure 15-10), bedpan or urinal by having him void directly into a specimen container or into a collection device. The specimen can also be collected by emptying urine from a portable commode, bedpan or urinal into a collection container.

Clean Catch, or Midstream, Urine Specimen Collection. A clean catch, or midstream, urine specimen is collected to determine whether the person has an infection, especially a urinary tract infection. The urine is analyzed for white blood cells and bacteria. Because the test is for bacteria, it is important that you do not touch and contaminate the inside of

the container, because contamination would affect the results of the lab test.

This type of collection is called a "clean catch" because the opening of the urethra is cleaned before the person starts to void. The cleaning removes any bacteria that may be around the opening so that it is not confused in the lab with the bacteria that may be in the urine. This type of catch is also called a "midstream" collection because the person starts to void (*not* in the container), then stops, then voids into the container. The initial flow of urine washes away additional bacteria around the urethral opening, giving the lab a more accurate specimen for the test. A clean catch specimen can be collected while the person is using the bathroom toilet, portable commode, bedpan or urinal.

24-hour Urine Specimen Collection. A 24-hour urine specimen is collected over 24 consecutive hours. The specimen is used to check for the pres-

ence of various chemicals in the urine, such as protein. For example, a person with kidney problems may have to provide urine over a 24-hour period so that the doctor can ask the lab to check for protein in the urine. Too much protein present in the urine shows that the kidneys are not working properly.

When you begin the collection, label and store the container according to your employer's policy.

Like a routine urine specimen, a 24-hour urine specimen can be collected while the person is using the bathroom toilet, portable commode, bedpan or urinal. Speak with your supervising nurse on ways to properly store the urine specimen.

Collecting Urine Specimens for People in Isolation. For people in isolation, take special precautions when collecting urine specimens. After putting on appropriate protective clothing, go into the person's room and place the labeled specimen container on a clean paper towel. Remove the lid of the container and place it on the paper towel. Collect the urine specimen and transfer the urine from the collection container into the specimen container, taking care not to touch the outside of the specimen container or to spill any urine on the outside of the specimen container. Use a clean paper towel to replace the lid on the specimen container. When you have finished the procedure, remove your protective clothing and dispose of it properly. Take the specimen container outside the isolation room and dispose of it according to the techniques indicated for the person's type of isolation. Put the specimen container in a designated area at the nurses' station, in the refrigerator or on a special tray, remove your gloves and wash your hands.

When collecting urine specimens, follow the specific procedure explained in Skill 47.

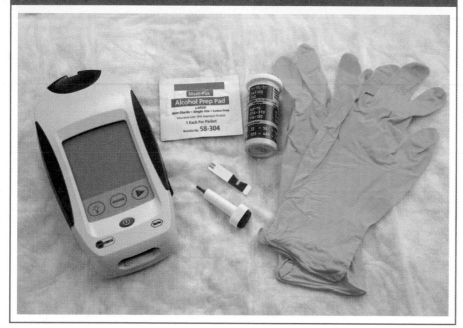

FIGURE 15-11 Using an electronic machine like this one is helpful in testing people who have diabetes, to determine the amount of glucose in their blood stream.

Straining Urine. The doctor may order that urine be strained. This is done primarily for a person suspected of having kidney stones and who may be passing stones in the urine. When straining urine for stones, follow the step-by-step procedure in Skill 48.

Testing Urine Specimens for Glucose and Acetone. Although there is not yet a cure for diabetes, it can be controlled through diet, exercise and medication therapy. Testing blood for glucose is the most common method for keeping track of the condition of someone with diabetes, but your facility may use other methods to test glucose levels in the body. (Figure 15-11). It is very important that you report glucose and acetone findings to your supervising nurse, because the person's diet and insulin dosage may have to be changed, depending on urine glucose and acetone results.

The doctor orders a test for glucose and acetone and specifies in the person's care plan what time of day to do the test, as well as how often to do the test. When testing urine for glucose and acetone, follow the procedure explained in Skill 49.

SPECIAL BOWEL ELIMINATION NEEDS

Because Mr. Rivera's stroke resulted in loss of feeling, he does not experience the urge to have a bowel movement, and as a result, he is often incontinent of stool, or feces. You have learned his bowel elimination pattern and are alert to when he normally has a bowel movement. Every other day, just after lunch, you ask him if you may help him to the bathroom or bring him the bedpan. He usually complains and says he does not have to go, but after you convince him to at least try, he admits that you were right.

Some people need assistance with special bowel elimination needs. As a nurse assistant, you play a key role in identifying potential bowel elimination problems by observing and reporting changes in elimination patterns. For example, you would alert your supervising nurse if someone in your care usually has a bowel movement every day after lunch and then does not have one for 3 days.

Because of problems with the digestive system, people sometimes suffer from constipation, fecal impaction, diarrhea or bowel incontinence, which are the most common bowel elimination problems. Also, because of these conditions and other health problems, some people need to have stool specimens collected and tested. When you respond to people who have special bowel elimination needs, it is important for you to remember that the people in your care cannot meet their own needs. They rely on you to help them and to offer support and encouragement.

Assisting People with Special Bowel Elimination Needs

Helping a Person Who is Constipated. The difficult elimination of a hard, dry stool is called **constipation**. It occurs when stool moves too slowly through the intestine and too much water is absorbed by the intestine. The following factors contribute to constipation:

- Not drinking enough fluid
- Ignoring the urge to eliminate
- Not exercising enough
- Changing the diet
- Aging
- Having certain diseases
- Taking some types of medication

A person who is constipated probably feels uncomfortable and may be irritable. He may complain that his abdomen feels hard. When he tries to move his bowels, he may feel pain, which is caused by straining to get the hard stool to move through the rectum and out the anus.

When a person in your care is constipated, offer him fluids frequently

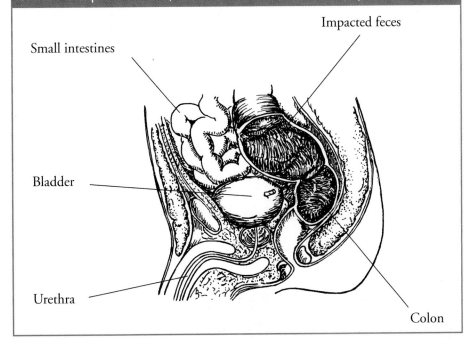

FIGURE 15-12 Fecal impaction is very painful. To reduce the possibility of fecal impaction, help the person maintain normal elimination patterns and, when instructed, treat constipation.

Small intestines

Impacted feces

Bladder

Urethra

Colon

and encourage him to eat high-fiber foods. Also encourage him to get more exercise and help him take more walks. In addition, help him maintain normal elimination patterns and report any changes to your supervising nurse. It may be necessary for the person to receive medication or an **enema** to help relieve constipation. As a nurse assistant, you may or may not be permitted to give someone an enema. When giving someone an enema, follow the procedures explained in Skills 50 and 51.

Helping a Person Who has Fecal Impaction. A more serious form of constipation is fecal impaction, a hard stool that remains in the rectum. It occurs when feces become too hard and too large to pass through the anus (Figure 15-12). A person with fecal impaction may have pain, discomfort and abdominal swelling. He also could have a mucus and water discharge

that looks like diarrhea, which occurs because liquid stool is oozing around the hard stool.

The nurse sometimes provides treatment for fecal impaction by manually removing stool. The manual removal of stool is called *disimpaction*. Sometimes fecal impaction is treated with an enema, which the doctor orders and the nurse or nurse assistant gives to the person with a fecal impaction.

Helping a Person Who has Diarrhea. When Josie had diarrhea, you reported this condition to your supervising nurse because diarrhea usually indicates that something is wrong. Diarrhea may be caused by a bacterial or viral infection, food allergies or poor nutritional habits. A person with diarrhea usually has frequent, watery stools, sometimes accompanied by cramping. She probably feels weak, tired, frustrated, embarrassed by the

smell and sore because of the irritation of the anus. Continued diarrhea can cause a serious fluid loss called **dehydration.**

Sometimes a doctor prescribes no medical treatment for diarrhea and simply lets it run its course. Other times a doctor may prescribe a clear liquid diet and a medication. Because Josie is so frail and cannot risk becoming dehydrated, the doctor prescribes medication for her diarrhea.

As a nurse assistant, you can help the person who has diarrhea if you understand the discomfort associated with it. Respond promptly to her call signal, place a portable commode by her bedside, offer clear liquids, provide good skin care and suggest more rest time. Keep her and her environment very clean. Make her room more pleasant by using a room deodorizer to mask unpleasant odors and by increasing air circulation with a fan or open window.

Report any occurrence of diarrhea to your supervising nurse. Because diarrhea can be contagious, pay special attention to the principles of Standard Precautions when helping a person who has diarrhea. Make sure the person understands and practices good personal hygiene, especially handwashing, as she cares for her own needs.

Helping a Person Who has Bowel Incontinence. Loss of control of the bowels, like loss of control of the bladder, is called *incontinence*. The following factors can lead to bowel incontinence:

- Damage to the brain that keeps the individual from feeling the urge to have a bowel movement
- Weakness of the anal sphincter muscle
- Medications
- Confusion about where to go to the bathroom
- Limited mobility that makes it hard to get to the bathroom

- Not having a call signal answered immediately
- Diarrhea
- Fecal impaction (liquid feces leak out from around the hard, impacted mass of feces)

Note: *Many of these factors are similar to those that lead to urinary incontinence.*

To help support a person who has bowel incontinence:

- Respond quickly to his elimination needs.
- Offer the person fluids frequently throughout the day. Increasing fluid intake decreases the problem of incontinence and may prevent stool from hardening and becoming impacted.
- Encourage a high-fiber diet.
- If the person has trouble rising or walking, help him get to the bathroom.
- Offer him frequent opportunities to go to the bathroom, particularly if he is confused.
- Give the person sufficient time and provide privacy.
- Learn his pattern of bowel elimination to determine how often you

should offer assistance. For example, one person's regular pattern may be daily. Another person's regular pattern may be every 2 to 3 days.

- Treat each person based on his individual needs.
- Be sensitive to the embarrassment a person may feel about being incontinent.
- If the person wears adult briefs, change them as soon as they become soiled to minimize skin irritation.
- Perform perineal care as often as the person needs it.
- Offer emotional support and encouragement.
- Assist with a bowel-training program. A doctor may sometimes recommend that a person participate in a bowel training program to help regain control of his bowel movements. As with a bladder-training program, the schedule for the program is written on the care plan. In addition to the steps above, you can help support the person in his bowel-training program by taking him to the toilet on

the regular schedule set up by the program.

Collecting Stool Specimens

A doctor orders a stool specimen to be collected when laboratory tests need to be run. The doctor uses the results of these tests to make decisions about a person's medical needs. Your responsibility is to collect the stool specimen. This can be done when the person uses the bathroom toilet, portable commode or bedpan.

Always observe the following precautions:

- Check with your supervising nurse to see whether he or she has specific instructions regarding the collection or handling of the stool specimen.
- Observe the principles of Standard Precautions and wear disposable gloves.
- Before collecting the stool specimen, have the person void first to avoid getting urine into the stool specimen.

When collecting stool specimens, follow the procedure explained in Skill 52.

Circle the correct answers and fill in the blanks.

1. _____ aids elimination by diluting the urine and keeping the stool soft.

2. Learn about the person's elimination pattern by asking him or a family member, or by checking his _____ to find out when and how often he urinates or has a bowel movement and whether there is anything special about his elimination habits.

3. Incontinence is the inability to control the release of:
   a. urine.
   b. feces.
   c. urine, feces and perspiration.
   d. urine or feces.

4. A portable commode is:
   a. a bedpan.
   b. a special toilet seat.
   c. a chair with a toilet seat and a container to collect waste.
   d. a collection container to put into a standard bathroom toilet.

5. When a person is sitting on a bedpan, it is important to help him into a position that best resembles sitting on a _____ and to check on him every _____ minutes.

6. Burning on urination, frequent but scanty urination, cloudy or dark-colored urine, or milky threads of mucus in the urine are signs of urinary _____

7. When a person in your care has a urinary catheter, prevent infection by providing _____ care on a regular schedule and whenever the person is soiled with secretions or feces.

8. An external catheter should be removed:
   a. once daily.
   b. only when the adhesive loosens and the catheter is ready to fall off.
   c. twice daily.
   d. every other day.

9. When testing a person's urine for glucose and acetone, check his _____ _____ to find out when and how often to do the test.

10. Symptoms of fecal impaction include:
   a. abdominal pain and a diarrhea-like discharge from the anus.
   b. burning on urination and an increased frequency to void.
   c. passage of hard dry stool and blood in the urine.
   d. excessive thirst and nausea.

1. When assisting a person onto the toilet or portable commode, how would you use good body mechanics?

2. How can you make someone feel safe and secure when you leave him alone to eliminate in private?

3. How can you make a person feel respected when you help him with elimination?

4. What can you do to help a person become more independent about his elimination needs?

5. What can you do to show your professionalism when you assist with elimination?

6. During one of Shirley McDay's incontinent times, you follow the care plan and put adult briefs on her. She begins to cry and says she does not want to be treated like a baby. What should you do?

7. You have helped Josie onto the portable commode. While you are waiting outside the curtain for her to signal that she is finished, her roommate asks you to help her get back into bed. What should you do?

8. Mr. Smith is expecting company. He is sitting in a wheelchair with his urinary collection bag hanging on the side. What can you do to enhance his self-esteem and protect his dignity and privacy?

9. What is different about collecting a urine specimen from Mrs. Wang, who is in isolation, and collecting a urine specimen from someone who is not in isolation?

10. You are changing Dominique's briefs when your nurse supervisor calls for you from the hall. What should you do?

Skill 39: Helping a Person Use the Bathroom Toilet

PRECAUTIONS

- Make sure the person in your care is safe before leaving him or her alone in the bathroom. Stay just outside the bathroom door.
- Check on him or her at least every 5 minutes to make sure he or she is okay and to see if he or she needs any assistance.

PREPARATION

1. Gather supplies:
   - Towel and washcloth (if you need to assist with perineal care)
   - Disposable gloves (if you need to assist with perineal care)
   - Plastic trash bag (if you need to assist with perineal care)
2. Follow Preparation Standards (see Chapter 7).

PROCEDURE

1. Assist the person in getting to the bathroom, either by walking or by wheelchair. ☐ ☐
2. Help the person adjust clothing and sit on the toilet. ☐ ☐
3. Make sure the toilet paper and call signal are within the person's reach (Figure 15-13). ☐ ☐
4. Make sure it is safe to leave the person alone. Close the door for privacy. ☐ ☐
5. Wait outside the door until the person has finished or return to the room when the person signals. ☐ ☐
6. Check on the person at least every 5 minutes. ☐ ☐

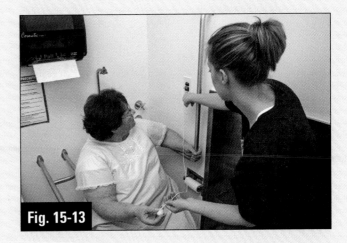

Fig. 15-13

7. Put on gloves and assist the person with cleaning herself with toilet paper, if necessary. ☐ ☐

8. Help the person get off the toilet, wash hands and return to the room. ☐ ☐

ADDITIONAL INFORMATION

Return to the bathroom. If urine was collected, follow the directions about what to do with the urine.

COMPLETION

Follow Completion Standards in compliance with your facility. For a complete list of those used in this course, see Chapter 7, "Controlling the Spread of Germs."

Skill 40: Helping a Person Use a Portable Commode

PRECAUTIONS

- Check with your supervising nurse before moving the person from the bed to the commode.
- Make sure the collection container is under the seat.
- If the commode has wheels, lock the wheels before moving the person from the bed to the commode.
- Check on the person at least every 5 minutes to make sure he or she is okay and to see if he or she needs any assistance.
    - Ask a co-worker to help, if needed.

PREPARATION

1. Gather supplies:
   - Disposable gloves
   - Plastic trash bag
   - Washcloth (for perineal care)
   - Towel (for perineal care)
   - Laundry bag (or plastic bag for wet or soiled laundry)
   - Collection container cover
   - Portable commode with collection container (if one is not already present in the room)
2. Follow Preparation Standards (see Chapter 7).

PROCEDURE

1. Move the portable commode to the side of the bed. Lift the lid of the commode and remove the pail cover. ☐ ☐

Skill 40: Helping a Person Use a Portable Commode—cont'd

2. Lower the side rail, if used, and help the person sit on side of bed. ☐ ☐
3. Transfer the person to the commode as you would transfer him to a chair (Figure 15-14). ☐ ☐
4. Make sure the toilet paper and call signal are within reach. ☐ ☐
5. Return to the room when the person signals. Check on him at least every 5 minutes. ☐ ☐
6. Assist the person to wipe and clean after eliminating, if needed. ☐ ☐
7. Assist the person to wash and dry his hands as needed. ☐ ☐
8. Help the person get off the commode. ☐ ☐
9. Help the person back into the bed. ☐ ☐

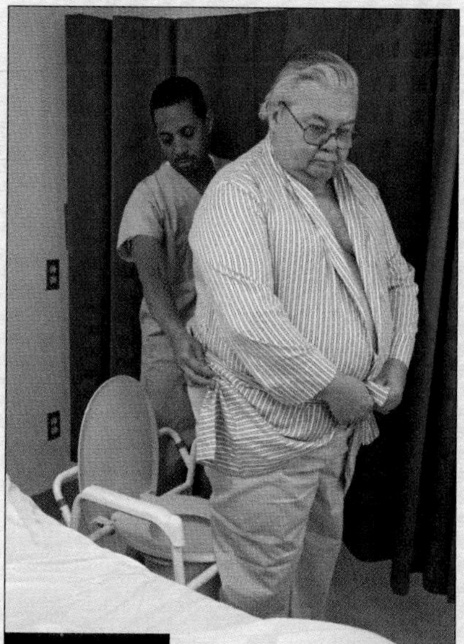

Fig. 15-14

ADDITIONAL INFORMATION

Remove the collection container from the commode, and replace the cover. Take the collection container to the dirty utility room or to the bathroom, empty it, and clean it.

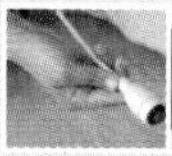

COMPLETION

Follow Completion Standards in compliance with your facility. For a complete list of those used in this course, see Chapter 7, "Controlling the Spread of Germs."

Skill 41: Helping a Person Use a Bedpan or Urinal

PRECAUTIONS

- Check a person who is sitting on the bedpan or using a urinal at least every 5 minutes to make sure he or she is okay or to see if he or she needs assistance. If the person is on the bedpan or has a urinal in place for longer than 5 minutes, he or she can develop pressure sores.

PREPARATION

1. Gather supplies:
   - Disposable bed protector
   - Disposable gloves
   - Plastic trash bag
   - Washcloth (for perineal care)
   - Towel (for perineal care)
   - Bedpan or urinal cover
   - Laundry bag (or plastic bag for wet or soiled laundry)
2. Follow Preparation Standards (see Chapter 7).

PROCEDURE

1. Lower the head of the bed so that the person is as flat as possible. ☐ ☐
2. If the person has no open sores on the buttocks, powder the rim of the bedpan to make it easier to put it under the person. ☐ ☐
3. Fold the top linens out of the way, keeping the person's legs covered. Be sure the person's clothing is also out of the way. ☐ ☐

4. Place the disposable bed protector under the person's buttocks. ☐ ☐

    For a bedpan: (Figure 15-15) Help the person onto the bedpan. Ask the person to bend her knees and raise her buttocks by pushing against the mattress with her feet (Figure 15-16, A). Assist, as necessary, by slipping your hand under the person's lower back and lifting slightly.

    If the person is unable to help, turn her onto her side away from you (Figure 15-16, B). Place the bedpan firmly against her buttocks. Gently turn the person back onto the bedpan.

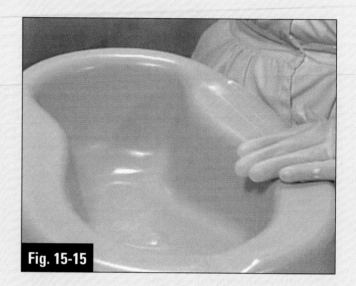

Fig. 15-15

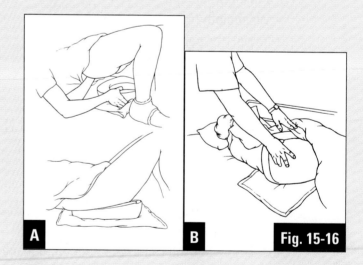

A   B   Fig. 15-16

For a urinal: (Figure 15-17) Give the urinal to a male. If he needs assistance, put the urinal between his legs and gently put his penis into the urinal opening.

5. Arrange the top linens back over the person and raise side rails if the person is in the bed. ☐ ☐

6. Raise the head of the bed so that the person is in a comfortable sitting position. Ask him to bend his knees, if possible. ☐ ☐

7. Make sure the toilet paper and call signal are within reach. Leave the room if it is safe to leave the person alone. Wait outside the door until the person has finished and signals (Figure 15-18). ☐ ☐

8. If the person cannot or does not signal, check on him at least every 5 minutes. ☐ ☐

9. When the person has finished eliminating, put on disposable gloves and help him off the bed pan. ☐ ☐

10. Help the person wipe and clean. Provide perineal care, as necessary. Always clean a female from front to back. Help the person wash their hands, as necessary (Figure 15-19). ☐ ☐

11. Remove disposable gloves and wash your hands. ☐ ☐

COMPLETION

Follow Completion Standards in compliance with your facility. For a complete list of those used in this course, see Chapter 7, "Controlling the Spread of Germs."

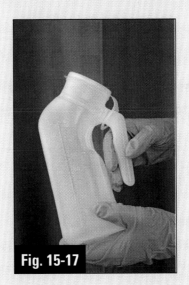
Fig. 15-17

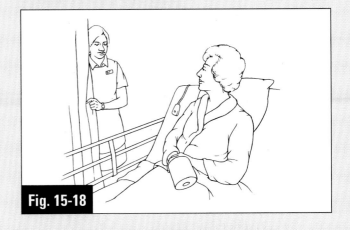
Fig. 15-18

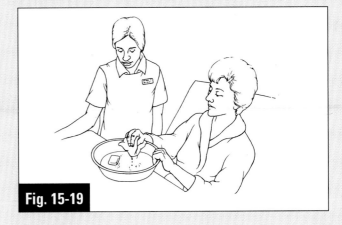
Fig. 15-19

Skill 42: Providing Perineal Care for a Person with a Urinary Catheter

PRECAUTIONS

- Always clean the perineum from the front to the back.
- Make sure the catheter tubing is taped or secured by a fastener to the inner thigh for security.
- Make sure the drainage bag is attached to the bed and that it is lower than the person's bladder.
- Make sure the tubing is not kinked.
- Make sure the drainage bag and tubing are not touching the floor.

PREPARATION

1. Gather supplies:
   - Bath blanket
   - Washcloth
   - Towel
   - Disposable bed protector
   - Disposable gloves
   - Paper towel
   - Plastic trash bag
   - Laundry bag (or plastic bag for wet or soiled laundry)
   - Cotton balls
2. Follow Preparation Standards (see Chapter 7).

PROCEDURE

1. Lower the head of the bed so that the person is lying as flat as possible on his back. ☐ ☐
2. Put the bath blanket over the person. ☐ ☐
3. Put a disposable bed protector under the person's buttocks. ☐ ☐

4. Drape the person's perineal area by doing the following:
   - Help the person bend his knees and spread his legs.
   - Place the bath blanket over the person like a diamond. Put one corner at the person's neck, a corner at each side and one corner between his legs.
   - Wrap each side corner around the person's feet. Bring each corner under and around a foot. This keeps the blanket from sliding off the person. ☐ ☐
5. Put on the disposable gloves. ☐ ☐
6. Provide perineal care.
   - Using separate cotton balls, clean and dry 4 inches of the catheter, starting where it comes out of the urethra.
   - Observe the area around the catheter for any signs of leaking urine.
   - Look at the person's skin for any signs of infection, such as redness, swelling, pus, drainage or crusting. ☐ ☐
7. Make sure the catheter tubing is taped or secured by a fastener to the person's inner thigh (Figure 15-20). Allow some extra tubing so that the catheter is not being pulled. Make sure the bag is attached to the bed, not the side rails. ☐ ☐

COMPLETION

Follow Completion Standards in compliance with your facility. For a complete list of those used in this course, see Chapter 7, "Controlling the Spread of Germs."

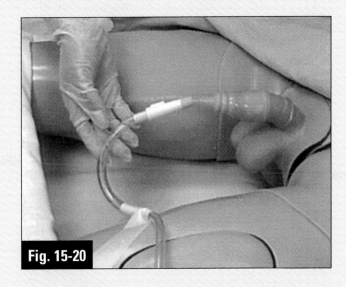

Fig. 15-20

Skill 43: Cleaning Around Tubes and Catheters

PRECAUTIONS

- Soap may irritate the skin.
- Do not pull on tubes or catheters because they might become dislodged.

PREPARATION

1. Gather supplies:
   - Washcloth
   - Lubricant, if needed
   - Disposable gloves
   - Cotton-tipped applicator, if needed
   - Antibacterial cream or lotion, if directed
   - Mild soap, if needed
   - Towel
   - Plastic trash bag
2. Follow Preparation Standards (see Chapter 7).

PROCEDURE

1. Drape a towel over the person's chest. ☐ ☐
2. Remove, with warm water and a washcloth, any mucus or secretions collected around tubing. ☐ ☐
3. Rinse the skin and dry with a towel. ☐ ☐
4. Apply lubricant, antibacterial cream or lotion, if instructed to do so. ☐ ☐

ADDITIONAL INFORMATION

Always wash around the tube without putting pressure on it (Figure 15–21).

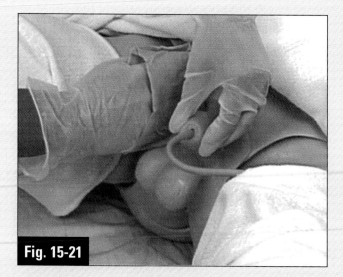

Fig. 15-21

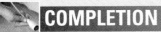

COMPLETION

Follow Completion Standards in compliance with your facility. For a complete list of those used in this course, see Chapter 7, "Controlling the Spread of Germs."

Skill 44: Changing an Ostomy Appliance

PRECAUTIONS

- Always follow universal precautions and use infection control techniques when changing an ostomy appliance.

PREPARATION

1. Gather supplies:
   - Two pairs of disposable gloves
   - Disposable bed protector
   - Toilet tissue
   - Washcloth
   - Towel
   - Stoma bag deodorant
   - Skin adhesive
   - Clean stoma bag, clamp
   - Scissors
   - Plastic trash bag
   - Mild soap, if needed
2. Follow Preparation Standards (see Chapter 7).

PROCEDURE

1. Lower the head of the bed so that the person is lying as flat as possible in a supine position. ☐ ☐
2. Put on disposable gloves. ☐ ☐
3. Drape the person to expose the stoma area on the abdomen. ☐ ☐
4. Remove the soiled appliance (stoma bag) from the person and place it in a bedpan. ☐ ☐

5. Wipe around the stoma with toilet tissue and then wash the area with warm water or mild soapy water. Pat skin dry. ☐ ☐

6. Place stoma bag deodorant in a new, clean stoma bag. Apply skin adhesive, if needed. Apply the new appliance over the stoma, making sure there are no wrinkles (Figure 15-22). ☐ ☐

7. Seal the bottom of the appliance with a clamp according to manufacturer's instructions. ☐ ☐

8. Dispose of stoma bag in a labeled biohazard bag. ☐ ☐

9. Remove disposable gloves and wash your hands. ☐ ☐

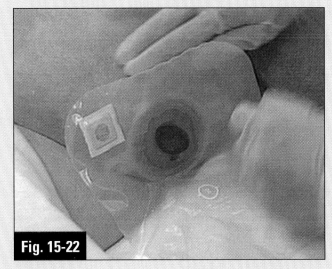
Fig. 15-22

ADDITIONAL INFORMATION

Follow specific manufacturer's instructions for applying and fitting the appliance over the stoma.

 COMPLETION

Follow Completion Standards in compliance with your facility. For a complete list of those used in this course, see Chapter 7, "Controlling the Spread of Germs."

Skill 45: Emptying a Urinary Drainage Bag

PRECAUTIONS

- Do not allow the end of the drainage tube to come in contact with anything except its holder.

PREPARATION

1. Gather supplies:
   - Disposable gloves
   - Graduate container to collect and measure the urine (if the person does not have one in the room)
   - Alcohol swab
   - Plastic trash bag
2. Follow Preparation Standards (see Chapter 7).

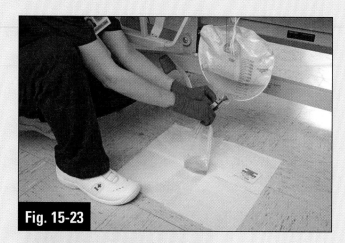

Fig. 15-23

PROCEDURE

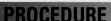

1. Put on disposable gloves. ☐ ☐
2. Place the graduate container underneath the drain on the drainage bag. ☐ ☐
3. Remove the drain from its holder on the side of the drainage bag and open the clamp on the drain. Allow the urine to flow into the graduate container (Figure 15-23). ☐ ☐
4. Close the clamp. Wipe the end of the drainage tube with an alcohol swab. Replace the drain inside its holder (Figure 15-24). ☐ ☐
5. Remove disposable gloves and wash your hands. ☐ ☐

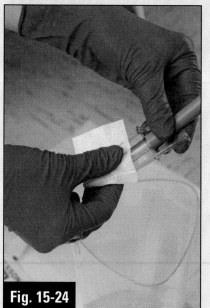

Fig. 15-24

COMPLETION

Follow Completion Standards in compliance with your facility. For a complete list of those used in this course, see Chapter 7, "Controlling the Spread of Germs."

Skill 46: Applying an External Urinary Catheter to a Male

PRECAUTIONS

- Make sure the tubing does not get twisted at the tip of the man's penis.
- Check the person frequently to make sure the condom is not too tight and that there is good circulation.

NOTE: *If you observe any swelling or color change, remove the condom and report your observations to your supervising nurse.*

- When transferring the person to a chair, move the drainage bag before moving the person and make sure the catheter is not pulled off his penis.
- Make sure the catheter tubing is taped or secured by a fastener to the person's inner thigh for security.

PREPARATION

1. Gather supplies:
   - Bath blanket
   - External urinary catheter and drainage bag
   - Tape or catheter fastener
   - Washcloth
   - Towel
   - Bandage scissors
   - Paper towel
   - Disposable bed protector
   - Disposable gloves
   - Plastic trash bag
   - Laundry bag (or plastic bag for wet or soiled laundry)

2. Follow Preparation Standards (see Chapter 7).

PROCEDURE

1. Provide perineal care. ☐ ☐
2. Put the head of the man's penis in the condom and unroll the condom over his penis (Figure 15-25, A). Secure the condom with the adhesive strip (Figure 15-25, B). Allow slack or room at the tip of his penis (Figure 15-25, C–D). ☐ ☐
3. Attach the condom to the drainage bag (Figure 15-25, E) Make sure the drainage bag is lower than the person's bladder (Figure 15-26), and hang it from the bed frame. ☐ ☐
4. Use a leg band, or loosely tape the tubing to the person's inner thigh. ☐ ☐
5. Remove the disposable bed protector. ☐ ☐

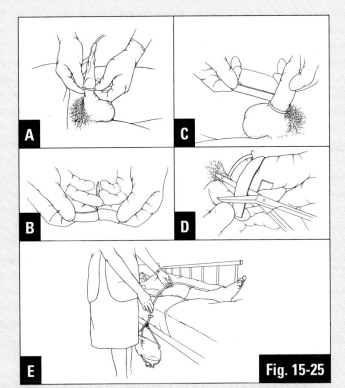

Fig. 15-25

ADDITIONAL INFORMATION

Record that you have applied an external urinary catheter to a male.

COMPLETION

Follow Completion Standards in compliance with your facility. For a complete list of those used in this course, see Chapter 7, "Controlling the Spread of Germs."

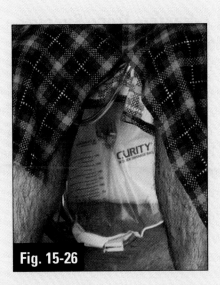

Fig. 15-26

Skill 47: Collecting Urine Specimens

PRECAUTIONS

- Always follow your supervising nurse's instructions for specimen collection.
- Remember the principles of infection control when collecting specimens.
- Always wear disposable gloves.

PREPARATION

1. Gather supplies:
   - Specimen cup labeled with the person's name, the date and time of the collection, the type of specimen (urine), your name and any additional information your employer requires
   - Disposable gloves
   - Urine collection "hat," if the person uses the toilet
   - Plastic trash bags
2. Follow Preparation Standards (see Chapter 7).

PROCEDURE

Method 1: Routine Urine Specimen Collection

1. Follow the procedure for using the bathroom toilet, portable commode, bedpan or urinal.
   - *Using the bathroom toilet.* Make sure there is a collection container for the person to use. This may be a specimen cup with a lid or a urine collection "hat" that sits on the rim of the toilet. If a collection hat is used, tell the person not to throw the toilet paper in the hat.

- *Using a portable commode.* Ask the person not to have a bowel movement and not to put the toilet paper in the commode. Put a disposable bag at the bedside for the used toilet paper.
- *Using a bedpan.* Do not powder the bedpan. Ask the person not to have a bowel movement and not to put the toilet paper in the bedpan. Put a disposable bag at the bedside for the used toilet paper.
- *Using a urinal.* No special considerations are necessary. □ □
2. Put on disposable gloves. □ □
3. After obtaining the urine specimen in the collection container, take it to the bathroom or dirty utility room. □ □
4. Pour about 60 cc of the urine into the labeled specimen cup. □ □
5. Place the lid on it and put the cup in the designated area in the nurses' station, refrigerator or special tray. □ □
6. Remove disposable gloves and wash your hands. □ □

Method 2: Clean Catch, or Midstream, Urine Specimen Collection

1. Open the clean catch kit and put it on a clean surface. □ □
2. Offer the person the opportunity to provide his or her own perineal care and to collect the urine specimen without assistance. Instruct the person to:
- Cleanse the perineal area with soap and water. Wipe the area three times with the cleansing wipes in the package or with

gauze squares soaked with povidone-iodine.

- *For males:* Cleanse the tip of the penis (Figure 15-27, A). (For uncircumcised males, retract the foreskin and keep it retracted.) Cleanse the tip of the penis with soap and water, and wipe three times with cleansing wipes or gauze squares soaked in povidone-iodine, moving in a circular pattern from the urethral opening outward, using a separate pad each time.
- *For females:* Cleanse the labia, urethral opening and vaginal area separately with a cleansing wipe or gauze squares soaked in povidone-iodine (Figure 15-27, B).
  - Separate the labial folds with the thumb and forefinger of one hand.
  - Wipe down one side with a wipe or gauze square and the other side with the second wipe. Throw each wipe or gauze square into a plastic trash bag.
  - Wipe down the center with a third wipe or gauze square. Throw away wipe or gauze square in a plastic trash bag.
  - Then wipe down the other side with a clean wipe or gauze square and throw it into a plastic trash bag. Always wipe from front to back.
  - Begin voiding and then stop long enough to place a sterile container under the stream to collect midstream urine (Figure 15-27, C).

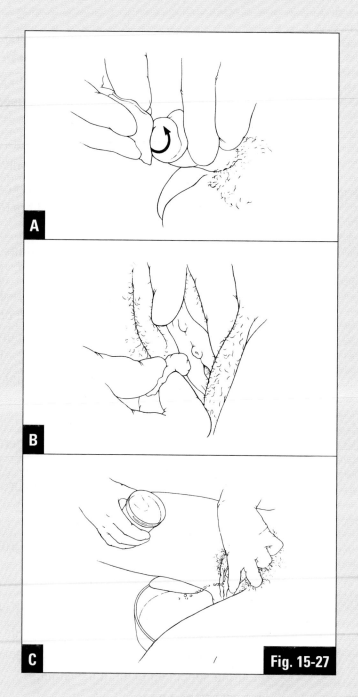

Fig. 15-27

- To keep the urine clean, separate the labia to protect the clean urethral opening.
  - Fill the container, remove it (Figure 15-27, D), and then finish voiding into the toilet, portable commode, bedpan, or urinal (Figure 15-27, E). ☐ ☐

3. If the person is unable to collect the specimen, put on disposable gloves and follow the previous steps to collect the specimen. ☐ ☐

4. After the person has finished voiding, cover the container. ☐ ☐

Method 3: 24-Hour Urine Specimen Collection

1. Explain 24-hour collection procedure to the person. ☐ ☐

2. Have the person void in a bedpan. When the person has finished, discard this specimen. ☐ ☐

3. Note the time that the person voided. The time you write down is the time the collection starts. ☐ ☐

4. Prepare 24-hour urine collection signs marked with the person's name, the date and time that the collection started and the date and time it will end. Put the signs in all appropriate areas. ☐ ☐

5. Put appropriate preservatives (if they are to be used) in the specimen collection container. Check with your supervising nurse for directions. ☐ ☐

6. Have the person notify you immediately each time she voids in the collection hat, portable

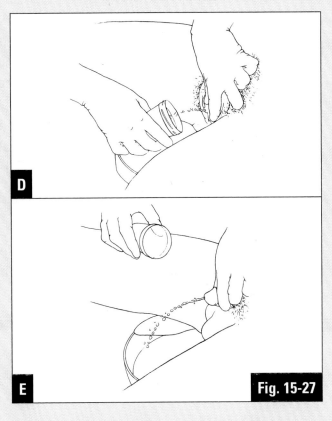

D

E

Fig. 15-27

commode, bedpan or urinal so that the urine can be emptied into the specimen collection container (Figure 15-28). ☐ ☐

7. Have the person void at the end of the 24 hours. Add this to the container. Tell the person this is the last collection for the 24-hour period. Remove all signs about the 24-hour collection. ☐ ☐

8. Put the specimen in the designated area in the nurses' station, refrigerator or special tray. ☐ ☐

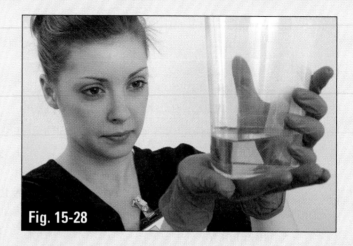
Fig. 15-28

COMPLETION

Follow Completion Standards in compliance with your facility. For a complete list of those used in this course, see Chapter 7, "Controlling the Spread of Germs."

Skill 48: Straining Urine

PRECAUTIONS
- Always follow universal precautions and use infection control techniques when straining urine.

PREPARATION
1. Gather supplies:
   - Bedpan or urinal and cover
   - Disposable strainer or 4 × 4-inch gauze squares and container for urine
   - Specimen container
   - Disposable gloves (two pairs if you will be assisting with perineal care)
   - Plastic trash bag
   - Washcloth (for perineal care)
   - Towel (for perineal care)
2. Follow Preparation Standards (see Chapter 7).

PROCEDURE
1. Have the person collect all his urine in a clean container, bedpan or urinal. ☐ ☐
2. Put on disposable gloves. ☐ ☐
3. Take the container with urine to the dirty utility room. ☐ ☐
4. Place the disposable strainer or 4 × 4-inch gauze onto the rim of the collection container. ☐ ☐
5. Pour the urine through the strainer or gauze into a graduate container if measuring urine. ☐ ☐
6. Pour the urine through the strainer into the toilet if not measuring. ☐ ☐

7. Place the strainer or gauze with crystals, stones or particles into a specimen container. Label the container and take to the designated location. ☐ ☐

8. Remove disposable gloves and wash your hands. ☐ ☐

ADDITIONAL INFORMATION

Ask women not to put toilet tissue in the bedpan.

COMPLETION

Follow Completion Standards in compliance with your facility. For a complete list of those used in this course, see Chapter 7, "Controlling the Spread of Germs."

Skill 49: Testing Urine for Glucose and Acetone

PRECAUTIONS

- Always follow your supervising nurse's instructions for specimen collection.
- Remember the principles of infection control when collecting specimens.
- Always wear disposable gloves. Include other protective equipment, if there is a risk of urine splashing.

PREPARATION

1. Gather supplies:
   - Labstix
   - Disposable gloves
   - Paper towel
   - Watch with a second hand
2. Follow Preparation Standards (see Chapter 7).

PROCEDURE

Method 1: Procedure for Using Labstix

1. Put on disposable gloves. ☐ ☐
2. Remove a test strip from the bottle and recap the bottle (Figure 15-29). Hold the end of the strip with the pads in the urine for 2 seconds and then remove it. Before the test, the pad for acetone is buff-colored and the glucose pad is blue. ☐ ☐

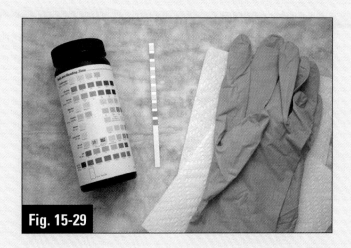

Fig. 15-29

3. Remove the strip and hold it horizontally. Wait 15 seconds before comparing the color of the strip with the color on the Labstix color chart. Write down the acetone result after 15 seconds and the glucose result after 30 seconds. ☐ ☐

4. Discard the urine specimen if it is not needed for another test. ☐ ☐

5. Remove gloves and wash your hands. ☐ ☐

Method 2: Procedure for Using Tes-tape

1. Put on disposable gloves. ☐ ☐

2 Remove a strip of Tes-tape about 4 inches long from the roll. ☐ ☐

3. Dip one end of the strip into the urine and remove it. ☐ ☐

4. After waiting 60 seconds, compare the darkest color of the tape with the Tes-tape color chart. Write down the reading. ☐ ☐

5. Discard the urine specimen if it is not needed for another test. ☐ ☐

6. Remove gloves and wash your hands. ☐ ☐

ADDITIONAL INFORMATION

Report obvious blood in urine.

COMPLETION

Follow Completion Standards in compliance with your facility. For a complete list of those used in this course, see Chapter 7, "Controlling the Spread of Germs."

Skill 50: Giving a Person a Tap Water or Soap Solution Enema

PRECAUTIONS

- If the person complains of pain when you are giving an enema, stop the procedure and wait until the pain goes away. Reassure the person and have him or her take deep breaths. If the pain continues, stop and report the situation to your supervising nurse.
- Take care when putting the tip of the enema container or enema tubing into the person's rectum because rectal tissue is very delicate. Put the enema tip in only about 2 to 4 inches.
- If you have difficulty putting the tip of the enema tubing at least 2 inches into the person's rectum, tell your supervising nurse.

PREPARATION

1. Gather supplies:
   - Disposable bed protector
   - Enema unit
   - Lubricant jelly
   - Bath thermometer
   - Disposable gloves
   - Plastic trash bag
   - Laundry bag (or plastic bag for wet or soiled laundry)
   - Bedpan cover
   - Washcloth
   - Towel
2. Prepare the enema solution by clamping the tubing and filling the enema container with the amount of water ordered by the doctor. The usual amount is 500 to 1000 cc.
3. Follow Preparation Standards (see Chapter 7).

Skill 50: Giving a Person a Tap Water or Soap Solution Enema—cont'd

PROCEDURE

1. Put on disposable gloves. ☐ ☐
2. Lower the head of the bed so that the person is flat. ☐ ☐
3. Cover the person with a bath blanket and have him remove pajama bottoms or underwear. ☐ ☐
4. Help the person turn onto his left side with the right knee bent (Figure 15-30, A). ☐ ☐
5. Place bed protection under the person's buttocks. ☐ ☐
6. Tear off a piece of toilet paper and squeeze a small amount of lubricating jelly onto it. ☐ ☐
7. Lubricate the tip (2 to 4 inches) of the tubing by rotating the tip in the jelly (Figure 15-30, B). ☐ ☐
8. Raise the person's upper buttock and insert the enema tip into his rectum no more than 2 to 4 inches (Figure 15-30, C). ☐ ☐
9. Open the clamp and, holding the bag no higher than 12 inches above the anus, allow the solution to flow slowly into the person's rectum (Figure 15-30, D). ☐ ☐
10. Remove the tube from the person's rectum and encourage him to hold solution in a side-lying position for as long as possible. ☐ ☐
11. Help the person onto the bedpan. Raise the head of the bed to a semi-Fowler's position and place toilet paper and the call signal within his reach (Figure 15-30, E). ☐ ☐

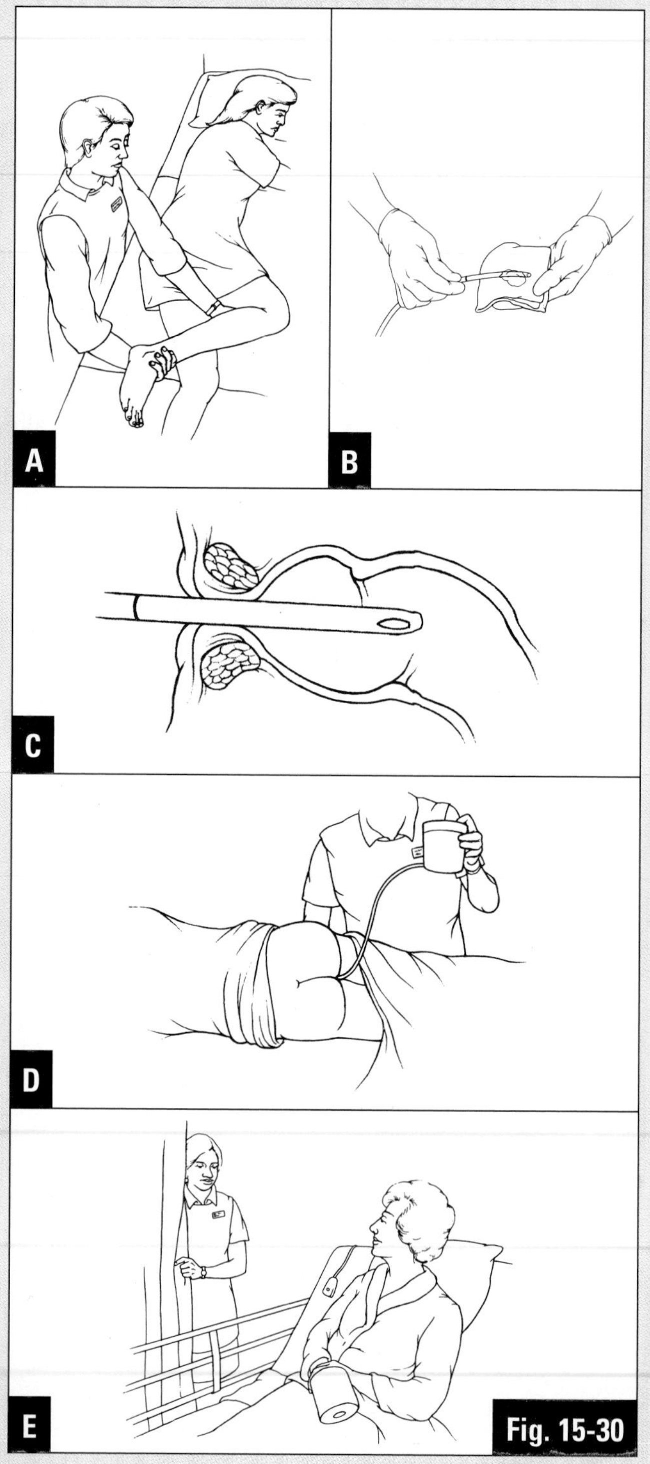

Fig. 15-30

12. Return to the room when the person signals. If the person cannot or does not signal, check on him at least every 5 minutes. ☐ ☐
13. When the person has finished eliminating, fill a washbasin with warm water and bring it to the bedside. Lower the bed and help the person off the bedpan (Figure 15-30, F). ☐ ☐
14. Help the person wipe and clean himself, if needed. Help the person wash their hands, as necessary. Always clean from front to back on a female. ☐ ☐
15. Remove bed protector. ☐ ☐

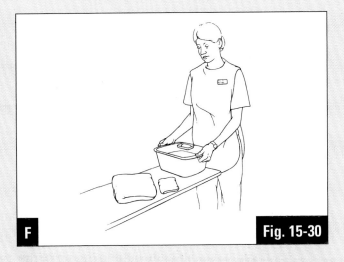

F   Fig. 15-30

COMPLETION

Follow Completion Standards in compliance with your facility. For a complete list of those used in this course, see Chapter 7, "Controlling the Spread of Germs."

Skill 51: Giving a Person a Prepackaged Cleansing or Oil-Retention Enema

PRECAUTIONS

- If the person complains of pain when you are giving an enema, stop the procedure and wait until the pain goes away. Reassure the person and have him or her take deep breaths. If the pain continues, stop and report the situation to your supervising nurse.
- Take care when putting the tip of the enema container or enema tubing into the person's rectum because rectal tissue is very delicate. Put the enema tip in only about 2 to 4 inches.
- If you have difficulty putting the tip of the enema tubing at least 2 inches into the person's rectum, tell your supervising nurse.

PREPARATION

1. Gather supplies:
   - Disposable bed protector
   - Disposable enema package
   - Disposable gloves
   - Portable commode, if used
   - Plastic trash bag
   - Cover for bedpan or commode container
   - Laundry bag (or plastic bag for wet or soiled laundry)
   - Towel
   - Washcloth
2. Follow Preparation Standards (see Chapter 7).

PROCEDURE

1. Put on disposable gloves. ☐ ☐
2. Lower the head of the bed so that the person is as flat as comfortable. ☐ ☐

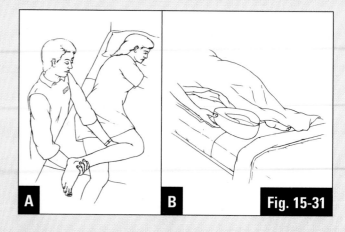

A   B   Fig. 15-31

3. Cover the person with a bath blanket and help remove pajama bottoms or underwear. ☐ ☐

4. Help the person turn onto her left side with the right knee bent (Figure 15-31, A). ☐ ☐

5. Place a disposable bed protector under the person's buttocks (Figure 15-31, B). Put the bedpan within easy reach. ☐ ☐

6. Open the enema package and take off the protective cover (Figure 15-31, C). ☐ ☐

7. Raise the person's upper buttock and insert the enema tip no more than 2 to 4 inches into her rectum (Figure 15-31, D). ☐ ☐

8. Squeeze the plastic bottle until all the enema solution is given (Figure 15-31, E). ☐ ☐

9. Remove the tube from the person's rectum, and encourage her to hold the solution in for as long as possible. ☐ ☐

10. Help the person onto the bedpan, commode or toilet (Figure 15-31, F). Raise the bed into a semi-Fowler position and place toilet paper and call signal within her reach. ☐ ☐

11. Wait outside of the person's door until she signals. If the person cannot or does not signal, check on her every 5 minutes. ☐ ☐

12. Fill a washbasin with warm water. ☐ ☐

13. Help the person off the bedpan. ☐ ☐

14. Help the person wipe and clean herself. Help the person wash her hands, as necessary. ☐ ☐

15. Remove disposable gloves and wash your hands. ☐ ☐

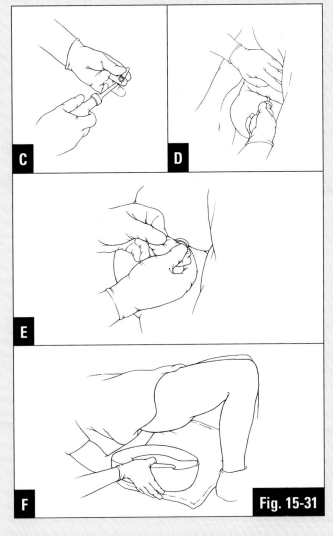

C   D

E

F   Fig. 15-31

Skill 51: Giving a Person a Prepackaged Cleansing or Oil-Retention Enema—cont'd

COMPLETION

Follow Completion Standards in compliance with your facility. For a complete list of those used in this course, see Chapter 7, "Controlling the Spread of Germs."

Skill 52: Collecting Stool Specimens

PRECAUTIONS

- Check with your supervising nurse to find out any specific instructions for collecting or handling stool specimens.
- Remember the principles of infection control when collecting specimens.
- Wear disposable gloves when handling a stool specimen.

PREPARATION

1. Gather supplies:
   - Disposable gloves
   - Specimen container
   - Two tongue depressors
   - Washcloth and towel
   - Plastic trash bag
   - Bedpan (use the person's bedpan)
   - Toilet paper
   - Washbasin
   - Soap
2. Follow Preparation Standards (see Chapter 7).

PROCEDURE

1. Explain that you need the person to use the bedpan, but that he should not void or put toilet paper into the bedpan. ☐ ☐
2. Lower the side rail (if used) on the side where you are working. ☐ ☐
3. Place the bedpan under the person's hips. ☐ ☐
4. When the person has finished his bowel movement, put on disposable gloves. ☐ ☐

Skill 52: Collecting Stool Specimens—cont'd

5. Remove the bedpan, cover it, and take it to the bathroom. ☐ ☐
6. Label specimen container with the person's name, the date, the time, specimen (stool), your name and any additional information your employer requires. ☐ ☐
7. Use the tongue depressors to remove 1 to 2 tablespoons of the stool from the bedpan, and place it in the labeled container (Figure 15-32). ☐ ☐

> **NOTE:** *Be careful not to contaminate the outside of the container with stool.*

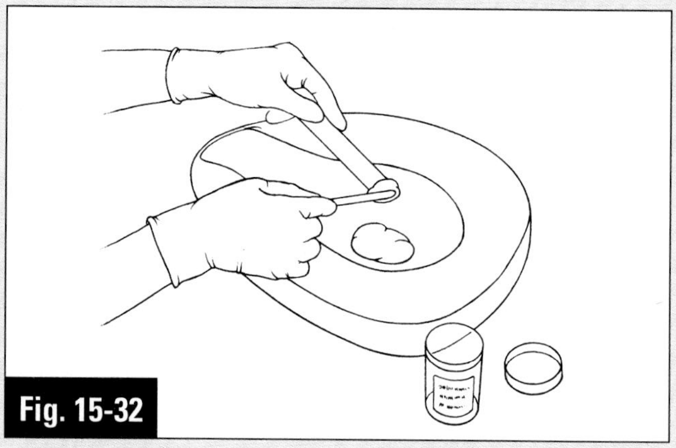

Fig. 15-32

8. Put the lid on the specimen container. ☐ ☐
9. Throw away tongue depressors in the plastic trash bag. ☐ ☐
10. Empty, clean and dry the bedpan. ☐ ☐
11. Remove disposable gloves and throw them in the plastic trash bag. ☐ ☐
12. Wash your hands. ☐ ☐
13. Put the specimen in the designated area. ☐ ☐

COMPLETION

1. Follow Completion Standards in compliance with your facility. For a complete list of those used in this course, see Chapter 7, "Controlling the Spread of Germs."

2. Report:
   - Color of stool
   - Consistency of stool
   - Odor of stool
   - Any difficulty in eliminating
   - Pain
   - Bleeding
   - Red or swollen areas

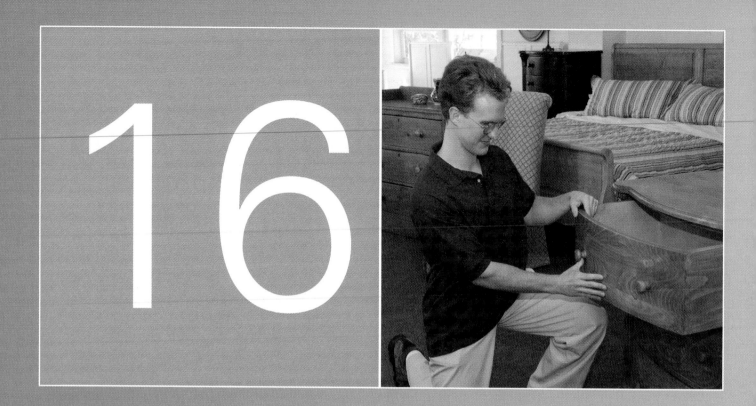

16

Providing Restorative Care to Help with Rehabilitation

GOALS

After reading this chapter, you will have the information needed to:

Promote independence, self-care and good health habits.

Help a person to be active.

After practicing the corresponding skills, you will have the information needed to:

Help a person walk with and without a cane, crutches and a walker.

Help a person with passive range-of-motion exercises.

A young man came to a master craftsman's shop, lugging behind him an old, water-marked chest of drawers. He leaned it up against the wall because it had a broken foot and could not stand well on its own. The chest was crafted from a beautiful piece of oak, but years ago it had been damaged in a flood. It also showed the signs of a fall, including a deep gouge in its left side. The five drawers either struck or fell open. Three of them were missing drawer pulls. "Please, sir," he asked the master craftsman, "could you possibly fix up this old chest? It was mine when I was a child, and now I would like to give it to my newborn son." The master craftsman grumbled and shook his head at the damaged piece of furniture and told the young man to come back in two weeks.

Later, when the young man returned to the shop, he could hear the sounds of the master craftsman gently sanding and rubbing in the back room. While he waited for the craftsman to come to the front of the shop, the young man looked around anxiously for his old chest of drawers. He hoped the craftsman had been able to repair the foot and fill in the gouge. He wondered whether he had been able to replace the drawer pulls. Soon he was filled with anxiety. He did not see his chest anywhere. Perhaps the master

craftsman had not had time to work on it. Perhaps it was too worn and old to be fixed.

Just then the master craftsman came into the front room and said, "Well, young man, what do you think of it?"

"Of what?" asked the young man.

"Of your chest of drawers, of course," said the craftsman, pointing to a beautiful, shining, smooth chest of drawers that stood proudly on its own feet in the center of the shop.

The young man could not believe his eyes. "This is it?" he stammered. "I can't believe it." He could see ever so slightly where the gouge had been. The drawer pulls were not an exact match, and one of the drawers still stuck a little when he opened it. But the rough edges had been smoothed, and the old dirt had been rubbed out with oil to make the inner color of the wood shine with a rich luster. "I was afraid that you couldn't fix it," the young man finally said.

"I didn't fix it," said the old man, with the same dignity that the chest now wore. "I restored it."

THE ART OF RESTORING

The master craftsman saw his task not as fixing, but as restoring. As a nurse assistant, your work is similar. You do

not merely patch up people and keep changing their bandages. Instead, you help people find their inner strength, stand on their own again and find dignity in their lives, even though they are not like new. This kind of caregiving is called *restorative care*. When you provide restorative care, your goal is to help a person become as fully functional as possible and to help him or her be able to enjoy life.

Restorative care is part of the basic nursing care that you apply every day as you perform your other duties. It is the extra effort that you give to help a person reach his or her highest level of wellness. When you follow the doctor's or supervising nurse's orders for the amount and type of restorative care for each person, you can prevent disabilities and promote self-esteem, independence and dignity in each person.

When a person functions as well as possible in all areas of life, she has reached her best overall health. By encouraging her to do as much for herself as possible, you help increase her self-esteem and sense of purpose.

HOW TO RESPOND TO THE PERSON'S NEEDS

When providing restorative care, also called *rehabilitation nursing,* you use rehabilitation techniques and procedures. In addition to monitoring the person's vital signs, you promote her independence in daily living and emphasize communicating with her. You also enable a person to enjoy life more fully. *Enable* is an important word in restorative care. Enabling a person gives her the power to do something (Figure 16-1). How do you give a person such power? If you apply the following principles of rehabilitation, you enable a person to stand on her own, just as the restored chest of drawers, in less than perfect condition, but shining and full of dignity. As a nurse

---

KEY TERMS

ambulation: (am-byoo-LAY-shun) the medical term for the act of walking.

atrophy: (AH-tro-fee) a condition in which a part of the body, such as a muscle, wastes away or shrinks as a result of disuse or inadequate nutrition.

contracture: (kun-TRACK-tyur) a condition in which unused muscles cause a person's joints to become permanently bent.

immobile: (im-MOW-bul) unable to move.

osteoporosis: (os-tee-oh-puh-RHO-sis) a disease that weakens bones, increasing the risk of sudden and unexpected fractures.

prompting: using a simple statement to help someone remember.

range of motion: the amount of movement possible in a joint.

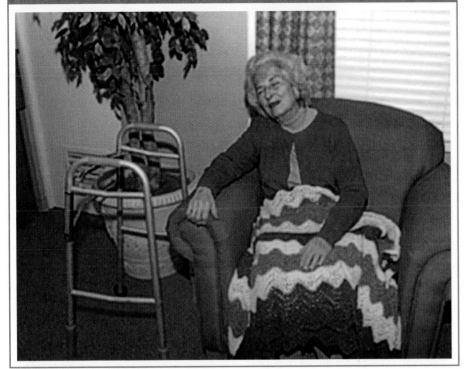

FIGURE 16-1 Enabling the resident, by ensuring that her walker is within reach, gives her the power to be more independent.

assistant, you enable a person when you:

- Emphasize her abilities rather than her disabilities. Recognize what she can do for herself and encourage her to do it.
- Begin her rehabilitation program early, according to the doctor's and supervising nurse's orders. Decreasing the amount of time she spends in bed prevents complications such as pressure sores; urinary tract infections; muscle weakness, tightening and shortening; **atrophy,** or disuse syndrome; and respiratory infections.
- Keep her active by helping with exercise whenever possible because activity strengthens and inactivity weakens.
- Treat the whole person, not just the affected part of her body. Consider her emotional, social, spiritual, vocational and physical being. Assist with developing her

care plan and make sure that it meets her specific needs.

PROMOTING A HEALTHY LIFESTYLE

Views on being healthy have changed during this century. People once believed that being healthy was a matter of luck. After the discovery of antibiotics and vaccines, people believed that taking these medicines was the way to control disease and illness.

Today, evidence shows that many diseases are caused by unhealthy habits, such as smoking cigarettes, lack of activity or eating improperly. Many things that affect health can be controlled. As a caregiver, you can help a person reach his best overall health by encouraging him to adopt good health and lifestyle practices. You encourage him by promoting independence, self-care, and good health

habits; teaching important skills to help him gain independence and measuring his progress in the areas of independence and self-care.

Promoting Independence, Self-Care and Good Health Habits

Because the process of restorative care requires the help of all the health care team members, many people are involved in helping the person in your care become healthier and more independent. The physical therapist and occupational therapist may be key players. A speech therapist, dietitian or other health care worker also may play active roles. All health care team members depend on you to report how the person progresses with activities and to reinforce what instructions have been put in place for restorative care. As a nurse assistant, you have many opportunities to encourage the person to take control of his life and health.

Independence. When you help a person do things for himself to gain independence, your goals are to teach, retrain, motivate and encourage him to do as much as he is physically and mentally able to do by himself. How can you promote independence in a person? In the following scenario, notice what the nurse assistant does to promote independence in this resident.

This resident has breathing difficulties and gets tired even when dressing. Although he moves very slowly, he likes to choose his own clothes and dress himself as much as possible.

The nurse assistant has six other people to help with dressing. She thinks she does not have time to stand by waiting for this resident to put on his robe. However, knowing how much it means to him to dress himself, the nurse assistant holds up the robe for the resident and asks him to put his arm in. Then the nurse assistant stands by ready to help the resident if needed. She notices that the resident becomes tired while putting on his robe (Figure 16-2).

The nurse assistant praises the resident for completing the difficult task of putting on his robe this far and asks him if he would like help to finish the task. He says that he would, and the nurse assistant finishes pulling down the robe and straightens the sleeves. She lets the resident rest a minute as she finishes making the bed and then helps him put on his shoes.

What did the nurse assistant do to promote independence for this resident?

- While giving care, she paid attention to the whole person—mind, body and spirit. She understood how much it meant to him to do things for himself. Because the resident felt physically able to take care of himself, it was important to encourage him to do so.

- The nurse assistant explained to the resident what she would do *for* him and *with* him.
- She encouraged and praised him for even his smallest successes.
- She focused on the resident's abilities, not his disabilities.
- She was patient.

Self-Care Through Personal Care. A person who is encouraged to help provide for his own personal care feels positive about becoming independent and improving his health and appearance. To maintain independence, a person may need to use certain self-help devices, such as the following commonly used personal care items:

- A toothbrush with a built-up handle that is easier for a person to grasp when brushing his teeth (Figure 16-3)
- A long-handled device with a hook on the end, designed to help a person take off his shoes (Figure 16-4)

- A zipper pull that attaches to a person's zipper, making it easier to grasp when she zips and unzips her clothes by herself (Figure 16-5)
- A long-handled shoe horn, which enables a person to put on his shoes (Figure 16-6)

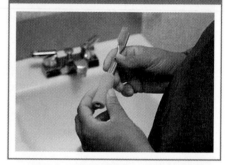

FIGURE 16-3 An inexpensive way to build up the handle of a toothbrush is to put a foam curler around the handle. This makes the handle larger and provides a nonslip surface.

FIGURE 16-4 A person who has difficulty bending over can use this device to help remove shoes.

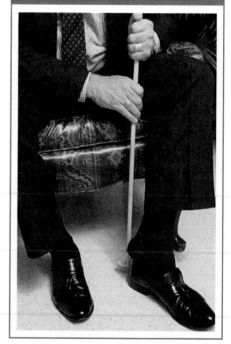

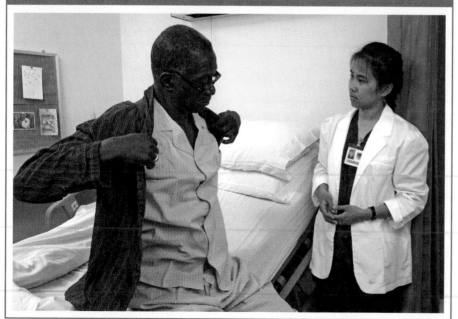

FIGURE 16-2 The nurse assistant encourages this resident to do all that he can for himself. She also notices when he gets tired and needs assistance.

FIGURE 16-5 A person who cannot grasp small items can attach a zipper pull to a zipper. She can then fasten the zipper by pulling on the zipper pull.

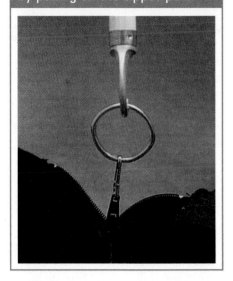

- A washcloth mitt made of self-fastening fabric, which enables a person to wash or bathe himself (Figure 16-7)
- A sock aid, which helps a person with weak hands and limited range of finger joint movement to put on socks (Figure 16-8)
- A grabbing device (long-handled, scissors-like device) that helps a person pick up things (Figure 16-9)

By encouraging people to use these self-help devices, you help them increase their independence. People who think they are becoming self-sufficient feel better about themselves, have improved energy levels and are happier because they believe their lives are more productive.

You may feel frustrated when it takes more time for a person to do something using a self-help device than it does when you provide the care. It is important to be patient because as a person becomes more

FIGURE 16-8 Using a sock aid helps people who have trouble bending over or who have hand problems to put on socks.

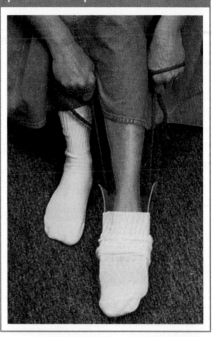

FIGURE 16-6 A person who uses a wheelchair or who has difficulty bending over can use a long-handled shoe horn to help put on shoes.

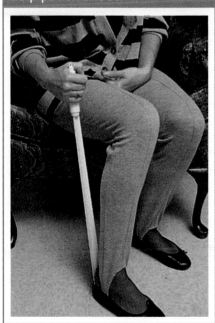

FIGURE 16-7 A mitt makes it easier for a person who does not have good control of his hands to wash by himself.

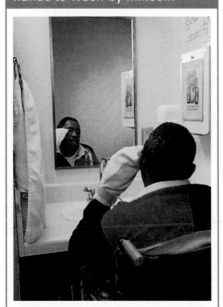

FIGURE 16-9 A person in a wheelchair or someone who cannot bend over can use a grabbing device to pick up things from the floor or reach light items on shelves.

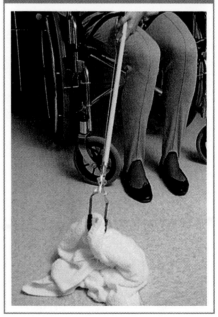

self-sufficient, the time he needs to do a task decreases. Both you and the person should feel very proud of this hard work and accomplishment. Of course, you may need to provide more help with certain tasks, such as putting on elastic stockings. Elastic stockings promote blood flow to the heart. Wearing these stockings will help prevent blood clots from forming. If a person has circulation problems or is bed ridden the doctor may order them to wear elastic stockings. To assist a person in putting them on, follow the procedure in Skill 53.

Good Health Habits. A person is never too young or too old to adopt good health habits. Everyone, including you and the people in your care, can benefit from making healthy lifestyle choices. What good health habits can you suggest to the people in your care? You can suggest that they gain control of their own well-being by following the ideas in Box 16-1.

Teaching Independence Skills

Some people need to learn new ways to do old things so that they can do as much for themselves as possible. For example, Mrs. Garcia needed to learn how to walk with a walker to maintain her independence. While certain members of the health care team may begin to teach or retrain a person, the nurse assistant is often asked to continue or reinforce the teaching. This is a very important and essential part of your job as a nursing assistant. You are the team member who spends the most time each day with the resident.

In Chapter 5, "Communicating with People," you read about effective teaching techniques. The same principles apply to helping a person learn how to maintain her or his independence.

- Explain the task you want a person in your care to complete. Use short, concise statements.
- Give clear instructions.
- Ask the person to repeat your instructions. (This feedback lets you know whether or not she understands.)
- Repeat the instructions, if necessary, using the same statements.
- Give an example, if necessary.
- Demonstrate the procedure.
- Explain why the activity is important.
- Ask the person whether she has any questions.
- Have patience. Progress may be slow, but if you become impatient, there may be no progress at all.

In addition, use a method called **prompting** to reinforce something that has been taught. It is a way of reminding a person what to do without actually telling her. For example, Mrs. Garcia is about to stand up by herself and use her walker. Her walker is to the left of where she is going to stand, not right in front of her (Figure 16-10). By asking Mrs. Garcia if her walker is where she wants it, you remind her that it is not in the right place. If a person hesitates to do something that you know she can do, it is better to prompt her than to do it for her.

Furthermore, when a person who is doing a task gives you a questioning look, do not assume she has forgotten what to do. She may be worried about doing the task wrong in front of you. Help by asking, "What do you think you should do next?" The person may tell you and then go on with the task. If necessary, tell her what step should come next, but encourage her to do the task independently.

Helping a Person Walk

Walking is good exercise. Because of a disability, someone may need to use a device that helps her walk, such as a walker, cane or crutches. Using such a device helps give the person a way to exercise independently. The physical therapist or nurse teaches the person how to use the device, and you reinforce what she learns, which is part of restorative care. A person in your care may need your assistance because she is learning how to use a device or because she may be unsteady when walking with a device. When a person is dizzy, sweaty, in pain or short of breath, encourage her to sit down and rest. When helping someone walk, follow the specific procedure that is explained step by step in Skill 54. If a person begins to fall, help that person by following the specific procedure that also is explained in Skill 54.

BOX 16-1

HOW TO MAINTAIN GOOD HEALTH HABITS

- Eat a well-balanced diet and drink adequate fluids.
- Exercise regularly.
- Do not smoke.
- Get yearly checkups from a doctor.
- Receive routine dental care.
- Examine your breasts or testicles monthly.

- Make time for daily relaxation.
- Visit with family and friends.
- Do rewarding activities.
- Talk about your feelings.
- Follow safety rules.
- Wear a seat belt when in a car.

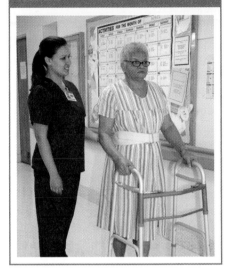

FIGURE 16-11 Many walkers have adjustable legs so that a walker can be fitted to a person's height.

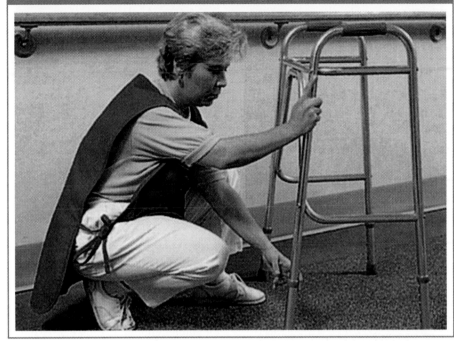

When a person has an IV or catheter, make sure this equipment is cared for properly so that treatment is not disrupted and the person is not harmed as you help her walk. Make sure an IV bag or bottle is always higher than the IV entry site. Also make sure a urinary catheter bag and tubing are always lower than the person's bladder.

Find out how the physical therapist taught the person to use the device to help her walk. Make sure the person's shoes or slippers fit well and have nonskid soles. Encourage her never to walk barefoot. Help her put on her footwear, if necessary.

Helping a Person Walk with a Walker. A person uses a walker when she needs support on both sides. When a person uses a walker, make sure the rubber tips are in good condition. The height of the walker should be at about the same height as the person's hip bones and should be adjusted by the physical therapy department or supervising nurse (Figure 16-11).

The person in your care may use one of the following three kinds of walkers:

- **Pick-up walker.** A person who is unsteady on her feet, but who does not need to lean heavily, uses this type of walker. She can pick up the walker when she does not need to lean on it.
- **Four-wheeled walker.** A person who needs constant support when walking uses this type of walker.
- **Semi-wheeled walker.** A person who lacks strength and endurance uses this type of walker, which has two front wheels and two back feet. The person can stop and lean on the walker. When she thinks she is ready, she can pick up the back feet of the walker and roll it forward on the wheels.

Helping a Person Walk with a Cane. A person uses a walking cane when he needs support on one side but is able to walk without much difficulty. When a person uses a cane, make sure the rubber tips are in good condition. Put the cane near the person's stronger hand. Ask him to put his hand on the cane handle. Be certain that when the cane is at his side, the top of it is even with his hip bone and the bottom is 6 inches to the side of his foot. Walk on the person's weaker side and help him, if necessary.

Figure 16-12 shows two kinds of walking canes.

FIGURE 16-12 Two types of walking canes are quad (left, with four legs) and single-tip (right).

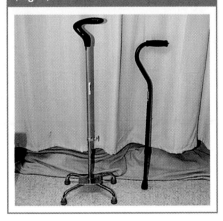

Helping a Person Walk with Crutches. A person uses crutches when he cannot use one leg or when both legs are weak and need support. The nurse or physical therapist adjusts the crutches to the proper height for the person (Figure 16-13). The person should not lean on a crutch with his armpit because he may injure himself. He can walk with crutches in several different ways, depending on how much weight he can bear on each foot and how strong his upper body is. The physical therapist teaches the person how to use the crutches, and you reinforce what he has learned.

Helping a Person Walk Without a Device. Put a safety belt on the person. (Review the information you read about safety belts in Chapter 10, "Positioning and Transferring People.") Never use a safety belt if the person has:

- Had a colostomy or ileostomy recently
- Severe heart problems

- Had abdominal, chest or back surgery recently
- Severe respiratory problems
- A fear of safety belts

If the person is weaker on one side than the other, stand on the weaker side, unless you are instructed otherwise, so that you can support the person's ambulation. Gradually increase the distance the person walks to help build his confidence. If no cane is used and person has a weak side you become the "cane" – thus you should walk on strong side.

PROMOTING ACTIVITY

Activity helps people attain or regain independence. Have you ever heard the expression, "Use it or lose it"? This condition really can happen. Many physical problems occur when people do not get enough exercise (Box 16-2). Their muscles become weak, flabby and tired; they can even develop atrophy. People may become **immobile** if muscles and joints are not used.

Lack of exercise also can cause problems in almost all the other body systems. For example, a person may become constipated when the movement of the intestines slows down, or he may develop pneumonia from secretions that pool in the lungs. When circulation slows down, a person may develop dangerous blood clots. Without exercise, bones lose minerals and become brittle, making it easy for them to break. The disease which causes this is known as **osteoporosis**. Even the immobile person who cannot move on his own needs to be active.

People feel better physically and emotionally when they exercise. Without exercise, people may feel depressed, angry, helpless and lonely. To help a person reach his highest capabilities, you must encourage and guide him to exercise. As a person exercises, he starts feeling better.

As a nurse assistant, you help a person stay active and mobile with range-of-motion exercises and **ambulation. Range of motion** is the amount of movement possible in a joint, such as the elbow, knee, or hip. It is also how far a person can move a joint comfortably. For example, one person may be able to bend his elbow and touch his shoulder with his hand and another person may only be able to bend his elbow an inch or two. The medical abbreviation for "range of motion" is *ROM*.

For the person in your care to get the most benefit, he needs to do each kind of exercise regularly. For example, you may help a person do range-of-motion exercises at least twice a day and help him walk several times a day. This regular exercise helps keep

FIGURE 16-13 Crutches fit properly when you can measure two fingers width of space between the person's armpit and the top of the crutch and when he can comfortably grasp the hand grip with his elbow extended.

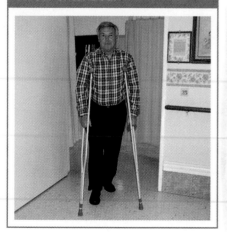

the person's muscles, joints and other body systems working.

Helping a Person with Range of Motion

The range of motion a person has can change within a day and from day to day. For example, a woman who has arthritis may not have much range of motion in the early morning because her muscles are stiff. But in the late morning, after her bath and after she had taken her pain medication, she may have more range of motion or mobility in her joints.

Range-of-motion exercises can be active, which means the person moves his joints. They also can be passive, which means another person moves the person's joints for him. You may be asked to help teach family members how to do passive range-of-motion exercises.

Passive range-of-motion exercises are important for people who cannot move much on their own. If you do not move the person's joints, his muscles shorten, which may cause the joints to become permanently bent. This condition is called a **contracture.** Bend your wrist so that your palm moves toward the inside of your arm. This bending is the position of a common contracture. Imagine what it would be like to try to eat, dress and go to the bathroom with your hands and arms bent in this position.

When helping someone with passive range-of-motion exercises, follow the specific procedure that is explained step by step in Skill 55 at the end of this chapter. When you do passive range-of-motion exercises, begin at the top of the person's body and work your way down. Exercise five sets of joints each time you do the exercises. Do all five sets of joints on one side of the person's body, and then move to the other side and start at the top again. Figure 16-14 shows how to make this activity pleasant. Smile!

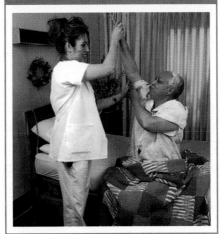

FIGURE 16-14 When helping someone do a specific number of passive range-of-motion exercises for each of the seven sets of joints, make this activity pleasant.

Measuring Progress

Rehabilitation can be a long, slow process. A key part of your job is observing even the smallest changes and improvements. Telling the person in your care about her progress encourages her to continue (Figure 16-15). Use your senses when observing a person for positive changes. What you observe depends on the goal of the restorative nursing care plan. You may have to watch to see how far a person walks, how well she eats or how far she can bend a joint. Listen to the person's descriptions of how much effort it took to do the task, or touch the person's skin to see whether it is warm, cool, moist or dry. Her skin can provide a clue about how much effort she exerted. For example, if she exerted a great deal of effort, her skin may be warm and moist.

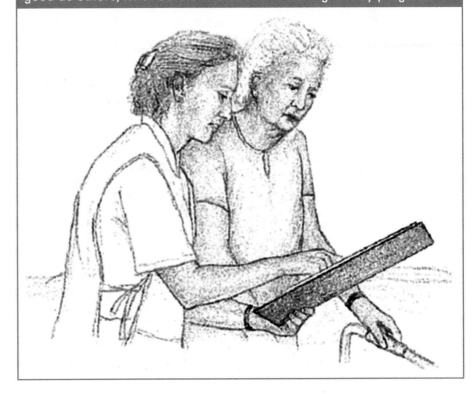

FIGURE 16-15 When she first entered the nursing home, Mrs. Garcia was a little depressed about the amount of progress she made while learning to walk better with her walker. The chart helps her keep track of her walking distance. Even though some days are not as good as others, Mrs. Garcia knows she is making steady progress.

Keeping track of small successes is important. If you say, "Mr. Lightfoot, you were able to do all but the sleeves on your turtleneck today, and last week you could only get it over your head before getting tired," he will probably want to try to pull on the entire turtleneck by next week. Your expressed observations encourage him to try harder.

Always remember to record your observations about the progress of the person in your care. This information helps the other health care team members.

INFORMATION REVIEW

Circle the correct answers and fill in the blanks.

1. To help people become as fully functional as possible and to help them to be able to enjoy life, you provide _restorative_ care.

2. To encourage a person's independence, you would:
   a. feed the person yourself so that his food does not get cold.
   b. set the food in front of him and leave the room.
   c. give him 5 minutes to feed himself and then feed him the rest of the meal to save time.
   d. encourage him to use a self-help eating utensil so that he can feed himself.

3. A built-up handle toothbrush, a long-handled shoe horn, a zipper pull and a stocking aid are examples of _self-help_ devices.

4. Inactivity can cause:
   a. atrophied muscles.
   b. blindness.
   c. fractures.
   d. arthritis.

5. Mrs. Clymer has arthritis and needs to do range-of-motion exercises. When you go to her room to help her, she says that she cannot do them today because she hurts too much. The best way to respond is to say:
   a. "You need to do them because the doctor ordered them. Let's just do them and get them over with."
   b. "If we do them quickly, we'll finish up faster."
   c. "Okay, we'll do them tomorrow."
   d. "It's so important for you to do these exercises to keep your joints flexible. Let's try to do them very slowly, and you can let me know when you need to rest or stop."

6. The physical therapist teaches a person how to use crutches, and the nurse assistant _reinforce_ what has been taught.

1. Mr. Rivera had a stroke, which resulted in left-side paralysis. What suggestions do you have for Mr. Rivera to help him increase his activity?

2. Mr. Roberts has severe arthritis in his hands. He struggles, but he usually manages to feed himself at breakfast and lunch using his adaptive fork. His wife feeds him dinner every night. What do you think you should do about this situation?

3. Ms. Jones complains about not being able to do things or get around like she did before the car crash that left her with a below-the-knee amputation. She has a prosthesis, but she does not like to wear it. She wants you to take her to the bathroom in her wheelchair. What do you think would be the best thing for you to do?

4. How can you help maintain independence for a person who needs to use a walker?

5. How can you help maintain good body mechanics for someone who uses a cane to walk?

6. Mrs. Garcia is upset because she couldn't reach the end of the hallway today. "Yesterday I walked twice as far with this stupid thing!" she says and angrily pushes away her walker. What can you do to help her feel better?

7. Name some of the body parts that are exercised when you help someone with passive range-of-motion exercises. Why are these exercises important for providing restorative care?

8. Why must you be especially careful to maintain the skin integrity of someone who uses crutches?

9. Ever since he developed contractures, Mr. Hudson has lost weight. "I'm just not as hungry as I used to be," he tells you at lunch. One day you overhear Mr. Hudson telling his roommate that he doesn't want to be a burden to anyone. What can you do to make sure Mr. Hudson receives adequate nutrition and maintains his independence?

Skill 53: Applying Elastic Stockings

PRECAUTIONS

- Apply elastic stockings when a person has been lying down for at least 15 minutes. The best time to apply elastic stockings is before the person gets up in the morning. If the person has been standing, have him or her sit in a chair with his or her legs elevated for 15 minutes before applying the stockings.
- Check the person's toes for circulation every hour. Look for coldness or a bluish color.
- Ask the person if he or she has numbness or tingling in the feet. Remove the stockings and report to your supervising nurse if these symptoms occur.

PREPARATION

1. Gather supplies:
   - Elastic stockings
2. Follow Preparation Standards (see Chapter 7).

PROCEDURE

1. Make sure the person is in a flat, supine position, if he can tolerate it. ☐ ☐
2. Pull the top sheet out from the bottom of the mattress and fold it back toward the person, exposing only his legs. ☐ ☐
3. Take one stocking and turn it inside out down to the heel. Put the stocking on the person's leg that is closest to you. Slide the stocking over the person's toes, foot and heel (Figure 16-16, A). Position the opening across the toes (Figure 16-16, B). ☐ ☐

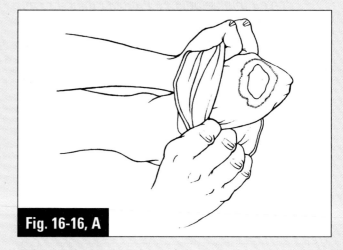

Fig. 16-16, A

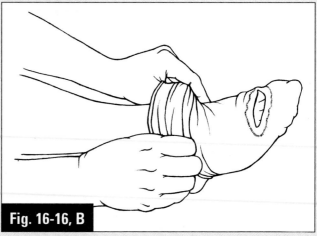

Fig. 16-16, B

4. Slide the rest of the stocking up the leg, smoothing out wrinkles (Figure 16-16, C–D). ☐ ☐

5. Check the stocking to be sure it is not too tight across the person's toes (Figure 16-16, E). ☐ ☐

6. Apply the second stocking to the other leg. ☐ ☐

ADDITIONAL INFORMATION

Elastic stockings come in various sizes. Check with your supervising nurse to be sure you have the correct size for the person.

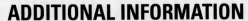

 COMPLETION

Follow Completion Standards in compliance with your facility. For a complete list of those used in this course, see Chapter 7, "Controlling the Spread of Germs."

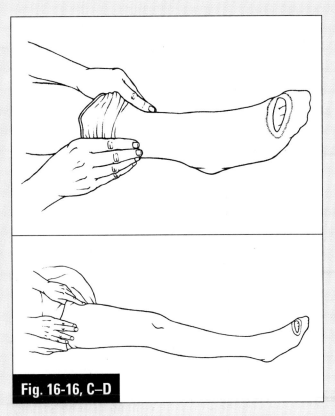

Fig. 16-16, C–D

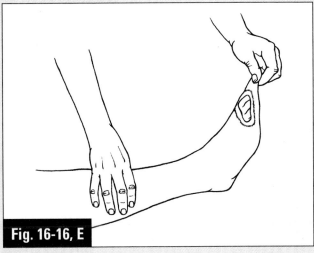

Fig. 16-16, E

Skill 54: Helping a Person Walk

PRECAUTIONS

- When a person is using a walker or cane, always be sure the rubber tips are in good shape.
- Always be sure to check how the person was taught to use the device to help him or her walk.
- Never use a safety belt if the person has:
  - A recent colostomy or ileostomy.
  - Severe heart problems.
  - Had recent abdominal, chest or back surgery.
  - Severe respiratory problems.
  - A fear of safety belts.
  - When a person has an IV or catheter, make sure this equipment is cared for properly so that treatment is not disrupted and the person is not harmed. An IV always should be above the catheter entry site. A urinary catheter bag and tubing always should be below the bladder.

PREPARATION

1. Gather supplies:
   - Walker, cane or crutches, if needed.
2. Follow Preparation Standards (see Chapter 7).

PROCEDURE

Option 1: Assisting a Person to Walk with a Walker

Make sure resident has non-skid foot wear on before assisting the person to walk.

1. Put a safety belt on the person. Grip the safety belt as needed to support the person. ☐ ☐
2. Put the walker directly in front of him. ☐ ☐
3. Help the person to stand. ☐ ☐
4. Ask the person to put his hands on the walker's handgrips, stand erect and slightly flex his elbows. ☐ ☐
5. Have the person lift the walker and put it down about 6 inches forward and then step into it. If the legs are weak, the person's arms should be used to support his weight. ☐ ☐
6. Encourage the person to walk normally, looking ahead, while using the walker (Figure 16-17).

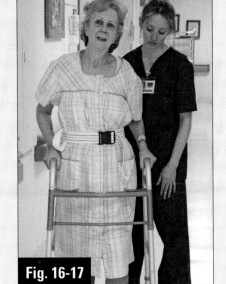
Fig. 16-17

Option 2: Assisting a Person to Walk with a Cane

Make sure resident has non-skid foot wear on before assisting the person to walk.

1. Put the safety belt on the person and assist to a standing position. ☐ ☐
2. Place the cane near the person's stronger hand. ☐ ☐

3. While the person is standing erect, place the stronger hand on the cane handle, with the elbow slightly flexed. Move the cane forward about 6 to 10 inches. □ □

4. Have the person use the cane for support while standing on the stronger side and moving the weaker leg forward until it is even with the cane (Figure 16-18). □ □

5. The leg on the cane side (strong side) is moved ahead of the cane and the weaker leg. □ □

6. Walk on the weaker side of the person to assist him or her as necessary. □ □

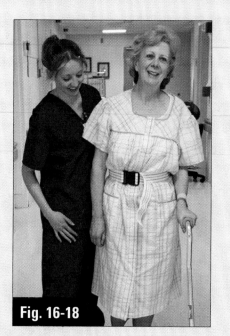
Fig. 16-18

Option 3: Assisting a Person to Walk with Crutches

Make sure resident has non-skid foot wear on before assisting the person to walk.

1. Put a safety belt on the person and assist to a standing position. □ □

2. Help him place a crutch under each arm. □ □

3. Tell the person to stand erect, place hands on handgrips and flex the elbows slightly. □ □

4. Instruct him to move forward, leaning on his hands and gripping the crutch between the chest and the inside of the upper arms. □ □

   If the person can bear weight on both feet, teach these steps:
   • Move the right crutch forward.
   • Move the left foot forward.
   • Move the left crutch forward.

- Move the right foot forward.
- Repeat these steps. ☐ ☐

If the person can bear weight on only one foot, have her:

- Move both crutches forward along with the weaker extremity.
- Move the strong leg up to the crutches. (If her upper body is strong, the person may be able to swing her body through the crutches and have her good leg land past the crutches.)
- Repeat these steps. ☐ ☐

5. Help the person practice the sequence. ☐ ☐

6. Remind the person to look ahead while using the crutches. ☐ ☐

Option 4: Assisting a Person to Walk Without a Device

Make sure resident has non-skid foot wear on before assisting the person to walk.

1. Put a safety belt on the person and help him to stand. ☐ ☐

2. Stand at the weaker side with your arm under the person's arm, holding his wrist while he or she gains a sense of balance. ☐ ☐

3. Hold the safety belt with an underhand grip or hold onto the back handles (Figure 16-19). ☐ ☐

4. Starting on the same foot as the person, walk on his weaker side and a little behind. ☐ ☐

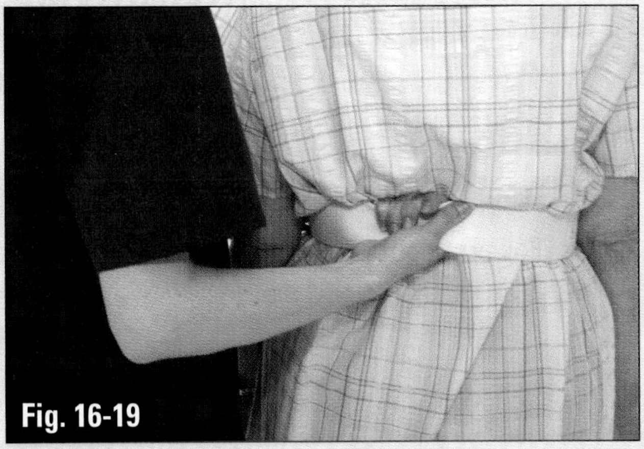

Fig. 16-19

Skill 54: Helping a Person Walk—cont'd

5. Remind the person to walk normally, looking ahead. ☐ ☐

6. Gradually increase the distance the person walks. ☐ ☐

   If the person in your care should fall:

   - Do not try to stop a fall; doing so may injure you and the resident. Use body mechanics to try to slow his downward moment to help prevent injury from the fall.
   - Put your arms around the person's waist or underarms, keeping him close to your body; bend your knees and lower the person slowly to the floor by sliding him down your leg.
   - Call for help.
   - Help make the person comfortable, reassure him and stay with him.
   - Do not move him until a nurse has checked him, and you have been told to do so.

ADDITIONAL INFORMATION

Review the section on first aid for falls in Chapter 8, "Keeping People Safe."

 ## COMPLETION

Follow Completion Standards in compliance with your facility. For a complete list of those used in this course, see Chapter 7, "Controlling the Spread of Germs."

Skill 55: Helping a Person with Passive Range-of-Motion Exercises

PRECAUTIONS

- Move each joint slowly, gently and smoothly.
- Support each joint during movement.
- Always move the joint only as far as the person can tolerate; never go beyond that point.
- Always watch the person's face, particularly the eyes, for any expression of pain. If the person has pain, stop the movement and report your observation to your supervising nurse.
- Always use proper body mechanics.

PREPARATION

1. Follow Preparation Standards (see Chapter 7).
2. *Position the person on his back (supine position) if he can tolerate it, and make sure his body is in proper alignment.*

PROCEDURE

Task 1: Exercising the Shoulder

1. With one hand, hold the person's wrist with his palm down and put your other hand under the elbow. Provide this support throughout the following motions. ☐ ☐
2. Raise the person's arm straight up and then move it alongside the ear (Figure 16-20). Then lower the arm to the side. Repeat 5 times. ☐ ☐
3. Move the person's arm out away from the body and return it to the side. Repeat 5 times. ☐ ☐
4. Carry the person's hand to the opposite shoulder, then back down to the bed. ☐ ☐

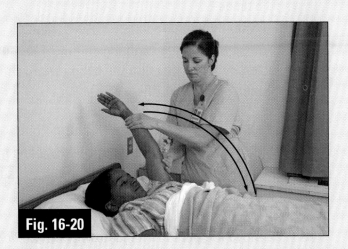

Fig. 16-20

5. Raise the person's elbow so that it is at the same height as the shoulder. Move the forearm up and down, as a police officer does when signaling a person to stop. Repeat 5 times. ☐ ☐

Task 2: Exercising the Elbow and Forearm

1. Hold the person's wrist with one hand and put your other hand under the elbow. Provide this support throughout the following motions. ☐ ☐

2. Bend the person's arm at the elbow so that the hand moves toward the shoulder on the same side (Figure 16-21). Then straighten the arm back down to the hip. Repeat 5 times. ☐ ☐

3. With the person's forearm at a right angle to the bed, turn the hand down toward the feet *(pronation)*. Then turn the hand toward the face *(supination)*. Repeat 5 times. ☐ ☐

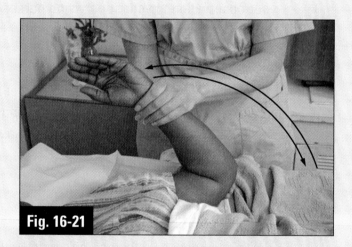

Fig. 16-21

Task 3: Exercising the Wrist

1. Hold the person's wrist with one hand and her fingers with your other hand. Provide this support throughout the following motions. ☐ ☐

2. Raise his hand off the mattress. ☐ ☐

3. Move the person's hand downward *(flexion)* and then straighten the wrist *(extension)*. Move the hand back *(hyperextension)* (Figure 16-22). Repeat 5 times. ☐ ☐

4. Straighten the wrist. Move the wrist from side to side *(abduction* and *adduction)*. Repeat five times. ☐ ☐

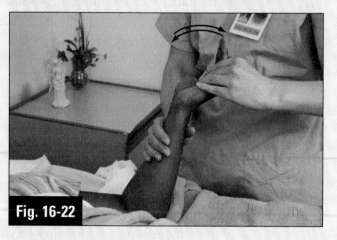

Fig. 16-22

5. Drop the wrist down, pointing the person's thumb toward her toes *(ulnar deviation)*. Then bring the thumb up toward the person's nose *(radial deviation)*. Repeat 5 times. ☐ ☐

Task 4: Exercising the Fingers and Thumb

1. Hold the person's hand with one of your hands and support her wrist with your other hand. ☐ ☐
2. Flex the person's fingers to make a fist with the thumb tucked under the other fingers. Straighten the hand by extending the person's fingers, including the thumb, one at a time. Repeat 5 times. ☐ ☐
3. Hold the person's thumb and index finger together in one of your hands. With the other hand, spread her middle finger away from her index finger. Move it to the index finger and hold the middle finger, index finger and thumb together. Move the ring finger away from the other three fingers (thumb, index and middle), then back to them. Hold all four fingers. Do the same with the little finger. Then hold the little finger and ring finger together and move the middle finger away and back. Complete with index finger and thumb. Repeat this exercise 5 times. ☐ ☐
4. Bend the person's thumb in toward the palm and back next to the index finger. ☐ ☐
5. Bring the person's thumb to the tip of each finger *(thumb opposition)*. Repeat this exercise 5 times (Figure 16-23). ☐ ☐

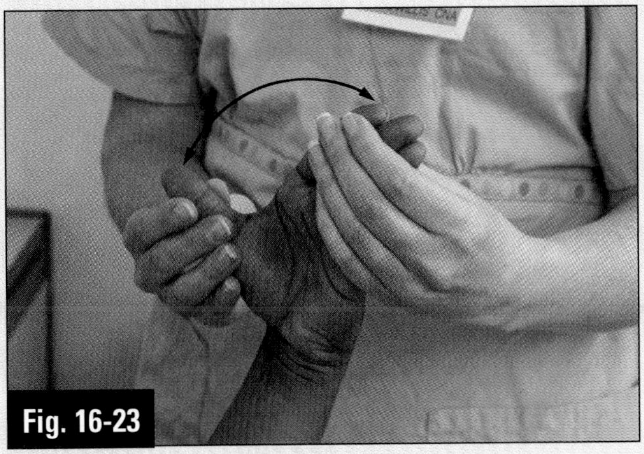

Fig. 16-23

Skill 55: Helping a Person with Passive Range-of-Motion Exercises—cont'd

Task 5: Exercising the Hip and Knee

1. Put one hand under the person's knee and your other hand under his ankle. Provide this support throughout the following motions. ☐ ☐

2. Bend the person's knee and move it up toward his head to flex his knee and hip *(flexion)*. Repeat 5 times, alternating with extension (as explained next, in Step 3) (Figure 16-24). ☐ ☐

3. Straighten the person's knee to extend his knee and hip. Lower his leg to the bed *(extension)*. Repeat 5 times, alternating with flexion (as explained in Step 2). ☐ ☐

4. Move the person's leg out away from his body *(abduction)* (Figure 16-25). ☐ ☐

5. Move the person's leg back to the center toward his other leg *(adduction)*. Repeat 5 times, alternating with abduction. ☐ ☐

6. Turn the person's leg inward and then out-ward to rotate the hip *(rotation)*. Repeat 5 times. ☐ ☐

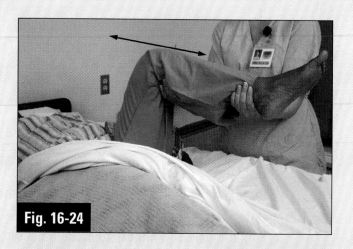
Fig. 16-24

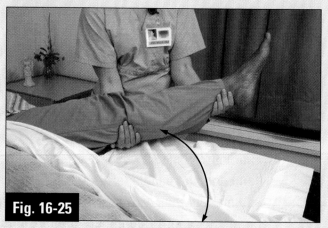
Fig. 16-25

Task 6: Exercising the Ankle

1. Put one hand under the person's ankle and grasp her foot with your other hand. Provide this support throughout the following motions. ☐ ☐

2. Push the person's foot forward toward her head *(flexion)* and then downward *(extension)*. Repeat 5 times (Figure 16-26, A–B).　☐　☐

3. Turn the person's foot inward *(adduction)* and then outward *(abduction)*. Repeat 5 times.　☐　☐

Task 7: Exercising the Toes

1. Put one hand under the person's foot and the other hand on the top of his foot over the toes.　☐　☐

2. Curl his toes downward *(flexion)* and then straighten them *(extension)*. Repeat 5 times.　☐　☐

3. Holding two toes, spread each toe in the same way that you spread the fingers *(abduction* and *adduction)* in Task 4 (Figure 16-27). Repeat 5 times.　☐　☐

Repeat the exercise in Tasks 1 through 7 on the opposite side of the person's body.

ADDITIONAL INFORMATION

Position the person on his back (supine position) if he can tolerate it, and make sure his body is in proper alignment.

COMPLETION

Follow Completion Standards in compliance with your facility. For a complete list of those used in this course, see Chapter 7, "Controlling the Spread of Germs."

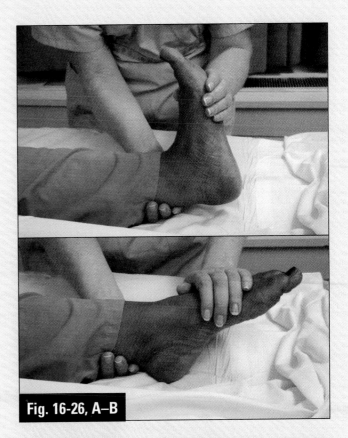

Fig. 16-26, A–B

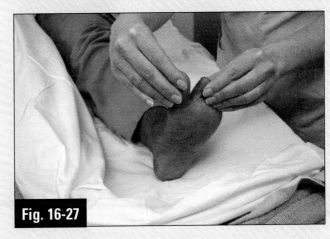

Fig. 16-27

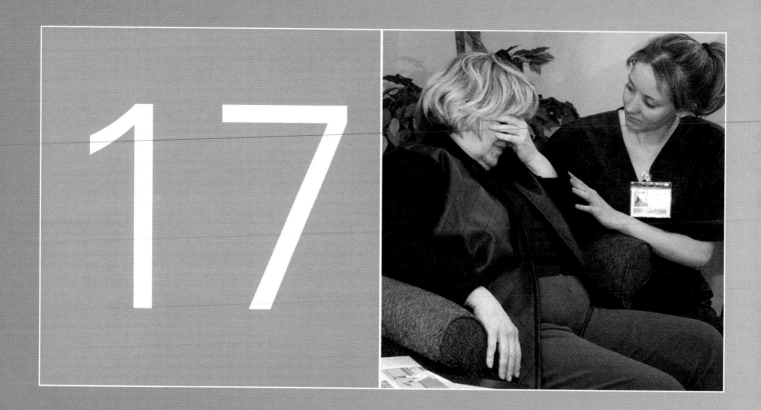

17

Providing Care for People with Specific Illnesses

GOALS

After reading this chapter, you will have the information needed to:

Describe the nature of acute and chronic conditions.

Describe common chronic conditions of several body systems.

Describe some of the characteristics or symptoms of several chronic illnesses.

Focus care to meet the specific needs of people with chronic illnesses.

Focus care to meet the specific needs of people who have cancer.

The first time you went to Gene and Sue Conrad's house to provide care for 63-year-old Mr. Conrad, he had recently been diagnosed with heart disease and needed help with personal care. When you arrived, you could see that Mrs. Conrad's eyes were red and puffy and that her eye makeup was smudged.

After hanging up your coat on the hall coat rack, you asked Mrs. Conrad what you could do to help her.

"Nobody can help me!" she said in a loud, high-pitched voice. Then she sat down in a chair and burst into tears. You put your hands on her shoulders to try to comfort her. When she calmed down, she said, "I'm sorry. It's just that Gene's disease has made everything so difficult. We can't go out together because I'm not strong enough to handle his wheelchair and oxygen tank, and I'm afraid to leave him alone. I feel like a prisoner. I never get out of this

house. All I do is take care of Gene. I don't mind taking care of him, because I love him. But I'm so tired. I don't see how we can continue to live like this."

As with many other families living with chronic disease, the Conrads had a hard time accepting a new lifestyle. However, over time, with help from several caregivers, the Conrads have adapted to living with Mr. Conrad's disease. He has learned how to do many things for

KEY TERMS

angina pectoris: (an-JY-nuh/PEK-to-ris) The medical term for *chest pain*.

aspiration pneumonia: Resulting from aspiration of food particles, vomit, water or infected material from the upper respiratory track.

benign: A tumor that grows slowly and within a localized area.

cannula: (KAN-you-luh) A tube placed under the nostrils to deliver oxygen.

cancer: Malignant tumor that can spread to other parts of the body.

cerebrovascular accident (CVA): (suh-ree-bro-VAS-kyu-ler) An interruption of blood flow to a part of the brain, which results in the death of a few or many brain cells. Also called a *stroke*.

chemotherapy: (key-mo-THER-uh-pee) Treatment with one or more drugs for the purpose of stopping cancer cells from multiplying.

chronic obstructive pulmonary disease (COPD): A condition of the respiratory system, that includes emphysema, asthma and chronic bronchitis—diseases that are long term and interfere with the body's ability to breathe efficiently.

coma: A state of deep prolonged unconsciousness in which an individual is incapable of sensing or responding to external stimuli.

congestive heart failure: (kun-JES-tiv) A condition of the cardiovascular system in

which weakened heart muscles prevent the heart from pumping blood effectively.

dialysis: A process that filters waste products from the blood.

edema: (uh-DEE-muh) Swelling of body tissue due to an accumulation of fluid.

end-stage renal disease (ESRD): Last stage of kidney failure, in which the kidney cannot get rid of waste products.

gait: The manner in which a person walks.

gestational diabetes: Diabetes developed during a mother's pregnancy.

glucose: End product in the blood after carbohydrate (sugar) metabolism (turning carbohydrates into energy the body can use).

homicidal: (hom-uh-SIDE-uhl) A tendency to harm other people with the intent to kill.

hyperglycemia: Too much sugar in the blood.

hypoglycemia: Too little sugar in the blood.

influenza (flu): A highly contagious infection of the respiratory tract transmitted by airborne droplets.

kidney failure: A condition of the urinary system that occurs when the kidneys no longer function and are unable to get rid of the body's waste.

malignant: A cancerous tumor that grows rapidly and spreads into other tissues.

metastasis: Spread of cancer to other parts of the body.

multiple sclerosis (MS): A chronic disease that gradually destroys the coating on nerve endings in the brain and spinal cord resulting in loss of muscle control, vision, balance, sensation (such as numbness) or thinking ability.

osteoporosis: (os-tee-oh-per-OH-sis) A condition of the skeletal system in which the bones become weak and fragile.

pneumonia: (nuh-MOAN-yuh) An infection in the lungs.

radiation: (ray-dee-AY-shun) Treatment in which x-rays are focused on the part of the body where cancer cells are growing.

suicidal: (sue-uh-SIDE-uhl) A tendency to intentionally and voluntarily harm oneself with the intent to take one's own life.

tumor: A new growth of cells. Tumors can be benign or malignant.

type 1 diabetes: (dye-uh-BEE-tez) A form of diabetes in which the pancreas produces very little or no insulin. Also called *juvenile-onset* or *insulin-dependent diabetes*.

type 2 diabetes: (dye-uh-BEE-tez) A form of diabetes in which the output of insulin from the pancreas is inadequate for the body's needs. Also called *maturity-onset* or *insulin-independent diabetes*, type 2 diabetes often develops later in life.

himself, and Mrs. Conrad arranges for help so that she occasionally can go out by herself, go to the store or enjoy a movie with her husband. They have learned how to adjust to their new lifestyle so that they can once again enjoy their life together.

PROVIDING CARE FOR PEOPLE WITH ACUTE AND CHRONIC ILLNESSES

Think about the last time you were sick. Did the illness occur suddenly? Perhaps one day you felt fine, and the next day you were ill with a cold or an infection. Or perhaps someone you know had surgery to remove an infected appendix (appendicitis). In both of these cases, the illness is considered an *acute* condition. That is, the illness happened fairly suddenly and lasted a short time. When your cold ran its course, you felt well again. Likewise, when the person received treatment for appendicitis, he felt well again.

Some other illnesses occur gradually and last a long time. These illnesses are *chronic* conditions. In many cases, a person who has a chronic condition lives the rest of his life with an illness or condition that never really goes away. Do you know someone who has a chronic condition, such as heart disease, diabetes or arthritis? Sometimes a person can have a chronic condition that continues for years without many serious symptoms, and then suddenly it flares up. When it flares up, the chronic condition is in an acute phase. The person feels ill and may need to consult a doctor. After treatment, the acute phase goes away, and the person continues to live with the chronic condition.

Think about some of the emotional events a person goes through when he has an acute condition. The illness disrupts his normal life. He cannot continue with daily activities. He may have to cancel plans or make an appointment to see the doctor. Has your life ever been disrupted by illness? Did

you go to the doctor for an examination and go home hoping the illness would go away soon? Did your family and friends support you and try to make you feel comfortable? If you had an acute illness, you probably were able to go back to your normal way of living after a few days or weeks.

What do you think it would be like to live with a chronic condition? A chronic condition lasts a long time, and may never go away. It often affects the activities of daily living. For example, a person who has arthritis may not be able to walk without a walker or cane, or a person who has heart disease may have to change his diet. A chronic condition also may impact a person's emotional health. He may be depressed or unhappy about not being able to do the things he once did, or he may be short-tempered because he is in pain. As a health care provider, you must focus your care so that you can help a person with a chronic condition to live the fullest life possible.

Family members and friends also are affected by a chronic condition. If a person's diet changes, his family may have to eat differently, too. If the person cannot move without help, he may need assistance with a variety of tasks. Family members and friends also may be sad, angry or depressed about the change in the person's health.

As you read this chapter, you will learn mainly about providing care for people with chronic conditions. Remember, it can be very difficult to cope day to day with a condition that may prevent a person from ever feeling really well.

CHRONIC CONDITIONS OF THE SKELETAL SYSTEM

Two chronic conditions that affect the skeletal system are arthritis and **osteoporosis**. When providing care, remember that a person with a bone disease has a chronic illness. She may feel depressed with her inability to move

without pain and her need to be more dependent on others. Your role is crucial. You can give her emotional support and encouragement.

Providing Care for a Person Who has Arthritis

Mrs. Chatterjee hardly looks up at you from her wheelchair. She rarely speaks and she eats little. You see on her chart that she is a 55-year-old woman who has had arthritis for the last 20 years. She has stiffness in her hips, knees and fingers, and these joints are tender and swollen. When she moves, she feels a great deal of pain. She often is depressed because of her inability to move without pain and because of how deformed her joints have become.

Characteristics and Symptoms of Arthritis. Arthritis is a condition of the skeletal system that causes joints to become inflamed, swollen, stiff and painful. A few or many joints may be affected. The smooth, slipping tissues that cover the ends of bones become rough or wear away, causing painful friction between bones when they move. The remaining tissues around the joints swell, which leads to stiffness. This stiffness makes normal movement difficult. Even an activity like unscrewing the lid of a jar or walking upstairs can be difficult and cause pain (Figure 17-1).

FIGURE 17-1 Adaptive devices, which make tasks easier, may be as simple as this rubber jar lid opener.

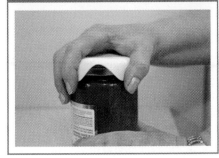

The Plan of Care. Mrs. Chatterjee's plan of care should focus on relieving her pain and helping her move. Imagine what it might be like being in constant pain or not being able to move without pain. When you provide care for a person with arthritis, such as Mrs. Chatterjee, focus on the following things:

- Let the person know that you know that movement is painful for her and that you are there to help her. Let her know you are concerned for her well-being. Ask her about the things that make movement easier for her.
- If the person takes medication, plan her daily morning care after she takes her morning dose. When she has less pain, she may be more in control and able to participate in her own care.
- Because warm water is soothing to the joints and helps reduce stiffness and pain, give her tub baths as often as possible. Make sure the water temperature is not too hot.
- To reduce stiffness and pain, encourage the person to wear warm clothing that covers the affected joints.
- Do gentle range-of-motion exercises to prevent contractures. Never move a joint that is painful, red or swollen.
- Handle the person's joints carefully and support the areas above and below the joint when you move her. This care decreases the pain that accompanies movement of the joints.
- Encourage her to exercise affected joints on her own. This activity promotes independence and keeps her joints more flexible.

A person who has an arthritic jaw joint may not be able to open her mouth or chew food comfortably. If she has arthritis in her hands, she may not be able to hold a toothbrush or comb. Personal care, especially mouth care, needs to be assessed for a person who has arthritis. Depending on which joints are affected, encourage a person with arthritis to maintain her independence through the use of the following joint-protection techniques:

- Attaching cloth loops to drawer handles to make them easier to open
- Pushing doors open with the side of her arm instead of her hand and outstretched arm
- Using the palms of both hands to lift and hold items such as cups, plates and pots and pans
- Using a cart to transport heavy items from place to place, instead of carrying them in her arms

Providing Care for a Person Who has Osteoporosis

When you first meet Charlotte Bryan, a delicate-looking woman of 68, she tells you how, for the past several years, she had been feeling pain in her back. "But I told myself, 'I don't have time to feel pain. I have too much to do.' So I ignored the pain," she said. "Then my favorite dresses seemed too long, and they didn't seem to hang right across my shoulders. 'Am I growing shorter?' I wondered. One sunny October morning, I began opening my bedroom window. Suddenly, I felt a great pain in my back and I fell to the floor. Slowly, I inched across the floor to the telephone and called for help.

"After doing a series of tests and x-rays, my doctor told me I had osteoporosis. He said that when I opened the window, the bones in my spinal column were not strong enough to support my muscles, and some of them broke. From now on, I have to be very careful not to fall because all the bones in my body have become weak and brittle."

Characteristics and Symptoms of Osteoporosis. *Osteoporosis* occurs mainly in women as they get older, often striking women who are in their 60s and 70s. The disease is caused by a gradual loss of minerals, especially calcium, in the bones. Calcium helps make bones hard and strong. When calcium is lacking, bones become soft and weak, and they break more easily. The spinal column of a person with osteoporosis shrinks, and the person becomes shorter. She may have a rounded upper back and stooped posture (Figure 17-2). As the disease progresses, she may have severe pain in the parts of the body that support her weight. She often tires easily and fears falling while walking.

The Plan of Care. Imagine how a person with osteoporosis might feel. Imagine how you would feel about losing the ability to move without pain, having to depend on others, and always fearing that you are going to break a bone. When providing care for a person who has osteoporosis, such

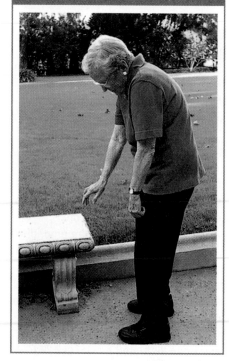

FIGURE 17-2 A person who has osteoporosis often has stooped posture. This happens when the bones of the upper spine weaken and collapse.

as Mrs. Bryan, focus mainly on safety. In addition, do the following things:

- Help the person exercise as much as she is able to do comfortably. Gentle exercise may help slow down bone loss.
- If the doctor orders a safety belt for the person, use it when helping her walk or move. The safety belt helps to support her and prevent falls. Use the belt very carefully. Remember, her bones are very fragile.
- Clear the paths and hallways near the person's room. Make sure that chairs are the proper height for her and that grab bars are fastened in appropriate places. These precautions help reduce the risk of injury.
- Help her choose clothes that do not emphasize posture changes.

CHRONIC CONDITIONS OF THE CARDIOVASCULAR SYSTEM

The cardiovascular system, using a pumping system of heart and blood vessels, transports nutrients and oxygen to all the tissues of the body and then carries away the wastes from these same tissues. You may know someone who has heart disease, because disease of the cardiovascular system is the leading cause of death in the United States.

Two chronic illnesses that result from poor functioning of the cardiovascular system are **angina pectoris** and **congestive heart failure.** Someone who has either of these illnesses may be afraid to do certain things, such as walking or working, for fear of making his or her chest pain and or shortness of breath worse. Your role is crucial because you can provide encouragement and help in alleviating fears. When providing care for someone who has a cardiovascular condition, you should always be on the lookout for the signs of a heart attack, which are described in Box 17-1.

Providing Care for a Person Who has Angina Pectoris

Today, when you go to 67-year-old Max Richardson's room, you knock on the door several times, but there is no answer. You knock again, call his name and go in. Inside, you find Mr. Richardson slumped in a chair, clutching his chest. You approach him, softly call out his name, touch him gently on the arm, tell him who you are, and ask him what is wrong and whether he is in pain.

Mr. Richardson whispers, "I need my medicine. I have pains in my chest." You signal your supervising nurse and tell her about Mr. Richardson. She brings the medicine, and Mr. Richardson places a tablet under his tongue. After a few minutes, you are relieved to see that he is sitting up and feeling better.

Characteristics and Symptoms of Angina Pectoris. Mr. Richardson suffers from angina pectoris, a condition that causes chest pain because the

---

BOX 17-1

SIGNS OF A HEART ATTACK

When providing care for people who have heart disease, it is especially important to recognize these signs of a heart attack:

- Persistent chest discomfort that lasts more than 3 to 5 minutes. It is not relieved by resting, changing position or medicating with nitroglycerin.
- Persistent chest discomfort that goes away and comes back.
- Discomfort, pain or pressure in either arm, back or stomach
- Discomfort, pain or pressure that spreads to the shoulder, arm, neck or jaw
- Dizziness, lightheadedness or loss of consciousness
- Trouble breathing, including noisy breathing, shortness of breath and breathing that is faster than normal
- Nausea
- Pale or ashen or slightly bluish skin
- Profuse sweating
- Change in pulse rate (faster, slower or irregular beat)

If you think a person in your care may be having a heart attack, stay with him and signal for help. The supervising nurse will assess the situation and use appropriate emergency procedures. If you provide care in a home to a client who is having a heart attack, call 9-1-1 (and follow your facility procedure). Help the person remain as calm and quiet as possible until help arrives.

If the person becomes unconscious with no signs of life (movement or breathing and no pulse) begin CPR and use an AED.

Notify your supervising nurse as soon as possible.

The American Red Cross strongly recommends that you take a CPR/AED course to learn how to perform CPR and how to use an AED.

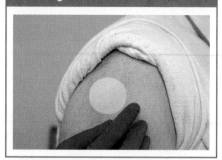

heart is not getting enough oxygen. An angina attack can be caused by activity, exercise or stress. The medication that Mr. Richardson takes to relieve the chest pain is nitroglycerin. He takes it in a pill form under the tongue, although some people take it in the form of a patch, which is applied to their skin (Figure 17-3). People suffering from angina who receive home health care usually have a supply of nitroglycerin with them and should know when to take it. In a hospital or nursing home, the medication policy of the facility may allow a person to keep his own supply of nitroglycerin.

The Plan of Care. When you provide care for an individual who has angina, encourage him to be as independent as possible without pain by doing the following things:

- Provide care in a relaxed and unhurried manner.
- Encourage the person to relax and breathe slowly if chest pain occurs. The increase of oxygen produced in the heart muscle reduces the pain.
- Tell him to stop an activity if he feels any chest discomfort. This decrease in activity reduces the need for oxygen.
- If he smokes, encourage him in his efforts to stop smoking.

Providing Care for a Person Who has Congestive Heart Failure

Sarah Rogers requires a great deal of care in the nursing home. When she walks from her bed to the chair in her room, when she tries to bathe herself, or even when she eats a meal, she becomes short of breath. Mrs. Rogers is a 60-year-old woman who, for the last 10 years, has lived with congestive heart failure.

Characteristics and Symptoms of Congestive Heart Failure. Congestive heart failure is a chronic heart disease. Because the heart no longer pumps strongly, the person with congestive heart failure may have high blood pressure and a build-up of fluid throughout her body. Some of the symptoms of congestive heart failure are difficulty in breathing, a weight gain due to fluid build-up and swelling of the feet, legs, hands and face. The person may feel anxious and restless as a result of her difficulties in breathing, and her symptoms may be worse at some times and milder at others.

The Plan of Care. When providing care for a person who has congestive heart failure, focus on helping her with her breathing and monitoring her fluid intake. In addition, do the following things:

- Provide frequent rest periods when helping the person with daily care activities. People with congestive heart failure often become tired after only a little exertion.
- Help her maintain a comfortable position, preferably a sitting position supported by pillows, that allows her to breathe more comfortably (Figure 17-4). Keep her legs elevated to reduce swelling of the legs and feet.
- Provide special mouth care. A person with congestive heart failure may breathe through her mouth or receive oxygen, which makes her mouth dry.

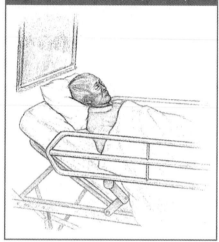

- Provide frequent opportunities for her to use the toilet. Medication for an individual with congestive heart failure can increase both urinary output and frequency of urination. As always, answer call signals immediately.
- Measure and record intake, output and weight every day. These measures are used to determine how well the person is eliminating excess fluid. A person with congestive heart failure may also have a fluid-restricted diet.

Because congestive heart failure is a chronic disease that Mrs. Rogers must live with for the rest of her life, she may be depressed sometimes. She needs encouragement and support. Involve her in her plan of care. Help her see that by pacing her activity during the day, she accomplishes more.

CHRONIC CONDITIONS OF THE ENDOCRINE SYSTEM

When glands in the endocrine system fail to function properly, certain conditions and diseases may result. One very common disease of the endocrine system is *diabetes* (sometimes called *diabetes mellitus*). There are three types of diabetes. In **type 1 diabetes,** the body does not produce enough insulin to break down, store and use sugars and starches. These sugars and starches are normally changed into **glucose** in the body and used for energy. In **type 2 diabetes,** the body may make enough insulin, but it cannot regulate its release accurately. In **gestational diabetes,** a mother develops diabetes during her pregnancy.

When providing care for a person who has diabetes, remember that she has a chronic disease. She may feel frustrated with the way her body fails to function properly, and she may have a hard time adapting to a new diet and demanding schedule. Your role is crucial. You are the one who can help assist her to deal with this intrusion on her life and make it into an acceptable way of living.

Providing Care for a Person Who has Diabetes

As a nurse assistant, you regularly care for Dorothy Roth, a 73-year-old woman who developed type 2 diabetes when she was 65 years old. This occurs when the body no longer accurately regulates insulin to break down blood glucose. Mrs. Roth says she has "sugar in the blood." She used to control her diabetes with a special diet, but recently she started taking an oral medication as well. Two of your responsibilities are to monitor what she eats and to provide good skin care.

Characteristics and Symptoms of Diabetes. Unlike type 2 diabetes, type 1 diabetes occurs when the body is not producing enough insulin to help it break down, store and use the sugar and starches in food for energy. As people grow older, they have a greater chance of becoming diabetic. There is no cure for diabetes, but it can be managed through diet, exercise and medication.

The medication may be pills that help the body produce and use insulin, or it may be insulin injections.

Several years ago, Mrs. Roth began feeling tired constantly, even though she was getting enough sleep. She always felt thirsty and needed to urinate more often than usual. She told her doctor about these symptoms and, after a few tests, he told her she had diabetes. Other symptoms of diabetes may include the following:

- Excessive thirst and hunger
- Increased urination
- Unusual weight loss or gain
- Fatigue
- Nausea
- Numbness in the hands and toes
- Slow healing of a sore or infection
- Blurred vision

Diet is the most important part of managing diabetes. Mrs. Roth, like all people with diabetes, is on a special diet that is low in carbohydrates (sugars) and fat. She must eat only foods specifically prepared for her. She should not have candy, cookies or other sweets, and she must limit her intake of carbohydrates like bread, potatoes, rice and pasta, which turn into sugar in the body. Her diet and medication help control the amount of sugar that is in her blood at any one time. This balance is important to her well-being. Too little sugar in the blood, called **hypoglycemia,** can cause:

- Dizziness
- Shakiness
- Sudden change in behavior (combativeness, argumentativeness, aggressiveness or anger)
- Cool, clammy skin
- Headache
- Seizures
- Unconsciousness

If you notice someone who has diabetes having any of these symptoms, tell your supervising nurse immediately.

Too much sugar in the bloodstream, called **hyperglycemia,** can cause:

- Weakness
- Thirst/Hunger
- Frequent urination
- Rapid weak pulse
- Headache
- Nausea and vomiting
- Seizures
- Dry mouth
- Breath that has a fruity smell
- Coma

If you notice any of these symptoms in someone who has diabetes, tell your supervising nurse immediately.

A person with diabetes can have many complications, such as vision problems and poor healing of any cut or wound, especially on the hands or feet.

The Plan of Care. When you carry out a plan of care for a person with diabetes, such as Mrs. Roth, focus your care on the following things:

- Provide good skin care to prevent pressure ulcers. Keeping the skin clean and dry is important.
- Provide good foot care. Examine her feet each day for small cuts or breaks in her skin. In people who have diabetes, cuts do not heal well because of decreased circulation, and even the smallest cut can become badly infected. The sensation of touch also may be impaired, and a person with diabetes may not feel an injury (Figure 17-5).
- Inform your supervising nurse when the person's toenails need to be cut. Because of the risk of injuring the person, only a doctor, licensed nurse or podiatrist may cut her toenails.
- Tell your supervising nurse if the person is not eating her food or is eating food brought in by friends or relatives. She should follow her diet strictly to avoid complications of the disease.
- If urine testing is ordered, make sure you test for sugar and acetone accurately and on time. Regular testing helps monitor sugar levels daily. Some people test their

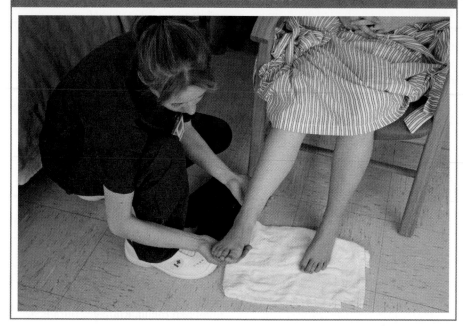

FIGURE 17-5 A person with diabetes often has poor circulation and may not realize that her shoes do not fit properly until a sore develops. To detect early signs of trouble, regularly inspect the tops and bottoms of her feet for red or sore areas.

blood for glucose levels at regular intervals during the day.

- Report any change in the usual amount of exercise, activity or stress in the person's life. Diet and dosage of insulin may have to be adjusted to help maintain balance.
- Encourage the person to exercise, because it improves circulation and helps the person keep a positive attitude.

CHRONIC CONDITIONS OF THE RESPIRATORY SYSTEM

Remember that in the respiratory system, the lungs supply your body with oxygen and rid your body of carbon dioxide. Disorders of the respiratory system include **influenza (flu), pneumonia** and **chronic obstructive pulmonary disease (COPD).** When providing care for a person with COPD remember that she has a chronic condition. She may be afraid because she

cannot breathe well. Your role is crucial, because you can help her stay calm and learn to live with her illness.

Influenza and Pneumonia

Influenza. Influenza is a highly contagious viral infection that affects the respiratory tract. The "flu" season is from November until April, with peak activity between late December and early March. In young adults and middle-aged people, the flu is usually a mild disease, but in older adults or people with chronic illnesses, the flu can be life-threatening. The best protection against the flu is prevention. It is highly recommended that residents in nursing homes receive a flu vaccine every year because it can reduce the risk of having to be hospitalized for the flu or the risk of getting pneumonia by 50 to 60 percent, and the risk of death by 80 percent (U.S. Department of Health and Human Services, Centers for Disease Control and Prevention, www.cdc.gov/flu). The older adult may not have the typical symptoms, but nurse assistants should

look for a change in behavior, subnormal temperature with low blood pressure, rapid pulse, fatigue and decreased appetite. The goal of care in nursing facilities is to prevent the spread of the infection. Encourage residents with the flu to rest in bed and have more liquids, such as water, juice and Jell-O™.

Pneumonia. Pneumonia is an inflammation of the lungs. Because of the inflammation the air sacs in the lungs begin to fill with fluid. Oxygen has trouble reaching the bloodstream. It can be a very serious illness in older adults because of normal age-related changes such as a weakened cough reflex and impaired mobility. This condition can result in death. Pneumonia may be caused by a virus (often a complication of the flu) or by bacteria. Bacterial pneumonia is treated with antibiotics. Older adults may also develop **aspiration pneumonia.** Residents who are in a coma or using feeding tubes are especially at risk for developing pneumonia.

The Plan of Care. When you carry out a plan of care for a person with flu or pneumonia, you should focus your care on the following things:

- Practice strict adherence to turning and positioning procedures.
- Encourage vaccinations for flu and pneumonia.
- Encourage the person to drink fluids.
- Encourage the person to rest.
- Encourage the person to cough.

Providing Care for a Person Who has COPD

You are ready to help a new patient, Mrs. Reilly, a 75-year-old woman who is being admitted to the hospital because she is suffering from dyspnea (difficulty breathing) and is perspiring. Both her feet are swollen, and she is afraid. You try to imagine what it would be like to have difficulty breathing and to be afraid that you are not going to be able to catch your next breath or that you may die. You know how important it is to try to calm Mrs. Reilly, because extreme fear increases shortness of breath and difficulty in breathing.

When you observe Mrs. Reilly, you notice cyanosis: her skin has a bluish-gray color, her fingernails look bluish and her lips look discolored. These signs mean that there is not enough oxygen circulating in her body.

Characteristics and Symptoms of COPD.

Mrs. Reilly has been diagnosed with an acute flareup of COPD. Many lung diseases are grouped together in this category, including chronic bronchitis, emphysema and asthma. Symptoms of COPD include the following:

- Coughing up a great deal of mucus
- A tendency to tire easily
- Loss of appetite
- Bent posture with shoulders elevated and lips pursed to make breathing easier
- A fast pulse
- Round, barrel-shaped chest
- Confusion (caused by lack of oxygen circulating in the body)

The Plan of Care.

Mrs. Reilly tells you that she has been a smoker for years. In fact, she still smokes. Even though she has great difficulty breathing, she tells you she would really like to have a cigarette. She tells you she has had chronic respiratory infections over the past 20 years and is now trying to live with COPD (Figure 17-6).

When providing care for a person who has COPD, focus on helping her breathe more easily and do the following:

- Encourage the person to take four or five deep breaths often during the day. Deep breathing helps fill the lungs with air and maintains flexibility in the chest wall.
- Encourage her to relax and breathe slowly but as deeply as possible. Relaxation and slow, deep breathing increase the flow of oxygen to the lungs. Often the person learns special breathing exercises that improve her ability to relax and breathe slowly.

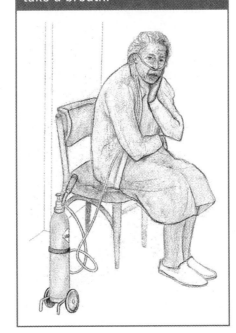

FIGURE 17-6 A person with advanced COPD spends much of her energy breathing. She may not be able to say long sentences or express an entire thought without stopping to take a breath.

- Provide special mouth care. A person with COPD may breathe through her mouth or receive oxygen, making her mouth dry.
- If a person is receiving oxygen therapy, check regularly to see that tubes are in place and not kinked. Follow your employer's rules about oxygen. If a person is using a nasal **cannula**, provide skin care to the skin around her nose.
- Provide a bedside commode when the person needs it. Sometimes using the commode is easier than getting to the bathroom when the person needs to conserve their energy or is experiencing shortness of breath. A commode is also more comfortable than a bedpan.
- Offer small, frequent meals, if necessary. This meal plan ensures adequate nutrition and reduces fatigue.

- Encourage a person with COPD not to smoke. Remind her that no smoking is permitted if a person is receiving oxygen.
- Encourage her to cough to help clear air passages of excess mucus.
- Elevate the head bed (Fowler's position) for comfort.

To help maintain her independence, let Mrs. Reilly set her own pace for activities. When she has some control over her life, she feels better about herself and is better able to cope with her illness.

CHRONIC CONDITIONS OF THE URINARY SYSTEM

The urinary system, the body's filtering system, eliminates waste in the form of urine. When that system fails to function properly, several conditions can result. **Kidney failure** is an example of a chronic condition of the urinary system. When providing care for a person who has kidney failure, remember that he has a chronic illness. He may feel depressed about his need for regular treatment. In your role, you can give him emotional support and encouragement to adapt to his illness.

Providing Care for a Person Who has Kidney Failure

Sam Green has had diabetes since he was 9 years old, and now, at the age of 75, he is in the early stage of kidney failure. The disease can be slowed by special diets, medication or both. If the disease progresses, Mr. Green may have to go on dialysis to filter waste from his blood.

Mr. Green often worries about his uncertain future and about the cost of the treatment and medications. Sometimes he resents the restrictions his illness places on his independence. He always talks to you about these feelings when you come to his room to provide care.

Characteristics and Symptoms of Kidney Failure. Kidney failure, also called *renal failure,* results from the kidney's inability to get rid of waste products. In its late stage, it is often referred to as **end-stage renal disease (ESRD).** Renal failure can be the result of an acute disease or of an injury that causes the kidneys to stop functioning temporarily. Renal failure also can be a complication of certain chronic diseases such as diabetes.

When waste products accumulate in the body, they produce some of the following symptoms:

- Fatigue, weakness and confusion
- Puffiness around the eyes and swelling in the hands and feet
- Pain in the kidney area
- Muscle twitching or cramping
- Nausea, vomiting and an unpleasant taste in the mouth, which often lead to poor nutrition
- Itching skin, often severe
- High blood pressure
- Extreme thinness with little muscle mass of extremities, if the renal failure goes on for a long time

People with advanced renal failure often need **dialysis**, a process that filters waste products from the blood using a special filtering solution. Two types of dialysis are peritoneal dialysis and hemodialysis. *Peritoneal dialysis* involves injecting a solution through the abdominal wall and then withdrawing it after a period of time. *Hemodialysis* uses a machine to clean the blood of waste products. Dialysis can be used to maintain the health of the person with renal failure in preparation for a kidney transplant. Dialysis treatment may be done a few times a week.

The Plan of Care. When providing care for a person with kidney failure, such as Mr. Green, focus on the following things:

- Encourage the person to rest.
- Carefully monitor and report his food and fluid intake. Encourage

his food intake in accordance with his diet plan.
- Plan activities of daily living to conserve the person's energy and to provide for periods of rest, because a person with kidney failure may frequently have periods of wakefulness at night.
- Take increased care to prevent infections. If the person is on dialysis, pay special attention to keeping the access site (either for peritoneal dialysis or hemodialysis) clean and dry. Keep his skin in good condition without breaks or sores that could become infected.

Help Mr. Green retain his independence by encouraging him to perform as many of his activities of daily living as possible. Encourage him and his family members to talk about their concerns.

CHRONIC CONDITIONS OF THE NERVOUS SYSTEM

One kind of problem with the nervous system occurs when it becomes impossible for messages to get back and forth from the brain to other parts of the body. This type of condition results from an interruption of activity in the nerves or spinal cord, usually caused by an injury. Parts of the brain also can be damaged.

Because they involve the brain, mental retardation and mental illness also are considered conditions of the nervous system. Alzheimer's disease is one of several diseases classified as cognitive impairment. These diseases impair a person's thinking and reasoning abilities. Other chronic conditions of the nervous system include multiple sclerosis, stroke, paraplegia, quadriplegia, Parkinson's disease and mental depression. When providing care for a person who has a disorder of the nervous system, remember that he has a chronic illness that may be difficult for him and his family to deal with. In your role,

you can support and encourage the person, as well as his family.

You have just finished visiting with Charlene Hunter, a 35-year-old mother who has had multiple sclerosis for the past 5 years. Mrs. Hunter has some difficulty walking, and she often loses her balance. She also has muscle tremors and muscle weakness, so sometimes she drops a plate or glass. Over the past few months, she has had problems with bladder control and she says she feels embarrassed when she loses control. Today she told you that the bladder problem is getting worse.

You think about how frustrating it must be for Mrs. Hunter to cope with this disease. She says she sometimes feels depressed. She knows the disease will get worse, and she says she feels helpless and out of control. She is afraid of becoming more disabled and unable to take care of her 2-year-old son.

Characteristics and Symptoms of MS. Multiple sclerosis (MS) is a chronic disease that gradually destroys the coating on nerve endings in the brain and spinal cord. This condition creates a situation similar to a short circuit or crossed wire. Nerves cannot communicate with each other or with the brain. MS is more common in females than males. A person has an increased risk of MS from teen years to age 50. What makes MS different from other diseases with similar symptoms is that the symptoms usually appear and disappear over a period of years. During the time that symptoms disappear, the person is said to be in remission. There is no cure for MS.

Symptoms of MS include the following:

- Feelings of numbness, tingling and burning
- Overwhelming fatigue at all times

- Vision problems (double vision, blurred vision or both)
- Insomnia
- Speech problems (slurring, using the wrong name for an object, slowness in replying to others)
- Bowel and bladder problems (constipation, incontinence)
- Fits of anger or crying (she may shut down her emotions to control her mood swings and may be intensely anxious or fearful)
- Paralysis
- Forgetfulness and slowness in understanding what is said to her
- **Edema** and cold feet due to lack of circulation (parts of the body affected by edema must be massaged to retain joint flexibility)

The Plan of Care. Your role is a challenging one as you carry out the plan of care for a person with MS. Focus on maintaining mobility and bowel and bladder control. Also help the person focus on what she *can* do, not on what she *cannot* do. Use the following caregiving techniques:

- Do passive range-of-motion exercises on the person's affected limbs, and encourage her to do active range-of-motion exercises when possible. Range-of-motion exercises prevent contractures and maintain joint mobility. Encourage her to actively help with exercises.
- Encourage the person to eat meals high in fiber. High-fiber foods help maintain healthy elimination. The use of laxatives also may be necessary.
- Encourage her to drink lots of fluids. High fluid intake increases urination and helps prevent bladder and kidney infections. High fluid intake is also important for bowel regularity. Often people with incontinence problems think reducing fluid intake solves the problem, but it does not. It causes *additional* problems.

- Encourage warm tub baths when possible, but make sure the water is not too hot. Warm water reduces muscle spasms (cramping), but hot water causes weakness and fainting.

Encourage the person to do as much as possible for herself so that she can be more independent. Remind her to pace herself and rest as needed so that she does not overdo it. Listen to the person and encourage her to talk with you about what is happening and express her feelings to you. Also encourage her to participate in activities and maintain friendships so that she does not isolate herself.

Providing Care for a Person Who has had a Stroke

You provide care regularly for Patricia Avery, a 55-year-old resident at Morningside Nursing Home. She had a stroke 5 years ago and, as a result, is paralyzed on her right side. You often think about how it must feel to be unable to move your arm and leg on one side of your body or how frustrated Mrs. Avery must feel when she wants to say something but the words won't come to her. Thinking about her feelings helps you understand why Mrs. Avery is often depressed.

Characteristics Resulting from a Stroke. *Stroke* is another term for a **cerebrovascular accident (CVA).** A stroke can cause paralysis, usually on one side. This condition is called *hemiplegia.* A stroke can result in weakness on one side instead of paralysis, a condition called *hemiparesis.* Other possible characteristics resulting from a stroke are the following:

- A decreased sense of pain, touch and temperature on the paralyzed side
- Bowel and bladder incontinence
- Difficulty speaking, reading or writing (she may want to say something, but the words won't

come to her, or she may not be able to understand what other people say—a condition called *aphasia*)

The Plan of Care. When carrying out the plan of care for a person who has had a stroke, such as Mrs. Avery, focus on the characteristics of her condition. This focus will help her regain function of her arm or leg. Also promote safety issues related to her loss of sensation, encourage her independence and do the following things:

- Perform passive range-of-motion exercises on the person's affected limbs. Range-of-motion exercises prevent contractures and maintain joint mobility. Encourage her to use the unaffected side of her body to exercise her paralyzed side as much as she is able (Figure 17-7).
- Supervise the person while she eats. If you have to feed her,

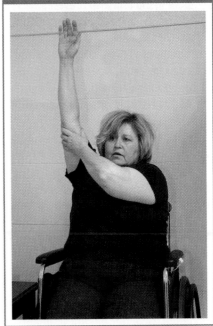

FIGURE 17-7 This resident, with paralysis on her right side, maintains her independence by taking responsibility for her range-of-motion exercises.

always put food in the side of her mouth that is not affected by paralysis. Make sure no food is left in her mouth after a meal is finished. Not being able to feel food in the mouth increases the risk of choking. Make sure she sits up while she eats so that she can swallow food more easily.

- Since the person may drool on the paralyzed side and her skin may become irritated, keep her face clean and dry. If possible, apply a protective skin cream.
- Supervise the person while if they shave. They may miss spots that they cannot feel, or may cut themselves and not feel it.
- Offer to help complete any personal care activities that may be difficult because of her weakness or paralysis.
- Help her walk, following the physical therapist's directions. She may need a walker or cane to steady herself.
- Raise the person's paralyzed arm on a pillow when she is in bed. Support the arm with a sling when she is out of bed. Paralyzed limbs have poor circulation, and raising the arm helps keep blood from pooling. Supporting the arm also prevents swelling and may help her feel that she has better balance.
- Put articles that the person needs, such as eyeglasses, hearing aid, telephone and a glass of water, within reach on her unaffected side.
- Put the call signal within reach on her unaffected side.

Encourage Mrs. Avery to do as much as possible for herself so that she can be more independent. If the dominant side of her body is affected, she may have to relearn how to do activities using her other hand. Encourage Mrs. Avery to use adaptive devices for eating, mouth care and other activities to maintain her independence. Give her encouragement and support. She needs to feel good about herself.

Providing Care for a Person Who has Paraplegia or Quadriplegia

When you visit Karen Bowman, she often asks you to turn the pages of her scrapbook, which is filled with pictures and mementos of her glorious days of swimming competition. She started competing in swimming events when she was 6 years old. Now, at age 22, she has been admitted to the subacute unit of the nursing facility—a quadriplegic, with no feeling in her arms, legs or lower trunk.

Some days, Miss Bowman becomes very angry and tells you about how stupid she was to go drinking and swimming with her sorority sisters. "If I hadn't been drinking, I would have noticed that the water was too shallow for diving. Now, look at me. Useless. Absolutely useless."

Characteristics of Paraplegia and Quadriplegia. Paralysis is a loss of the ability to move parts of the body that results from a brain or spinal cord injury. Paralysis can affect one side of the body (*hemiplegia*), two legs and the lower trunk (*paraplegia*), or both arms, both legs and the lower trunk (*quadriplegia*), depending on the location of the damage to the spinal cord or the brain and the severity of the damage. An injury in the lower back or at waist level can result in paraplegia. An injury in the neck or upper back can result in quadriplegia.

Often brain or spinal cord injuries occur suddenly, as in an automobile collision. Many spinal cord injuries also result from other activities such as diving into shallow water. If a person breaks her neck, her spinal cord can be severely damaged, although her brain may be uninjured and her thinking unimpaired. However, the brain cannot send messages to the body, and it cannot receive messages from the body.

If a person has paralysis, the affected parts of the body lose some or all of the following body functions:

- Sensation (pain, temperature, pressure, touch, vibration)
- Fine motor movement (small movements, such as writing, sewing and using a fork and knife)
- Gross motor movement (large movements, such as lifting arms or legs)
- Ability to maintain body temperature
- Balance
- Bladder and bowel control
- Breathing, without some form of assistance

The Plan of Care. When providing care for someone with paralysis, focus your caregiving on promoting independence and safety related to the person's difficulty in movement and loss of sensation. Also do the following things:

- Keep the skin clean and dry, and use lotions on rough or irritated areas. Provide good skin care to prevent pressure sores. Turn or reposition the person every 2 hours. Ensure proper body alignment. Be sure to elevate the hand of the affected arm above the elbow. Use rolled towels or a pillow to ensure that the affected leg does not rotate outward. Use footboards or special boots when necessary.
- Be aware that the person's sense of touch is impaired. She is unable to recognize pain and temperature and loses awareness of how her affected body parts are positioned.
- Encourage a person with paralysis to use self-help devices for eating, walking or mouth care. She may have a spoon or fork with a special grip, or a brace or splint on a

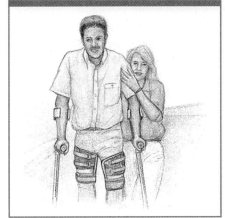

FIGURE 17-8 After strengthening his arms and shoulders, a person with paraplegia may be able to walk with crutches.

paralyzed limb. Using a cane or a walker also may help (Figure 17-8).
- Help with a bladder- or bowel-training program. (See Chapter 15, "Elimination," for more information on bladder- and bowel-training programs.)
- Encourage a person with paralysis to do as much as possible for herself so that she can be as independent as possible.
- Provide emotional support.

Providing Care for a Person Who has Parkinson's Disease

Patrick O'Malley is a 70-year-old man who has had Parkinson's disease for the past 20 years. He has muscle weakness, and his arms shake (muscle tremors). Also, he has a tremor that causes his hands to move in a "pill-rolling" motion. His posture is slumped, he bends forward and he shuffles when he walks. Because his balance is poor, he falls frequently.

When you first provided care for Mr. O'Malley, he was able to do many things for himself, although with great difficulty. Now his hands shake uncontrollably, and he can barely grasp or

hold on to anything. He also drools and has difficulty chewing his food.

Characteristics and Symptoms of Parkinson's Disease. Parkinson's disease is one of the most common nervous system disorders affecting older adults. In Parkinson's disease, the parts of the brain that control movement are gradually destroyed. A person with Parkinson's disease has stiff muscles, moves very slowly and has muscle tremors, which cause shaking or repetitive motions of the muscles, especially those of the hands, while the person is at rest. As the disease progresses, the person's **gait** is affected, and greater physical effort is required to complete even the smallest task. As a result, the person easily becomes tired and frustrated. The disease usually appears when a person is in his 50s or 60s. No one is sure exactly why this happens.

Symptoms of Parkinson's disease include the following:
- Uncontrolled movement of head, torso and extremities
- Lack of facial expression
- Difficulty chewing and swallowing
- Drooling
- Low-pitched, soft, slow and monotonous speech
- Constipation
- Confusion
- Mood changes
- Depression and loss of interest

The Plan of Care. When providing care for a person who has Parkinson's disease, such as Mr. O'Malley, think about his symptoms and focus your caregiving on safety, good nutrition and mobility by doing the following things:
- Encourage the person to rest often. Resting prevents him from getting too tired or frustrated.
- Avoid rushing him. Muscle tremors increase when the person becomes anxious.
- Give him warm tub baths to help relax his muscles and reduce muscle spasms.
- Encourage the person to use any self-help devices he may have for activities of daily living (Figure 17-9).

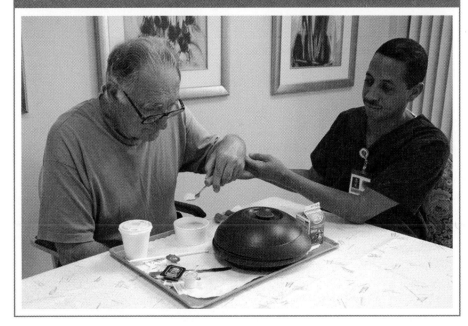

FIGURE 17-9 Even though a person may have constantly shaking hands, he can feed himself with an assistive device and a little help from the nurse assistant.

For example, he may have a comb, razor or toothbrush with an extended handle or grip.

- When he is walking, remind him to think about standing tall, swinging his arms, raising his feet and putting his feet down on the ground heel first and then rolling up to the toe. A person with Parkinson's disease has to make a conscious effort to do what comes naturally to people who can control their movement.
- Use a high toilet or elevated toilet seat set on top of a regular toilet seat equipped for use by people with disabilities, because a person with Parkinson's disease may have difficulty changing from a standing to a sitting position.
- As the person eats, remind him to think through the process of swallowing. For example, you might say, "Try keeping your lips and teeth closed" or "How about changing the side that you chew on so that one side does not get too tired?" or "Try lifting your tongue up and back, and swallow."
- Offer small, frequent meals and snacks. People with Parkinson's disease usually lose weight because they become tired before they finish a meal. They also may be embarrassed by the mess they make or by how slowly they eat, and they may lose interest in eating.
- Provide emotional support and be especially patient with his self-help efforts.

Providing Care for a Person Who has Mental Depression

Letitia Carpenter never talks to you when you go to her room to provide care. When you try to involve her in conversation, she just turns her head away. Most of what you know about Mrs. Carpenter's condition you learned from her son LeMar. He told you that every January Mrs. Carpenter, who is now 70 years old, became depressed but always "snapped out of it" with the

first signs of spring. But this year nothing seemed to help—not sunshine, not warmth, not flowers.

Characteristics and Symptoms of Mental Depression. Depression is a common mental disorder. It can be defined as a persistent feeling of sadness. Sometimes the depression can be triggered by an event, a trauma or a loss, but often it is not related to a single event. Signs of depression may be similar to those of a physical illness, and often the person is treated for the physical illness while the depression goes untreated. If a person becomes extremely depressed, she may try to take her own life. Depression is a common problem in older adults and often is mistaken for confusion or Alzheimer's disease.

Signs of depression include the following:

- Sadness
- Crying spells
- Decreased memory
- Inability to concentrate
- Low energy
- Fatigue
- Sleeping problems (too much or too little)
- Eating problems (too much or too little)
- Isolation and unwillingness to participate in social activities
- Irritability
- Feelings of helplessness
- Feelings of hopelessness
- Expression of wanting to kill oneself
- Headaches, muscle aches, backaches, abdominal pain or nausea
- Preoccupation with bodily functions and illness

The Plan of Care. For a person with depression, a mental health worker usually directs the efforts of the staff. When providing care for a depressed person, such as Mrs. Carpenter, focus on maintaining her safety and increasing her self-esteem. To accomplish this:

- Give the person appropriate positive feedback and reinforce her accomplishments.

- Help her express her own strengths and functional abilities.
- Work with the person to set simple, attainable goals. Be sure to praise her when she meets the goals.
- Listen when she expresses sadness (Figure 17-10).
- Provide time for the person to cry.
- Because her energy level is low, schedule rest periods throughout the day.
- Monitor her food intake to make sure that nutrition is adequate.
- Provide fluids frequently, because the person may not drink enough fluids on her own.
- Report all complaints of pain so that her symptoms do not get overlooked.
- Encourage the person to use a prescribed hearing aid or eyeglasses so that she is more in touch with the world around her.
- Encourage her to participate in activities, especially those that involve contact with another person and those that are physical, within her limitations. Avoid overly stressful or tiring activities.
- Encourage independence to try to build her feeling of self-worth.

Take all comments about suicidal thoughts seriously and report them to your supervising nurse. Also report

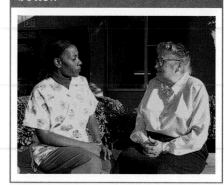

FIGURE 17-10 If you sit and listen, you may be able to help a person who is depressed feel better.

any of the following occurrences to your supervising nurse:

- The person shows a dramatic change in mood or behavior, such as increased withdrawal or elevation of mood. Sometimes a person who is deeply depressed and struggles with thoughts of suicide does not have enough energy to carry out a suicide plan. However, once she has finally made the decision to commit suicide, she may feel temporary relief and increased energy so that she can actually follow through with her plan.
- The person hoards medication or purchases a gun or other weapon.
- She gives away her belongings.
- She increases her use of alcohol.
- She becomes preoccupied with inner thoughts.
- She becomes secretive.

Report any sign of these to the supervising nurse. Do not conclude that a suicide threat or attempt is just a way to get attention. Especially vulnerable are the very old, a person who has just been diagnosed with a terminal illness, such as cancer or AIDS or a person who has suffered a severe loss or multiple losses.

Providing Care for a Person Who Might Cause Harm. To ensure the safety of some people with mental illness who may be at risk of harming themselves or others when left alone, you may be required to provide continuous observation. This is commonly called *one-to-one observation.* A person who needs one-to-one observation may be confused, **suicidal** or **homicidal.** Being sensitive to the person's feelings is important. Think of how you would feel if you were alone with a person you did not know who was watching you constantly. Talk to him calmly and treat him with respect. Explain that you are staying with him to ensure his safety. If he feels like talking, encourage him to talk. Allow him quiet time if he prefers. Be a good listener and observer.

Always be aware of the person's actions. If you observe any potentially harmful behavior, act to prevent it. If you think you cannot succeed alone, call for assistance immediately.

Be ready to give your supervising nurse your report when she arrives to check on the person (every 1 to 2 hours). Contact your supervising nurse more frequently if you think it is necessary.

Remember, you are doing a lot more than just sitting. Your continuous observation and reporting are crucial to the care and safety of the person.

Review your employer's policy with your supervising nurse before providing care for the person. Learn the following guidelines for a person on one-to-one observation:

- Always stay with the person— never leave him alone for any reason. If a person is suicidal, you must be close enough to him to reach out and touch him. You must escort him to the bathroom and stay with him.
- Inspect the person's belongings for potentially harmful objects. Remove and label them, and store them in a secure place out of his room.
- Remove all potentially harmful objects and substances from the area, including objects the person might throw. Examples of potentially harmful objects are scissors, razors, matches, belts, glass objects and all liquids.
- Make sure visitors have checked in with the nurse before visiting. Make sure all packages and items are inspected for potential risks. Your supervising nurse will tell you who may be alone with the person. This may be a family member who has a full understanding of the person's condition.
- Use only plastic forks and spoons at mealtime. Never give any type of knife to suicidal or homicidal people.

- Allow smoking only in designated smoking areas and only with staff supervision. Never allow the person to have matches or a cigarette lighter.
- Make sure the person wears a hospital gown and slippers.
- Make sure a suicidal or homicidal person stays in his room. If he must leave his room for a procedure, you or another person must accompany him.
- Give your complete attention for one-to-one observation. Avoid activities that distract your attention, such as reading or watching television.

CANCER

Providing Care for a Person Who has Cancer

As Elizabeth Little is recovering in the hospital from surgery, she begins to talk to you about her illness. "One day, while bathing, I found a lump in my breast and immediately went to my doctor. After a series of tests, the doctor determined that the lump was a malignant tumor. I felt shocked and angry. I'm just 34 and I eat properly and exercise every day. I love my job and I'm good at it. My fiancé and I planned to get married next month. I just felt good about my life. I don't deserve this."

Characteristics and Symptoms of Cancer. There is a good chance that you know someone who has or has had cancer, because this disease is the second leading cause of death in the United States. **Cancer** is the abnormal growth of new cells that can spread and crowd out or destroy other body tissues. The abnormal growth can be in the form of a malignant tumor, a solid mass or a growth of abnormal cells that can grow anywhere in the body. A **tumor** can be noncancerous (**benign**) or cancerous (**malignant**). Benign tumors usually grow slowly and do not spread to other areas of the body. Malignant tumors can spread, or **metastasize**, to other parts of the body.

Malignant tumors can grow fast and invade and destroy other body tissue. In the early stages, a malignant tumor does not cause pain or other symptoms, and the person may not suspect she has cancer. Sometimes cancer is detected during a routine physical examination. If a cancer is detected before it has begun to spread, there is a good chance that growth of the cancer can be controlled or stopped.

Typically, cancer is treated in one of three ways, depending on the kind of cancer, the location and whether or not the cancer has spread. Often the first treatment may be to remove the tumor surgically. The other two treatments are **chemotherapy** and **radiation**. A doctor determines the best treatment for each person and sometimes prescribes all three methods.

A doctor prescribes chemotherapy in the hope that the drugs can stop or slow the rate of growth of the cancer cells. The drugs used to treat cancer are so powerful that they affect all the systems in a person's body. As a result, the person may feel far worse than he felt before he was given the drugs. Common side effects include nausea, diarrhea, loss of hair and extremely dry skin. A person having chemotherapy may have some or all of these side effects.

The goal of radiation treatment is to destroy the cancer cells through the use of x-rays. A person usually does not feel pain during the treatment, but she can experience unpleasant side effects from it. The type of symptoms will depend on which part of the body is being treated and the type of radiation used. However, many people will experience skin burns, fatigue and possibly nausea and vomiting. Some people may have hair loss as a result of the radiation treatment. When caring for someone having radia-

tion therapy, provide good skin care. Most important, be available to give emotional support to the person you are caring for.

With her doctor's guidance, Ms. Little had decided to have surgery and a combination of radiation and chemotherapy to treat her breast cancer, but she felt frightened and worried. How would her fiancé react to the news? Would he still feel the same way about her after the surgery? Would she be able to wear the beautiful new bathing suit she had bought to wear on her honeymoon? What if the chemotherapy caused her hair to fall out? Would her job be held for her while she was recovering from surgery? Would she feel well enough during chemotherapy and radiation treatment to keep working? What if the treatment did not work and she died?

The Plan of Care. When providing care for a person who is being treated for cancer, such as Ms. Little, carry out the prescribed plan of care and incorporate the following suggestions:

- The most important thing for you to do is to be there for the person, listen to her, support her and show her you care by being positive and hopeful. Many people believe that having a positive, hopeful attitude helps in the healing process.
- During your caregiving, remember that infection control becomes of utmost importance. Chemotherapy and radiation affect a person's immune system, the system responsible for fighting off infection. Exposure to germs may cause infection. Therefore, follow strict hand-washing guidelines and Standard Precautions.
- Provide good mouth care to reduce the spread of germs. Perform mouth care every 2 hours, because some drugs can cause a person to have a very dry mouth or serious oral infections. A doctor may recommend the use of an antibacterial mouth rinse.

- Observe the mouth and other parts of the body for redness or irritation.
- Maintain adequate nutrition and proper rest.
- Generally, a person receiving treatment loses her appetite. For a day or so after the person has chemotherapy, she often has nausea and diarrhea.

Chemotherapy also can affect the person's sense of smell and taste so that nothing seems appetizing. However, she still needs nutritious foods to aid in the healing process and to give her strength. Here are some ways to provide good nutrition to a person who has lost her appetite: provide fluids frequently, especially nutritious fluids such as milk shakes and broth; provide good, nutritious foods anytime a person feels hungry; make sure food looks appetizing; make mealtime as pleasant and relaxing as possible; provide small, more frequent meals; offer snacks frequently; offer foods the person enjoys.

- *Never* provide care for a person who is receiving cancer treatment if you have a cold or flu, because you may pass your illness on to the person.
- You can help a person who begins to lose her hair feel better about herself by reassuring her that her hair will grow back after treatment is completed. Suggest that she wear a scarf, wig or even a favorite hat if she wishes (Figure 17-11).
- If the person receiving chemotherapy or radiation treatment feels tired, explain to her that she feels tired because of the treatment. (Sometimes when you know *why* you feel a particular way, you cope with your feelings better and allow yourself to rest.) She may be on a treatment schedule that lasts weeks or months. It takes a great deal of physical and emotional energy for her to fight the disease.

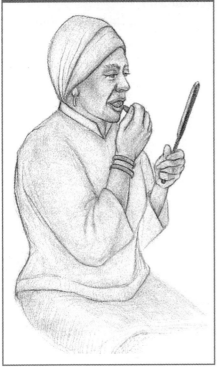

FIGURE 17-11 A common side effect of chemotherapy is hair loss, which may lead to self-image problems. To help maintain her self-esteem, encourage a person receiving chemotherapy to try new styles and to maintain her appearance.

- Encourage the person to rest more, take naps or go to bed earlier than usual. You may want to ask whether you can help her into a comfortable position to maintain proper body alignment and comfort.
- If the person's skin changes and she gets a rash from a drug she has received, or she reddens or burns from radiation treatment, provide good care by inspecting her skin often and keeping it clean. Also, give her frequent backrubs, especially if she is in bed a great deal, which help her relax. A backrub increases circulation to the skin. *Never* massage the area that receives the radiation treatment. Often this area has semipermanent marks on it that the radiologist put there to focus the x-rays. To prevent pressure ulcers and to avoid undue pressure, reposition the person frequently.

When providing care for a person who has cancer, report any changes to your supervising nurse without delay. Chemotherapy and radiation can cause a variety of side effects, which may alter the plan of care. The plan of care differs for each person, based on the person's special needs.

The most important thing to remember when providing care for a person with cancer, such as Ms. Little, is that she needs a positive attitude and kindness. She is going through an extremely stressful time, as are her family members, friends and also the health care team members who have grown to love and provide care for her. A great many support services are available for people with cancer. Your supervising nurse or the social worker can find out what is available in your community.

Sometimes a person completes the treatment only to find out that the cancer has reappeared or spread to different areas of the body. Depending on the nature of the recurrence, this situation may be particularly difficult for the person and family to accept. Often they believe that the person might die, and they take steps to deal with the possibility.

As you will read in Chapter 20, "Providing End-of-Life Care," a person goes through many stages when she faces a terminal illness, often moving in and out of these stages. Your support, compassion and skillful care are essential to providing comfort to the person and her family.

INFORMATION REVIEW

Circle the correct answers and fill in the blanks.

1. Someone with arthritis should be encouraged to:
   a. avoid the pain by not moving.
   b. take cold showers to reduce swelling of joints.
   c. exercise strenuously to keep joints flexible.
   d. do active or passive range-of-motion exercises regularly. *(circled)*

2. All of the following are signals of an impending heart attack *except:*
   a. pain in the lower legs. *(circled)*
   b. persistent chest pain that is not relieved by changing position, resting or medicating with nitroglycerin.
   c. shortness of breath.
   d. sweating.

3. A person with congestive heart failure generally is most comfortable when he is:
   a. lying flat.
   b. sitting up. *(circled)*
   c. lying on his left side.
   d. lying on his right side.

4. Someone with diabetes:
   a. needs to eat extra sugar and protein to maintain his strength.
   b. may have reduced sensation in his feet. *(circled)*
   c. needs to eliminate exercise completely.
   d. needs to have the nurse assistant cut his toenails daily so that they do not become too long.

5. Someone with COPD should be encouraged to:
   a. eat one large meal per day instead of several smaller meals.
   b. lie flat after eating.
   c. breathe deeply often during the day. *(circled)*
   d. smoke to relieve tension.

6. When providing care for someone who has had a stroke, you must:
   a. place the call signal within reach on the person's unaffected side. *(circled)*
   b. position the person so that he is lying flat when he eats, since he may have paralysis and may drool.
   c. place food in the person's mouth on the affected side.
   d. keep the paralyzed arm or leg lower than the rest of his body to keep blood flowing into it.

7. When providing care for someone with paralysis, focus your caregiving on promoting _independence_ through the use of assistive devices.

8. When a person is depressed, he may have thoughts about suicide. You must report any of the signals of suicide, such as dramatic _change_ in mood or behavior, giving away _possessions_, preoccupation with _____ thoughts, or hoarding _____.

9. A person who is being treated for cancer may have a decreased ability to fight off _disease_.

1. Today, while you are providing care for Mrs. Roth, who has diabetes, her hands start shaking. You ask her whether she is okay. "I'm fine!" she snaps, "So leave me alone!" What do you think might be happening? What should you do?

2. Martha Boswitch has MS. When you bring her breakfast tray one morning and ask her how she slept, she replies that her feet and hands were cold all night. What should you do?

3. Mrs. Reilly, who has COPD, is very short of breath. She has difficulty with any amount of exertion and needs to rest frequently. Today Mrs. Reilly's daughter is bringing her 6-month-old son to visit at 10:30 A.M. Mrs. Reilly wants to look especially nice, but she also doesn't want to be too tired to enjoy the visit. How would you help her plan her morning care so that she can accomplish both goals?

4. Do you know anyone who is quadriplegic? How does the person spend his day? If you do not know anyone with quadriplegia, imagine how you would spend your day if you had no feeling in your arms and legs and had to remain in a wheelchair?

5. Ruth Linquist is a new resident at Morningside Nursing Home. Because of her depression, she often doesn't sleep at night. When her husband stops by for afternoon visits, she usually is too tired to spend time with him. What might you do to make this situation better?

6. If you were told today that you had an illness that would require you to change your lifestyle completely, how would you react? Think of some possible changes and how you would respond.

18

Providing Care for People with HIV/AIDS, Hepatitis and Tuberculosis

GOALS

After reading this chapter, you will have the information needed to:

Explain what HIV is.

Explain what AIDS is.

Explain how HIV infection and AIDS are related.

Identify behaviors that can transmit HIV, the virus that causes AIDS.

List behaviors that are often mistakenly thought to transmit HIV, HAV, HBV and HCV.

Describe some medical problems of people who have AIDS.

Describe principles of care for someone who has AIDS.

Explain the difference between HAV, HBV and HCV, and their modes of transmission.

Describe some medical problems of people who have hepatitis.

Describe how tuberculosis is transmitted.

Today you go to the home of Mary Hill to provide care for her. Mrs. Hill's mother answers your knock at the door and explains that her daughter is having a bad day. You can smell the odors of vomit and diarrhea. In the living room, Mary rests on a makeshift bed made up on the sofa. Her ankles appear swollen, as well as the glands in her neck. You observe how dry and sore her mouth is as she speaks.

"I'm so glad you're here," Mary says. "I don't have the strength to even get out of bed. I feel so helpless. I can't even hold my baby." In the next room, you can hear Melissa fussing in her crib. Mary's mother heads toward the baby's crib to take care of her while you get ready to help Mary.

Before beginning Mary's personal care, you ask her what she would like to drink. When she says she doesn't want anything to drink, you suggest that she try sucking on some ice. You explain that fluids will help her dry mouth feel better and will also help reduce her bouts of diarrhea. She agrees to try the ice.

As you provide personal care for Mary, you handle her skin with extreme gentleness because you know how fragile it has become. After you complete her bed bath, help her dress in a clean sweat suit and put fresh linens on the sofa, Mary thanks you. "I feel so much better now that I'm fresh and clean. But I'm so tired."

FACTS ABOUT AIDS

Mary Hill has acquired immunodeficiency syndrome, or AIDS. Her husband Glen died a few months ago from an **opportunistic infection.** Mrs. Hill was infected with HIV through vaginal sex with her husband. She was pregnant when she was diagnosed with HIV, and her daughter Melissa tested positive for HIV **antibodies** in her blood when she was born.

The condition later to be known as HIV was first identified in 1981. It kills men, women and children everywhere in the world. The cumulative estimated number of diagnoses of AIDS through 2005 in the 50 U.S. States and District of Columbia was 956,666. People in every country are affected by AIDS.

People with AIDS need the care, kindness and compassion of health care workers who are not afraid to help them. One of the greatest obstacles to fighting fears about AIDS patients is the number of myths surrounding its transmission. One false idea is that you can get AIDS from insects. Another is that you can get it from your pets. These statements are not true, but they frighten many people. People are less afraid when they know the facts about HIV and AIDS (Box 18-1). Here are a few facts that are worth expressing:

- You *cannot* get AIDS from a drinking fountain.
- You *cannot* get AIDS from the sweat of an infected person.
- You *cannot* get AIDS from hugging someone who has AIDS.

The more you know about AIDS, the virus that causes it and how the virus spreads, the more in control you are of your own life and health.

KEY TERMS

anonymously: (uh-NON-uh-mus-lee) Without being identified by name.

antibodies: (AN-ti-bah-dees) Special proteins or chemicals the body produces when an infection is present.

candidiasis: (kan-de-DYE-uh-sis) The growth of painful white patches in the mouth, throat or vagina caused by a fungus called *Candida*.

cirrhosis: Liver disease that usually leads to liver failure and, eventually, death.

HIV wasting syndrome: An opportunistic condition characterized by the loss of 10 percent or more of total body weight over a short period of time.

Kaposi's sarcoma: (KAP-oh-sees/sar-KO-muh) A rare kind of skin cancer that may attack the skin, mucous membranes and lymph nodes.

occupational exposure: Exposure to disease in the workplace.

opportunistic infection: (op-or-too-NIS-tik) An infection caused by germs that normally would not make a person sick. Any person whose immune system is weakened may develop opportunistic infections.

placenta: (pluh-SEN-ta) A blood-filled structure through which the unborn child receives oxygen and nourishment and through which it gets rid of carbon dioxide and its other wastes.

***Pneumocystis carinii* pneumonia (PCP):** (NEW-mo-sis-tis/kuh-REE-nee-eye/new-MOAN-yuh) A parasitic lung infection that makes breathing very difficult. PCP is the leading cause of death for people who have AIDS.

prophylaxis: Preventive or protective measure.

sharps container: Special, protected container for disposal of used needles and other sharp objects.

syndrome: (SIN-drohm) Several signs and symptoms that occur together and characterize a disease.

BOX 18-1

MYTHS AND FACTS ABOUT HIV AND AIDS

Myth
You can get HIV from mosquitos.
Men cannot get HIV from women.
Only gay men are at risk for HIV infection.
HIV was created in the laboratory.
Sharing food can transmit HIV.

Fact
Latex condoms help prevent the spread of HIV.
HIV is not spread by casual contact.
Abstinence is the most effective way to prevent the spread of HIV infection.
Donating blood does not spread HIV.
There is no cure for HIV.

Because AIDS begins with HIV, let's look at HIV transmission first.

WHAT IS HIV?

HIV is the abbreviation for *h*uman *i*mmunodeficiency *v*irus, the virus that causes AIDS. HIV is passed from one person to another through blood-to-blood and sexual contact. In addition, infected pregnant women can pass HIV to their babies during pregnancy or delivery, as well as through breast-feeding. People with HIV have what is called *HIV infection*. Most of those people will develop AIDS as a result of their HIV infection.

How HIV is *Not* Transmitted

HIV is not spread through casual contact. Therefore, most interactions between people do not have to change. People cannot get HIV from simply being around someone who has tested positive for HIV infection. Specifically, HIV infection is *not* transmitted by any of the following behaviors:

- Hugging, close-mouth kissing or holding hands
- Rubbing the shoulders, massaging the body or touching an infected

person in a casual way (not in a sexual way)
- Sharing food or beverages, pencils, books, tools, eating utensils or clothes
- Being in the same room, sitting on the same chair or touching the same things

Doing these things can spread some other viruses, but HIV cannot be spread in these ways.

How HIV *is* Transmitted

HIV is not easy to get. It is transmitted through blood and a few other body fluids, the most important of which are semen, vaginal fluids, breast milk or bodily fluids containing blood. HIV is spread in three major ways—through sexual intercourse with an infected partner, from an infected mother to her baby and through exposure to infected blood.

From an HIV-infected Person to a Sexual Partner When Semen or Vaginal Fluid is Exchanged. The use of latex condoms can help prevent the spread of HIV during oral, anal or vaginal sex.

From an HIV-infected Mother to Her Unborn Baby During Her Pregnancy or During Childbirth. The virus is so tiny that it can pass through the membranes of the **placenta** and infect the blood of the developing fetus. Some babies who initially have a false positive reading for HIV antibodies may test negative when they get older as they lose the effects of the maternal antibodies. Other babies who test positive may actually be infected with HIV (Figure 18-1). An HIV-infected mother also may pass the virus to her nursing baby through breast milk. The virus can be present in breast milk and can enter the baby's system through the mucous membranes of the baby's mouth. Reported 33% of perinatal HIV transmissions worldwide are attributed to breast milk. In most instances, a mother who is HIV-positive should bottle-feed rather than breast-feed her infant. Without antiretroviral therapy, approximately 25% of pregnant HIV-infected women will transmit the virus to their child. ACTG protocol 076 showed that ZDV (also know as AZT) therapy was associated with a 67.5% reduction in the risk of HIV transmission from mother to child.

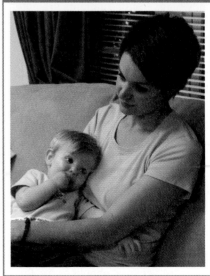

FIGURE 18-1 A mother who is HIV-positive can pass HIV antibodies and the virus to her baby. This can happen during pregnancy or during delivery of the baby.

From an HIV-infected Person to Anyone Who Shares a Needle with that Person. Whenever two people use the same needle to inject drugs, get a tattoo or pierce their ears, they risk spreading HIV if one of them is infected with the virus. Some infected blood may remain on the needle and can be passed from one person to another. If you use drugs, get the necessary help to stop using them. If you know people who inject drugs, warn them never to share needles with another person.

From HIV-Infected Blood Given to a Recipient. Organizations that collect blood donations have been testing blood for the virus since 1985. If they find antibodies to HIV, they destroy the blood.

How HIV is Transmitted in the Health Care Setting

Worldwide studies of people who provide care for those who have AIDS show that **occupational exposure** is not a primary means of HIV transmission. Since 2001, there have been 57 documented cases of health care workers who have contracted HIV as a result of exposure in the workplace. The best way to prevent health care workers from occupational exposure is to follow infection control precautions. This requires the health care worker to assume that the blood and other body fluids from *all* patients are potentially infectious. These precautions include routinely using barriers such as gloves and/or goggles when expecting contact with blood or body fluids, immediately washing hands and other skin surfaces after contact with blood or body fluids and carefully handling and disposing of sharp instruments during and after use.

Safety devices also have been developed to help prevent needle-stick injuries. Remember, if you see needles or syringes lying around, do not recap the syringe. The needles should be disposed of in a **sharps container.** If an exposure accident should occur, the

facility exposure plan should be activated. In most cases, it is recommended that a regimen of two anti-HIV medications be given as a post exposure **prophylaxis**, AZT (ZDV). When an HIV-infected health care worker does not use Standard Precautions, he or she can infect the person receiving health care.

Testing for HIV

A person can be infected with HIV without knowing it. A simple blood test can detect antibodies in the blood. If the test detects HIV antibodies, it is said to be *positive*, which is why someone who is infected with HIV is referred to as *HIV-positive*.

Many people who think they may have been infected may be afraid to have an HIV test because of what they might find out (Figure 18-2). Or they may be afraid that their employers or family members and friends might find out about the behaviors that put them at risk. They also may be afraid that they might lose their jobs if their test results are positive. People who have HIV often suffer discrimination, but local, state and federal laws can provide some legal protection. The Americans with Disabilities Act protects many people who have disabilities, including those who have HIV.

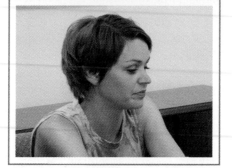

FIGURE 18-2 It may be very hard for someone to decide to have an HIV test done because of fear about what the results will be.

A person who may have been exposed to HIV must have the courage to be tested, because the sooner she knows she is infected with HIV, the sooner she can begin treatment that may prolong the time before she develops AIDS.

Facts About Testing. A person should keep the following things in mind when considering being tested for HIV:

- Testing may be done **anonymously** or confidentially. In an anonymous test the person is identified only by a number. In a confidential test, the name of the person being tested is provided but the results are kept private. A person's test results are confidential. They are identified by a number, not by a name.

- A positive HIV test does not mean that a person has AIDS or might develop AIDS any time soon. It simply means the person has been infected with HIV. A person infected with HIV should see a doctor immediately, because early treatment can slow the development of the disease and contribute to better-quality and longer life.

- A person recently infected with HIV still may have a negative result when tested. It takes from 6 weeks to 3 months after exposure (being open to the risk) for the antibodies to the virus to be detected in a person's blood. If a person whose test results are negative thinks that they may have been exposed to HIV, they should have the test repeated after 3 months. In the meantime, the person should prevent the spread of the virus by using latex condoms for every sexual encounter and, if injecting drugs, by not sharing needles.

- Getting a negative test result does not protect a person from becoming infected in the future. It means only that the person probably was not infected at the time of the test.

- In health care settings, when a worker experiences an occupationally related exposure such as a needle stick, policies may include immediate blood testing and then periodic blood tests in the following months. If a health care worker learns that she is infected with HIV, she can begin receiving early treatment that may delay the development of AIDS by months or even years.

When Test Results are Positive.
There are a number of tests available today to detect the presence of HIV. The standard test for HIV analyzes samples of blood or body fluid for antibodies to HIV, rather than the actual virus itself. Antibodies are substances the body makes to defend itself when it is invaded by germs. People who have antibodies to HIV have been infected with HIV.

If a person is found to have antibodies to HIV, the results still need to be confirmed by another test, which usually takes 1 or 2 weeks. There the person receives the test results and is given the opportunity to talk with a counselor (Figure 18-3). The counselor is trained to give necessary support and guidance to help the person deal with the information, receive appropri-

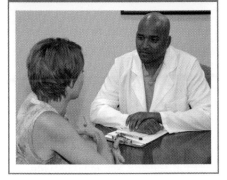

FIGURE 18-3 When Mrs. Hill found out she was HIV-positive, she had many questions for the counselor. She was very concerned about her baby's health and her own.

ate medical care and to educate the person on adopting sexual and drug use behaviors that protect others from becoming infected. The counselor reinforces the fact that the person is infected with the virus but does not yet have AIDS, if that is the case.

The counselor also advises the HIV-positive person to tell sexual partners and others who may have been infected so that they can be tested as soon as possible. If the person is embarrassed about telling others, she can ask the counselor for help.

WHAT IS AIDS, AND WHAT CAUSES IT?

Acquired immunodeficiency syndrome (AIDS) is a condition that results from HIV infection. By the time people with HIV develop AIDS, their immune systems have become damaged and may no longer be able to fight off other infections. This makes them vulnerable to diseases referred to as *opportunistic infections* that most healthy people usually resist or control, such as thrush, certain pneumonias or recurrences of childhood infections. They may also suffer from cancers rarely found among people with healthy body defenses. With medicine, many of these infections can now be prevented or treated. Because the virus can enter the brain and other organs throughout the body, people with AIDS may have trouble with movement, memory and body functions.

A person who is infected with HIV may look and feel healthy and lead a productive life for many years. However, during this time the virus is breaking down the person's immune system.

How Does AIDS Affect the Health of an Infected Person?

When a person is exposed to HIV, the virus enters his body, multiplies in the blood and other organs, and damages

his immune system. It may take a long time for the virus to destroy enough of the immune system to cause sickness. The person can be infected with HIV for 10 or more years without showing any signs or symptoms of AIDS, but he still is able to infect other people during that time.

Symptoms of AIDS

Health professionals believe that most people who are infected with HIV will eventually develop AIDS. Their symptoms may vary, but most experience at least several of the symptoms that are associated with AIDS. Not only do symptoms vary from one person who has AIDS to another, but also one person's symptoms and conditions can change from day to day. As a person's HIV infection worsens and the immune system weakens, any or all of the following symptoms can occur:

- White spots in the mouth or vaginal discharge (signs of yeast infection or **candidiasis**)
- Repeated episodes of diarrhea
- Dry cough or shortness of breath
- Swelling in the glands that does not go away
- Continual feelings of tiredness
- Fevers that occur again and again
- Night sweats
- Unexplained weight loss of 10 pounds or more (possible **HIV wasting syndrome**)
- Memory loss or confusion
- Pain and difficulty when moving
- Red or purplish spots on the skin

Some of these symptoms also occur in other illnesses, so they are not always signs of AIDS. But if a person has any of these symptoms for more than 2 weeks, he should consult a doctor.

Infections and Diseases Associated with AIDS

The most common opportunistic conditions that are seen in people when HIV infection has weakened their immune systems include ***Pneumocystis carinii***

FIGURE 18-4 (A) The Healthy Immune System: A healthy immune system is very effective at fighting a variety of illnesses and infections, including PCP and cancer (CAN). **(B)** The Immune System Infected with HIV: HIV has destroyed most of the special cells in the immune system that alert the body to invasion of disease. The body can no longer fight off diseases like PCP and CAN. It can sometimes, but not always, fight common colds and flu.

FIGURE 18-4 (A) The Healthy Immune System: A healthy immune system is very effective at fighting a variety of illnesses and infections, including PCP and cancer (CAN). **(B)** The Immune System Infected with HIV: HIV has destroyed most of the special cells in the immune system that alert the body to invasion of disease. The body can no longer fight off diseases like PCP and CAN. It can sometimes, but not always, fight common colds and flu.

FIGURE 18-5 Only a few people come to visit this resident, and he often feels isolated. When he feels down, he really appreciates the nurse assistant listening and expressing kindness toward him.

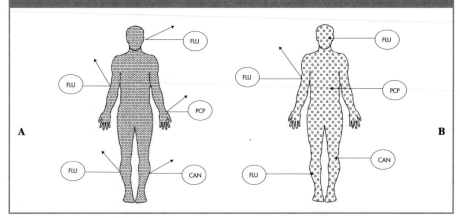

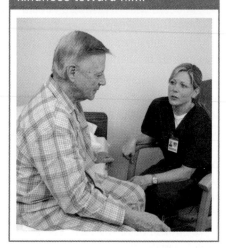

pneumonia **(PCP)**, tuberculosis and cancers such as **Kaposi's sarcoma** or invasive cervical cancer. A person with a healthy immune system would not become severely ill with these conditions, as happens in a person who has AIDS. Their bodies would be able to fight off any infections in time. Figure 18-4 shows what happens to people who have healthy immune systems and to those whose immune systems have been weakened by HIV.

Considering that the AIDS virus is a relatively new virus, the progress made in developing treatment therapies has been remarkable. Doctors are combining these drugs to more effectively treat people. These combined drugs are referred to as *drug cocktails*. Although not a cure, this therapy brings hope and new strength to many people with HIV.

PROVIDING CARE FOR A PERSON LIVING WITH AIDS

People who are living with AIDS need you to provide the same type of thoughtful caregiving that you provide to every sick person. They need you to help with things they cannot do for themselves. They need you to be the best nurse assistant you can be for them. Because they have a disease that has no cure and that often isolates them from other people, they may need more emotional support than some other people in your care. Remember to be kind and warm to all people in your care (Figure 18-5).

The one big difference in providing care for someone with AIDS is that you must remember that AIDS is a **syndrome,** a collection of different symptoms that may change from day to day. As the person's condition changes, you must change the types of care you provide.

Practicing the Principles of Care

When providing care for a person living with AIDS, all of the principles of care are important, but four principles need special consideration.

Dignity. The person in your care may have been treated unfairly or unkindly because of her disease. Dignity, self-respect and feelings of self-esteem may have been damaged. You can help restore her dignity by showing respect, compassion and concern for her feelings and needs while you provide personal care.

Communication. People living with AIDS may be cut off from friends and family by the disease or by the attitudes of people around them. They may need to talk with someone about their fears and feelings of loneliness. One of the most important things you can do as you provide care is to be a good listener. Think back to the communication bridges you learned about in Chapter 5, "Communicating with People." What are some things you can do to communicate more effectively when you provide care for someone with AIDS?

Independence. Often a person with AIDS loses control over many things in her life. Because of the disease, she may have lost her job, her home, her friends and family and many of her physical abilities. You must provide care in a way that encourages her to stay as independent as possible. You can help her keep as much control as possible over her daily life, but also save as much strength as possible. She needs her strength to fight off the next opportunistic infection.

Infection Control. Practicing proper infection control is very important to the well-being of the person with AIDS because of her weakened immune system. You must be especially careful not to spread germs that could cause the person to develop an infection.

Some people who work with those who have AIDS are afraid of becoming infected. Standard Precautions were designed to protect health care workers and the people for whom they provide care from contact with possibly infectious body fluids. You must practice Standard Precautions when you provide care for someone who has AIDS, just as you should practice those standard precautions when you provide care for anyone. You do not have to do anything differently for a person with AIDS than you do when you provide care for anyone else. You can safely touch, help and hug the person, as well as laugh and talk with her.

Dealing with the Symptoms of AIDS

Several symptoms commonly occur when a person has AIDS. Descriptions of these symptoms appear in Table 18-1, along with the physical and emotional care you may have to provide. In addition, as the level of the person's health changes and she spends more time in bed, keep the following suggestions in mind:

- Change the person's position in bed often at least every 2 hours.
- Monitor her skin condition and prevent bedsores.
- Maintain body movement as much as possible. Do gentle, passive range-of-motion exercises as needed.

- Provide general comfort measures, such as giving a backrub or placing a bell to ring within easy reach.

Risks of Physical Contact for a Person Who has AIDS

A person who has AIDS is particularly susceptible to infection caused by contact with people who have illnesses (especially chicken pox), foods that have not been handled safely and pets.

Risks of Contagious Illnesses. If someone living in the home with the person in your care has a contagious illness such as a cold, respiratory flu, stomach flu or diarrhea, you and the person who has AIDS should avoid close contact with that person. Your supervising nurse should remind all people living in the home to make sure their immunizations are up to date.

If the person who has AIDS has not had chicken pox in the past, he should avoid any contact with a person who has the disease, because it can be deadly for a person with AIDS. The person in your care should avoid contact with:

- A person with active chicken pox.
- A person recently exposed to chicken pox. He should not be in the same room with that exposed person from the 10th to the 21st day after exposure.
- A person who has not had chicken pox and who *may have been* exposed recently.
- A person who has shingles, because that disease may cause chicken pox in the person who has AIDS.

If you learn that the person in your care is exposed to chicken pox, report this information to your supervising nurse, who will recommend that the person see her doctor immediately.

Risks of Infections Through Touch. When providing care for a person who has AIDS, you can help protect

her from infections by doing the following:

- Wash your hands frequently.
- Do not touch the person or her personal items if you have skin infections, such as boils, cold sores, impetigo or shingles.

Risks of Infections Through Food. As you learned in Chapter 11, "Providing Care for the Person's Surroundings," and Chapter 14, "Healthful Eating," handling food properly is vital for preventing infection and contamination. This proper handling is especially important for a person who has AIDS, because some bacterial infections carried by spoiled food are fatal to a person who has a weakened immune system.

When Providing Home Care. When preparing food for a person who has AIDS, be sure to heat leftovers and other foods until they are steaming hot. Separate uncooked foods from cooked and ready-to-eat foods, and do not leave foods out of the refrigerator for more than 2 hours. Advise the person to avoid prepared foods from a delicatessen and soft cheeses such as feta, Brie, Camembert and blue-veined cheeses like Roquefort. Also advise her to avoid Mexican-style cheeses sold as "queso fresco" and "queso blanco." Have the person avoid raw, unpasteurized milk and products made from it, but let her know that cottage cheese, yogurt and other pasteurized products are safe to eat. Be sure to check "use by" dates on food labels and discard any food items with expired dates.

Foods such as organic vegetables and raw meats are very susceptible to bacteria. Either avoid these foods or handle them with great care. For example, thoroughly wash all fresh fruits and vegetables. Peel the skin of all fruits and vegetables, and avoid them if the skin cannot be peeled. Cook all poultry, beef, pork and eggs until they are well done. Use two separate cutting boards: one for fruits and vegetables and one for meat and fish.

TABLE 18-1 SYMPTOMS THAT MAY OCCUR WITH AIDS

Symptoms and Description	Physical Care	Emotional Care
Mouth infection Sores or white patches in the mouth may cause pain and make it difficult for the person to eat or drink. (candidiasis)	Provide frequent mouth care by using a soft toothbrush, a disposable mouth sponge or a special solution ordered by the doctor or supervising nurse. Leave sores and white patches alone. Trying to scrub them off may cause bleeding. Report to your supervising nurse if the person has difficulty swallowing. She may suggest changing the person's diet to include foods that are easier to chew and swallow and that contain fewer spices. Offer water if the person's mouth is irritated by juice or soda.	Be compassionate. Remember how you felt at a time when you had a cold sore in your mouth, or a toothache, and were unable to eat.
Diarrhea The person may not be able to control frequent,watery stools.	Provide good skin care. Keep the skin clean and dry. Offer liquids often and encourage the person to drink extra liquids to replace the lost fluids. Report to your supervising nurse the frequency of the diarrhea, as well as the color and consistency.	Because being unable to control the bowels is embarrassing to the person receiving care, reassure her that you understand and are not upset by her loose or uncontrollable bowels. Act calm and tell the person it is not a problem for you to help her to the bathroom or help with cleaning after an incident. Encourage the person to talk to you about what is happening and how she feels.
Nausea and vomiting An infection or a medication used to treat the person may cause nausea or vomiting.	Make the person as comfortable as possible. Ask what things would help her feel more comfortable. Reduce odors in the room, if possible. If the person wishes you to, gently wipe her face with a cool, slightly damp cloth. Provide mouth care as often as the person wants it. Wait until the person feels ready before offering food or liquid. Give clear liquids, such as ginger ale or gelatin, in small amounts to a person who is ready to eat again. Report to your supervising nurse whenever the person feels nauseated or has vomited, because she or he may be able to arrange for a medication that can help. Also be especially careful to report whether the person takes fluids and how much.	Reassure the person you are nearby to help if she needs anything. Reassure the person that you understand and are not upset if she vomits.

TABLE 18-1 SYMPTOMS THAT MAY OCCUR WITH AIDS continued

Symptoms and Description	Physical Care	Emotional Care
Breathing problems A person may have difficulty breathing and may be very nervous because of it.	Limit the person's activity if she has difficulty breathing. Check the person's position frequently. Sitting in an upright position makes breathing easier. Be sure nothing, such as tight pajamas or heavy bedclothes, blocks the person's breathing. Follow the doctor's orders if oxygen is required to help the person breathe. Encourage the person to stay out of areas where people are smoking.	Stay with the person during an episode of difficult breathing. Sit or stand calmly and quietly by the person. Your calmness may help her become calm. Be aware that anything upsetting may make the person's breathing more difficult. Anxiety causes difficulty in breathing, and the difficulty in breathing causes the person to become even more anxious.
Swelling (edema) Swelling may occur in different parts of the body, including the face.	Apply cool compresses to the swollen area as directed by the doctor or your supervising nurse. Raise the head of the bed or help the person lie on several pillows if her head and face are swollen. Check with your supervising nurse about placing pillows under the person's swollen arms, legs, hands or feet. Raising a swollen part of her body higher than the level of her heart helps reduce swelling. Observe the person's skin frequently. The skin over a swollen area may become stretched or torn. Provide good skin care by gently applying lotion to the swollen area. This may help keep her skin from drying and tearing.	Be compassionate. Think how you would feel if your face were swollen and misshapen. Tell the person you care, and encourage her to talk to you about what is happening and her feelings.
Chronic fatigue Feeling constantly tired is a common symptom of AIDS.	Ask the person how you can help. Involve her in planning her care. Ask what tasks she would like to help with and what tasks you should plan to do. Offer as much assistance as possible with personal care activities so that the person can save her energy. Offer frequent rest periods during activities such as walking or bathing. Plan your care so that the person can be rested and alert at times when there are things she wants to enjoy during the day, such as visitors or a special activity.	Reassure the person that you understand her tiredness is caused by the disease and that you want to help as much as possible. Be compassionate. Imagine how you would feel if you were so exhausted you were barely able to brush your own teeth.

Continued

TABLE 18-1 SYMPTOMS THAT MAY OCCUR WITH AIDS continued

Symptoms and Description	Physical Care	Emotional Care
Fever Many opportunistic infections may cause a low-grade fever in the afternoon and evening or may cause night sweats.	Encourage the person to drink liquids to replace fluids lost during sweating. As directed by the doctor or your supervising nurse, give a lukewarm sponge bath to help reduce the fever, but keep the person from becoming chilled. Keep her covered with a light blanket during the bath. Change linens and clothing frequently when sweating occurs. Use ice packs when directed by your supervising nurse. Place these in a face cloth or towel (never directly on the skin) and then in the person's armpits or near the genital region, or in both areas. Take the person's temperature often if she receives medications that are supposed to bring the temperature down.	Encourage the person to talk about feelings of anxiety or fear.
Muscle loss Many people with AIDS lose as much as 20 percent or more of their body weight, which includes both body fat and muscle. This loss makes them even more susceptible to infections and skin problems.	Add high-calorie and high-protein extras such as butter or margarine to foods. Spread peanut butter on apple slices or bananas and add honey to tea. Have the person maintain an intake of 2000 to 2700 calories per day. Good nutrition is very important in helping to strengthen the immune system and to counteract weight and muscle loss. To help tone and strengthen the person's muscles, help her with range-of-motion exercises that you learned in Chapter 16, "Providing Restorative Care to help with Rehabilitation." Because the person may have little fat or muscle between her skin and bones, reposition her every 2 hours to prevent decubitus ulcers, and give good skin care to prevent skin breakdown.	Help the person look her best by helping her with grooming and dressing. Encourage family members or friends to purchase new clothes in smaller sizes, if possible, so that the weight loss is less noticeable.
Mental difficulties Because HIV often infects the person's nervous system, she may become confused.	Make sure the environment is safe and restful. Decrease clutter and noise. Speak in short sentences and use simple statements. Use memory cues, such as clocks and calendars, to help the person keep track of the time and date.	Stay calm, since your calmness has a tranquil effect on the person.

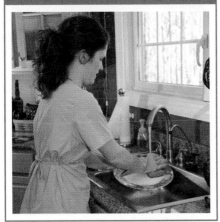

FIGURE 18-6 A person with AIDS does not require separate dishes or eating utensils, and dishes used by a person with AIDS do not require special methods of cleaning.

Remember, a person with AIDS does not require separate dishes or eating utensils, and dishes used by a person with AIDS do not require special methods of cleaning (Figure 18-6).

The person with AIDS can prepare food for others, provided that she does not have diarrhea caused by a germ that can be spread by food. Anyone preparing food should wash her hands before beginning the preparation and avoid licking her fingers or spoons used during preparation.

Risks of Infections Through Pets. When providing home care for a person who has AIDS, help protect her from infections through pets by having her avoid all contact with litter boxes or animal stool, bird cage droppings and water in fish tanks.

Risks of Infections Through Personal Items. It is especially important that a person with AIDS not share razors, toothbrushes or other disposable items that sometimes draw blood. She also should not share other personal items such as tweezers, cuticle scissors and pierced earrings that sometimes draw blood.

Providing Emotional Care to a Person Who has AIDS

It is important to provide emotional care to a person who has AIDS, but it also may be difficult. The following tips may help you:

Be a Good Listener. Try to stop what you are doing, no matter how important it is, and listen to what the person says. Talking may be the person's greatest need at that moment.

Be Trustworthy. Do not gossip about the person with your family or friends. Living with AIDS is difficult. Respect the privacy of the person in your care.

Be Dependable. Do what you say you are going to do, when you say you will do it. The person with AIDS has much uncertainty in her life. It helps if she can count on you to be dependable.

Be Positive. Always try to point out any improvement in the person's health, outlook, energy level or capability. At the same time, if she is concerned about something, stay in touch with her feelings. Do not over look something that is very important and serious to her.

Do Not be Fooled by Anger. Remember that the person you are providing care for may be angry at AIDS, not at you. Do not take the anger personally, and do not let it affect the kind of care you give.

Keep Your Own Emotions Out of the Way. You may develop strong emotions as you provide care for a person who has AIDS. You may watch the person waste away and die. You may feel sorrow, frustration or anger about someone going through such pain, but you must save your feelings for another time and place. Find someone you can talk to, such as your supervising nurse, a social worker or a counselor in a community organization that helps people who live or work with people who have AIDS.

Think about all you have learned about providing care for a person who has AIDS. What things could you do to help Mrs. Hill live more comfortably? How can you provide for her physical needs? How can you provide care for her emotional needs, especially for her need to be a caring mother for Melissa? What things can you do to protect yourself from infection while providing care for them?

When a Person with AIDS Dies

The person with HIV infection or AIDS may go through several episodes of "near death." He may have all the signs of approaching death and then recover. In some cases, the person remains weak, but in others, he may recover enough to provide for his own care. This "roller coaster" ride of events causes emotional turmoil for the person, as well as for his caregivers. The person may repeatedly move through emotional stages of dealing with dying.

Because of his changing health status, a person with AIDS may begin making plans for his death and funeral, plans that would not otherwise have occurred until a later time in his life. You already read that talking about death can be uncomfortable, but you must be open to the person and listen to him. It is important for him to be able to make his desired plans and discuss these plans in advance. Your role as a nurse assistant is to provide emotional support as the person and his family make difficult decisions. As the person approaches death, continue to provide care to him and his family, practicing the principles of care, especially focusing on dignity, privacy, independence and infection control.

The person with AIDS who is dying will experience many of the same signs of approaching death as those listed in Chapter 20, "Providing End-of-Life Care." The care that you provide will focus on:

- Continuing personal care activities; keeping the person's skin clean and dry.
- Continuing communication; speaking calmly, slowly and reassuringly.

- Keeping the person from getting too hot or too cold.
- Elevating the head of the person's bed if breathing is difficult for him or her or if the person experiences an increase in secretions.
- Changing the person's position in bed frequently and using pillows for support.
- Frequently moistening and cleaning the person's mouth.
- Monitoring the person's urinary output, since kidney function decreases and fluid intake may have lessened.

If the person dies in the hospital, nursing home or at home, follow your employer's policy and procedures. Discuss these topics with your supervising nurse.

Discuss your fears and feelings about death with your supervising nurse and seek support for your own grief.

THE CONTINUED AIDS CRISIS

During the 1990s, the epidemic shifted steadily toward a growing proportion of AIDS cases in African Americans and Hispanics and in women, and toward a decreasing proportion in men who have sex with men (MSM). The incidence of infections with MSM has increased in recent years. African Americans and Hispanics have been disproportionately affected since the early years of the epidemic. In real numbers, African Americans have out-numbered whites in new AIDS diagnoses and deaths since 1996 and in the number of people living with AIDS since 1998. The proportion of women with AIDS in 2005 was 26%, and the proportion infected heterosexually has also increased, passing the proportion infected through injecting drug use. As more effective treatments have become available, a decrease in the incidence of AIDS and AIDS-related deaths has resulted.*

*For a complete list of sources for these statistics, see the sources listed at the end of this book.

BOX 18-2

CURRENT HIV AND AIDS INFORMATION

Toll-Free
1-800-CDC-INFO
or
1-800-232-4636
TTY
1-800-232-6348
In English, en Espanol
24 Hours/Day
http://www.cdc.gov/hiv

You can learn more about AIDS from the National AIDS Hotline (Box 18-2) or the American Red Cross.

PROVIDING CARE FOR A PERSON WITH HEPATITIS

What is Hepatitis?

Hepatitis is a disease caused by a virus that infects the liver. Hepatitis A, B and C are the most common types, and hepatitis D and E are the least common. Hepatitis B, C and D can lead to severe illness, life-long disease, scarring of the liver, liver failure, liver cancer or even death.

Hepatitis A Virus (HAV)

Hepatitis A, the least serious, is a liver disease caused by the hepatitis A virus. HAV can affect anyone. In this country, HAV can occur as a single case of the disease or be a widespread epidemic. During epidemic years, 35,000 cases of HAV have been reported. However, in the late 1990s, the HAV vaccine became more widely used, and the number of cases reached historic lows. As more and more people are vaccinated against

---

HAV, the number of cases reported will continue to be significantly lower. You may be at risk of getting HAV if you:

- Travel to a place where food and water are not clean
- Share dirty needles
- Are a man who has sex with other men
- Live in the same house with some-one who has HAV
- Have a child who goes to the same day care facility with some-one who has HAV

How is HAV Transmitted?

HAV is found in the stool of persons infected with HAV. It is usually spread from person to person by putting something in the mouth that has been contaminated with the stool of a person with hepatitis.

Prevention. The best protection is per-forming proper handwashing and to get the hepatitis A vaccine (Figure 18-7). If a person has been exposed to HAV or expects possible exposure, such as when traveling to a country where HAV is common, short-term protection is available from immune globulin.

Hepatitis B Virus (HBV)

Hepatitis B (HBV) can be transmitted to anyone, including those who already have other forms of hepatitis. The num-

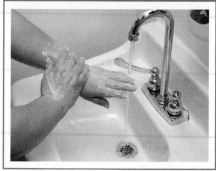

FIGURE 18-7 The best protection from hepatitis is performing proper handwashing and to get the hepatitis A vaccine.

ber of new infections per year has declined from an average of 260,000 in the 1980s to about 60,000 in 2004. One out of 20 people in the United States will get hepatitis B some time during their lives. (The risk increases for people who fall within the categories listed below.) HBV is spread by blood, semen or vaginal fluids from an infected person. It is transmitted in the same manner as HIV. You are at risk for infection if:

- You have sex with an infected person.
- Your mother had hepatitis B when you were born.
- You shared personal items that had infected blood on them, such as toothbrushes or razors.
- You share needles and other equipment used for injecting illegal drugs.
- You are a health care worker and were exposed to infected blood.
  The risk is also higher if your parents were born in Southeast Asia, Africa, the Amazon Basin in South America, the Pacific Islands and the Middle East.

How HBV *is* Transmitted

Hepatitis B is transmitted by direct contact with the blood or body fluids of an infected person. If you have unprotected sex with an infected person or you share needles with an infected person, you are at high risk for getting HBV. A baby can get hepatitis B from an infected mother during childbirth. As you can see, HBV is transmitted in the same ways as HIV. People who do not practice safe behaviors are at risk for both infections.

How HBV is *Not* Transmitted

HBV is not transmitted by casual contact. You will not become infected by hugging, talking or shaking hands. HBV is *not* spread through food or water.

Signs and Symptoms of HBV

A person may have HBV (and be spreading the disease) without know-

ing it. Only a blood test can tell for sure. Sometimes, people who are infected with HBV never recover fully from the infection; they carry the virus and can infect others for the rest of their lives. About one million people in the United States are carriers of HBV. Many people *do* have symptoms that may include:

- Yellow color to the eyes or skin (jaundice)
- Loss of appetite
- Possible nausea, vomiting, fever, stomach or joint pain
- Extreme exhaustion, making it impossible to work for weeks or months

Is There a Cure for HBV?

There is no cure for HBV, which is why prevention is so important. The best protection against HBV is the hepatitis B vaccine. Three doses are needed for complete protection. Health care workers are *highly* encouraged to receive the hepatitis B series. Your employer must provide the vaccination free to employees whose job puts them at risk of being infected (jobs that create the possibility of contact with blood and other body fluids.) The health care worker may decline the vaccination, but doing so increases the risk of infection with HBV.

Hepatitis C (HCV)

Hepatitis C is a liver disease caused by the hepatitis C virus (HCV), which is found in the blood of persons who have this disease. The infection is spread by contact with the blood of an infected person. HCV can be spread by sex, but this is rare.

How HCV is *Not* Spread

Even though HCV is not often spread by sex, safe sex practices should still be followed. That is, use latex condoms correctly every time. You will not get HCV through casual contact. Hepatitis C is *not* spread by any of the following:

- Breast-feeding
- Hugging

- Food or water
- Sharing eating utensils or drinking glasses
- Sneezing
- Coughing

Treatment for Hepatitis C

Hepatitis C is serious for some persons, but not for others. Most persons who get hepatitis C carry the virus for the rest of their lives. Most of these people have some liver damage, but many do not feel sick from the disease. Some persons with liver damage due to hepatitis C may develop **cirrhosis** of the liver and liver failure, which may take many years to develop. A blood test can determine whether you have hepatitis C. There are medications available for the treatment of HCV, but there is *no* vaccination or cure.

WHAT IS TUBERCULOSIS (TB) INFECTION?

Tuberculosis (TB) is a bacterial infection of the lungs. In most people who breathe in TB bacteria and become infected, the body is able to fight the bacteria and keep the bacteria from growing. The bacteria become inactive, but they remain alive in the body and can become active later. This condition is referred to as *TB infection*. Although people with TB infection usually have a positive skin test reaction, they have no symptoms, do not feel sick and cannot spread TB to others; however, they can develop TB disease later in life if they do not receive preventive therapy. Many people who have TB infection never develop TB disease. In these people, the TB bacteria remain inactive for a lifetime without causing disease. In other people, especially people who have weak immune systems, the bacteria become active and cause TB disease.

How TB is Spread

TB is a contagious disease that is spread through the air from one person to another. TB in the lungs or throat can be infectious. People with TB disease are most likely to spread the disease to people they spend time with every day, including family members, friends and co-workers. The bacteria are put into the air when a person with TB disease of the lungs or throat coughs or sneezes (Figure 18-8). People nearby may breathe in these bacteria and become infected. When a person breathes in TB bacteria, the bacteria can settle in the lungs and begin to grow. From there, they move through the blood to other parts of the body, such as the kidney, spine and brain. TB in these other parts of the body is usually not infectious.

Signs and Symptoms of TB

Symptoms of tuberculosis depend on where in the body the TB bacteria are growing. TB bacteria usually grow in the lungs, where they may cause pain in the chest, a bad cough that lasts longer than 2 weeks and the coughing up of blood or sputum (phlegm from deep inside the lungs). The procedure used to collect sputum specimens is explained step by step in Skill 56. Other symptoms include the following:

- Weakness or fatigue
- Weight loss
- No appetite
- Chills
- Fever
- Sweating at night

Providing Care for a Person with TB

Because TB is highly contagious, you should follow Isolation Precautions.

- Wear a mask when assisting with personal care. Wearing a gown is not necessary unless your clothing might possibly be contaminated.
- Ask the person to cover his mouth with a tissue when coughing so that bacteria are not sprayed into the air. Have him discard the tissue into a plastic bag. Arrange for the contents to be burned.
- Early in his treatment, have the person wear a mask when he is in

close contact with other people. This mask prevents droplets from being spread into the air, where they can be breathed in by someone else.

- Install and use a window fan to circulate the air in closed rooms—pulling fresh air into the room—not out.
- Practice good handwashing techniques.
- Make sure the person's plan of care includes good nutrition and adequate rest.
- Make sure his diet is well balanced and adequate in calories to promote healing and rebuilding of lost body mass.
- Plan rest periods for the person during the day to minimize fatigue.

People may have fears and misconceptions about TB. These feelings and ideas may interfere with their following the doctor's instructions about treatment and follow-up. By encouraging the person and the family to talk about their fears, the caregiver may be able to identify and correct misconceptions and lessen fears.

How Can I Get Tested for TB?

A TB skin (referred to as a mantoux skin test) test is the only way to find out whether you have TB infection. You can get a skin test at the health department or at your doctor's office. You should get tested for TB if you have spent time with a person with infectious TB, if you have HIV infection or another condition that puts you at high risk for TB disease, if you are from a country where TB disease is very common or if you simply think you might have TB. You can get a TB skin test from your personal health provider or your local health department. A TB skin test will be either positive or negative for TB *infection only*. Many people who have TB infection never develop TB *disease*. A chest x-ray and a laboratory test will confirm whether you have *active* tuberculosis. This testing is a requirement in many

states prior to being employed as a health care professional.

TB and Older Adults

In the United States, more older adults live in nursing homes than in any other type of residential institution. Such concentrations of older adults, many of whom are infected with *tubercle bacilli* or other infections, and some whose immune systems are not working well, create high-risk situations for disease transmission.

Elderly nursing home residents are at greater risk for tuberculosis than are elderly persons living in the community. Nursing home employees are also at increased risk for tuberculosis when compared with other employed adults. Each facility should ensure that appropriate tuberculosis prevention and control measures are undertaken to protect residents and staff.

In large facilities, an infection control committee will usually be responsible for operating the tuberculosis prevention and control program. Skin tests should be administered to all new residents and employees as soon as their residency or employment begins, unless they have documentation of a previous

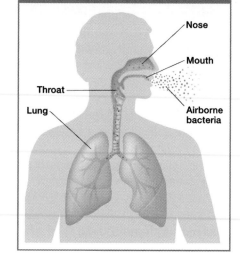

FIGURE 18-8 The bacteria are put into the air when a person with TB disease of the lungs or throat coughs or sneezes.

Nose

Mouth

Throat

Lung

Airborne bacteria

positive reaction. Each skin test should be administered and read by appropriately trained personnel and recorded in the person's medical record. All persons with a reaction of greater than or equal to 10 mm should receive a chest x-ray to identify current or past disease. TB screening requirements vary by state, by facility and by physician.

INFORMATION REVIEW

Circle the correct answers and fill in the blanks.

1. Which statement is true? You can get AIDS if you:
   a. share eating utensils with an infected person.
   b. are bitten by an infected dog.
   c. share needles with an infected drug user.
   d. come into contact with someone's sweat during a basketball game.

2. AIDS is:
   a. a syndrome that results from HIV infection.
   b. a type of virus that infects only homosexual men and IV drug users.
   c. a type of bacteria that you can get in foods.
   d. an illness that you can catch by breathing certain germs in the air.

3. The abbreviation HIV represents three words: _____ immunodeficiency _____.

4. The use of latex _____ during vaginal, anal and oral sex can help prevent the spread of HIV.

5. To find out whether she is infected with HIV, a person has a simple test that checks for antibodies in the _____.

6. The best protection from getting hepatitis B is to get a series of _____.

7. Medication is available for hepatitis C.
   a. T
   b. F

8. People infected with HCV can carry the virus for the rest of their lives.
   a. T
   b. F

9. Hepatitis _____ is the least serious condition among hepatitis A, hepatitis B and hepatitis C.

10. Tuberculosis:
    a. is always fatal.
    b. is spread by touching the person.
    c. always requires hospitalization.
    d. is spread by breathing in droplets that have been sprayed into the air by an infected person's coughing, laughing or sneezing.

11. A TB _____ test is a way to find out whether you have TB infection.

QUESTIONS TO ASK YOURSELF

1. A friend tells you that he tried shooting up drugs a few years ago, but he no longer uses drugs. He says he is afraid to get tested for AIDS for fear he might find out he is going to die. He also is afraid that his employer might find out about the test and fire him. How would you feel? How would you help him decide what to do?

2. Mrs. Hill is expecting visitors. She has lost a lot of weight and her clothes no longer fit. What can you do to help her look her best?

3. Mrs. Hill yells at you for fixing her hair wrong. You think she is being unfair and you are tempted to yell back at her. What things would you do to help calm yourself and Mrs. Hill?

4. A person with AIDS cuts himself while trying to shave. What precautions would you take before trying to help him?

Skill 56: Collecting Sputum Specimens

PRECAUTIONS

- Always follow universal precautions and use infection control techniques when collecting sputum.

PREPARATION

1. Gather supplies:
   - Mouthwash solution
   - Labeled specimen container
   - Protective eyewear (optional)
   - Disposable gloves
   - Plastic trash bag
   - Towel
2. Follow Preparation Standards (see Chapter 7).

PROCEDURE

1. Help the person into a sitting position and place a towel on her chest. ☐ ☐
2. Place an emesis basin under the person's chin and have her rinse her mouth with mouthwash solution. ☐ ☐
3. Have the person take one or two breaths, cough deeply and expel sputum into a specimen container (Figure 18-9). ☐ ☐
4. Cover the container. Provide mouth care for the person. ☐ ☐
5. Put the specimen in the designated area. ☐ ☐
6. Make sure it is labeled correctly—according to your nursing supervisor's instructions. ☐ ☐
7. Follow completion steps. ☐ ☐

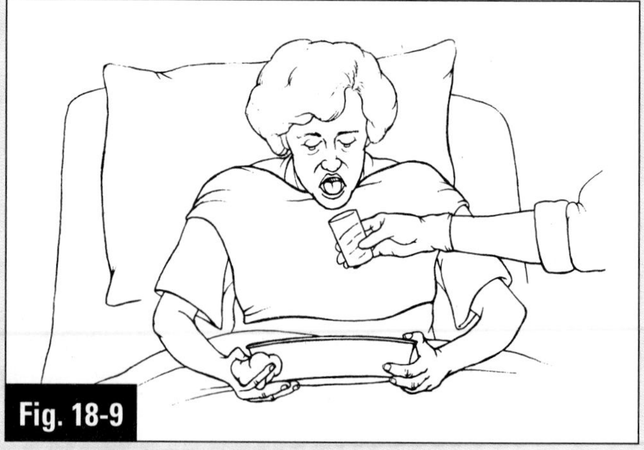

Fig. 18-9

ADDITIONAL INFORMATION

Make sure that the person understands that sputum comes up from the lungs when she coughs and is not the same as saliva that is formed in the mouth.

 COMPLETION

Follow Completion Standards in compliance with your facility. For a complete list of those used in this course, see Chapter 7, "Controlling the Spread of Germs."

19

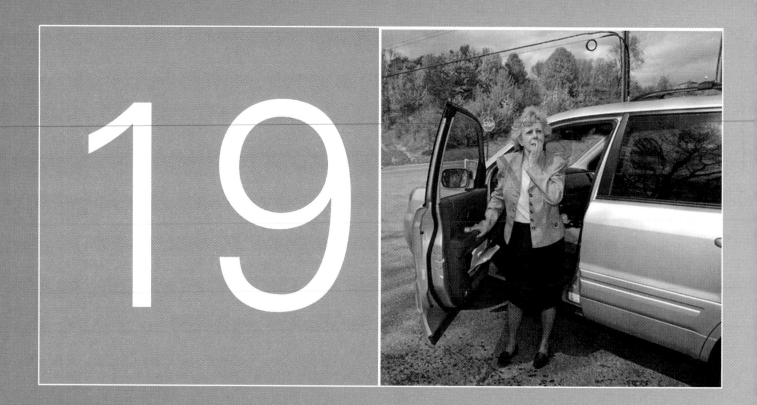

Providing Care for People Who Have Alzheimer's Disease and Related Dementias

GOALS

After reading this chapter, you will have the information needed to:

Discuss cognitive impairment and dementia, including Alzheimer's disease.

Discuss how to meet the needs and respond to the behavior of a person who has dementia.

Identify the needs and behaviors of a person who has Alzheimer's disease.

Identify ways that caregivers can make a difference when providing care for a person with Alzheimer's disease.

Discuss the challenges caregivers face when providing care for a person who has Alzheimer's disease.

Demonstrate an appropriate response to a person whose behavior is dysfunctional.

Discuss how to communicate with a person who has Alzheimer's disease.

Identify the needs of a caregiver who provides care for a person who has dementia.

One day, Shirley McDay's husband asks whether you have time to talk. You sit in the nursing home dayroom and listen as he tells you about the person Mrs. McDay once was. "By the time Shirley was 50 years old," he says, "she owned and operated an up-and-coming flower shop with a greenhouse filled with beautiful flowers and plants. She supervised two gardeners, an accountant, a receptionist and a driver. Sometimes during busy seasons, she also helped make deliveries. She loved being her own boss.

"Three years later, she moved to a larger shop, where she eventually supervised 15 employees. She was more successful than she had ever dreamed. But, little by little, she also became more and more forgetful. Often, she misplaced her keys and forgot to keep appointments. She must have wondered what was happening.

"By the time she was 55, Shirley was acting more and more confused. She accused me and her employees of taking her eyeglasses, jewelry and other items she couldn't find. She couldn't manage her business, and we became concerned about her driving.

"Shirley always used the same route to drive to the flower shop. But one day she got lost and must have become very frightened. When a police officer saw her weaving in and out of traffic, he pulled her over and asked to see her driver's license. In his report, he wrote that my wife didn't seem to understand what he meant. When he asked Shirley her name, she started questioning him: 'What are you saying? What are those lights on your car? Why did I hear sirens?'

"She agreed to be admitted to the hospital for tests and evaluation. While waiting for the results, we were standing in the room by her bed—my two daughters, my son and myself. Shirley was sleeping, when suddenly she opened her eyes and looked around at each of us, searching our faces. When she looked at me, I said, 'Hello, Shirley.' She sat up in bed and kept saying, 'Who are you? Who are you?' I said I was her husband, John. She said, 'No, you're trying to trick me. I don't know you. Where is John? He'll be here. I know he will.' I couldn't believe what I was hearing."

Mr. McDay stops talking and begins to cry.

WHY DO PEOPLE BECOME CONFUSED?

A person becomes confused when her ability to know, think, understand, remember, believe, solve problems, learn and create decreases. These mental activities are cognitive functions. Confusion is a symptom of memory loss, a condition that occurs when a person experiences **cognitive impairment.**

Some people assume that confusion from memory loss is a condition of old age. But most adults over the age of 65 do not behave in a confused way. In general, healthy older people are able to think and remember about as well as they did when they were younger. The majority of middle-aged and older adults retain their abilities to learn, remember and solve problems. A normal adult may forget something, then realize that she has forgotten, and later remember whatever it was that she forgot.

Cognitive impairment, exhibited by memory loss, is **not** a normal part of the aging process but the result of changes in a person's body. For example, a person may become confused when taking a particular medication.

KEY TERMS

anxious: (ANGK-shus) The state of being extremely nervous or agitated.

CAT scan: Computerized axial tomography, a form of x-ray that produces a three-dimensional picture of sections of the brain or other parts of the body.

catastrophic reaction: (kat-uh-STROF-ik) Violent and sudden behavior that disrupts order.

cognitive impairment: A decreased ability to know, think, understand, remember, believe, solve problems, learn and create.

coping: (KOPE-ing) The ability to deal with problems and difficulties.

dementia: (de-MEN-she-uh) An incurable disorder of the brain in which there is a progressive loss of memory and other cognitive (thinking) functions.

disoriented: (dis-OR-ee-en-ted) A condition in which a person is unsure of who she is, where she is and what day or time it is.

dysfunctional: (dis-FUNK-shun-uhl) Functioning in a way that is not normal.

frontotemporal lobe dementia: A type of dementia that usually has a slow onset characterized by changes only in personality for some time.

Lewy body dementia: A condition characterized by progressive loss of memory, language, calculation and reasoning, as well as other higher mental functions. This disease may worsen more quickly than Alzheimer's.

social facade: (fuh-SOD) In a social setting, pretending to know or recognize an unfamiliar person or thing.

vascular dementia: A condition identified by an advancing decline of the intelligent functioning of the brain, accompanied by excessive changes in behavior and personality.

Similarly, someone who has not eaten for a long time may become confused and forgetful. Someone who suffers from a vitamin deficiency also may suffer memory loss. All these kinds of cognitive impairment can be reversed. The doctor can change the person's medication, health care workers can give nutrients to the person who has not eaten and the doctor can provide vitamin therapy to someone with a vitamin deficiency. When these physical needs are addressed, the person's memory generally returns, and she no longer acts confused.

In addition, cognitive impairment can be caused by certain illnesses, such as lung infections, stroke, heart attack, depression, hypothermia, hypoglycemia, brain tumors and alcoholism. When these conditions are treated properly, many of the symptoms of memory loss decrease.

Some kinds of cognitive impairment are chronic and cannot be reversed. These chronic medical conditions are commonly called *dementias*. **Dementia** is an illness characterized by the loss of powers of the mind, the ability to remember things, to think things out and to understand things. With dementia, the mind gradually ceases to function as it once did. An affected person exhibits changes in personality, becomes confused and has difficulty carrying on a sensible conversation. The person may behave oddly and become difficult. It is not unusual for the person to get very anxious or aggressive. The person becomes increasingly unaware of her surroundings and ultimately becomes unable to perform normal tasks. About 50 percent of all people admitted to nursing homes suffer from some type of dementia.

FACTS ABOUT DEMENTIA

Dementia refers to any chronic brain disorder that affects normal thought processes and that cannot be reversed. The most common symptoms are memory loss, personality changes and problems with reasoning, orientation and personal care. In some forms of dementia there are indications that the disorder may be inherited. Dementia is not caused by stress or a crisis, but it is often *during* a time of crisis that others may notice something is wrong—the person gets confused. Dementia is not caused by too much or too little mental activity, and it is not a normal part of growing older. However, the older you are, the more likely you are to develop dementia. It is estimated that about 6 to 10 percent of people aged 65 years or older have dementia. The prevalence of dementia increases with age. About 30 percent of people 85 or older develop dementia.

Dementia cannot be cured at present, but treatment may be possible to relieve some of the symptoms. With Alzheimer's disease, as people become more aware of the symptoms and seek out treatment earlier, the average time of survival becomes longer, increasing to as many as 10 years or more from the time of diagnosis. Categories of dementia are related to the part of the brain affected and the age at which symptoms occur. The main types are **vascular dementia, Lewy body dementia** and **frontotemporal lobe dementia.** Of all the people diagnosed with dementia, the majority suffer from a condition called *Alzheimer's disease.*

ALZHEIMER'S DISEASE

When Mr. McDay regains his composure, he asks if he may tell you more about what happened to his wife. You take time to listen.

"My family and Shirley's co-workers were the first to notice that things weren't exactly 'right' with her," Mr. McDay says. "Her forgetfulness and irritability were not typical of her usual behavior. But none of us realized how serious it was until she was unable to understand and communicate with the police officer. In the hospital, the doctor examined her family history, performed a physical examination, tested her memory and reasoning power and looked for symptoms of some underlying condition, such as vitamin deficiency. He ordered laboratory tests and x-rays, including a **CAT scan** (Figure 19-1). The CAT scan showed signs of brain shrinkage, which explained why she was less and less able to reason and understand. It also explained why her personality had changed—so much that not only did she not recognize her family members, but we didn't recognize the person she had become. The doctor said Shirley had Alzheimer's disease."

Responding to People Who have Alzheimer's Disease or Other Dementias

A person who has dementia such as Alzheimer's disease (AD) has the same basic needs as other people. Because of situations created by her condition, her capacity for meeting these needs often becomes limited, and her behav-

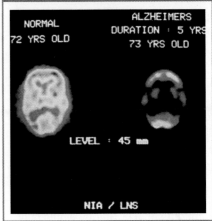

FIGURE 19-1 Alzheimer's disease is characterized by the death of nerve cells, which causes slight to severe memory loss, depression, confusion and difficulty thinking.

ior becomes **dysfunctional** and may seem inappropriate to you. As a nurse assistant, you must understand these needs and behaviors, and you must know how to respond appropriately to them so that you can ensure the well-being and comfort of a person with Alzheimer's disease.

When you see someone behaving dysfunctionally, think of the behavior as a form of communication. The person is trying to tell you in the only way she can that something is wrong. Your job is to observe and think about the behavior to find out what she is trying to communicate so that you can provide appropriate care.

A person who is confused because of memory loss may behave in ways that seem strange to you. But the dysfunctional behavior of a person who has Alzheimer's disease has some common patterns. She may put up a **social facade,** pace or wander, rummage and hoard, have extreme **catastrophic reactions** or become more and more restless and confused as evening approaches. She may say things that do not make sense, see or hear things that are not real, or believe things that are not true. She may be depressed, angry or suspicious of people.

Some people who are confused because of simple memory loss may occasionally exhibit some of the same dysfunctional behaviors as people with Alzheimer's disease. If you know how to respond to these behaviors, you can provide better care. In spite of her dysfunctional behaviors, a person with Alzheimer's disease, as well as any person who is confused, still must be treated with dignity and respect.

Social Facade. Mr. McDay continues to pour out his story about his wife's illness. "You know, at first she was just a little forgetful," he says. "But, now that I look back on it all, I realize that her forgetfulness and confusion gradually were getting worse. When we went out socially, Shirley would only

pretend to know the familiar people who talked with her. Soon it became obvious to me that she didn't remember any of them. I guess she put up a front to 'save face' and to hide the fact that she couldn't remember."

Think of a time when you may have pretended to remember someone who recognized you. Why do you think you pretended? Some people, especially those in the early stage of Alzheimer's disease, pretend to remember because they feel this will help them maintain their dignity and self-respect. In the earlier stage of her illness, Mrs. McDay was aware of her disability and tried to hide it. She put up a *social facade*. Because she did not look ill, she often was able to hide her illness.

It is important to know how to respond to a social facade. At a social event you may meet an old friend who only pretends to remember you. How should you respond? An inappropriate response would be: "You don't really remember me, do you?" A more appropriate response would be: "You may not remember me. I'm Chris Johnson. We haven't seen each other since our last high school reunion."

If you know a person has Alzheimer's disease, you can promote good communication by making eye contact. Speak slowly, ask general questions and use simple sentences. Give her information that she needs to respond appropriately. For example: "Mrs. McDay, your husband is coming down the hall. He looks well today." Keep the conversation brief.

Pacing and Wandering. Sometimes a person who has Alzheimer's disease displays a behavior called *pacing and wandering*. She walks aimlessly in an area and then walks away. Pacing and wandering may be the result of several causes: the person may be overstimulated by too much talking or noise around her; she may feel uncomfortable, **anxious** or **disoriented;** she may

be looking for someone or something; or she may not like what is happening where she is. Her behavior is a form of communication, but it could be unsafe.

When responding to pacing and wandering behavior, use some of the following suggestions:

- Reassure the person. Listen for a clue to what her behavior communicates. Gently ask, "May I walk with you?" and guide her back to where she should be (Figure 19-2).
- A distraction may help. Offer her a snack, take her for a walk, or do something she likes to do to help stop the pacing before her anxiety gets worse.
- Take her to use the bathroom. She may have a full bladder and not realize it.
- Try to help her remove her shoes. Removing her shoes may prompt an old memory that taking off

FIGURE 19-2 If someone who has Alzheimer's disease wanders toward an unsafe area, try to redirect her by suggesting she do something else, such as take part in an activity in the dayroom.

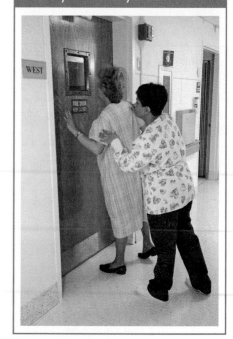

shoes means a person should sit or lie down. (For safety reasons, replace her shoes if this action does not stop her pacing behavior.)

- Observe her for signs of anxiety (restlessness, fidgeting). Give her a ball or another smooth object to manipulate in her hands.
- Talk to her and listen to what she has to say.
- At her room entrance, place a familiar object (perhaps dried flowers or a photo from her past) to help her locate her room.
- Take steps to prevent the person from leaving. Some health care facilities have special safety doors to indicate when the door is being opened by a person who is wearing an ankle or wrist bracelet that triggers an alarm as she approaches the door.
- If you provide home health care for a person who has Alzheimer's disease, have her wear a medical ID bracelet or necklace imprinted with her name, address, phone number and the words *memory impaired*. Or place a card in her pocket with all this information written on it.

Table 19-1 contains ideas to discourage people from wandering into inappropriate areas or from leaving the building. You remember one of the ideas suggested during a meeting with your supervising nurse, and you decide to try it. You get a piece of adhesive-backed black felt from the arts and crafts cart, cut a large circle from the felt and place it on the floor in front of the storage room door. You walk with the resident toward the door. She stops at the black circle. After studying it for a moment, she turns and walks away. It works! (Figure 19-3).

Rummaging and Hoarding. Mrs. McDay has begun going into other people's drawers and closets, taking items and hiding them. These activities are called *rummaging and hoarding*. A person who has Alzheimer's disease may rummage and hoard because she is feeling generally lost and confused, or she might not be able to find an item that she wants.

When you respond to Mrs. McDay's rummaging and hoarding

TABLE 19-1 WAYS TO DISCOURAGE PEOPLE FROM WANDERING

Take This Action	Why
Place a dark mat, felt circle, or grid made of masking tape on the floor in front of doorways	People who have impaired thinking often stop and will not use the doors, because they think there are holes or puddles in front of them.
Cover doors with wallpaper or curtains.	Covering the doors makes them less noticeable.
Place mirrors on doors.	Cognitively impaired people often stop when they see the reflection of a person in a mirror, because they do not recognize themselves.
Place a stop sign on a door.	Cognitively impaired people have better long-term memories and respond well to brightly colored safety signs that they remember from the past.
Use self-adhesive fabric to attach an 18-inch strip of fireproof fabric to a doorframe, or hang cafe curtains that swing open.	A cognitively impaired person often stops when he sees the fabric and will not cross through the door.
Encourage a person in your care to help you with simple tasks such as folding napkins, sorting papers, decorating a bulletin board and pushing a beverage cart.	Keeping busy helps a person feel useful and active.
Suggest that your employer install alarms on all doors leading to the outside or to dangerous areas; or suggest the use of a movement sensor or alarm signal attached to the person's body or clothing.	Alarms will alert health care workers if someone is trying to leave.

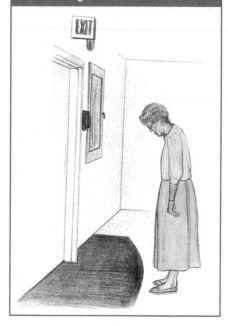

FIGURE 19-3 The staff in this nursing home painted a black band in front of each exit door to prevent a confused person like Shirley McDay from wandering outside.

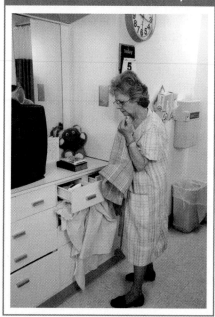

FIGURE 19-4 A nurse assistant placed common items in this drawer to satisfy Mrs. McDay's desire to rummage. The nurse assistant learned several of Mrs. McDay's hiding places so that items could be returned to the drawer when necessary.

behavior, use some of the following suggestions:

- Do not scold her, because she may become fearful of you as her caregiver.
- Try distracting her. Offer her another activity or a snack. Reorient her to the location of her own personal belongings.
- Take her to the bathroom. (She may have been searching for it when she wandered into someone else's room.)
- Learn her hiding places so that you can find lost items.
- Use your sense of fun and humor to help Mrs. McDay enjoy her environment, but be careful not to laugh at her behavior.
- Label all of her personal items and provide specific places for them. Put valuables away.
- Keep a spare set of keys in a safe place.

- Provide a rummaging drawer (Figure 19-4).

Catastrophic Reactions. When you greet Mrs. McDay this morning, she ignores you and seems restless. You explain to her that you want to give her a tub bath. After you gather supplies and prepare the bath, you approach Mrs. McDay. You mention again that you are going to help her with her bath. She begins to yell and lash out and then tries to hit you.

Mrs. McDay is having a *catastrophic reaction*. Whenever a situation overwhelms her ability to think or react, she tends to overreact because she has lost the ability to control her impulses. At times she may strike out at people around her. When such situations occur, what should you do?

When responding to a person in your care who is having a catastrophic reaction, first identify yourself as you approach her. Look for nonverbal cues to her behavior. What nonverbal cues indicate that Mrs. McDay might be uncooperative? Do not take the attack personally. Avoid arguing with her. Keep routines as structured, predictable and orderly as possible.

Although Mrs. McDay's behavior during a catastrophic reaction cannot be controlled, the situation can. Stay calm. Prevent Mrs. McDay from injuring herself or anyone else, but do not restrain her. Acknowledge her anger by saying something such as, "You seem very upset. What is upsetting you?" or "Things can get pretty scary when you're alone. What is frightening you?" or "You seem to be uncomfortable. What is making you uncomfortable?" or "Where do you have pain? Let's see what we can do to make you feel better." After each question, wait for a verbal or nonverbal response. What are some ways you can help Mrs. McDay if she is afraid, uncomfortable or in pain?

Reassure Mrs. McDay that you aren't going to hurt her and won't allow her to hurt anyone. Let her know the limits by saying something such as, "It's not okay to hit someone. It hurts." Distract her with her favorite activity. If she remains unable to respond to your request, try giving her a bath later.

Sundowning. As late afternoon or evening approaches, you may notice that a person who has Alzheimer's disease gets more and more restless or confused. She may become more demanding, upset, suspicious or disoriented. The person may be experiencing a behavior called *sundowning*, which is common to people with Alzheimer's disease. What do you think would cause a person's spirits to go down and anxiety go up when the sun goes down?

During the day, as the hours pass, a person with Alzheimer's disease may

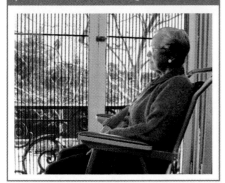

FIGURE 19-5 Agitation is one aspect of sundowning. Relaxing or taking an afternoon nap may give a person more energy later in the day and prevent sundowning.

become tired or less able to handle stress or may have difficulty **coping** with things. Approaching darkness may cause her to feel confused or afraid (Figure 19-5). Instead of communicating her needs, she may exhibit some of the following signals:

- Restlessness, anxiety
- Worried expressions
- Reluctance to enter her own room
- Reluctance to enter brightly lighted areas
- Crying
- Wringing her hands
- Pushing others away
- Gritting her teeth
- Taking off her clothing

These signals may represent real physical needs, such as needing to use the bathroom or being hungry, uncomfortable or in pain. On the other hand, they may represent the need for loved ones who once shared her evenings, other human contact or control over something. What are some ways you can identify the person's needs?

It is important to know how to respond to a person who is experiencing sundowning. After determining that the person does not have physical needs to be met, look for other clues that could tell you what her emotional needs might be. She may have a wor-

ried look on her face. She may be frightened of the dark or of unfamiliar sounds, or she might be afraid of being left alone. Accept her feelings.

Provide a night light for the person to see her surroundings, avoid glaring, bright lights. Offer to stay and visit with her. Talk softly to her and rub her arm or back. Comfort her with something to cuddle, and play soothing music. Try to keep bedtime at the same time each evening. Developing a bedtime routine may help.

If Mrs. McDay experiences sundowning, try giving her some flowers to arrange to remind her of her former work in the flower shop. These measures should improve her feeling of security. If her reaction to approaching darkness includes pacing, provide a secure, visible place in which she can safely pace, or take her for a walk.

Find out when Mrs. McDay normally rested and try to follow that pattern. Before she had Alzheimer's disease, Mrs. McDay worked hard all morning in her shop and usually put her feet up after lunch. To follow that pattern, keep Mrs. McDay active in the morning and let her rest after lunch. Plan fewer activities in the evening. Don't argue and don't ask her to make decisions during her anxious times. A person experiencing sundowning needs to feel calm and secure.

A person displaying any or all of these behaviors is responding to something in her environment. You must remember that she is not behaving this way on purpose to make her caregiver's job difficult. Patience and understanding are vital for providing care for people who have Alzheimer's disease.

MAKING A DIFFERENCE WHEN PROVIDING CARE FOR A PERSON WITH ALZHEIMER'S DISEASE

Alzheimer's disease and the other dementias progress through predictable stages and worsen over time. People who have the early stages of

the disease may be able to receive health care at home. However, demands on the caregiver's time increase as the person becomes less and less independent.

Providing care for a person with Alzheimer's disease is a stressful and challenging task. Understanding the disease and the behaviors that accompany it helps you provide care for the person compassionately and safely.

A person with Alzheimer's disease still needs joy and pleasure in her life. Simple pleasures such as a warm comfortable bed, a gentle massage, soft music, sweet smells and bright colors can add to the quality of the person's life. Even when people are confused and out of touch with reality, compassionate care helps them feel more secure. Always remember to celebrate the person's life by looking beyond the disease and seeing the person inside.

When you provide care for a person who has Alzheimer's disease, it is important to remember that:

- The person does not act the way she does deliberately. It is the condition that causes her behavior.
- The person is an adult and must be treated with respect and dignity. Even though her behavior seems childlike, never laugh at inappropriate language or speech. Never talk about her as if she were not there.

When you provide care, keep the following overall guidelines in mind:

- Be creative and flexible. Something that works well for one person who has Alzheimer's disease may not work for another. If one thing does not work, try something else. Also, after a while, a particular technique may no longer work with the same person.
- Avoid situations that call for the person to make difficult choices or those that require the person to explain "why."

- Keep the environment calm and organized.
- Talk about pleasant past events.
- Be patient.

Caregiving Tips

Here are some additional tips to remember when you provide care for a person who has Alzheimer's disease.

Tips for Communicating.

When speaking to the person:
- Stand directly in front of her and maintain eye contact. Touching her arm or shoulder gently may help keep her attention focused.
- Speak softly, slowly and clearly, using simple words and sentences. If she doesn't understand, repeat the same words. Avoid talking to the person with AD like a baby.
- Use direct statements when you want her to do something. For example: "It's time to eat breakfast now."
- Minimize distractions and noise—such as the television or radio—to help the person focus on what you are saying.
- Call the person by name.
- Allow extra time for her to understand and answer. Don't expect a quick response to a question or statement. If you don't get an answer, ask the question again using the exact same words, or come back in 5 or 10 minutes to ask again.
- Try to frame questions and instructions in a positive way.
- Because a person who has Alzheimer's disease is more comfortable in her own reality than in the present, don't argue with her or confront her. If she believes that it's 1956 and she's 19 years old, don't tell her she's wrong. Respond to the emotions she expresses.
- To help orient her when she is confused, remind her about where she is, what time of the year it is and what day it is (Figure 19-6). For example, your resident may asks why her mother hasn't come home yet. You know her mother passed away 30 years ago. If you tell her that her mother is dead—it will feel to her like this is the first time she has heard this news. Instead ask her about mother, what kinds of things she bought at the store, the color of her favorite dress etc.

Tips for Responding to Behavioral Problems.

When the person exhibits behavior that seems inappropriate to you:
- Don't accuse her of lying or stealing. Her understanding of the world is different from yours.
- Use distraction. A temporary change of subject or scene often solves the problem. Often, distracting the person may cause her to forget what caused the problem.

Tips for Maintaining an Orderly and Safe Environment.

To keep the person's surroundings and activities orderly and safe:
- Follow a simple, set routine. Introducing change can be confusing for her.
- Avoid situations that could make her angry or frustrated.
- Show her how to do things. For example, move your arm in an appropriate motion to demonstrate tooth brushing.
- Do activities in small steps. Remember that she is able to pay attention for just a short time.
- Remove safety hazards (Box 19-1).

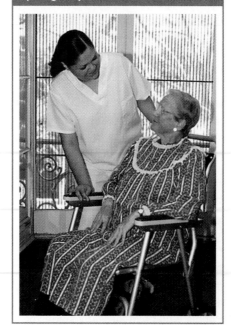

FIGURE 19-6 In the morning, to help orient someone who is confused, say, "Good morning, Mrs. Jones. Today is Tuesday, and it's a warm, beautiful spring day."

Tips for Promoting Dignity and Independence. To show respect for the person and to promote her dignity and independence:

- Help her dress independently. Set out her clothes in the order in which she will put them on (Figure 19-7).
- Praise her actions as often as possible.
- In a nursing home, try to get her involved in scheduled activities that occupy her time, calm her and give her a feeling of purpose and accomplishment.
- Make sure she gets enough exercise.

Caregiving Techniques for Helping with Daily Activities

Use the following techniques when helping a person who has Alzheimer's disease with bathing, oral hygiene, dressing and grooming, mealtime and elimination.

Bathing. A person who has Alzheimer's disease may refuse to bathe because it seems too complicated. Furthermore, the person may believe that her privacy is being

invaded. Respect her need for privacy and dignity.

- Find out the person's bathing schedule and stick to it.
- Have everything ready before starting. Be calm and unhurried. Avoid discussing whether the person needs a bath. Use expressions such as, "It feels good to be clean."
- If the person resists, try distraction or wait and try again later. Never use force.
- Avoid using a shower. Water coming from above may frighten her.
- Use only a few inches of water in the tub. If the person objects or seems unhappy, adjust the water level according to her comfort. Keep the bathroom very warm because people who have Alzheimer's disease get chilled very easily. Make sure safety mats, side rails and grab bars are available.
- Remove locks from the bathroom door. Remove electrical appliances such as hair dryers and curlers, electric razors and radios from the bathroom.
- Never leave the person alone in the bath or shower.

Oral Hygiene. Often a person with Alzheimer's disease doesn't brush her teeth or allow anyone to help her brush them. If she fights the procedure, stop and try again later. Use motions and gestures to encourage her to do it alone (Figure 19-8). In some cases, mirror the movements: pick up a toothbrush to prompt her to do the same, or move a toothbrush in your mouth so that she will do the same. Sometimes seating the person in a recliner and standing to the side while giving mouth care may make her feel less threatened.

Dressing and Grooming. A person with Alzheimer's disease may not know what clothing is appropriate to wear, which garments to put on first or

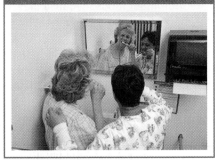

FIGURE 19-8 Sometimes showing a person who has Alzheimer's disease how to do a very common task is enough to trigger her memory of how to complete the task.

how to fasten clothing. She may become frustrated with trying to dress or groom herself.

- Try to have the person get dressed at the same time each day so he or she will come to expect it as part of the daily routine.
- Encourage the person to dress himself or herself to whatever degree possible. Plan to allow extra time so there is no pressure or rush.
- Allow the person to choose from a limited selection of outfits. If he or she has a favorite outfit, consider buying several identical sets.
- Arrange the clothes in the order they are to be put on to help the person move through the process.
- Provide clear, step-by-step instructions if the person needs prompting.
- Choose clothing that is comfortable, easy to get on and off and easy to care for. Elastic waists and Velcro enclosures minimize struggles with buttons and zippers.
- Have her wear shoes with nonskid soles (not backless shoes, however, because they may cause the person to trip or fall).
- Go slowly. Come back to an activity if it becomes too frustrating.

FIGURE 19-7 Encourage a person who has Alzheimer's disease to choose between two clothing options, and lay the garments out in the order in which she should put them on. Place outer garments on the bottom and underwear on top.

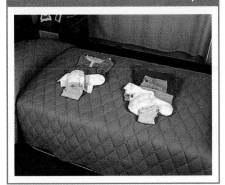

Mealtime. A person who has Alzheimer's disease may not remember whether she has eaten, how much she has eaten or what she has eaten. She may not remember how to use eating utensils and may have to be fed or reminded to chew or swallow.

- Offer finger foods, because they may be easier for the person to handle and less messy.
- If the person chokes easily, grind or chop the food.
- Try to serve foods that the person likes.
- Have healthy snacks on hand. To encourage eating, keep the snacks where they can be seen. Use straws or use cups with lids to make drinking easier.
- Use self-help devices to help the person feed herself. (See Chapter 14, "Healthful Eating.")
- Serve food warm. Make sure it is not too hot or too cold.
- Provide a limited number of choices of food and serve small portions.
- Put only one food in front of the person at a time.
- Use simple instructions such as, "Pick up your fork. Put the food on it." Repeat as necessary.
- Remind the person to chew and swallow.
- Avoid placing things like ketchup, salt or pepper on the table until the person asks for them, because she may use them inappropriately, or they may distract her.
- Keep things that might look like food (dog biscuits, flower bulbs, marbles, beads etc.) out of sight.

Elimination. Think about all the activities that you do in the bathroom— telling a person "it is time to go to the bathroom" can be very confusing. A person with Alzheimer's disease may not recognize the signals that tell her she needs to use the bathroom. She may not remember where the bathroom is or what to do once she gets there. It may help to do some of the following things:

- Post a picture of a toilet on the door of the bathroom to help the person recognize it (Figure 19-9). Use reflective tape around the door to help her see at night.
- Set a regular schedule for going to the bathroom, and include using the bathroom as a regular activity after she has eaten. Maintain a regular routine for using the toilet for as long as possible to minimize and delay the need to use catheters and adult briefs.
- Watch for signs such as restlessness that may indicate that the person needs to go to the bathroom.
- When helping a person get to the bathroom, turn on the light before she enters the room.
- A person with Alzheimer's disease may not want to enter the bathroom. She may think her reflection in the mirror is another person. Try removing or covering the mirror.
- Help the person remove or adjust clothing as necessary.
- Respect the person's need for privacy.
- Encourage the person to eat a high-fiber diet to help prevent con-

stipation. (See Chapter 14, "Healthful Eating.")
- To help prevent nighttime accidents, limit certain types of fluids—such as those with caffeine—in the evening.

Helping People Who are Agitated, Confused or Wandering

You must have reliable information to find successful ways to help a person with dementia. A person in your care may communicate this information to you verbally or through her behavior and facial expression. The information also might come from family members and friends. As you gather information, look for clues and ask questions (Table 19-2).

Focus on the Environment. Create a restful, stress-free environment for the people in your care to reduce some of the reasons for using restraints. Part of creating such an environment is establishing good communication. As you read in Chapter 5, "Communicating with People," people who cannot speak often communicate through their behavior and facial expressions.

Focus on Kindness. People who have severe cognitive impairment respond better to caregivers who treat them gently, sensitively and with respect. As a nurse assistant, you can provide better care for these people if they know that you care about them, are trying to understand them and are willing to help them.

Focus on Quiet. When providing care for an agitated or confused person, talk softly and eliminate as much extra noise as possible. Playing the person's favorite kind of music at a low volume on the radio may help.

Focus on Calmness. To help an agitated or wandering person relax and to help satisfy her need for motion, encourage her to sit in a comfortable rocking chair. Give her something soft

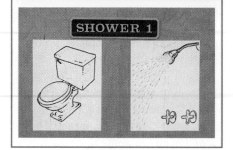

FIGURE 19-9 Placing pictures on a door shows a person who has Alzheimer's disease what is behind the door. Visual prompts help a person who may be unable to read written signs.

TABLE 19-2 LOOKING FOR BEHAVIORAL CLUES

General Question	Specific Question
What problem does the person in my care have?	Is the person's wandering a problem for her?
Is there a need behind this problem?	Why does the person need to wander? What is she looking for? Does she need to see that everyone is safe?
When does this behavior happen?	Is there a pattern or routine? Does the person's wandering happen at certain times every day?
What circumstances make this problem worse?	Does the person seem especially restless after taking a certain medication? (If so, perhaps the supervising nurse needs to discuss this reaction with the doctor.)
If a behavior pattern is the problem, is there a connection with a behavior from the person's life in the past?	Is this behavior similar to the behavior the person had in a job she held in the past?
What is the problem for the health care team involved in providing care for this person?	Is the problem that the person might fall, get lost or upset other residents?
Can the health care team members accept her behavior and ensure her safety?	Can they put her needs before theirs? Can the health-care team accommodate the person's need to "make rounds"? Are there ways to let the person wander without endangering herself or others?

to hug, such as a stuffed animal; this also may help calm her.

Focus on Familiarity. Encourage family members to bring in items that are familiar to the person in your care. Although it is true that even confused people living at home may wander, a person's desire to wander may decrease if she feels at home in her room.

UNDERSTANDING THE NEEDS OF FAMILY CAREGIVERS

Most dementias, including Alzheimer's disease, are chronic conditions that last for the rest of an affected person's life. A disease of this kind may be overwhelming to the person who has the condition and to her family. The loss of the ability to

think and reason causes dysfunctional behavior that is difficult for family members to understand. To be able to cope with the person's behavior and celebrate the person's life, family caregivers must take care of their own needs.

The family is an important part of the care that this person receives. Get the family involved in the planning of the person's care when possible.

Circle the correct answers and fill in the blanks.

1. Loss of the ability to think and reason is called _dementia_.

2. Of the people diagnosed with dementia, the majority suffer from _Alzheimer's_.

3. Behavior is a form of _communication_. The person is trying to tell you something.

4. Early in the disease process, a person with Alzheimer's disease may pretend to remember someone or something when in fact she does not. This behavior is called putting up a _social facade_.

5. Mrs. McDay keeps wandering into other people's rooms and taking their personal items. You often find the missing items in Mrs. McDay's dresser drawer. What is the best response to this behavior?
   a. Scold Mrs. McDay so that she will understand that she cannot take other people's things.
   b. Have Mrs. McDay return the items and force her to apologize for stealing.
   c. Return the missing items to their owners yourself, and try to determine when Mrs. McDay is most likely to wander into someone else's room and the reason why she behaves this way.
   d. Keep Mrs. McDay confined to her room so that she does not have the opportunity to take things.

6. Mrs. McDay's behavior described in question 5 is an example of _____ and _hoarding_.

7. Mrs. McDay becomes very upset and starts to scream at you and other staff members when you ask her to sit down for breakfast. Her extreme reaction is an example of:
   a. pacing.
   b. catastrophic reaction.

   c. sundowning.
   d. social facade.

8. Which is the best response to Mrs. McDay's behavior?
   a. Restrain her so that she does not hurt herself or someone else.
   b. Walk away.
   c. Tell her that you understand that she is upset and offer to walk with her for a while.
   d. Insist that she sit down because she should know better than to behave like that.

9. Which of the following would be most useful in helping Mrs. McDay find her own room?
   a. Placing a recent picture of her on the door.
   b. Writing her name on a sign on the door.
   c. Placing a picture of her family on the door.
   d. Placing a picture of her as a young woman on the door.

10. Mrs. McDay confronts Mrs. Morgan in the hall and accuses her of wearing her clothes. What is the best thing for you to say?
   a. "You both have such good taste in clothes. I think it's time for lunch now. Come with me."
   b. "Don't be ridiculous. You know that she wouldn't even be able to fit into your clothes."
   c. "Mrs. Morgan, tell Mrs. McDay that you are not wearing her clothes."
   d. "You're absolutely right. I'll make her take them off immediately."

1. How would it feel to provide care for someone who paces and wanders and has to be watched constantly?

2. How would you feel if you were unable to control your bowels and bladder?

3. What things could you do to give dignity and respect to a person with Alzheimer's disease? How could you give her joy and pleasure?

4. What are some things you can do to prevent a person who has impaired thinking from leaving a room?

20

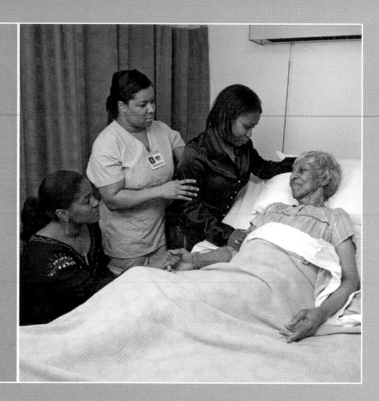

Providing End-of-Life Care

GOALS

After reading this chapter, you will have the information needed to:

Define *palliative care.*

Define *hospice care.*

Discuss factors that influence a person's reaction to death.

Discuss the five emotional stages of death.

Describe what is important to persons who are dying.

Describe your role in providing for the needs of a person who is dying.

Recognize pain and nonpain symptoms experienced at the end of life.

Discuss the needs of the family and friends of someone who is dying.

Recognize signs of approaching death.

Recognize signs that death has occurred.

Discuss the bereavement process for family, friends and staff.

After practicing the corresponding skill, you will have the information needed to:

Provide postmortem care.

Josie Miller has been a resident of your skilled nursing facility for the past 2 years. She has advanced heart and lung disease that limits her ability to care for herself. She is no longer able to walk in her room because of shortness of breath and severe arthritis. During the past 6 months Josie has been hospitalized for pneumonia and congestive heart failure three times. After the last time, Josie told her family that she doesn't want to go back to the hospital again. She signed an advance directive saying that she wants to be kept comfortable but does not want any special measures taken to prolong her life.

Over the past few weeks Josie's condition has gotten worse. She has trouble eating and is losing weight. She does not want to get out of bed because of pain and feels that she is too weak to sit in her chair. Her doctor gently told Josie that there is no treatment that will cure her condition. He let Josie and her family know, however, that there are many things that can be done to keep her very comfortable; this is called *Palliative* or Comfort Care.

As a nurse assistant, you help people as they deal with illness, injuries and medical conditions. You work with people to help them gain strength and to encourage them to become as active as they can be so that they can improve their health and, if possible, become well again. But illness is not always followed by improved health or recovery. Some-

times death occurs suddenly, and sometimes it comes at the end of a long struggle.

Because you may have to face the death of a person in your care, it is important for you to understand certain things about death and dying. You must recognize feelings you may have, and you must have particular information so that you can help someone through the dying process and provide emotional support to grieving family members and friends.

PALLIATIVE CARE

Palliative care is the term used to describe a special approach to care at the end of life. It is the active total care of patients whose disease is not responsive to curative treatment. The focus of care is on controlling pain and other symptoms and includes care for psychological, social and spiritual problems. The goal of palliative care is to help dying persons and their families have the best possible quality of life.

Some terminally ill people receive palliative care through a health care delivery system known as *hospice care*. Many years ago, the word *hospice* simply meant a place of hospitality and caring for travelers. Today, *hospice* refers also to the philosophy of giving special care to those who are dying. Hospice care is a system of providing the dying with care by health care teams and volunteers.

Central to the hospice way of thinking are the ideas that the dying

person is an individual who should not be separated from the family or support system and that dying is a normal and expected part of the life cycle. The family is encouraged and trained to participate in the care. The focus is on keeping the person as comfortable and pain-free as possible, because the fear of pain greatly contributes to the stress of the person, his or her family and the caregivers. The emphasis is not on curing the illness, but rather on providing physical, emotional, social and spiritual comfort to the dying person. The hospice philosophy also provides practical assistance, emotional support and **bereavement care** to the dying person's family.

The hospice philosophy also allows the person to die in her own way, surrounded by the people she loves. The person is able to participate in the rituals that hold special meaning for her. Most hospice programs provide care for the dying in their homes, in the nursing home in which they live or in special facilities in which care is provided. Some hospitals and nursing homes have hospice units. The principles of hospice and palliative care are important to practice with all persons who are dying, even those not enrolled in a formal hospice program.

Factors that Influence a Person's Reaction to Death

How do you think you might feel if someone you know were to die? You might feel sad, angry, powerless or guilty. When you have these feelings, you might try to ignore them because they make you uncomfortable or because they are too painful to deal with. It is a natural and normal reaction to want to distance yourself from the things that make you sad or uncomfortable or give you pain.

During past centuries, most people died at home with their families around them. Death and dying were considered normal parts of life. Many popular stories and songs were writ-

---

KEY TERMS

bereavement care: (buh-REEV-ment) care provided for people who are grieving after someone dies.

lividity: (luh-VID-uh-tee) dark discoloration of a dead person's skin as a result of blood pooling.

rigor mortis: (RI-ger/MOOR-tis) rigid extremities, which occurs 6 to 8 hours after death.

taboo: (tah-BOO) forbidden.

ten about the death of a loved one. In this century, though, as doctors learned more and more ways to save lives, many people began thinking of death as unnatural and frightening. Talking about death became **taboo.** It was almost as if people believed they could keep death from happening if they did not talk about it. How healthy do you think this attitude is?

Before the 1960s, health care workers were not trained to talk about death with people in their care. As a result, people with terminal illnesses often felt isolated in a health care setting. In fact, they frequently were put in private rooms so that their dying would not upset other people receiving care. Health care workers did not tend to stop by to visit with them as they might with people who were getting better. Dying people were sometimes viewed as the failures of the medical profession. As a result, a dying person felt uncomfortable about discussing her or his feelings about death and dying with caregivers. During the 1960s, health care professionals began to realize that people needed help in dealing with these feelings; thus the "death awareness" movement began.

Death, like birth, is part of life. Dying can take place in the presence of loving family, friends and health care workers. Or a person may die alone. As a nurse assistant, you may be the only one with the person who is dying. The person may not have a family, her relatives might live too far away or she may no longer be close to them.

Age. Many people are exposed to death for the first time when an older person dies, such as a grandparent who has lived a long life. With advances in medicine, Americans now live well into their 70s and 80s. Death in the later years of life is much more expected, accepted and understood, and it generally causes less stress for

family members than the death of a younger person or a child. As you read in the section on human development (Chapter 4, "Understanding People"), dealing with death is something that an older person attends to in that part of the life cycle. However, it is not something young adults, adolescents or children normally deal with.

Death can occur at any stage of the life cycle and can be either expected or sudden and unexpected. Although the death of an older person—especially if she has had a long, debilitating illness—is not pleasant, the death of a newborn, child or young person is generally seen as an unjust tragedy.

Talking about death is frightening to some people because it is so final and because it causes them to think about their own dying (Figure 20-1). The more you understand your feelings about death, the better prepared you are to help others make the transition from life to death. Being comfortable with your own feelings about death might help you to listen, touch

and respond appropriately to the dying person and to the family and friends who also may be struggling with painful feelings.

The age of a terminally ill person is one factor that influences how a person reacts to being told of her own approaching death or that of a loved one. Some other factors that may influence her reaction are her culture, sense of fulfillment, religion and family and friends. To gain insight about how the person feels about death and how you feel about death, ask yourself the questions listed after each of the following factors.

Culture. What stories about dying did the person learn when she was growing up? Was she taught that death is part of life or that it is to be feared? *How do people in your family talk about death?*

Sense of Fulfillment. Did the person live her life fully, with little regret? Were her basic needs met? Was she able to fulfill her hopes and dreams? Was her life purposeful, meaningful

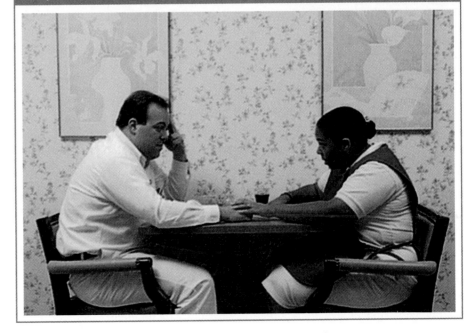

FIGURE 20-1 Talking with friends or co-workers can help you sort out your feelings about death.

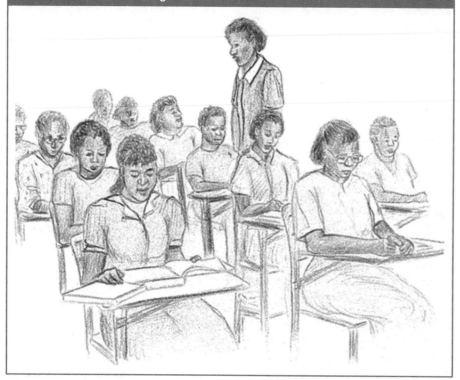

and rewarding? (Figure 20-2) *Are you doing what makes you feel good about yourself and your life?*

Religion. Does the person hold a belief in a spiritual being and an afterlife, which provides additional support and meaning? Or does this belief (or lack of it) cause a feeling of dread for what comes after death? *What do you and the people in your family believe about an afterlife?*

Family and Friends. Does the person feel loved and connected? Has she been able to finish any "unfinished business" in her life? If not, does this situation make her feel angry about death? "Unfinished business" may include needing to talk about unresolved guilt, regret or resentment; sharing messages of love and appreci-ation with significant others; or just simply saying good-bye to someone. *What unfinished business would you want to take care of with the people who are important in your life?*

Five Emotional Stages of Dealing with Dying

The factors that you just read about show how our past experiences with living affect our view of death. Dr. Elis-abeth Kübler-Ross, an early pioneer in the death awareness movement, iden-tified five stages of emotions that the dying person may experience: *denial, anger, bargaining, depression* and *acceptance.* Each person may go through these stages at his or her own pace and may move back and forth among them instead of progressing straight through them.

Denial. Denial means that the dying person cannot accept that something so terrible is happening to her. For example, she cannot accept that she has a terminal illness. A period of denial is a time when the shock of the information makes the dying person put it away so that she can delay deal-ing with it until she is more emotionally ready. Sometimes a person starts out by acknowledging her illness and the likelihood of death and then slips into denial, which becomes a crutch that supports her until she is ready to deal with this harsh and frightening reality. Some people move back and forth between denial and reality.

Anger. What kinds of things do you say when you are angry? Often the dying person expresses anger, which is an expression of other underlying emotions: fear, resentment and frustra-tion. If her anger seems to be directed toward you, it is important that you do not take her emotional expressions personally. She may really be angry at her situation, not at you. She may not be able to express her angry feelings to her family, and so she goes through this critical stage by expressing her anger at you or other caregivers, per-haps over some insignificant thing you said, did or did not do. It is most help-ful to try and look *beyond* the anger to the emotion that is behind it. Looking at the underlying emotion may give you a better understanding of what she is really expressing and may help you to know how to handle it best.

Another person may become angry with the higher spiritual being that she worships. She may ask, "Why me?" or "What did I do to deserve this? Am I being punished?"

Bargaining. A person may try to bar-gain for more time by making a deal, usually with her higher spiritual being. For example, she may think or say, "If I just make it to my daughter's wed-ding, I'll be ready to go. I won't ask for anything else." The specific nature of the promise, however, is not important. What is important is that the person uses this time to take care of unfinished business. Listen to what the dying person says but make no judgments.

Depression. If you have ever felt depressed, what did you think about during that time? Depression in this stage of the dying process can take two forms: (1) grief over past losses, disappointments and unfulfilled dreams; and (2) preparation for the losses to come. For example, Rodney Britten wants to talk with you about the losses he feels as his death approaches. It is important to listen to and accept this sorrow, because it is a sad time. A time of depression is not the time to try to cheer him up, to try to distract him from his grief or to try to convince him that he has much to be

grateful for in his life. You may be the only person the dying person can talk to about preparing to die, because his family may not be available or may be fearful of talking about the person's death (Figure 20-3).

Another behavior you begin to see at this stage is withdrawal or detachment. The person's interests begin to decrease. He may no longer show an interest when people talk about home, politics or business. He gradually loses interest or detaches from everything around himself except for his needs for comfort and his concern for the people he loves. This stage may be harder for some men who are dying, because they may believe that they do not have permission to cry or grieve.

Acceptance. Think back to a time in your life when you may have finally accepted something after a difficult

struggle. This acceptance may have been a time of calm for you. That does not necessarily mean that you were happy, but perhaps you felt more peaceful. The dying person feels peaceful when she reaches this emotional stage in the dying process. Her acceptance allows her to "let go" of the need to fight the inevitable movement from life into death. It is a time of peaceful resignation.

Not all people go through all five of these stages, and even if they do, they may move back and forth among the stages. It is not your job to help the person move through these stages toward acceptance. Your role as a nurse assistant is to listen, be kind, accept the person's feelings and try to be understanding. Helping a person who is dying means providing her with emotional support while she deals with this tragedy in her own personal way and at her own emotional speed.

Elisabeth Kübler-Ross said that dying people teach us how to live, how to look at our own lives and how to see every day as a precious gift. This is what we receive from the people in our care.

When a Person is Dying

The approaching death of a person affects many lives. Family members and friends begin to experience their own grief. Caregivers, particularly those who spend a great deal of time with the dying person, also experience feelings about the impending death. All these feelings must be recognized and dealt with so that they do not interfere with the quality of care the dying person receives.

What is Important to Dying Persons?

Recently there has been an increased focus on improving the care of dying person and their families. Studies have been done to learn from those who are dying what health care workers can do to help them. One of the most

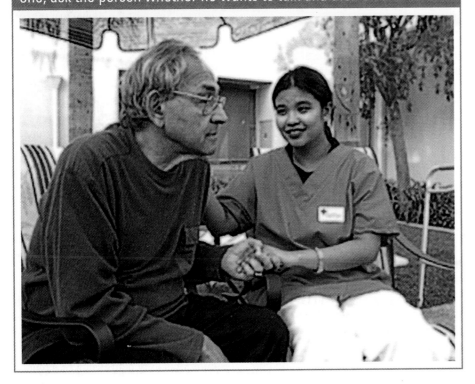

FIGURE 20-3 A person who wants to talk about his approaching death may not give you many verbal cues. When you think you hear one, ask the person whether he wants to talk and then sit and listen.

BOX 20-1

HOPES AND WISHES OF A DYING PERSON*

1. To be kept clean
2. To name a decision maker
3. To feel comfortable with my nurse
4. To know what to expect about my condition
5. To have someone listen to me
6. To maintain my dignity
7. To trust my doctor
8. To have financial affairs in order
9. To be free of pain
10. To keep a sense of humor
11. To say goodbye to important people
12. To be free of shortness of breath
13. To be free of anxiety
14. To discuss my fears with my doctor
15. To have a doctor who knows me as a person
16. To resolve "unfinished business"
17. To have people touch me
18. To know that my doctor feels comfortable talking about dying
19. To share time with close friends
20. To know that my family is prepared for my death
21. To feel prepared to die
22. To have my family with me
23. To have my treatment preferences in writing
24. Not to die alone
25. To remember my life accomplishments
26. To receive care from my regular doctor

*Steinhauser, K.E., Christakis, N.A., Clipp, E.C., McNeilly, M., McIntyre, L., and Tulsky, J.A. Factors considered important at the end of life by patients, family, physicians, and other care providers. *JAMA* 2000; 284:2476–2482.

important things is to know what is important to a person as they get closer to death. Box 20-1 lists some of their hopes and wishes.

Providing for Needs of the Dying Person

From reading Box 20-1, it is clear that your role as a nurse assistant is very important in responding to the needs of a dying person. You spend so much of your time providing the very intimate and personal care that can mean so much to someone who is dying. By applying the principles of care and your knowledge about what the person and her family are experiencing and by expressing your compassion, you can make a difference in how people experience the dying process. Table 20-1 lists the principles of care and some examples of what you can do for the dying person.

Common Symptoms Experienced by Persons Who are Dying

Although certain diseases may cause particular symptoms, there are many symptoms that are commonly experienced by persons who are dying. As a nursing assistant, it is important that you become familiar with these symptoms, recognize when they occur, and report them promptly in order for the dying person to receive the necessary treatment.

Pain. Pain is the most common and most feared symptom that occurs when someone is dying. Many people think that uncontrolled pain must always be part of the dying process. However, even severe pain can be managed. Letting a dying person and their family know this helps to decrease their anxiety. Your role is to ask frequently whether the person you

are caring for has pain and to learn what makes it better and what makes it worse. Some of the daily care tasks you must perform may be associated with pain or discomfort. Alerting the nurse to this is important so that pain medication may be given before the painful activity takes place. Some dying persons have problems communicating, which may limit their ability to report pain. Therefore, it is helpful to look for other signs that might show whether the dying person is in pain. Crying, grunting, pained facial expressions and resisting care are some examples of nonverbal signs of pain.

Shortness of Breath. Another symptom that occurs among persons who are dying is shortness of breath, which may be caused by heart failure, lung diseases, neurologic disease and complications from other diseases. This symptom is very distressing to a dying

TABLE 20-1 DOING YOUR BEST FOR A DYING PERSON

Principle of Care	What You Can Do
Communication	Talk about what the person wants to talk about. Be open and accepting of beliefs and ideas that may be different from your own. Respect the person who may not want to talk at all, recognizing that your nonverbal communication becomes even more important than usual. Make eye contact and stay in touch by making physical contact. When you stand at the bedside, put your hand on her hand, arm or shoulder. Talk in a normal tone of voice and avoid whispering. Even if the person is unconscious, don't say anything you would not want her to hear. Listening and touching are your two most important tools. Do not isolate the person or leave her alone for long periods of time. She may feel that you have given up on her if she finds herself alone. However, ask occasionally to see whether she *wants* to be alone, because a person who is dying may want time alone to think or pray.
Dignity	Treat the person as an individual. Continue to offer choices and ask permission to provide care. Consider and respect the person's religious and cultural preferences. She may or may not wish to have a priest, rabbi or minister present. She may wish to have a favorite passage from a book read to her or a favorite piece of music played. Specific rituals may have to be performed before or at the time of death. A person of the Roman Catholic faith who is near death may want to have a priest called in to administer the Catholic ritual for the dying. If the person is an Orthodox Jew, it is important to know that the body must not be handled or touched after death until after the prescribed ritual is performed by a rabbi. Many religions and cultures have their own customs and rituals relating to death. Ahead of time, be sure to ask the person in your care or her family members whether something special needs to be done and make sure this information is recorded in her care plan. If the religious or cultural practices are not followed, the family members may experience additional unnecessary grief. Not only will they have to deal with the loss of a loved one, but they may also feel guilt or anger associated with not performing a required ritual.
Independence	Give the person the opportunity to do as much for herself as she is able and willing to do. A dying person does not lose her sense of pride or her need to be in control.
Privacy	Provide care quickly and efficiently to allow her maximum private time with her family and with her clergy, if requested.
Safety	Provide care as usual. Even though the person may not be as mobile as before, you must make sure that she is safe. Keep the room comfortable, lighted, well ventilated, clean and neat.
Infection Control	Practice Standard Precautions as always. You can prevent unnecessary discomfort by providing proper skin care and by meeting the person's nutritional and elimination needs. Provide excellent personal care, especially mouth care, because the person's mouth may be extremely dry.

person and their family. You may provide relief for mild shortness of breath through proper positioning and helping individuals with relaxation and special breathing techniques. Sometimes increasing air circulation with a fan in the room provides comfort for those who feel breathless. Severe shortness of breath may require medication such as morphine and the use of oxygen.

Pressure Ulcers. The dying person may also experience pressure ulcers or bedsores. To prevent or reduce their occurrence, you may need to change the person's position in bed more often than every 2 hours. Ask your supervising nurse whether a special mattress can be used to help protect the skin.

Other symptoms that may occur include decreased appetite, depression, constipation, nausea/vomiting and anxiety. Ask yourself what you can do to help relieve some of these symptoms. Most important, keep the person as comfortable as possible.

PROVIDING FOR NEEDS OF THE FAMILY

When dealing with the approaching loss, family and friends experience emotional stages similar to those of the dying person. They may feel denial, anger, resentment, a need to bargain, depression and ultimately, acceptance and recovery. This grieving process often begins before the loss occurs and continues for many months afterwards. In the case of the loss of a spouse or a child, the grieving period may take years. The person who is grieving eventually begins to resume normal activities, but the grieving process continues.

You must accept and not judge the family members' feelings of sadness, anger or relief. You can be supportive by listening and giving physical comfort and by asking about their personal needs for food, water, coffee or tea or rest. Encourage family members to talk with you about their feelings for the person. Let them know that other members of the health care team, such as social workers, also are available to talk and listen.

Encourage family members to touch the dying person. Your comfort and ease in touching the person as you provide care is an example that the family may follow. Even an unconscious dying person can still hear and feel and may find it very consoling if family members hold her hand and talk about happy times they shared with her. As a nurse assistant, you can help family members feel comfortable about sharing memories by asking questions about the dying person's life. You might encourage them to bring family photos in so that everyone can see the photos and talk about them (Figure 20-4). This activity helps the dying person and the family to review the accomplishments and happy times of her life.

As a nurse assistant, you have an opportunity to provide needed attention and support to a dying person, as well as to her family and friends. Your caring should focus on the person's basic human needs and respect their dignity, privacy and individuality. You may feel rewarded and fulfilled knowing that you have helped others through a difficult time.

Working with the dying person, their families and their friends also can be stressful and can trigger many feelings. To help others effectively, you must understand your own feelings about death. Just as you encourage people to talk about their feelings, you also must talk about your feelings. You may have formed a close relationship with the dying person and her family, and you may experience the loss with sadness or relief. Talk with your supervising nurse or social worker, and after the person dies, attend memorial services, if possible.

When Death Comes

Josie Miller has died from complications of heart and lung disease. After a few minutes of crying, Josie's daughter Sheila asks whether you would help her select a dress for Josie's burial. You tell Sheila that you will and say that you know how much choosing a pretty dress would please Josie, since she was always so particular about her appearance (Figure 20-5). Sheila says, "I know my mom was angry and difficult when she first moved in here. After she was diagnosed with the heart condition, she hated leaving her apartment and didn't want to admit that she couldn't take care of herself anymore. The doctor told her she probably didn't have long to live. She didn't believe him and did not like this place or anybody in it. But you were the first one to win her over. You were

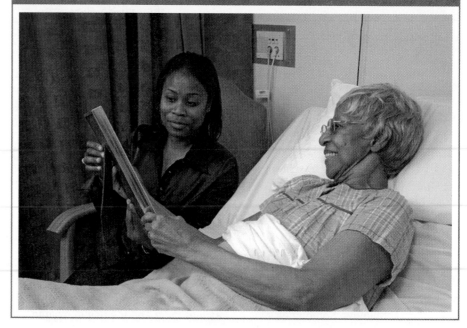

FIGURE 20-4 Josie and Sheila look over their family photo, from Sheila's wedding.

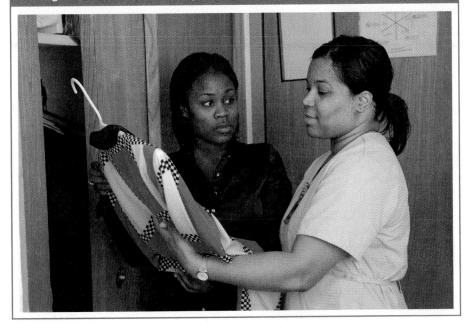

FIGURE 20-5 As Sheila begins to think about making funeral arrangements, she asks for your help in choosing a dress for Josie.

so patient and understanding of her feelings."

Signs of Approaching Death. As death approaches and the body systems of the dying person shut down, you begin to see many changes. These changes may occur gradually or rapidly. The signs may not necessarily occur in the order listed in Box 20-2, and not all the signs may occur in everyone.

Signs that Death has Occurred. A person is considered to be dead only after a doctor has examined her and pronounced her dead. When a person has died:

- She has no pulse, respiration or blood pressure.
- The pupils of her eyes are fixed (no movement) and dilated (widened).
- Her skin shows areas of dark discoloration as the blood pools on the side on which she is lying. This condition is called **lividity.**
- Her body becomes cold.
- Her bladder and bowels may empty.

- Her extremities become rigid within 6 to 8 hours. This condition is called **rigor mortis.**

Providing Postmortem Care. The word *postmortem* means "after death." Even after a person dies, she and her family have the right to be treated with dignity and privacy. It is very important to respect the family's need to have time with the person who has died before any postmortem care is started. Some families may not want to see the body at all after death, but some may need time to be with the body. This need should be respected, and family members should not be rushed.

Handle the person's body with care and respect. If someone is helping you to provide this special service, your conversation should be respectful and appropriate. Sometimes when people are uncomfortable with a new situation, they may laugh or joke as a way of dealing with their feelings. If you are uncomfortable, be sure to talk to your supervising nurse and ask for assistance if necessary. Feelings are not right or wrong, but as a good nurse assistant, you do not want your feelings to get in the way of doing your job well. It is helpful to think of what the loss of this person's life means to the family and the community.

When providing care for the body of a person who has died, you must know the policies and procedures followed by your employer. When provid-

---

BOX 20-2

SIGNS OF APPROACHING DEATH

- Elevated temperature
- Rapid, weak or irregular pulse
- Decreased blood pressure
- Cool, moist and pale skin
- Cold and pale hands and feet
- Increased perspiration
- Incontinence
- Periods of increased, shallow respiration followed by

periods of decreased respiration
- A gargling sound with breathing caused by mucus in the airway.
- Loss of, or a drifting in and out of, consciousness
- Loss of movement
- Loss of the ability to communicate

ing care for a dead person's body, follow the specific procedure that is explained step by step in Skill 57. You also must be sensitive to the feelings of others who share the room with the one who just died. They may feel frightened and sad and may need your attention and reassurance.

Bereavement for Family, Friends and Staff

After you and Sheila select a dress for Josie to wear for her burial, Arlene looks at the picture of Mr. Williams and Josie on Josie's nightstand. "And you were the one who brought Jack in to meet her," Arlene says to you, smiling.

You say that you think it was love at first sight with Mr. Williams and Josie and you chuckle.

"They were quite a pair, weren't they? They were always together," says Arlene. Suddenly, Arlene says, "Oh no, poor Jack. He doesn't know Josie has died. He'll be heartbroken." She says that she'll go and tell him right away, before he finds out from somebody else.

With tears welling up in her eyes, Arlene takes the framed picture of Josie and Mr. Williams off the nightstand and says, "I know Josie would like Jack to have this picture." Arm in arm, you and Arlene walk together toward the dayroom, where

Mr. Williams spends much of his time. You wait a few minutes to watch as Arlene gently breaks the news to Mr. Williams.

The death of a person in a nursing home can greatly sadden staff and other residents, as well as their families and friends. The residents know each other and usually have had time to develop friendships (Figure 20-6).

As a nurse assistant in a nursing home, you probably are one of the people who know the dying person very well, and the person may feel closer to you than to other people in the facility. Therefore, you may have both a personal and a professional desire to provide care for the dying resident. It is a special privilege for a

nurse assistant to help a resident come to the end of her life with peace, dignity and a feeling that someone cares. You may experience anger about the person's extended suffering, relief that her suffering has ended and sadness at the loss of a relationship. If you cannot work through these or other feelings, or if old memories of your own have been triggered, talk about them with your supervising nurse or social worker. Coming to terms with these feelings within yourself is important so that they do not interfere with your ability to support and help dying residents.

Be sure to tell other residents that the person has died so that they do not wonder and worry. Encourage residents to talk about their memories of the person who died and help them to remember the good things. When you give information about the person's death to other residents, you may say whether she died peacefully, where she died, what she was doing at the time of death and who was with her. Encourage other residents to talk about their own fears about death or their sadness about losing a friend, and encourage them to attend religious or memorial services, if possible. Those residents affected by the death may pass through the emotional stages of grieving and need your ongoing attention.

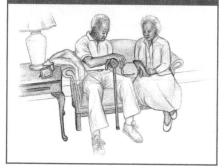

FIGURE 20-6 Mr. Williams is very shaken over Josie's death. He knew she had been very ill, but the news is still hard for him to handle.

INFORMATION REVIEW

Circle the correct answers and fill in the blanks.

1. Factors that influence how a person reacts to being told of her own approaching death or that of a loved one are:
   a. listening, touching and responding.
   b. the presence of health care workers and family members.
   c. death awareness and taboo.
   d. age, culture, fulfillment, religion and family and friends.

2. ___Palliative Care_____ is a term used to describe a special approach to care at the end of life.

3. The five emotional stages of dealing with dying are:
   a. denial, anger, bargaining, depression and acceptance.
   b. denial, delivering, bargaining, esteem and acceptance.
   c. preparing, experiencing, depression, elation and acceptance.
   d. posturing, preparing, anger, knowing and acceptance.

4. People in the denial stage of dealing with their own impending death may:
   a. acknowledge that they are going to die but feel that they need more time to finish writing a will and settle financial affairs.
   b. express outrage at the unfairness of having a terminal illness.
   c. express that they have finished up old business and are ready to die.
   d. state that their doctors are wrong and have made a mistake.

5. Family members of a person who is dying should be:
   a. encouraged to talk about their feelings and their needs.
   b. discouraged from participating in the care of the person, because it is too upsetting.
   c. encouraged to visit with the person who is dying for only a few minutes because it is too tiring for her or him.
   d. discouraged from expressing how they feel.

6. Some terminally ill people receive care at home through a health care delivery system called ___Hospice___.

7. Skin discoloration caused by pooling blood after death is called ___Lividity___.

8. Providing care for a person's body after death is called ___postmortem___ care.

9. The body of a person who has died should be handled with care and _____.

1. *How do you think Mr. Williams will react to the news of Josie's death? What are some things you can do to help him with this loss?*

2. *Mr. Williams discusses Josie Miller's death with a group of residents the day after her death. You notice that Mrs. Casey looks very upset and doesn't say anything. What should you do?*

3. *After Josie's death, Arlene calls the nursing home director to ask whether she can bring the flowers from Josie's funeral to the nursing home. How do you think the other residents will react? Arlene also asks whether it would be a good idea to have a short memorial service in the dayroom for the residents who knew Josie. What do you think about Arlene's idea?*

4. *Mr. Calloway, a 90-year-old nursing home resident, is dying after a long illness. He is a widower whose three children visit him at various times. Two of the children visit regularly to talk with him and comfort him. The third child, a son named Mike, seldom visits, seems quiet and withdrawn and stays for only a short time. One day when you are bathing Mr. Calloway, he says he is concerned about Mike. He says that Mike does not seem to care that he is dying, but that he often seems to be hurt, angry or upset. How would you respond to Mr. Calloway? What, if anything, would you report to your supervising nurse about Mr. Calloway's conversation? Why do you think Mike is behaving the way he is?*

Skill 57: Providing Postmortem Care

PRECAUTIONS

- Always follow universal precautions.

PREPARATION

1. Gather supplies:
   - One or two pairs of disposable gloves
   - Disposable bed protector
   - One or two completed identification tags
   - Clean sheet
   - Washcloth
   - Soap
   - Shroud—a baglike garment used to hold a dead person's body (optional)
   - Plastic trash bag
   - Laundry bag (or plastic bag for wet or soiled linens)
2. Follow Preparation Standards (see Chapter 7).

PROCEDURE

1. With approval from the nurse supervisor, remove any equipment, tubes, clothing or jewelry from the person (Figure 20-7, A). ☐ ☐
2. Replace dentures if approved by the nurse supervisor. ☐ ☐
3. Close the person's eyes and mouth and clean her body (Figure 20-7, B). ☐ ☐
4. Place bed protector under the person's buttocks and cover the body with a clean sheet. ☐ ☐
5. Put an identification tag around the person's ankle (Figure 20-7, C). ☐ ☐
6. Allow the family to view the body, if permitted. ☐ ☐

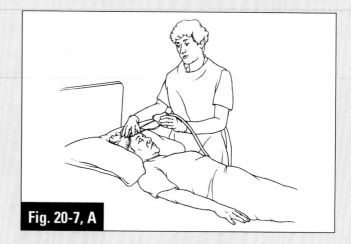

Fig. 20-7, A

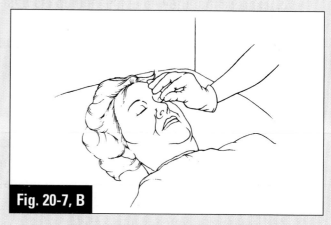

Fig. 20-7, B

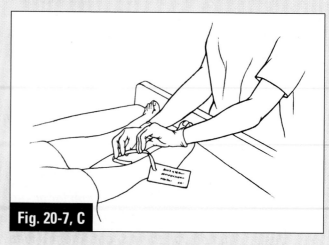

Fig. 20-7, C

7. Wrap the person's body in a shroud (if used) (Figure 20-7, D) and fold as follows:
   - Fold the top down over the person's head.
   - Fold the bottom up over her feet.
   - Fold the sides over the person's body and tape the ends together (Figure 20-7, E).
   - Attach an identification tag to the shroud. ☐ ☐

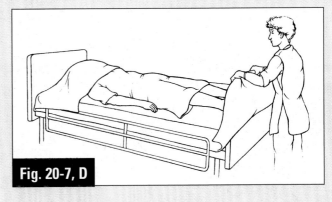
Fig. 20-7, D

 COMPLETION

Follow Completion Standards in compliance with your facility. For a complete list of those used in this course, see Chapter 7, "Controlling the Spread of Germs."

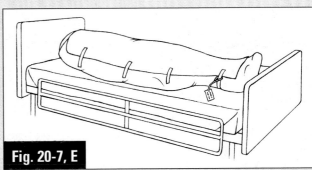
Fig. 20-7, E

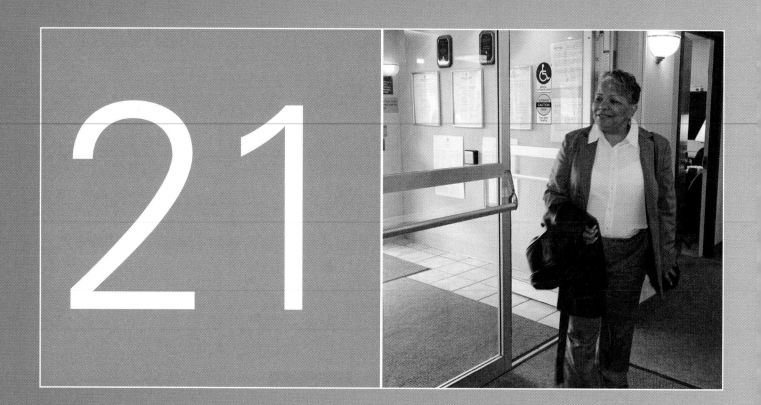

Chapter 21

Life Skills Training

GOALS

After reading this chapter, you will have the information needed to:

Do a job search.

Fill out a job application.

Design a résumé.

Interview effectively.

Prioritize your work time.

Use critical thinking skills.

Demonstrate how to cope with stress and anger.

Betty steps down off the bus on a winter day and wonders, "Am I ready for this?" She looks around her, takes a deep breath and pulls her coat tighter around her. She begins to walk, studying the addresses on the buildings she passes.

Betty feels as if she has become an expert at scanning the classifieds and filling out job applications. She has proofread her résumé over and over. But now she has an interview, and she wonders, "Will I know how to answer each question? Will they ask me any 'trick' questions? If someone asks me to describe my best skills, I don't know what I'll say! How can I talk about myself without looking as if I am bragging? What in the world makes a 'good interview'? Or is there even such a thing!"

Betty finds the building where she will soon have her interview. When she looks at her watch, she doesn't know whether it's good news or bad news that she is thirty minutes early. To calm herself down, she steps into a warm coffee shop next door and orders a soothing mug of herbal tea. And as she sits at a cozy booth, she goes over in her mind every challenging question she can think of and realizes—she has practiced ways of answering every question on her list.

She can approach this interview with confidence!

Betty is facing one of the greatest challenges anyone faces in looking for a new job. The interview. Most of us will have at least one job interview in our lives—and some of us will have

many! There is, after all, more to finding a job than reading the papers, filling out applications or mailing in a résumé. There is also the interview!

Even with all that, Betty knows, getting a job is one thing. But keeping a job involves strategy and planning, too.

How prepared are you?

LOOKING FOR A JOB AND GETTING A JOB

During your training you have been given the skills to become a nurse assistant. Some nurse assistants will choose to keep and enjoy this profession for years to come. Some will go on to become licensed nurses. Some will choose to leave the medical profession altogether. Whatever you choose to do, you are now ready for a major change in your life; this change is called a *transition*. You are now ready to make the transition from student, to applicant, to employee.

Many nurse assistant training programs are offered in a long-term care facility, which then may become the student's employer after graduation. Other programs are independent training schools. The information in this chapter will be of immediate help to you regardless of whether you have been trained in a facility or a school.

TRANSITION—FROM STUDENT TO APPLICANT

Identifying the Right Job for You

Once you have graduated from your program and passed your state certification test, you will start looking for a job. Before searching, it is important to ask yourself a few very important questions:

- What kind of job are you going to look for?
- Where do you want to work? Acute care, skilled nursing, office, clinic?

- When is the best time for you to work? Day, evening or night shift?
- What kind of job will fit you best?
- How are you going to get the job?

It will be important to know where, how and when to look for a job. Most people start looking for a job without a plan, which can result in wasted time and a feeling of frustration. You can avoid this—and increase your chances of success—by making a plan. Being organized will help you make the most of your search and find the job that is right for you. Once you have decided where, when and what you want, you are ready to make the first part of your transition from student to applicant.

The Job Search

Where to Look. There are many resources to help people who are looking for a job. Most people will begin with newspaper advertisements in the area where they want to live (Figure 21-1). You may know people who are already nurse assistants, and they can tell you about the places they work. There are employment agencies that know where open positions are posted. Some agencies do not charge applicants; they are paid instead by the employers. State and county offices of unemployment often have job listings, and the Internet can lead you to jobs and employment agencies.

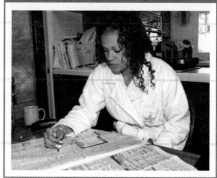

FIGURE 21-1 To begin your job search, look for jobs in the newspaper.

Here are the top seven resources that will help as you look for employment:

1. Ads in newspapers
2. Direct employer contact
3. Yellow Pages
4. School career centers
5. Internet
6. Library
7. New business openings

Additional resources include the following:

8. Job hotlines
9. Bulletin boards
10. Employment development department (unemployment department)
11. Personal business cards
12. Job fairs
13. Internship/volunteer work
14. Job shadowing
15. Trade journals
16. Chambers of commerce
17. Hidden job market
18. Newspaper
19. Local community colleges
20. Employment agencies

When to Look. Although nursing is not a seasonal job, there are certain times of the year when more positions open up. For example, many schools close for the summer, and this is when people with children tend to move, so there are usually more jobs available in June and July than in December when many people are celebrating the holidays.

How to Look: Reading Job Advertisements. Before you can begin to look for a job, you need to know how to read a job advertisement. You must be able to understand what the abbreviations in the ad mean. Table 21-1 lists common abbreviations

TABLE 21-1 COMMONLY USED ABBREVIATIONS IN EMPLOYMENT ADS

Abbreviation	Definition	Abbreviation	Definition
AA	Associate of Arts degree	EOE	Equal opportunity employer
Acct.	Accounting	Econo	Economical
Ad.	Advertisement	Exp.	Experience
Addl.	Additional	Flex.	Flexible
Apps.	Applications	FT	Full-time
Asst.	Assistant	HHA	Home health aide
Attn.	Attention	HS	High school
Avail.	Available	HR.	Hour
BA	Bachelor of Arts degree	Immed.	Immediate
Ben.	Benefits	K (as in $10K)	Thousand
Bkpg.	Bookkeeping	Max.	Maximum
BS	Bachelor of Science degree	Mgmt.	Management
Btwn	Between	Mgr.	Manager
CNA	Certified nursing assistant	Min.	Minimum
Co.	Company	M–F	Monday through Friday
Cust.	Customer	Mo.	Month
DMV	Department of motor vehicles	Non Smkg	Nonsmoking
ECE	Early childhood education	OT	Overtime

TABLE 21-1 COMMONLY USED ABBREVIATIONS IN EMPLOYMENT ADS—cont'd

Abbreviation	Definition	Abbreviation	Definition
PC	Personal computer	Sal.	Salary
Plyr.	Player	Sec'y	Secretary
Pos	Positions	SRV	Service
PT	Part time	Tel.	Telephone
P/U	Pick up	w/	With
Pref.	Prefer/preferred	Wk	Work/week
RE	Real estate	WPM/W.P.M.	Words per minute
Ref.	References	Yr/Yrs	Year/Years
Req'd/Req.	Required		

BOX 21-1

SAMPLE ADS

RECEPTIONIST
Ad agency seeks F/T hard wrkng, energetic individual for entry-level position. PC exper. a must. BA helpful. Fax (310) 555-1222.

NURSING CNA
All shifts. Student applications accepted. Early mornings, must be avail. Tues.–Sat. Paid wkly. (818) 555-9299.

NURSE ASSISTANT
FT. M–F nights. Sal $15/hr. Good ben. Exp. Pref. (319) 666-5555.

PART-TIME DRIVER
Floral deliveries. Good DMV record. Car insur. a must. $10.00/hr. to start. Well-organized w/ability to handle multiple tasks. Good communication skills and friendly. O.T. avail. Call Mr. Fred Potter. (818) 555-0000.

MEDICAL ASST.
Immediate FT/PT position. Must be pleasant & motivated. Span. Spkg pref'd M–F 40 hrs. per wk. No tel. calls please. Résumé/apply in person: Dr. Robert Jones, M.D. Attn: Lucy Smith, 111 Walnut Street, Pasadena, California.

used in job ads; compare these with the sample ads in Box 21-1.

The Effective Application

So now that you have found a job you want, what will be the best way to get the job? Filling out applications can be intimidating. Some of these forms are two or three pages long, and they often ask difficult questions. It is important to be honest in answering all the questions. As a new graduate, you will probably not have any experience in the health field. However, you may have learned skills in other jobs that your potential employer will find valuable. Think about those skills or talents, and make sure they are included on the application. All applicants are trying to impress the employer; but never lie or mislead on the application.

Always be neat in your handwriting, or if possible, type the application (Figure 21-2). Remember, the application is your introduction to the employer. You have only one chance to make a first impres-

FIGURE 21-2 Your job application must be complete and neat.

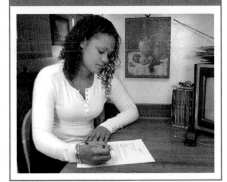

sion. When the employer is reviewing two applications—one written neatly and the other scrawled over the page—it is obvious which application will get the first interview.

Some employers will ask you to attach a résumé to the application. A résumé is usually a one-page document highlighting previous experience, education, personal information or qualifications. The most important thing to remember about a résumé is to keep it brief.

Designing Your Résumé

Résumés have several different formats, but all are in some way similar to the résumé in Box 21-2. Most will emphasize either employment history or prior job duties, qualifications and abilities. It is impossible to say which format is superior. This can be determined on an individual basis. If you have held a wide variety of jobs (i.e., delivery driver, fast-food worker, telephone solicitor), then focusing on the different experiences may be preferred. If your employment experience includes only one or two prior jobs, then focusing on their stability would work best. The most common format for a résumé begins with the individual information (name, address, telephone number, e-mail address) in the upper left corner or centered. This is usually followed by a one-line statement of the

---

BOX 21-2

SAMPLE RÉSUMÉ

Below is a sample résumé format:

Name _____
Address _____
City, State _____
Home phone _____
Cellular phone _____
E-mail address _____
Job Objective: Offering excellent skills in resident care and communications, seeking position as a nurse assistant.
Education: American Red Cross, Los Angeles, CA
- Precertification Nurse Assistant Program, June 2007
- Home Health Aide Program, June 2007

Work Experience:
Skills and Abilities:
- Bilingual: English/Spanish
- Proficient in taking accurate vital signs
- Skilled in resident assessment
- Conscientious
- Punctual
- Honest

Certifications:
- Certified Nurse Assistant, State of California
- Home Health Aide Certification, State of California
- BLS-CPR Certified
References upon request

---

type of job desired (i.e., "Seeking full-time employment as a ..."). This is followed by a statement of educational history, then employment history (or skills), and finally, a short statement of personal history or community involvement (e.g., volunteer at American Red Cross). Résumés serve as a "capsule" of the employee and should be limited to no more than two pages.

Interviewing for the Job

Interviews can be a stressful experience. It's important to reassure yourself that the employer wants to fill the job with the best possible candidate. They want you to do well in the interview, and most will try to put you at ease and make the process easy for you. Essentially, they are already on your side (Figure 21-3). Of course, there are specific things you can do to

---

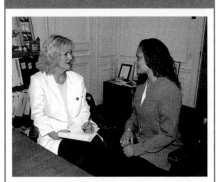

give yourself the best possible chance of getting the job.

When you get a phone call setting up an interview, make sure you learn all you can about what will be expected and how the interview will be conducted. What documents will they want to see? Who will interview you? Some interviews are done by one person, such as the Director of Nursing or the Staff Developer. Other interviews are conducted by a panel of two or three people. Sometimes there will be a "serial interview" in which you are interviewed by the Staff Developer first, then the Director of Nursing, then the Administrator. By knowing what to expect, you can be fully prepared.

Examine Box 21-3, a sample evaluation form. Note the criteria that interviewers are looking for; then read the sample interview questions below.

Practicing before an interview can be very helpful.

- Tell me about your past work experience and/or training that will help you with this job.
- Why did you want to become a nurse assistant?
- What do you like most about your job as a nurse assistant?
- Why did you choose this facility to look for employment?
- What are your career goals in 5 years?

The night before your interview, prepare yourself so that your morning will go smoothly. Select professional-looking clothing, making sure everything is neat, clean and pressed. It would not be appropriate to show up for your interview in either a party dress or a T-shirt, shorts, and sandals. Put together all the paperwork you will need for your interview and have it organized and ready to go with you. Get a good night's sleep.

On the morning of the interview, make sure you have everything you need before going out the door. Plan a little extra time to get there. It is always better to be 15 minutes early

---

BOX 21-3

MOCK INTERVIEW EVALUATION FORM

NAME OF APPLICANT (LAST, FIRST, MIDDLE INITIAL)
SPECIFIC JOB OBJECTIVE

Directions: Please rate the performance of the person being interviewed, using the criteria listed below. For each item, rate the person on a scale of 1 to 3, with 3 being the highest rating. Record each rating in the "Rating Selected" column. Add the ratings to get the total score.

Criteria	Rating Selected	Comments
1. Eye contact with interviewer		
2. Voice: consistent volume, appropriate tone		
3. Facial expressions		
4. Mannerisms: body movements, posture		
5. Appropriate dress and grooming		
6. Goal-oriented		
7. Appropriate responses to questions asked		
8. Effectiveness in describing strengths, skills and abilities in relation to the job		
9. Knowledge of company/job title		

WHAT DID YOU LIKE ABOUT THE APPLICANTS PERFORMANCE?

WHAT WOULD YOU SUGGEST FOR IMPROVEMENT?

Total Score _____   Maximum Score = 27

than to be 15 minutes late. If you plan to take a cellular phone, make sure it is "off" or on vibrate mode. You do not want a call to interrupt your interview.

When you meet the person or people who will be interviewing you, remember that manners count. Employers need to know that you will treat your patients, families, co-workers and managers with dignity and respect. A firm handshake is a great introduction. Be calm and at ease. If the employer likes you at the interview and you are selected for this job, everybody wins.

The interview begins. Listen carefully to each question. Make sure you understand exactly what has been asked. Keep your answers brief and to the point. Stay relaxed and focused. Do not get too intense, and remember to smile. Some questions may be very complex or difficult. It is all right to ask the interviewer to clarify the question. This is your chance to show the interviewer that you can "think on your feet"—that is, to adapt to the conditions of the interview. You can have a great interview and set the standards for everyone else who wants your job. Always think of it as *your* job. This shows you have self-confidence.

At the end of the interview, thank the interviewer(s) for the opportunity to come in. Each interview you go through will add to your experience and will make you better at the next interview. In the next day or two, call the interviewer, e-mail them or send a thank-you card. If the employer has narrowed the choice down to you and one other applicant, this follow-up call or card could make the difference. Take a little time to think about how you felt the interview went and whether there are things you can do better next time. Always make the interview a learning experience.

A successful applicant will have a good chance to receive a job offer. This is frequently done over the telephone. If you receive a job offer, get as much information about the position as possible. Ask about pay scale, benefits, hours, starting date, appropriate attire and who your supervisor will be. Remember, choose the job you think fits you best.

TRANSITION—FROM APPLICANT TO EMPLOYEE

The employer has made a decision and has called to offer you the job. Now you are ready to make the transition to employee and complete the process. All your hard work in school is now paying off. You have been a successful student and a successful applicant; now you have the opportunity to be a successful employee. Preparation will be the key to success.

Just as you prepared for the interview, you must prepare for work. Have appropriate clothing (usually a uniform) ready, neat and clean for every day you will work. Be mentally prepared to work hard, and enjoy what you do.

The first day in any new job will be the **orientation.** Federal law (and in most states, state law) mandates a certain number of hours to be spent in orientation. This includes filling out personnel forms (W-2s, emergency contact etc.), going over facility policies and procedures and so forth. During orientation it is also important to ask about the location and proper usage of emergency equipment such as fire extinguishers.

Understanding Expectations

Being a successful employee means understanding what is expected from your employer. During your orientation, you will learn about the job performance expectations. Employers should provide a written job description; this is your first opportunity to discover how, where, when, what and why things must be done a certain way. The employer will explain the hours of operation, attendance and behavior policies and define the employer expectations. Each workplace has its own "personality." That is, each facility operates the way the management wishes and in compliance with federal and state regulations and laws.

Employer Expectations. Here are some common expectations of employers:

- Show up on time and ready to work.
- If you will not be at work, call your supervisor or the designated person as soon as you know that you will not be coming in—at least 2 hours before your shift begins.
- Take breaks only when assigned. Follow these guidelines for taking a break:
  - Be sure your residents are safe.
  - Tell your supervisor where you are going and when you will be returning.
  - Tell co-workers to check on your residents for you.
  - Return within the time agreed upon.
- When your shift is over, report to your supervisor before leaving the floor.
- Clock in and out only on *your* time card; do not have *anyone else* clock in or out for you.
- Follow directions. If you do not understand, ask.
- Complete tasks. If you are not able to complete something, tell your supervisor.
- Document your actions. Remember this saying: "*It is not done if it is not documented.*" Documented means written down. If it was documented (legally), it was done.
- Be honest.
- Be loyal.
- Assist when needed.

Employee Expectations. Just as employers have expectations, any employee has a right to expect certain things from an employer. These expectations may include the following:

- Orientation
- Adequate staffing
- Mentoring
- Allowance for breaks and meal(s)
- Job duties within job description
- Safe work environment
- Adequate notice of shift changes
- Employee handbook that outlines and explains policies/procedures
- Positive work environment
- Explanation of emergency procedures
- Adequate notice of assignment changes

Probationary Period

Some jobs have a **probationary period,** which provides the employer time to evaluate job performance and potential—and gives the employee time to evaluate the employer. The lengths of probationary periods vary: some end after 90 days (3 months), whereas others may last up to a year. Some states and even some facilities have stopped the probationary period, in which case the employer has the right to dismiss an employee at will. Normally, at the end of the probation period, the employee's supervisor will complete a performance evaluation and discuss it with the employee. A decision on whether to continue or terminate employment will then be made.

Teamwork: Putting Yourself in Another's Shoes

During the first few days or weeks of employment, you will begin to fit into your job as a new employee. At first, you will notice differences between the classroom setting and the work setting. As you become more comfortable with your place on the team, your transition will be easier.

It is important for you to follow the directions of the supervisor responsible for orienting you to the facility. This may be the Director of Staff Development or a floor supervisor, who will be a licensed nurse. You may be assigned to work with another, more experienced nurse assistant who will act as a mentor. This person is essential in helping you to make a smooth transition. It will be important for you to learn as much as possible from these resources. The directions and information you receive during this period will help you as you become a team member. Fitting into a new situation can be difficult, tense and intimidating at times. Every new employee goes through this, and most are able to make the adjustment in time.

Managing Your Time

Time management is one of the most challenging tasks you face as a busy adult—particularly if you are a parent. You may ask yourself, "How do I juggle my job(s), time with my children and my spouse, time to do the laundry and house cleaning, time with my friends, time to pay bills and get groceries, and time for myself?" The Time Management Checklist, Box 21-4, will help you assess your own time management skills. In the meantime, here are some tips to help you manage all the things you must do: (Figure 21-4)

1. Plan ahead for each day. Prioritize your activities, allow plenty of time and have a backup plan (especially for child care).
2. Always plan to report to work at least 15 minutes before your shift starts.
3. Record all appointments and coordinate them with your work schedule.
4. Check your phone messages and write them down. Open mail daily.
5. Make sure you have a reliable alarm clock.

6. Have reliable transportation, either your own car, a car pool or public transportation.
7. Keep a monthly calendar of work and personal/family activities both at work and at home.
8. Share household duties with your spouse and children.
9. Establish set times for daily activities such as homework, baths and bedtime.
10. Pay bills twice a month (e.g., on the 1st and the 15th of each month).
11. Keep ongoing grocery lists and shop once a week for the entire week.

What other ideas do you have? Remember that backup plans are crucial to an initial plan. Always be able to answer questions such as "What if my child care provider is closed for the day or can no longer keep the kids? What if my car breaks down? What is my plan for when my children are ill?" Making a list of daily activities, planning times and ensuring backup plans are all essential in helping you keep your job, reduce your stress and accomplish your daily activities.

Knowing Certification and Renewal Requirements

Keeping your nurse assistant certification up to date is also essential to keeping your job. Although each state has different renewal requirements, the following documents and information are most commonly needed to renew your certification:

1. Proof of work
2. Inservice requirements/continuing education
3. Renewal fee
4. Application
5. Directions on where to send renewal forms and fees

Remembering your time-management skills are important in the renewal process. You have to plan ahead to have your inservice hours

BOX 21-4

TIME MANAGEMENT CHECKLIST

Answer *yes* or *no* to each statement in this time management checklist.

		Yes	No
1.	I get to work 15 minutes early so that I can plan my workday before it begins.	____	____
2.	I know what I want to accomplish each day.	____	____
3.	I list tasks that need to be done each day and check them off as they are completed.	____	____
4.	I take big jobs and break them into smaller pieces.	____	____
5.	I don't take too much time away from my work by continually listing and planning.	____	____
6.	I do the most difficult and least interesting jobs first thing in the morning.	____	____
7.	I don't put off tasks; I do them *now*.	____	____
8.	I avoid letting one day's work carry over to the next day.	____	____
9.	I make full use of each day to complete that day's work.	____	____
10.	I sometimes evaluate myself to find out where I lose time.	____	____
11.	People compliment me on my use of time.	____	____
12.	I don't spend too much time on the phone.	____	____
13.	I watch and learn from the people around me who always seem to be ahead of schedule.	____	____
14.	I look for ways to use my time wisely each day.	____	____
15.	I group tasks logically.	____	____
16.	I listen carefully when someone explains a task.	____	____
17.	I set deadline dates for myself.	____	____
18.	I stick to self-imposed deadlines and to those imposed by my boss.	____	____

Total the "Yes" and the "No" columns: ____ ____

completed, your renewal fee saved and your application completed and submitted before your certification expires. Remember: keeping your job means keeping your nurse assistant certification.

SURVIVING THE JOB

Using Critical Thinking Skills

To "survive" your job and all the tasks and activities you juggle among work, home and your social life, you need to use critical thinking skills. This process involves five easy steps:

1. Identify the problem.
2. List alternatives to solve the problem.
3. List the pros and cons of each alternative solution.
4. Decide on the solution.
5. Evaluate: Is the problem solved?

These critical thinking steps will help you in your everyday life and work.

Part of surviving a job means recognizing conflict and what actions are appropriate and what actions are not. Certain actions are never tolerated in the workplace. Violence or the threat of violence, resident abuse, sexual harassment, possession of weapons or illegal drugs, intoxication and theft are each considered grounds for immediate termination by most employers. Should you either witness or be subjected to any of these circumstances,

report them immediately to the supervisor or other administrative staff and complete an incident report.

What about other conflicts in the workplace? Conflict always has a negative impact at the job. It is important to remember that every member of the nursing staff, from the nurse assistant to the Director of Nursing Services, should demonstrate professionalism. Professionalism does not require staff members to like every other member of the team, but it does require all employees to work as part of the team. This means treating every member of the team (as well as patients and visitors) with dignity and respect. Even if a team member is rude to you, it is not

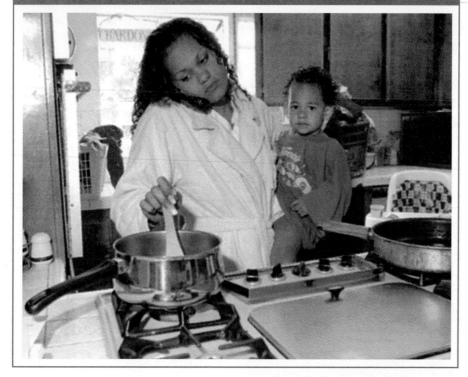

for me to want to work with you. I really don't like feeling this way." This statement expresses how the other person's behavior affects you; it is nonthreatening, and it invites conversation, which can lead to settlement. The two of you can discuss what is not right and decide how you can work together to make the situation better for both parties.

Most conflict can be resolved between the two parties involved. If you believe you have honestly tried, but failed, you can then bring the problem to the attention of your supervisor. All employers have a chain of command to follow. You do not have to like everyone you work with, but you have to work with everyone at your job. Always try to create a "win-win" situation.

Following the Chain of Command

Sometimes, even with your best efforts, the conflict cannot be

appropriate for you to be rude in return. To be a valued member of the team, the nurse assistant must have strong interpersonal skills and be able to resolve conflicts (Figure 21-5).

Creating the "Win-Win" Situation

It is always best to solve conflict as quickly as possible so that both parties have a more positive attitude about the future. This is the "win-win" solution. It is also best to confront the source of the conflict directly, but this does not mean attacking the other person. If you feel that another team member has been rude, it will most likely make matters worse to say, "You are really rude to me and everyone else; nobody likes being around a jerk like you." This will probably provoke the other person to counterattack. Rather, try saying something such as, "When you talk to me like that, it makes me feel bad, and it is difficult

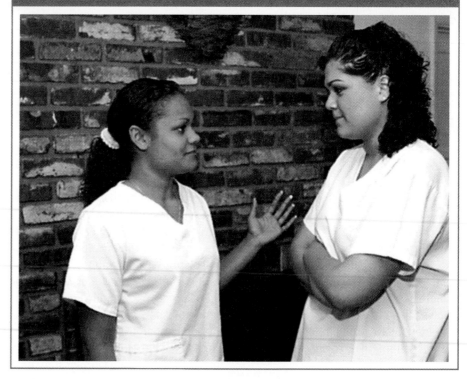

FIGURE 21-5 If there is a conflict, confront the source in a positive manner.

resolved between two persons. At that point, it is appropriate and necessary to involve someone else to try to resolve the problems. This person will usually be your immediate supervisor; however, this depends on the particular "chain of command" at your workplace. A common chain of command moves upward from employee to immediate supervisor to department head to assistant administrator to administrator to owner. Sometimes conflict resolution will involve every member of the chain of command; other times the conflict will be resolved in the first step. Regardless of how many members are involved in the resolution, it is vital that once the conflict is resolved, the central parties agree to "let it go."

Coping with Stress

Another important skill in surviving a job is your ability to recognize and cope with stress in your personal life and at your workplace. Recognizing your limitations and responsibilities and setting "rules" will help you cope with stress. Try the following coping skills:

1. Know your limitations; set limits for work, home and elsewhere.
2. Say no when you need to.
3. Stay within the scope of your job/practice (do not do something you have not been trained to do).
4. Identify responsibilities at work and home.
5. Get enough sleep (6 to 8 hours/night).
6. Eat healthy food; be aware of good nutrition.
7. Take time for yourself.
8. Exercise: walking, swimming, bicycling.
9. Organize your time.
10. Keep a sense of humor.

These steps will not take stress away, but they will help you cope with stress.

How do you recognize that you may be experiencing stress? Here are some signs of stress to watch out for:
- Muscle tightening
- Crying
- Headache
- Raising of voice
- Stomach ache
- Anger
- Change in eating patterns
- Sleeping problems
- Heart palpitations
- Inability to focus

Understanding Anger

Anger is a natural human response to stress. Anger is neither better nor worse than any other human emotion. Anger is important to human survival; it evokes the "fight or flight" response. Fight or flight response begins with a sudden release of hormones (adrenaline, norepinephrine and endorphins) in response to a perceived threat. Physical symptoms include elevated heart rate and central blood pressure, flushing of the cheeks, rapid breathing and decreased blood flow to the skin. Emotionally, this is the point at which a person feels the desire either to attack or run away. Some people report "seeing red." Have you ever felt that way? It is not important *whether* you get angry (everyone does at some point in their lives). The important thing is how you *handle* it. This is crucial to surviving your job and managing your personal life. The first step in managing anger is understanding why the behavior occurs. Let's explore a number of reasons:

Physical Conditions. Sometimes illness affects residents' behavior—illness such as dementia. Residents can become aggravated because of pain. They are not purposely trying to be mean. Co-workers also may exhibit negative behavior, especially if they are not getting enough sleep or nutrition, or if they suffer from migraine headaches or mental strain. These conditions make people less tolerant

of everyday experiences and they become angry more easily.

Life Experiences. Sometimes residents or co-workers learn aggressive or otherwise inappropriate behavior throughout their lives and continue this behavior when in a nursing facility.

Environmental Factors. When people feel out of control or frustrated, they may exhibit anger. This happens most often to residents who are receiving direct care, since this level of care may be confusing or humiliating for residents who were previously able to care for themselves.

Managing Anger

Remembering the following advice will help you to handle anger more effectively:
- Do not take it personally.
- Seek causes for the behavior, and watch for physical clues.
- Check to be sure signs of infection and/or injury are absent.
- Talk about the situation.
- Sit down and act calmly with the person exhibiting anger.
- If you are getting angry yourself, take deep breaths, take a walk or leave the situation—as long as the resident is safe.
- Talk in a calm, nonthreatening tone.
- Get at eye level with the person.
- Avoid touching someone if he is very angry.
- Do not get too close; this may be threatening to the person.
- If someone is angry about what you are doing, stop the task and give the person time to cool off.
- Ask for help if you need it.

WHEN IS SCHOOL OVER?

Learning begins at about the time the umbilical cord is cut. By the age of 1 to 2 weeks, an infant can distinguish his mother's voice from other voices. Similarly, you have been taught the basic skills and techniques to become a certified nursing assistant. Once on the job, you will continue to learn new skills and additional techniques to be a better nurse assistant. This process will continue for the rest of your life.

Much of what you will know 5 years from now will be "OJT"—that is, on-the-job training. You will have the chance to learn new skills, new methods, new science and new interpersonal skills. It is crucial to keep up to date with caregiving practices and to incorporate the constant flow of new information that you will receive during your lifetime and career.

Becoming a nurse assistant may be only a first step in your career. Some nurse assistants go on to become technicians, nurses, administrators, physicians or other types of health care professionals. Some will discover that being a nurse assistant is exactly what they want to do. Perhaps you will find the greatest satisfaction doing exactly what you have been trained to do here. Maybe you will decide that health care is not going to satisfy you, and you will move on to a completely different field. No matter how you decide your career

should proceed, you will experience life-long learning and skills that will help you in your career and your life. As you become successful in your job, those you are caring for will receive the care they need, and you will experience satisfaction from it.

WHAT'S THE BEST REWARD?

If you have decided to be the best nurse assistant you can, to give the best care you can, to be the best member of the team you can, then something wonderful will happen to you.

It might happen when you are discharging a patient home. It might happen after giving a distressed family member some time and comfort. It might happen when a former patient comes back just to see you. That person may look into your eyes and take your hand. There may be tears in the person's eyes. There may be tears in your eyes. Then the most wonderful thing that can happen to a nurse assistant will happen to you. The person will say "Thank you. You made it easier. You are a great nurse assistant."

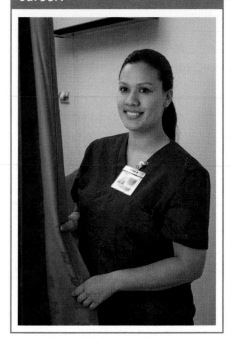

FIGURE 21-6 Being a nurse assistant is a rewarding career!

The reward is that you are giving care that someone needs, and without you, the care the person deserves may not happen (Figure 21-6).

You are critical to all you care for …

1. To practice applying for your first job as a certified nurse assistant, go to several different agencies and facilities and ask them for an application. Make several photocopies of each so that you can practice filling them out neatly. Keep these on file to help you organize your thoughts when you fill out others.

2. Using the list of criteria given in Box 21-3, practice your interviewing skills in front of a mirror, rating yourself on each item. After practicing, exchange lists with a friend, rating each other on these same areas.

3. Look at the list of bulleted questions on page 468. Try answering each of them until you feel confident you will not be caught off guard—but do not memorize your answers!

22

Managing Your Time

GOALS

After reading this chapter, you will have the information needed to:

Describe how to schedule your time each working day.

Discuss how to adjust your time if unplanned events occur.

Explain how to communicate clearly to help you stay in control of your time.

"I hate days like this," Nora Fuentes says to her friend and neighbor, Sylvia, as she sinks into a seat on the bus. "Why can't I get my act together? Just when I think I have a morning routine all worked out and I'm feeling like a super single mom, something unexpected happens. First the iron stops working before I've finished ironing my uniform. Then Ginny says her sweater doesn't match her pants and she needs me to help her pick out another outfit. Eight years old and she's already worrying about how she looks! Then, to top it all off, Emmy throws up her breakfast—everywhere. All over the kitchen floor. All over her clothes. And then, after I clean her up, she insists on getting dressed and going to school, because the first-graders have a special program today.

"Right now it seems almost impossible that I'll be able to concentrate on the residents in my care today. What if the school nurse calls to say that I need to pick up Emmy, who shouldn't have been sent to school in the first place? And if Ginny is clothes-conscious now, what will she be like when she's a teenager? And where am I going to find the money to pay for a new iron?

"All this when I woke up feeling great about beginning my second month as a nurse assistant. I sure hope I can manage my day at the nursing home better than I've managed my time at home today. It's a miracle that I'm even on the bus!"

LOOKING AHEAD TO THE WORKING WORLD OF CAREGIVING

While you are in training as a nurse assistant, someone else plans your work time for you. When you work as a nurse assistant, however, you plan much of your own time. In training, you provide care for a few people. In your work experience, you may have to juggle your time to provide care for many people at once. As you gain experience, you perform your duties more quickly and with more confidence. Learning to make the most of your time enables you to give people the best care possible.

The world of learning and the world of work are different. They *must* be different. When you learn new ideas and skills in a training program, you learn to perform every step of a task—such as giving a complete bed bath—in a specific, uninterrupted way. By learning the ideal way to perform these skills, you master how to perform each step.

When you work in a health care setting, the situations are not so specific and ideal. They become more complex. For one thing, other people and situations influence how you use your time. For example, someone else makes decisions about how many people are in your care. How much time

you spend caring for each person is also determined by factors outside your control—for instance, the person's medical condition and level of mobility (Figure 22-1). Finally, unplanned events happen when you least expect them. For example, you may be giving a bed bath when the person you are bathing becomes *nauseated* and begins to vomit. You have to stop what you are doing and sit the person up or turn his or her head to the side. Then, once the person is no longer vomiting, you must make sure he or she is okay, report the situation to your supervising nurse, and decide what new actions to take. In addition, you may have to consider the safety hazard of *vomitus* on the floor, the person may have to be bathed again, and the entire bed may have to be changed. You must make new decisions based on each new situation. No matter what you decide, this bed bath will take longer than normal.

Each day you make many decisions that affect the care you give and the time you have planned for the tasks you must perform. Your responsibility is to plan how to get all your work done as effectively as possible, regardless of the number and needs of people in your care.

As you move from the role of student to employed nurse assistant, you move into areas of greater responsibil-

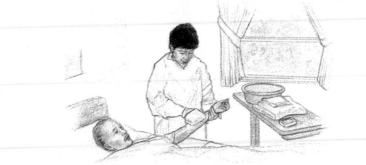

FIGURE 22-1 It takes more of your time to provide care for a person who must stay in bed than to help someone who is somewhat mobile and can do some things for him- or herself.

ity. You must handle this transition thoughtfully and carefully. You can make this transition smoothly if you know how to:

- Plan your time.
- Balance your scheduling needs and the needs of the people in your care.
- Stay in control of your time.

PLANNING YOUR TIME

Every day on your new job, you have many tasks to complete and details to remember. So far, you have been learning specific skills. Now you have to know how to put them all together. You must create a **schedule** to guide you through the day. At first, scheduling your time seems difficult. As you gain experience, you will find the best way to plan your day.

In a nursing home setting, at the beginning of each shift, you find out how many people are in your care and who they are. The nursing care plan and a verbal report from either the caregivers who worked on the previous shift or from your supervising nurse give you information about the kind of care that each person needs or changes to the existing care plan. You also learn about prescheduled activities or treatments. As you listen to the report, take notes, being careful to write down the following:

- Daily tasks that have to be done at specific times, such as measuring vital signs, providing treatments, serving meals and turning and positioning
- Daily tasks that must be done but have no set time, such as bathing, dressing and oral hygiene
- Special things that have to be done or considered that day for the people in your care, such as a nursing home resident's scheduled trip to the beauty shop, a person's appointment with the physical therapist or an appointment for an electrocardiogram

After listing the tasks that you must do that day, think about the order in which to do things and write down a tentative schedule. Often you will feel pressured to begin the day's activities without planning, but it will save you time in the end if you take a few minutes to create a plan before you start.

Some tasks might involve important preparation steps. For example, you may have to schedule time to use the tub room before you can give a person a tub bath. When you make your schedule, be sure to include each step in the larger tasks.

Your employer may provide a worksheet on which you add notes to remind yourself of each person's needs. For example, you may want to note that Mr. Wilson had an upset stomach yesterday or that Mr. Britten is worried because his partner is flying to Australia on business today. You may want to note the tasks that will require the assistance of your co-workers. You need the help of one or more nurse assistants or special equipment when you transfer a person who:

- Weighs a lot
- Is frail, weak or in pain
- Is much taller or larger than you
- Has pressure ulcers
- Is unable to bear his or her own weight

You also may need a supervisor's assistance when you do not have the experience needed to work with a specific person.

After you finish your schedule, put a star next to each task that must be done at a specific time. Then **prioritize** the remaining tasks by marking the most important ones to remind you to do them first, if possible. Now, when you look at your schedule, you know *what* must be done and *when* it must be done. Unscheduled events always occur. But when you know what *has* to be done, it is easier to readjust your schedule.

As a nurse assistant, you spend a great deal of time with the people in your care. Because of this constant involvement, you often are the person most familiar with their desires and special needs, and you learn how to fit their needs into your schedule. For example, you may have learned that Mrs. McDay becomes agitated if she is rushed through her morning care or if her usual routine is changed; in addition, you know that when Mrs. McDay becomes agitated, it takes much longer to provide comfort and care for her. So it makes sense to stick to her routine as much as possible and to be relaxed when providing care for her.

What do you do when you need additional time to care properly for Mrs. McDay? How do you cope when an assignment is too risky for you to handle alone or too time-consuming for you to do your best job? How might you feel when it seems as if you are being asked to do the impossible, or when asking for help seems like "dumping" on co-workers who already are dealing with their own heavy loads? These questions are difficult to answer, but in the real world, these situations do happen.

If members of the health care team are dependable and honest in handling their responsibilities, it makes it easier to handle unexpected situations. For example, when one member of the team decides to "play hooky" or calls in sick, or when she does not "pull her weight," her workload has to be split up and given to the team members who are there until a substitute becomes available. This places an unfair burden on everyone and causes resentment. On the other hand, sometimes a health care team member really *is* sick and needs an unexpected day off. If each team member is honest and considerate at times when special needs arise, the other members of the team should willingly work harder to carry the work load.

When an assignment seems too risky to handle alone or too time-consuming for you to do a thorough job, it is important that you discuss this problem with your supervising nurse. Perhaps your supervising nurse does not realize how much time you must have for the special needs of a person like Mrs. McDay. Or perhaps you do not realize that another member of the team has just called in sick. Sharing information with your supervising nurse and other team members helps the health care team work well together so that everyone can enjoy a sense of satisfaction from a job well done.

Resolving Schedule and Needs Conflicts

Mr. Rivera usually likes to receive his complete bed bath immediately after breakfast. After breakfast today, though, he says he wants to rest for about a half hour. Knowing how important his needs are, you let him rest and plan to come back in a half hour to give him his bath. If you had written a schedule for the day and Mr. Rivera's needs changed, what would you do with that half hour's time?

Every day, no matter how well you plan things for yourself, people's needs change—and so does your schedule. You may ask, "Why bother to make a schedule if I can never stick to it?" The answer is that the schedule is an important tool that reminds you of *what* you have to do, *when* you must do it, and *which* things are most important for you to do.

Working in a health care setting is much like traveling by car. No matter how well you map out your trip, you are bound to make some detours along the way. Your schedule is like a road map that helps you find an alternate route to your destination (Figure 22-2).

Staying in Control of Your Time

You have just finished helping Mr. Wilson brush his hair and shave. You're ready to leave his room to attend to the next thing on your schedule when

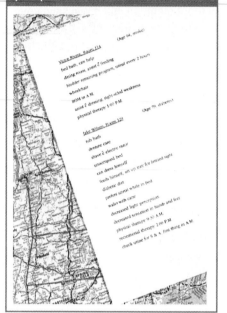

FIGURE 22-2 Think of your schedule as a road map that helps you "plan" your route as you provide care.

he says, "Before you leave, could you do one quick favor for me?" You say that you would be happy to do something for him. Then he says, "Please make me a nice cup of tea and some dry toast. I'm hungry, but I just couldn't eat breakfast. I don't want to wait for an order to come up from the kitchen."

You want to be able to do this special task for Mr. Wilson, but you think to yourself that his quick favor is not going to be quick at all. You know that this task may take 20 minutes of your time. What can you do now? What could you have done to anticipate this situation? How would you handle a similar situation in the future?

Sometimes, unplanned events can be handled by taking charge of your time from the beginning. When you first go into Mr. Wilson's room, check to see what has to be done and let him know how long you are going to be there this time. Also, let him know when you plan to come back. Before you start your tasks in Mr. Wilson's room, ask him whether he thinks he

might need anything special. If, at the beginning of your time with Mr. Wilson, he says he wants tea and toast, you can adjust the time that you spend on other planned tasks to include his special request. If you wait until the end of your time with Mr. Wilson to find out that he has special needs, these last-minute requests may affect the rest of your schedule.

If you communicate your plans clearly to the person in your care, you may lessen the number of unplanned events during the day. What you say through verbal communication is important, and *how* you express it with your face and body through nonverbal communication is equally important. The following tips will help you remember to communicate your message clearly and, in the end, may save time:

- When you assist a person, even on a very busy day, try to be relaxed. Remember that the person in your care is your reason for being there. If you seem to be hurried and stressed, the person also may become stressed, which may require you to spend more time with him.
- If touching is acceptable to him, touch the person you provide care for. Placing a hand on the person's shoulder or holding his hand is calming and helps him know that you care. Showing the person that you care about him may help him feel more secure and help you spend your time more efficiently and effectively.
- When you help a person, take time to speak with him and really listen to what he has to say. Sometimes the simple act of stopping and listening to the person shows that you are available. This action can reduce his anxiety and perhaps even save you time in the long run.

Planning your time well, knowing how to adjust your schedule and communicating your plans clearly to the person in your care may help you to control your time and, as a result, enjoy your job more and be more successful.

NORA'S DAY

In the following scenario, you will observe a day in the life of Nora Fuentes as she begins her second month of work as a nurse assistant at Morningside Nursing Home. The scenario does not provide all the possible types of decisions that you make as a nurse assistant, but it does show how one nurse assistant manages her time on one given day.

Nora arrives for work promptly at 7 A.M. She has been getting to know the residents at Morningside Nursing Home and is beginning to feel good about the way she performs her job. Some days, however, she finds it challenging to get everything done. Although she has been providing care for just five people, she knows that her load soon will increase to at least eight. Therefore, she feels a need to focus on how she manages her time.

Morning Report

Today, in morning report, Nora learns that she has five residents in her care: Rachel Morgan, Victor Rivera, Jake Wilson, Shirley McDay and Rodney Britten (Figures 22-3 through 22-7).

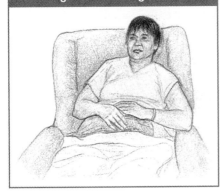

FIGURE 22-3 Rachel Morgan has multiple sclerosis. She lives in Room 121 at Morningside Nursing Home.

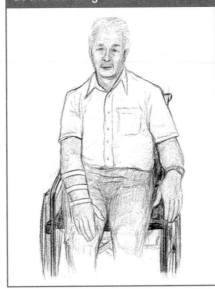

FIGURE 22-4 Victor Rivera had a stroke. He lives in Room 114 at the nursing home.

Nora already knows four of these residents well, but Mr. Britten has been at the nursing home just a few days. She looks at the quick, abbreviated notes she has written during report and reads:

Rm. 121 *R. Morgan*, 45, M.S. (un-bed)
- Can feed self (DR)
- Help with: bed bath—dressing—bedpan—transfer to WC—ROM
- Blurred vision—tires easily
- *PT—1 P.M.

Rm. 114 *V. Rivera*, 78, stroke (un-bed)
- Help with: bed bath—dressing—elec razor—urinal (7, 9, 11, 1)—feeding (DR)—transfer to WC
- L-sided weakness—*ROM in A.M.
- *PT—1 P.M.

Rm. 120 *J. Wilson*, 79, diabetes (un-bed)
- Can: dress—feed self (DR)—walk/cane—tub
- Help with: dentures—elec razor
- Sight—light perception—sensation: hands & feet
- *PT—10:30 A.M. Rec.T—2 P.M.
- *Urine S&A early A.M.—diabetic diet

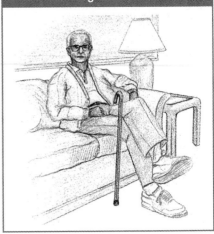

FIGURE 22-5 Jake Wilson has diabetes and lives in Room 120 at the nursing home.

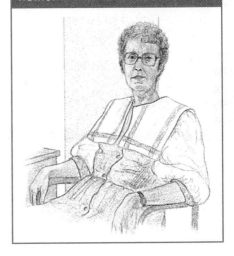

FIGURE 22-6 Shirley McDay, who has Alzheimer's disease, lives in Room 119 at the nursing home.

Rm. 119 *S. McDay*, 55, Alzheimer's (un-bed)
- Can: feed self (DR)—OOB BR—walk with assist
- Help with: tub—remind her to use the toilet—incont. care—dressing
- Wanders A.M. & P.M.—rummages and hoards

*Indicates that the task must be done at a particular time.

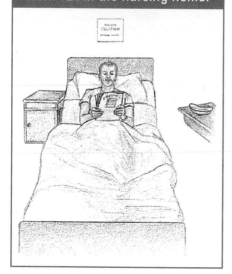

Rm. 124 *R. Britten*, 41, AIDS, wound isolation (oc-bed)
- Help with: bed bath—soft foods and liquids—bedpan
- Vomiting and diarrhea
- *V.S. in A.M.

Planning the Day's Schedule

After reading the morning report, Nora creates a schedule for the day's activities similar to the one shown in Table 22-1.

She looks over her schedule and notes that she needs help lifting Rachel Morgan and Victor Rivera into and out of bed. Nora decides to talk to her friend Arthur Cid to see whether he might be able to help her. Arthur has been working as a nurse assistant for 2 years, and Nora always learns so much from him. Arthur and Nora compare assignment sheets and realize that they are working in nearby rooms and that they both will need help with lifting, so they arrange to work

*Indicates that the task must be done at a particular time.

together. They also realize that they have the same lunch break.

Following the Schedule

Nora's first stop is Room 121, where she offers Rachel Morgan the bedpan. "I'll be back shortly to help you with your bed bath and dressing," Nora says before she leaves the room.

Nora's next stop is Room 114. She offers Victor Rivera his urinal. Because Mr. Rivera had suffered a stroke and is on a bladder training program, he must be offered his urinal every 2 hours. "I'll be back with your breakfast tray, Mr. Rivera," Nora says. Nora washes her hands after exiting Mr. Rivera's room.

She then heads to Room 120. Because Jake Wilson is diabetic, he has to have his urine checked for sugar and acetone first thing in the morning. He knows the routine well, so he urinated once earlier in the morning and then again later to provide a sample. Nora thanks him before asking how his favorite football team did in the game last night.

"The Redskins beat the Cardinals 34 to 10! You should have seen it!" Mr. Wilson says, his eyes sparkling. "I played some football myself when I was a young fellow."

Using Standard Precautions, Nora tests the urine for glucose and acetone and records the results, which she later reports to her supervising nurse.

"How are my 'levels' this morning?" asks Mr. Wilson.

Nora reassures Mr. Wilson that the test results are normal. She washes her hands and then walks with him to the tub room. While Nora helps Mr. Wilson with his dentures and shaving, they discuss his activities for the day.

"Today's my session with the physical therapist," he says. "I want to be on time for her."

"Don't worry, Mr. Wilson," says Nora, as she walks him back to his room. "You'll be there on time." She

then goes to Rachel Morgan's room to set up her A.M. care.

"I think I can wash myself today, but it may take me awhile," Mrs. Morgan says.

Nora smiles at her. "You just do what you can, Mrs. Morgan," she says at the door, "and I'll be back to help you finish your bed bath."

Nora puts on a gown and gloves before going into Mr. Britten's room to take his vital signs and provide A.M. care. Mr. Britten, who has AIDS, has developed a staph infection in an open wound on his arm and must remain in wound isolation until the infection is gone.

"Hello, Ms. Fuentes," Mr. Britten says quietly. Nora greets Mr. Britten and begins wrapping the blood pressure cuff around his unaffected arm. She asks him about his partner's trip to Australia.

A smile tugs at the corners of his mouth. "Owen leaves for Sydney today," he says. "Would you believe I already miss him? He'll be gone for 2 whole weeks." Nora records Mr. Britten's vital signs, which are normal.

"Maybe he'll bring you a kangaroo," she says.

"If he does, I'll name it 'Nora'," he says with a grin.

Nora discards her gown and gloves and washes her hands before going to Room 119, where she greets Shirley McDay, who has Alzheimer's disease.

"Hello, Mrs. McDay, I'm Ms. Fuentes, your nurse assistant. Today is Tuesday, it's 7:45, and it's time for your morning bath," says Nora. After the bath, Nora helps Mrs. McDay get dressed.

"I think I'll wear this outfit today," says Mrs. McDay, selecting a green blouse and an orange skirt from her closet. The blouse and skirt don't match, but Nora knows that green and orange are Mrs. McDay's favorite colors.

TABLE 22-1 SAMPLE CAREGIVING SCHEDULE

	Rachel Morgan	Victor Rivera	Jake Wilson	Shirley McDay	Rodney Britten (Reverse Isolation)
7:00 A.M.	Bedpan Set up A.M. care, bed bath, help dress	Urinal	Urine S&A Tub 7:15 Assist dentures/shave	Tub 7:45 Help dress	V.S. A.M. care (gown/gloves)
8:00 A.M.	Rest Up to w/c to DR (need help)	Tray setup/ Assist feed	Assist walk to DR	Assist walk to DR	Tray setup Assist feed Oc-bed
9:00 A.M.	Un-bed DR—back	Urinal A.M. care, help dress, ROM	DR—back	DR—back	Rest
10:00 A.M.	Rest in bed (need help) ROM	Up to w/c (need help) Un-bed	*10:30 PT Un-bed	Un-bed	
11:00 A.M. 11:30 lunch	Rest	Urinal		Check incont.	Check diarrhea
12:00 noon	Up to w/c to DR (need help)	Tray setup Assist feed	Assist walk to DR	Check incont. Assist walk to DR	Tray setup Assist feed Rest
1:00 P.M.	*1:00 w/c DR to PT	Urinal *1:00 PT	DR—back	DR—back	Check diarrhea
2:00 P.M.	Rest in bed (need help)	Rest in bed (need help) Wife visits	*2:00 RecT	Check incont.	V.S.
3:00 P.M. Report Charting		Urinal			Check diarrhea Remove trash and linens (need help)

* Indicates that task is to be done at a specific time.

Wanting to say something positive, Nora says, "That blouse looks so nice on you." Mrs. McDay smiles shyly (Figure 22-8).

Then Nora returns to Mrs. Morgan's room to help her finish her bed bath and get dressed. Because Mrs. Morgan tires easily, Nora helps her get comfortable in her bed so that she can rest before going to the dining room for breakfast.

Next, Nora washes her hands, puts on a gown with gloves and enters Room 124 (Isolation Room) with Mr. Britten's breakfast tray. She suggests that he start eating the breakfast himself while she helps the other residents to the dining room for breakfast. Nora assures him that she will come back to help him finish his breakfast.

Nora removes and discards the gown and gloves and washes her

FIGURE 22-8 Her outfit may be unusual, but Mrs. McDay feels good about being able to select her own clothing.

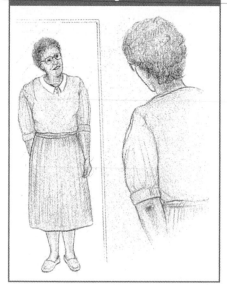

hands before enlisting Arthur's help with getting Mrs. Morgan out of bed and into the wheelchair. As she pushes Mrs. Morgan to the dining room, she stops along the way and invites Jake Wilson and Shirley McDay to walk with her and Mrs. Morgan to the dining room.

After getting the three residents settled in the dining room, Nora takes a breakfast tray to Mr. Rivera who, until his condition worsened this week, had been eating regularly in the dining room. She helps him with his breakfast by placing her hand over his hand on the spoon. He has difficulty chewing and swallowing, so it takes a long time to help feed him. "My wife is coming to visit me today," says Mr. Rivera, dribbling oatmeal out of his mouth. "I can hardly wait." Nora gently wipes his chin and discusses the visit with him.

Observing Isolation Precautions when she returns to Mr. Britten's room, Nora apologizes for taking so long. Much to her surprise, she finds that Mr. Britten has eaten all his breakfast by himself.

"I'm so tired, I just want to sleep now," he says. Nora leaves Mr. Britten's room. She removes and discards the gown and gloves and washes her hands.

While Mrs. Morgan eats breakfast in the dining room, Nora changes the linens on her bed. Then she washes her hands before she goes into Mr. Rivera's room and offers him the urinal.

"One of these days I'm going to be regular like a clock," Mr. Rivera jokes. Nora helps him with his bed bath and helps him brush his teeth. While helping him dress, Nora encourages Mr. Rivera to fasten as many buttons as possible with his "good hand."

"You did more buttons today than you did yesterday," she says when he becomes tired. "You're really making good progress." Mr. Rivera beams. When Mr. Rivera is dressed, Nora helps him slowly complete his range-of-motion exercises. Nora washes her hands after leaving the room.

On her way to the dining room, Nora smiles at Arthur, who is leading an elderly woman back to her room.

In the dining room, Nora greets Rachel Morgan and wheels her to the elevator.

"How was breakfast?" Nora asks.

"Today they had pancakes, which I just love," says Mrs. Morgan. When they reach Room 121, Nora tells Mrs. Morgan that she'll be right back with someone to help transfer her into her bed.

"All right, dear," says Mrs. Morgan. Nora steps into the hall and sees Arthur carrying bed linens.

"Arthur, could you please help me transfer Mrs. Morgan into her bed?" she asks.

"Comin' right up," says Arthur. "Let me just put these linens down in Mr. Lightfoot's room, and I'll be right there" (Figure 22-9).

After Mrs. Morgan is comfortably settled in bed, Nora heads back to the dining room, where Mr. Wilson and Mrs. McDay have finished breakfast. As the three near the elevator, Mr. Wilson mentions that he's going to visit a friend on the second floor. Nora glances quickly at her watch and

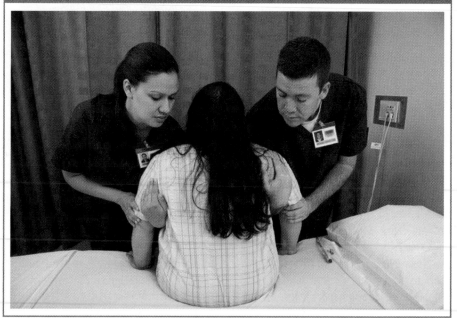

FIGURE 22-9 Nora and Arthur work well together. They know that they can always count on each other to be good team members.

reminds him about his physical therapy appointment.

"I'll be back in time," says Mr. Wilson. Nora walks Mrs. McDay back to her room.

"Is this my room?" Mrs. McDay asks as they near the supply closet.

"No, here we are," Nora says at the door to Room 119. She encourages Mrs. McDay to sit in a chair while Nora changes the linens on her bed. After the bed is made, Mrs. McDay climbs onto the bedspread and reaches for a magazine.

Nora sighs as she walks to Mr. Britten's room. She puts on a gown and gloves and enters the room. Mr. Britten is awake and is glad to see her. Nora gives him his bed bath, moving him as gently as possible to protect his fragile skin. She makes sure he is comfortable before leaving the room.

Getting Assistance

Nora washes her hands and heads toward Room 120 to see whether she can find Arthur. He is in the room finishing Stephen Lightfoot's personal care. Arthur is ready to move Mr. Lightfoot out of bed, and he needs Nora's help.

"Arthur, I'll help you move Mr. Lightfoot *and* change his bed if you will help me move Mr. Rivera and change his linens," Nora says.

"You've got a deal," says Arthur.

As both nurse assistants lift Mr. Lightfoot into the bedside chair, he complains of extreme shortness of breath. First, Arthur makes sure that Mr. Lightfoot's oxygen tubes are not kinked anywhere. Then, so that Mr. Lightfoot doesn't hear, he quietly consults with Nora to see whether she also noticed the blue color around his lips. Arthur decides to report Mr. Lightfoot's condition to his supervising nurse. First he takes Mr. Lightfoot's pulse and respiration and asks Nora to stay with him while he reports his vital signs and change in color to his supervising nurse.

After the supervising nurse attends to Mr. Lightfoot's breathing problem, Nora and Arthur go to Mr. Rivera's room. It is now about 10:15 A.M. They move him into his wheelchair and change his bed.

After leaving Mr. Rivera's room, Nora passes Mr. Wilson in the hall on the way to his physical therapy appointment. She then goes directly to Room 121 to help Rachel Morgan with her range-of-motion exercises.

"Both of my arms are kind of stiff today," says Mrs. Morgan, as they begin the exercises. Nora gently moves her wrists back and forth.

"We'll do everything slowly," she says, "and you tell me when to stop."

After completing the exercises, Mrs. Morgan rests in her bed.

Adjusting the Schedule

At 11:00 A.M., Nora finishes changing the linens on Mr. Wilson's bed when she remembers that it is time to offer Mr. Rivera the urinal again.

"Gosh, I've gotta go check on Mr. Britten, too," she thinks to herself as she rushes toward Mr. Rivera's room.

Halfway down the hallway, Nora notices that Mrs. McDay's call signal is on. "I'll be right there," she calls to Mrs. McDay. In her nervous state, Nora bumps into Arthur in the hall.

"Arthur," she says, "I don't know what to do first! Mr. Rivera, Mrs. McDay, and Mr. Britten all need my help at the same time!"

"Calm down, Nora," says Arthur. "Let me see your schedule."

Down the hallway, Mrs. McDay cries out for her mother.

"I'll offer Mr. Rivera his urinal and then check on Mr. Britten while you take care of Mrs. McDay. Sounds like she really needs you," says Arthur.

"I don't know what I'd do without you!" Nora calls over her shoulder.

When Nora steps into Room 119, she sees that Mrs. McDay has wet the bed. Mrs. McDay rocks in her bed, scolding herself and picking at her bedspread. "I'm nothing but a baby! A baby!" she mutters under her breath.

Nora sighs to herself as she helps Mrs. McDay out of bed, removes the wet linens, and puts them in the hamper. As she helps Mrs. McDay wash and dress, she reassures her that the incontinence is not her fault and tells her that she doesn't mind helping her clean up. She continues to comfort Mrs. McDay as she makes her bed.

After a few minutes, Mrs. McDay asks, "Can I go to the dayroom?"

After helping Mrs. McDay to the dayroom, Nora goes to Room 124 and changes Mr. Britten's bed linens. She knows that he feels lonely in isolation and that he enjoys visiting with her while she provides care. However, Nora is scheduled for lunch at 11:30, and she's very hungry. She doesn't know how she's going to make it.

Controlling Time

After heating her soup in the microwave, Nora joins Arthur at a table where he is sipping a cup of coffee. It's 11:40 A.M., and Nora has just 20 minutes to relax before she will have to begin taking people to the dining room and helping feed lunch to the people in her care.

"I always seem to be running late," Nora says.

"Some days are like that," Arthur agrees. Then he suggests that they review Nora's schedule to see whether she could have made any changes.

Arthur looks over Nora's schedule. "It seems to me that you have everything well organized," he says. "But people aren't like puzzle pieces, you know, that always fit into place. They don't always fit into our plans." Nora smiles.

"What do you do at home when things don't work out as planned with your kids' schedules?" Arthur asks.

Nora laughs, tells him about her crazy morning, and confesses that she tries to stay flexible and roll with the punches. "After Emmy threw up, I just wanted to cry. But eventually everything works out, most of the time," Nora says.

Arthur laughs. "That's what they mean by experience being the best teacher," he says. "It takes a while to learn how to balance the needs of each person with all the things that you have to get done. Do you think you could have done anything differently this morning?" (Figure 22-10).

Nora thinks back on her morning. "I guess I could have checked on Mr. Britten before I did Mrs. Morgan's range-of-motion exercises. But I didn't know that Mrs. McDay would need me just when I had to offer Mr. Rivera his urinal. I was so worried that I would mess up his bladder training program. I can't thank you enough for helping me today."

When Nora finishes talking, Arthur asks her what she has accomplished that morning. As Nora begins to list the many things that she accomplished, she begins to relax, realizing that she has successfully completed all her morning tasks. Feeling renewed, she

goes back on the floor and helps everybody get lunch.

Focusing on Each Person in Your Care

It is 12:30 P.M. when Nora brings Mr. Britten his lunch tray. Instead of hurrying out, she stops to talk for a few minutes. Mr. Britten tells her about how hard it is for him to be in the nursing home while his partner is traveling on business.

"I worry about him, and I would feel better if I were at home," he says. "He's the only friend and family I have."

"Owen sounds like a very special person. I hope I get to meet him," says Nora. She tells Mr. Britten that she'll be back later to check on him. Nora washes her hands before leaving the room.

Nora stops by Rachel Morgan's and Victor Rivera's rooms to make sure that they are ready for their physical therapy appointments at 1:00 P.M. She offers Mr. Rivera his urinal before leaving.

At 1:15, Nora finds Mrs. McDay sitting by the window in her room. Nora asks her whether she would like to talk for a while. Mrs. McDay looks up at Nora and yells, "I just want to be alone!" Then she begins to cry. Nora recognizes that Mrs. McDay is probably having a catastrophic reaction. The earlier incontinence has upset her more than Nora realized.

Nora walks over to Mrs. McDay, sits next to her and speaks to her in a calm voice. After a while, Nora comments to Mrs. McDay that the brightly colored afghan spread across her lap is very pretty. Mrs. McDay smiles a little. "My sister made this afghan for me when I got married," she tells Nora (Figure 22-11).

At a few minutes before 2:00 P.M., Nora stops in Room 120 to check on Mr. Wilson before his recreational therapy appointment. A physical therapy aide brings Mr. Rivera into his room and helps Nora move Mr. Rivera into his bed so that he can rest before his wife comes to visit. The physical therapy aide returns to the hall with Mrs. Morgan and again helps Nora as they transfer Mrs. Morgan out of the wheelchair and back into bed.

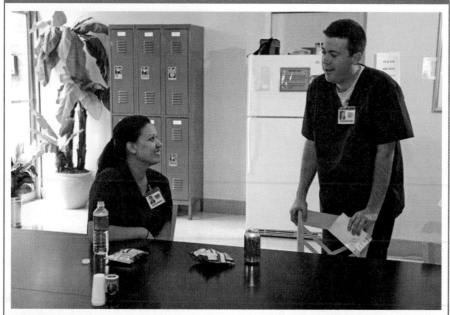

FIGURE 22-10 Arthur is right when he tells Nora that experience is the best teacher. As a seasoned nurse assistant, he knows that coping with conflicts and crises is part of an ordinary work day.

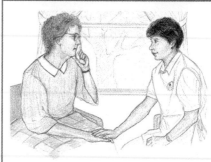

FIGURE 22-11 Nurse assistants know how important it is to take time out from their busy schedules to comfort patients, like Mrs. McDay, who is having a catastrophic reaction.

"Those physical therapy sessions always wear me out," Mrs. Morgan says as Nora tucks the sheet around her shoulders. A few minutes later, Mrs. Morgan is fast asleep.

Nora's shift is over at 3:00 P.M. Before leaving, Nora and Arthur go to Mr. Britten's room. Nora checks his vital signs, and then she and Arthur double-bag and transfer his soiled linens and trash. After saying good-bye to everyone, Nora completes her charting and makes her report to the team for the next shift. She includes a description of Mrs. McDay's catastrophic reaction in her report.

As she leaves the floor, Nora waves to Mr. Wilson, who is returning from recreation therapy. She smiles and feels very satisfied with herself.

On her ride home on the bus, she again meets her friend Sylvia. "Did your day get any better?" Sylvia asks.

"What? Oh, I barely thought about all that happened this morning," says Nora. "There was so much happening at the nursing home today. It's good for me to have a place of my own to go, where I can get away from all the responsibilities of being a single mother. Not that I don't have a mountain of responsibilities at work!

"I learned a lot today. I learned that people—me, my family and the people in my care—aren't puzzle pieces that fit neatly into my plans—I also really saw the value of making a schedule. Finally, and perhaps most important, I learned how important it is to be relaxed and flexible."

FICTION AND REALITY

Nora's day is fictional, although it may seem very real. It represents what a nurse assistant's typical day may be like. However, no two days are the same for anyone. These situations show how a nurse assistant, who has responsibilities that are similar to the ones that you may have, planned her day and controlled her time, yet

responded to the needs of the people in her care. If you try to stay organized and plan your day, as well as remain flexible and responsive to unexpected situations as they arise, you too can manage your time effectively.

You should also remember that once you begin working, you will have the opportunity to work on different shifts. Your duties will be different depending on which shift you are assigned. Look at Table 22-2 to see the

various tasks you may do on different shifts. Because the work load is usually more time-consuming on the day shift, you will probably have more residents assigned to you on the afternoon or midnight shifts than you will on the day shift. If you work the afternoon shift, you will have more opportunity to meet the residents' family members. You can use this time to get to know them and to learn their concerns. You can also take this opportunity to learn

TABLE 22-2 COMPARISON OF JOB TASKS FOR DAY, AFTERNOON AND MIDNIGHT SHIFTS

Day Shift	Afternoon Shift	Midnight Shift
*7:00 A.M.–3:30 P.M.	*3:00 P.M.–11:30 P.M.	*11:00 P.M.–7:30 A.M.
Greet residents	Greet residents	Look in on residents
A.M. care	Pass water	Pass water
Assist with elimination	Assist with elimination	Position residents every 2 hours
Breakfast	Position every 2 hours	
Pass water	Prepare for (supper) dinner	Clean w/c or special equipment
Shower/bath	Assist in passing trays	Showers (if needed)
Dressing	Undressing	Monitor residents
Prepare for treatments	Vital signs	Vital signs (if needed)
	Perineal care	Measure intake and output
Vital signs	Pass HS snacks	
Prepare for lunch		
Measure intake/output	Measure intake/output	Chart
Chart	Chart	

* Shift time varies depending upon where you work.

more about each resident, visiting and helping him or her to reminisce. It is a good idea to start a journal or notebook and write some of what you learn about each resident. This is especially helpful when talking to residents who have trouble remembering things, but it can also be helpful for keeping track of all your residents.

Whatever shift you decide to work, remember that it is always important to maintain a balance between planning a schedule and staying flexible: people are not puzzle pieces!

INFORMATION REVIEW

Circle the correct answers and fill in the blanks.

1. Which of the following are legitimate factors that influence how you use your time as a nurse assistant?
   a. The number of people in your care, their medical conditions, the kind of care they need and their mobility
   b. How many staff members are out sick
   c. How you spent your time before work and how well you coped with your prework activities
   d. Whether you wore your watch and remembered to set the time correctly

2. Your work day will go more smoothly if you plan a _____ of tasks that you must do.

3. When planning your schedule in a nursing home setting, you should consider which of the following factors? (Select two.)
   a. How many people have been assigned to your care
   b. What you are wearing that day
   c. What time your favorite program is on TV
   d. How quickly and efficiently you can get the job done

4. When you identify the most important tasks to be done and list them in order, you _____ the tasks.

5. When other co-workers ask for your assistance, you should:
   a. stop whatever you are doing and help them.
   b. refuse to help if your schedule does not allow time for such an interruption.

   c. work this request into your schedule as well as possible.
   d. report the request to your supervising nurse.

6. If your day's assignment seems impossible to complete, you should:
   a. do the best you can and not worry about it.
   b. ask for assistance from your co-workers.
   c. speak to your supervising nurse immediately.
   d. feel angry about being taken advantage of and leave at the end of your shift, even if the work is not done.

7. What is the best way to handle unexpected events? (Select two.)
   a. Rearrange your schedule the best you can.
   b. Ignore the events.
   c. Ask for help, if you need it.
   d. Ignore your schedule for the rest of the day.

8. Now that you have read this chapter, you have the information to _____ your time each working day, _____ your time if unplanned events occur and _____ clearly to help you stay in control of your time.

1. How would you have planned your schedule if you were Nora? Were there some things that Nora could have communicated to the people in her care that would have helped her stay in control of her time?

2. You have established your schedule for the day at the nursing home where you work. In your care are two people who need complete bed baths, one person who takes a tub bath, three people who take showers and one person who can do her own partial bath. How would you schedule your time to complete these baths?

3. You are serving dinner to the residents of a nursing home. You realize that Mr. Harris and Miss Yarnell both need a lot of assistance with eating tonight. You provide care for both of them and for one other person who needs help with eating. What would you do so that each of these residents has the chance to eat a hot dinner?

4. Remembering the six principles of care—safety, privacy, dignity, communication, independence and infection control—when and how did Nora practice these principles during the day?

Word Element Usage

WORD ELEMENTS—PREFIXES

Prefix	Prefix Meaning	Combined Form
a-, an-	without, not	an/esthesia (without sensation)
ab-, abs-	away from	ab/duction (move away from)
ad-	toward, near	ad/duction (move toward)
anti-	against	anti/inflammatory (substance used to fight infection)
brady-	slow	brady/cardia (slow heart rate)
circum-	around	circum/oral (around the mouth)
contra-	against, opposite	contra/ception (preventing conception, or pregnancy)
de-	down	de/pendent (hanging down or below)
di-	two	di/plopia (double vision)
dys-	abnormal, difficult, bad	dys/function (not functioning properly)
erythro-	red	erythro/cyte (red blood cell)
ex-	out, out of, from	ex/crete (discharge, get rid of)
hyper-	over, excessive	hyper/active (overly active)
hypo-	under, decreased	hypo/thyroid (underactive thyroid)
in-	within or not	in/continent (not able to control the release of urine or feces)
		in/dependent (not dependent)
mal-	bad, abnormal	mal/nourished (poorly fed)
non-	no, not	non/poisonous (not poisonous)
peri-	around, covering	peri/osteum (covering of the bone)
post-	after, behind	post/operative (after an operation)
pre-, or pro-	before, in front of	pre/operative (before an operation)
re-	again, back	re/port (speak or write about a previous event)
semi-	half	semi/conscious (half-conscious or alert)
tachy-	fast, rapid	tachy/cardia (rapid heart beat)

WORD ELEMENTS—ROOTS

Root	Root Meaning	Combined Form
arthr/o	joint	arthr/itis (inflammation of the joint)
bronch/o	bronchus, bronchi	bronch/itis (inflammation of the bronchus)
cephal/o	head	en/cephal/itis (inflammation of the brain)
cholescyst/o	gall bladder	cholecyst/ectomy (removal of the gall bladder)
col/o	colon, large intestine	col/ostomy (surgical opening into the colon)
crani/o	skull	crani/otomy (surgical opening into the skull)
cyan/o	blue	cyan/osis (having a blue color)
dermat/o	skin	dermat/ology (study or science of the skin)
fet/o	unborn child	fet/us (unborn child)
gastr/o	stomach	gastr/itis (inflammation of the stomach)
glycos/o	sugar	glycos/uria (sugar in the urine)
gynec/o	woman	gynec/ologist (one who studies diseases of women)
hemat/o	blood	hemat/uria (blood in the urine)
herni/o	rupture	herni/orraphy (surgical repair of a hernia)
hyster/o	uterus	hyster/ectomy (removal of the uterus)
lapar/o	abdomen, or flank	lapar/otomy (surgical cut into the abdomen)
lith/o	stone	chole/lith/iasis (having stones in the gallbladder)
mamm/o, mast/o	breast, mammary gland	mamm/orgam (diagnostic picture of the breast)
men/o	menstruation	men/opause (cessation of menstrual activity)
my/o	muscle	my/algia (muscle pain)
narc/o	numbness, stupor, or sleep	narc/otic (producing numbness, stupor or sleep)
necr/o	death	necr/osis (death of tissue or bone)
ophthalm/o	eye	ophthalm/oscope (instrument for examining the eye)
oste/o	bone	oste/oarthritis (inflammation of the bones and joints)

WORD ELEMENTS—ROOTS (Continued)

Root	Root Meaning	Combined Form
path/o	disease	path/ogen (disease-causing organism or substance)
ped/o	foot, child	ped/al (pertaining to the foot)
phleb/o	vein	phleb/itis (inflammation of the veins)
pneum/o	lung/air	pneum/othorax (air in the chest cavity)
proct/o	rectum	proct/oscope (instrument for examining the rectum)
psych/o	mind	psych/ology (study of the mind)
pulmon/o	lung	pulmon/ary (pertaining to the lung)
rect/o	rectum	rect/ostenosis (narrowing of the rectum)
ren/o	kidney	ren/opathy (disease of the kidney)
sept/o, sept/i	poison, infection	sept/icemia (poison in the blood)
therm/o	heat	therm/otherapy (application of heat for treatment)
thorac/o	chest	thorac/otomy (surgical incision into the chest)
thromb/o	clot	thromb/olytic (destruction of a clot)
tox/o, toxic/o	poison	tox/emia (poisonous substance in the body)
ur/o	urine	ur/ology (study of the urinary system)
urethr/o	urethra	urethr/itis (inflammation of the urethra)
uter/o	uterus	uter/ovaginal (pertaining to the uterus and vagina)
vertebr/o	spine, vertebrae	vertebr/al (pertaining to the spine)

WORD ELEMENTS—SUFFIXES

Suffix	Suffix Meaning	Combined Form
-al	pertaining to	therm/al (pertaining to heat)
-algia, -algesia	pain	an/algesia (without pain)
-cide	kill	germi/cide (substance that kills germs)
-cise	cut	ex/cise (to cut out)
-ectomy	excision, removal of	append/ectomy (removal of the appendix)
-emia	blood condition	hypo/glyc/emia (low blood sugar)
-esthesia	sensation	an/esthesia (without sensation)
-gram	printed record	mammo/gram (diagnostic picture of a breast)
-graph	device for recording	electro/cardio/graph (machine for recording the activity of the heart)
-itis	condition of inflammation	phleb/itis (inflammation of the veins)
-iasis, -ism	having the characteristics or condition of	dwarf/ism (having the condition of, or being, a dwarf)
-logy	the study or science of	neuro/logy (the study or science of the nervous system)
-meter	measuring instrument	thermo/meter (instrument that measures temperature)
-oma	tumor	hemat/oma (tumor caused by an accumulation of blood)
-pathy	disease	cardio/myo/pathy (disease of the heart muscle)
-phasia	speaking	a/phasia (unable to speak)
-phobia	an exaggerated fear	photo/phobia (fear of, or intolerance to, light)
-plegia	paralysis	quadri/plegia (paralysis of all four extremities)
-rrhage, -rrhagia	excessive flow	hemo/rrhage (excessive flow of blood)
-rrhaphy	surgical repair of	hernio/rrhaphy (surgical repair of a hernia)
-rrhea	profuse flow, discharge	rhino/rrhea (nasal discharge)
-scopy	examination using a scope (instrument to enable one to see)	endo/scopy (examination of internal cavities by the use of a scope)
-stomy	creation of an opening	colo/stomy (surgically created opening into the colon)
-tomy	surgical cutting	utero/tomy (surgical incision into the uterus)

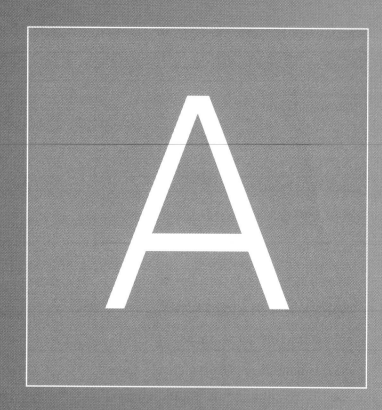

Medical Terminology— Supplemental Activities

GOALS

Upon completion of this module you will have the information needed to:

Define basic prefixes used in medical terminology.

Define basic suffixes used in medical terminology.

Define basic combining forms used in medical terminology.

Analyze medical words by identifying the prefixes, suffixes and combining forms.

Use combining forms, suffixes and prefixes to build medical words.

Define terms that apply to various chapters in the rest of the textbook.

FORMING MEDICAL TERMS

For students who have never worked in a health-care setting, learning medical terms may seem to be an overwhelming task. Some of the words are long, some are difficult to pronounce and spell and many of them are not used in everyday conversation. Nevertheless, mastery of medical terminology can be achieved. The following tips may help you with your task:

- Instead of trying to memorize the terms, learn the meaning of each part of the word.
- Try to relate the medical term to the corresponding structure or function of the human body.
- Be aware of word similarities. Some words are spelled similarly but are pronounced differently and have separate meanings.

ADDITIONAL PRACTICE FOR CHAPTER 6, THE LANGUAGE OF CAREGIVING

The first step in learning a medical term is understanding how to divide the word into its component parts. The component parts of a medical term are the *root, combining vowel, prefix* and *suffix*. The root is the foundation of the word. All medical terms have one or two roots. A prefix is a part *sometimes* added before a root to change its meaning. A suffix is a part *sometimes* added at the end of a root to change its meaning. The combining vowel links the root to either another root or a suffix and is usually the letter *o*. The combining vowel has no meaning of its own; it only joins one part of a word to another.

The second step is to define each separate component part of the word. Finally, determine the meaning of the complete term by reading the meanings of the individual word parts backwards—from the suffix to the prefix. Let's apply these steps in defining the following medical term:

HYSTERECTOMY

The root is *hyster* and means "uterus."

The suffix is *-ectomy* and means "removal of."

The complete word *hysterectomy* means "removal of the uterus."

As you can see, there is no combining vowel in the word *hysterectomy*. The combining vowel is almost never used if the suffix begins with a vowel, as in *-ectomy*. Let's try another example. Can you identify the root, suffix, and combining vowel in the following term?

CYSTOGRAM

1. The root is _____ and means _____.
2. The suffix is _____ and means _____.
3. The combining vowel is _____.
4. The complete word means _____.
   Let's try one more example.

CHOLECYSTECTOMY

5. The root is _____ and means _____.
6. The suffix is _____ and means _____.
7. The complete word means _____.

Now that you understand how roots, suffixes and combining vowels are used to form medical words, we will look more closely at using two additional word parts frequently found in medical terms: prefixes and combining forms. You already know what a prefix is; the combining form is the root plus the combining vowel. Combining forms can be used with a variety of suffixes.

CYSTITIS

8. The root is _____ and means _____.
9. The suffix is _____ and means _____.
10. *Cystitis* means _____.
    Let's do another example.

HEPATITIS

11. The root is _____ and means _____.
12. The suffix is _____ and means _____.
13. *Hepatitis* means _____.

Now let's look at some prefixes in use.

HYPOGLYCEMIA
The prefix is *hypo-* and means "under."
The root is *glyc* and means "sugar."
The suffix is *-emia* and means "blood disorder."
The complete word means "low blood sugar."

HYPERGLYCEMIA
The prefix is *hyper-* and means "above."
The root is *glyc* and means "sugar."
The suffix is *-emia* and means "blood disorder."
The complete word means "high blood sugar."

As you can see, these words are similar but have different meanings. Consult the Word Element Usage if you need help with the meaning of a word part.

ADDITIONAL PRACTICE FOR CHAPTER 7, CONTROLLING THE SPREAD OF GERMS

Instructions: Give meanings for the following terms.

1. antiseptic _____
2. antibodies _____
3. antimicrobial _____
4. contagious _____
5. contaminated _____
6. disinfect _____
7. germ _____
8. infection _____
9. infection control _____
10. infectious _____
11. microorganisms _____
12. pathogen _____
13. Standard Precautions _____

ADDITIONAL PRACTICE FOR CHAPTER 9, MEASURING LIFE SIGNS

Instructions: Complete the following questions by filling in the blanks or circling the correct answers.

1. *Auscultate* means to listen for sounds produced by _____.
2. The thin disk of a stethoscope that is placed on the skin to hear body sounds is called the _____.
3. T   F   *Diastolic* describes the pressure of blood against the walls of the arteries when the heart relaxes; this pressure is the first sound heard when taking a blood pressure.
4. The gauge on a sphygmomanometer that measures systolic and diastolic blood pressure is called the _____.
5. What two instruments measure blood pressure? _____
6. What is the stethoscope used for? _____
7. T   F   *Systolic* describes the pressure of blood against the walls of the arteries when the heart pumps; this is the first pumping sound heard as air is released from the blood pressure cuff.

ADDITIONAL PRACTICE FOR CHAPTER 10, POSITIONING AND TRANSFERRING PEOPLE, AND CHAPTER 16, PROVIDING RESTORATIVE CARE TO HELP WITH REHABILITATION

Instructions: Match each of the following terms with its correct meaning on the next page.

alignment	flex	physical restraint	restraint
ambulation	gait	rehabilitation	supine position
contracture	mobility	restorative services	turgor
epidermis	range-of-motion		

1. Any device used to limit movement of a person or to control mood or behavior _____
2. The ability to move _____
3. To bend _____
4. The outer protective layer of skin _____
5. Correct positioning to keep the spine straight and to avoid any twisting, straining, pressure or discomfort _____
6. The process of regaining physical health _____
7. The ability of the skin to return to its normal shape when it is squeezed or gently pinched _____
8. Activities or devices that help a person improve, maintain or regain physical functions _____
9. The medical term for *walking* _____
10. A device that physically prevents a person from moving freely _____
11. A position in which a person lies flat on his or her back _____
12. The way a person walks _____
13. The movement of a person's joint as far as it will go in every direction possible for that joint; may be performed by the individual or by another person _____
14. A condition in which unused muscles cause a person's joints to become permanently bent _____

ADDITIONAL PRACTICE FOR CHAPTER 14, HEALTHFUL EATING

Instructions: Match each of the following terms with its correct meaning.

appetite   dehydration   hypoglycemia   nutrient
atrophy   digestion   nausea   nutrition
cholesterol   hyperglycemia   NPO   obesity

1. An abnormally low amount of sugar in the blood _____
2. Indicates that a person is to take nothing by mouth, including food and fluids _____
3. A white, fatty substance that occurs naturally in the blood and tissues of the human body and that also is found in meat, egg yolks, liver, most dairy products and animal fat _____
4. A substance that the body needs to grow, maintain itself and stay healthy _____
5. The desire to eat and drink _____
6. A feeling of sickness in the stomach _____
7. Not having enough water in the body _____
8. An abnormally high amount of sugar in the blood _____
9. Having too much body fat _____
10. The process of breaking down food into a form that can be absorbed in the body _____
11. A condition in which a part of the body, such as leg muscle, wastes away or shrinks because of disuse or inadequate nutrition _____
12. The total of all the processes involved in taking in and using food and fluids for the health and maintenance of the body

_____

ADDITIONAL PRACTICE FOR CHAPTER 15, ELIMINATION

Instructions: Match each of the following terms with its correct definition.

1. abdomen _____   a. Another term for solid body waste or feces
2. anus _____   b. A thin layer of body tissue that lines the inside of body passages and cavities that communicate directly or indirectly with the outside of the body, such as the inside of the mouth, nose, eyes, vagina or rectum

3. constipation ____
4. defecate ____
5. diarrhea ____
6. eliminate ____

7. enema ____
8. fecal impaction ____

9. feces ____
10. incontinence ____
11. mucous membrane ____
12. perspiration ____
13. perineal care ____
14. rectum ____
15. stool ____
16. urinate ____
17. urine ____

c. To get rid of
d. Liquid body waste from the kidneys and bladder
e. The part of the body between the ribs and groin
f. A condition in the bowels in which elimination is difficult or infrequent and results in hard, dry stool
g. Body waste eliminated through the skin
h. A solution introduced into the rectum and lower colon to relieve fecal impaction or constipation
i. The opening at the end of the rectum through which feces pass
j. To eliminate liquid waste from the bladder
k. The frequent passage of liquid feces
l. A condition of the bowels in which hard stool is wedged in the rectum
m. To eliminate solid waste from the body
n. Lower portion of the large intestines just inside the anal opening
o. A nursing procedure in which a person's body is cleaned from the genitals to the anus
p. Solid body waste
q. The inability to control the release of urine or feces

ADDITIONAL PRACTICE FOR CHAPTER 17, PROVIDING CARE FOR PEOPLE WITH SPECIFIC ILLNESSES

Instructions: In each of the following groups of words, circle the term that is spelled correctly. The meaning of the term is provided.

1. The medical term for heart pain
   angia pectoris   *angina pectoris*   *angio pectores*
2. Hardening and thickening of the arteries
   arteriosclerosis   *ateriolerosis*   *arterosleroses*
3. Any of the branching blood vessels carrying oxygen-rich blood from the heart to all parts of the body
   artere   *aretory*   *artery*
4. An interruption of blood flow to a part of the brain, which results in the death of a few or many blood cells
   cerebrovascular accident   *cerebro accident*   *cerovascular accident*

Instructions: Fill in the blanks in the following sentences to complete each medical term.

5. A condition caused by the human immunodeficiency virus that results in a breakdown of the body's defense systems is **acquired** ____ ____.
6. Hardening and thickening of the arteries is _____ **-sclerosis.**
7. Treatment with one or more drugs that stop cancer cells from multiplying is _____ **-therapy**.
8. An incurable disorder of the brain in which there is a progressive loss of memory and other cognitive (thinking) functions is **dem-** _____.
9. A disease in which the pancreas does not secrete enough insulin and the body is not able to use all the carbohydrates, resulting in a high concentration of glucose in the blood, is **dia-** _____.
10. An ongoing condition of the brain marked by changes in the level of consciousness and/or abnormal muscle or sensory activity is **ep-** _____.
11. Swelling of the body tissue due to an accumulation of fluid is **ed-** _____.

12. A disease or condition marked by an inflammation of the liver is **hep-** _____.

13. The microscopic organism that causes AIDS is the human _____ virus.

14. A condition of the skeletal system in which the bones become weak and fragile is **osteo-** _____.

Instructions: For each of the following terms, write a sentence in which the term is correctly used. Answers will vary. Ask your instructor to check your work.

15. abnormal _____

16. abrasion _____

17. abuse _____

18. adapt _____

19. admit _____

20. auscultate _____

21. biology _____

22. cognitive _____

23. cognitive impairment _____

24. communication _____

25. compression _____

26. disoriented _____

27. dysfunctional _____

28. grooming _____

29. resident _____

Instructions: Match each of the following terms with its correct definition.

30. asphyxiation _____   a. The condition of having difficulty breathing

31. aspirate _____   b. To breathe in

32. cannula _____   c. An odorless, tasteless gas that a person breathes into the body through the respiratory system; essential for maintaining life

33. cyanosis _____   d. A tube placed under the nostrils to deliver oxygen

34. dyspnea _____   e. A condition characterized by blue or gray coloring of the skin, caused by lack of oxygen in the blood

35. oxygen _____   f. Suffocation caused by a lack of oxygen

APPENDIX A ANSWER KEY

Additional Practice for Chapter 6, The Language of Caregiving

1. cyst; bladder
2. gram; printed record
3. o
4. diagnostic record of the bladder
5. cholecyst; gallbladder
6. -ectomy; removal of
7. removal of the gallbladder
8. cyst; bladder
9. -itis; inflammation
10. inflammation of the bladder
11. hepat-; liver
12. -itis; inflammation
13. inflammation of the liver

Additional Practice for Chapter 7, Controlling the Spread of Germs

Answers should approximate these:
1. A substance that stops the growth of germs.
2. Special proteins or chemicals the body produces when an infection is present.
3. Capable of killing or slowing the growth of pathogens.
4. Easily transmitted from one person to another by direct or indirect contact.
5. Containing dirt or disease-causing germs.
6. To remove disease-causing germs.
7. A tiny living organism that cannot be seen by the eye.
8. A harmful condition caused by the growth of germs in the body.
9. Action taken to control the spread of germs.
10. Spreading or capable of spreading rapidly.
11. Tiny living things that can be seen only with a microscope.
12. A harmful germ or microorganism that causes disease.
13. Special infection control procedures that health professionals use to protect themselves and the people in their care from potentially infectious body fluids.

Additional Practice for Chapter 9, Measuring Life Signs

1. the heart
2. diaphragm
3. F
4. manometer
5. sphygmomanometer and stethoscope
6. listening to heart and lung sounds
7. T

Additional Practice for Chapter 10, Positioning and Transferring People, and Chapter 16, Providing Restorative Care to Help with Rehabilitation

1. restraint
2. mobility
3. flex
4. epidermis
5. alignment
6. rehabilitation
7. turgor
8. restorative services
9. ambulation
10. physical restraint
11. supine position
12. gait
13. range-of-motion
14. contracture

Additional Practice for Chapter 14, Healthful Eating

1. hypoglycemia
2. NPO
3. cholesterol
4. nutrient
5. appetite
6. nausea
7. dehydration
8. hyperglycemia
9. obesity
10. digestion
11. atrophy
12. nutrition

Additional Practice for Chapter 15, Elimination

1. e	5. k	9. p	13. o	17. d
2. i	6. c	10. q	14. n	
3. f	7. h	11. b	15. a	
4. m	8. l	12. g	16. j	

Additional Practice for Chapter 17, Providing Care for People with Specific Illnesses

1. angina pectoris
2. arteriosclerosis
3. artery
4. cerebrovascular accident
5. immunodeficiency syndrome
6. arterio-
7. chemo-
8. -entia
9. -betes
10. -ilepsy
11. -ema
12. -atitis
13. immunodeficiency
14. -porosis

Note: *For questions 15 through 29, answers will vary widely. Ask your instructor to check your work.*
30. f   31. b   32. d   33. e   34. a   35. c

B

Body Basics

GOALS

After reading this module, you will have the information needed to:

Describe each body system.

Identify the major parts of each body system.

Describe how the body systems work together.

OUR BODIES AND BEHAVIOR

Our behavior is affected by our bodies and how well they function. If our bodies are strong, we can work and exercise. If our bodies look physically fit and attractive, friends and strangers notice and admire us. When our bodies are in proper working order, we can take walks, enjoy meals, watch movies and engage in countless other activities. However, when we are ill or our bodies are injured, our behaviors change.

Ten systems of organs work together to make the body function. Each system plays an important part in daily activities. The bones of the *skeletal system* give structure to the body. The *muscular system* moves the body in many different directions. The skin, or *integumentary system,* protects the body from cold and germs in the outside world. Food moves through the *digestive system* to nourish the body and to rid it of indigestible material. The *urinary system* rids the body of harmful wastes. The lungs work in the *pulmonary system* to bring oxygen into the body. The heart and blood work together in the *cardiovascular system* to distribute oxygen from the lungs, as well as nutrients from food, to every cell in the body. The *reproductive system* gives the body the ability to produce children. The *nervous system* and *endocrine system* coordinate the other systems, but in very different ways. For example, the endocrine system sends hormones through the bloodstream to regulate a wide variety of ongoing functions, while the nervous system sends messages to various parts of the body by electrical impulses sent through nerves.

Our bodies change as we age. Aging is an ongoing, natural and expected process. Throughout life, our bodies replace old cells with new ones. As we age, this process of cell replacement slows down, resulting in body systems that do not work as they used to. Our body systems grow and change until they reach their peak, and then they start to decline. Various systems reach their maximum ability at different times during life. For example, the muscular system reaches its peak of ability when we are in our 20s.

Aging is a normal part of life, not a disease. Some people appear to grow older more rapidly than others because of heredity, and others age faster because they live in an unhealthy environment or ignore their health. Positive behaviors like exercise and nutritious eating can slow down the aging process, but nothing can make it stop. You can keep your body healthy by adopting positive behaviors. Also, by encouraging positive behaviors among the people in your care, you can help keep them as healthy as possible.

As you learn about the body systems you will be able to identify health conditions that affect certain body systems and how body systems relate to one another.

THE NERVOUS SYSTEM

The nervous system coordinates our responses to what goes on in the world around us, as well as what is happening inside of us. No other animal can think, speak or act as a human, because the human nervous system is more complicated than that of any other creature.

Our senses serve as our window to the outside world. We see with our eyes, hear with our ears, smell with our noses and taste with our tongues, because these organs have nerves that carry sensations to our brains. Nerves located in our skin give us a sense of touch and balance.

An adult's brain weighs about 3 pounds. It is made up of several types of cells, including neurons, which look like flowers on a stem. Resembling a large, gray acorn squash divided by many hills and valleys, the brain processes all information from the outside world, as well as sensations from inside the body, such as pain and hunger.

The brain sends information about how the body should respond. Messages travel through nerves that go to the spinal cord, a bundle of nerves protected by bones called *vertebrae,* or the backbone (Figure B-1). More nerves run from the *spinal cord* to the arms, legs, chest and abdomen. We get messages from the brain that tell us to run, kick up our heels, eat a hamburger or respond in any of a million other ways that make us human. Here's a fascinating fact—nerve cells coming together at junctions called *synapses* do not actually touch. The transmission from one cell to another is carried out by chemicals that "ferry" the impulse across the synapse.

How the Nervous System Ages

A person is born with as many neurons as he or she will ever have. After age 25, the body experiences a slow, but steady, loss of nerve cells. That loss causes no change in behavior or function unless a person has an injury, a disease or poor nutrition. The rate at which messages are sent from the body to the brain also slows down, causing the body to react more slowly. For example, it may take longer for the hand to receive the message that it is touching something hot (Figure B-2). The rate of learning may also slow down.

THE ENDOCRINE SYSTEM

Many glands located throughout the body make up the endocrine system (Figure B-3). Each gland secretes one or more substances called *hormones.* Hormones travel through the blood or through specific tubes called *ducts* to an organ called the "target." Hor-

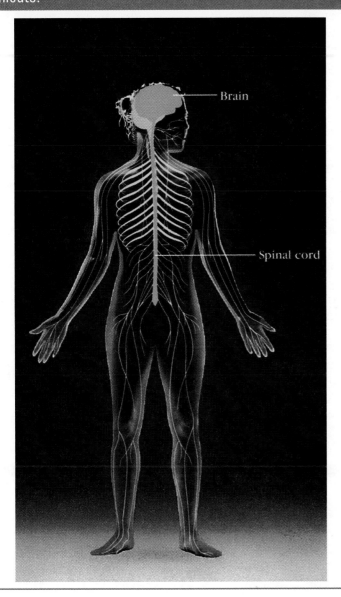

FIGURE B-1 Messages travel through nerves that go to the spinal cord, which helps the brain and other parts of the body communicate.

Brain

Spinal cord

the pancreas does not secrete enough insulin, the body develops diabetes.

Four small parathyroid glands and the larger thyroid gland are all grouped together in the neck in front of the windpipe. Parathyroid hormone controls the level of calcium in the blood and bones. Thyroid hormone is the key in regulating metabolism, which is the rate at which the body turns food into energy.

Two other glands that influence metabolism are the adrenal glands, situated on the top of each kidney. Adrenal hormones control the amount of salt, potassium and water in the body; they also constrict blood vessels and make the heart pump faster.

Testes and ovaries are part of the reproductive system, but the hormones they secrete are part of the endocrine system. For instance, men's testes secrete androgens such as testosterone, the hormones responsible for male sex characteristics. Women's ovaries secrete estrogen and progesterone, the hormones that influence menstruation and pregnancy.

Finally, the pituitary gland, the master gland situated deep in the brain, controls all other glands in the body and secretes growth hormone. Abnormalities of the pituitary can produce extreme results.

How the Endocrine System Ages

In the endocrine system, the most striking effects of aging are seen in women who have reached their "change of life," or menopause, when the ovaries stop producing the hormones estrogen and progesterone. When this happens, the woman no longer menstruates and her ability to have children ends. Testosterone production in men slows with aging but does not stop. Most other hormones are not affected by aging.

mones tell their targets just what to do, when to do it and how much they should do.

The endocrine system cannot work alone, however. It works closely with several other body systems. The nervous system, for example, regulates glands by letting them know how much hormone to secrete, and the

cardiovascular system helps carry the hormones to their targets.

The largest gland is the pancreas, located in the abdomen near the stomach. Scattered throughout the pancreas are cells called *islets of Langerhans,* which secrete insulin, the hormone that regulates the amount of sugar in the bloodstream. If

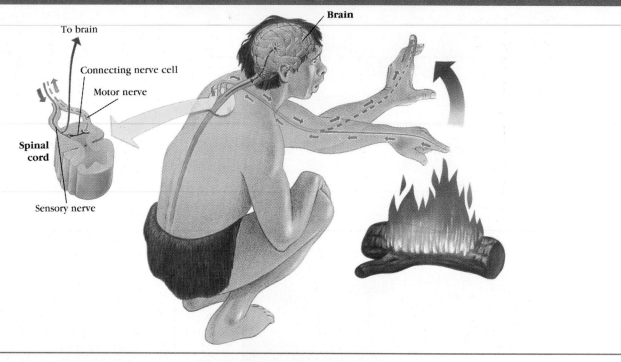

To brain

Connecting nerve cell

Motor nerve

Spinal cord

Sensory nerve

Brain

FIGURE B-3 Many glands located throughout the body make up the endocrine system.

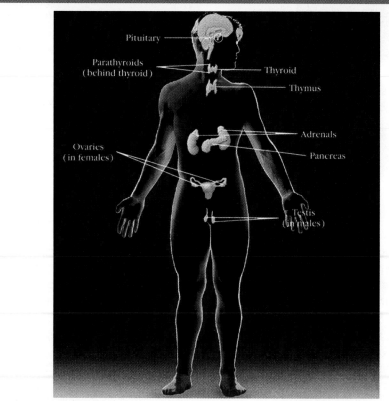

Pituitary

Parathyroids (behind thyroid)

Thyroid

Thymus

Adrenals

Pancreas

Ovaries (in females)

Testis (in males)

THE REPRODUCTIVE SYSTEM

Humans reproduce when a man's sperm joins with a woman's egg. The resulting embryo grows for 9 months in the woman's uterus before it makes its appearance in the world. The process may sound simple, but the human reproductive system is a complex set of organs inside and outside the male and female bodies (Figure B-4).

The male reproductive organs are situated mostly outside the body. Urine is carried from the body through a tube in the penis called the *urethra*. Behind the penis hangs the scrotum, a pouch of loose skin that holds the testes, the rounded organs, about 1½ inches long, that produce sperm and hormones. Loose channels inside the penis fill with blood when it is erect. When a man ejaculates, semen, the fluid that carries sperm, also flows through the urethra. Urine and semen do not flow through the urethra at the same time.

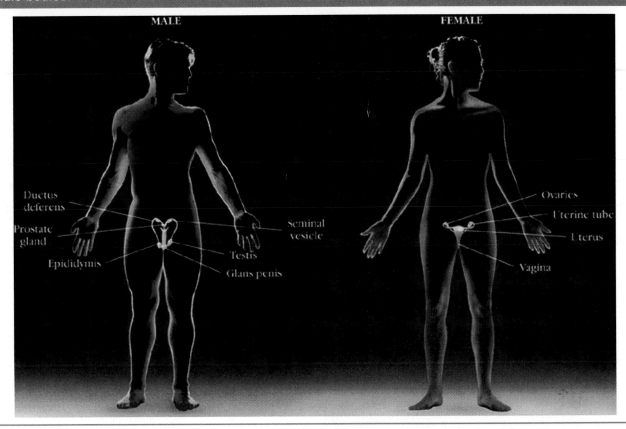

The female has two almond-shaped organs called ovaries. An ovary is on each side of the uterus in the abdominal cavity. The ovaries produce ova or eggs and hormones during a female's reproductive years.

There are two fallopian tubes, one on each side of the uterus. The tubes are attached at one end to the uterus. The egg travels through the fallopian tubes to the uterus. The uterus is a hollow, muscular organ. It is located inside a woman's abdomen. The uterus serves as the home of the growing fetus for 9 months.

The cervix of the uterus opens up into a passage way extending from the uterus to the outside of the body called a vagina. The labia majora and labia minora are two sets of folds on either side of the vagina. These provide pro-tection for the uterus and the urethral and vaginal openings.

How the Reproductive System Ages

As the body ages, the most important change that may occur in the male reproductive system is the enlarge-ment of the prostate gland, which squeezes the urethra and interferes with the passage of urine. A man also may have increasing difficulty main-taining an erection, and he may pro-duce fewer sperm and less seminal fluid, but he can still father a child in later years. A woman, on the other hand, stops producing eggs and hor-mones when menstruation ceases in menopause. This change occurs nat-urally from the mid-to-late 40s to the early 50s, or earlier if the woman has had her ovaries and uterus surgi-cally removed. Both men and women can enjoy sexual activity well into older age.

THE CARDIOVASCULAR SYSTEM

Life depends on a heart that pumps blood. Using blood vessels as its vehi-cle, blood travels throughout the body, making its first stop at the lungs to pick up oxygen for delivery to every cell. During the blood's return trip to the heart, the liver and kidneys filter out harmful and useless waste (Figure B-5).

The heart, made mostly of thick muscle, is about the size of a man's fist and weighs about 12 ounces. It is divided into four compartments, called

Carotid artery

Jugular vein

Brachial artery

Superior vena cava

Pulmonary artery

Heart

Aorta

Inferior vena cava

Radial artery

Femoral artery and vein

tiny blood vessels called *capillaries* that connect these arteries and veins. Capillaries are so small that red blood cells, visible only through a microscope, have to squeeze through them in single file. The blood itself is made of cells and plasma, the fluid that carries the cells. Red cells carry oxygen, white cells fight infection and platelets help the blood to clot.

How the Cardiovascular System Ages

As people grow older, their veins and arteries lose some of their elasticity, so blood pressure may rise, and circulation may decrease. Poor eating habits, little exercise and a family history of heart disease increase an older person's chance of having a heart attack.

THE RESPIRATORY SYSTEM

The human body depends on oxygen to live. Without it, the heart could not beat, the stomach could not digest food, and hair would not grow. Air containing oxygen enters the body through the respiratory system.

When a person inhales, air enters the body through the mouth and nose (Figure B-6, A). It swirls through the sinuses, the hollow spaces in the skull, and then makes its way through the trachea, or windpipe, the thick tube that leads from the throat to the lungs (Figure B-6, B). On its trip to the lungs, tiny hairs called *cilia* warm and clean the air.

This warmed air continues along the trachea, which splits into two slightly smaller tubes called *bronchi*, which enter the right and left lungs. The bronchi divide again and again like branches of a tree, becoming smaller and smaller tubes that end in little air spaces called *alveoli* (Figure B-7).

Each lung has millions of alveoli that conduct the real business of respiration, the exchange of life-giving oxygen and body waste called *carbon*

chambers, which are separated by small valves that act like miniature swinging doors to keep blood flowing in one direction. Several blood vessels supply the heart with blood.

Blood vessels called *arteries* carry blood away from the heart. The largest artery, the aorta, has strong, elastic walls that will not tear under the high pressure of the blood as it is pumped from the heart. Arteries that carry

blood to the internal organs and arms and legs are smaller; and smaller still are the arterioles that carry blood to individual cells. Blood vessels called *veins* carry blood on its return trip to the heart. Veins are thinner than arteries because they carry blood under less pressure.

So how is blood transferred from the outgoing arteries into the returning veins? Well, our bodies have 10 billion

FIGURE B-6 Air enters and exits the body through the mouth and nose (A), traveling through the trachea or windpipe, whose bronchial tubes lead into the lungs (B).

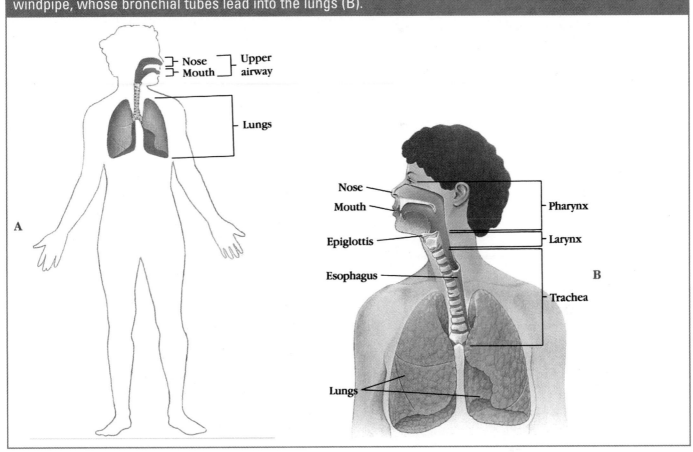

FIGURE B-7 Bronchi divide into smaller and smaller branches that end in little air spaces called *alveoli*.

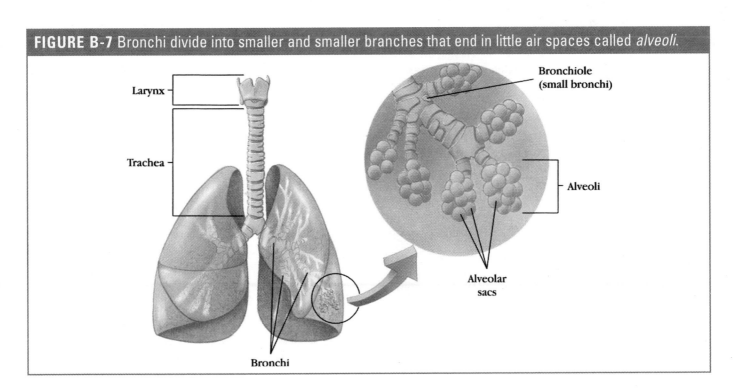

dioxide. Blood flows past the alveoli and picks up oxygen from the air in the lungs. Then the alveoli remove the body's wastes from the blood, and the person blows out these wastes by exhaling air through the same path as the air that was inhaled.

Imagine this: We each have 300 million alveoli, a number that is greater than the population of the United States. If one person's alveoli were opened up and spread out flat, they would cover an area equal to about eight room-size carpets.

How the Respiratory System Ages

As people age, their lungs become less elastic, and their rib cage muscles may become weak, resulting in shallow breathing and a greater chance of developing pneumonia or other lung infections.

THE INTEGUMENTARY SYSTEM

The human body has a covering of skin, hair and nails, together called the *integumentary system,* which protects the body from the outside world. The skin acts as a barrier to bacteria, keeps water inside the body, contains sense organs that allow people to feel and regulates body temperature (Figure B-8).

The skin, which is more than a simple protective sheet, is made up of several parts. The outer layer, called the *epidermis,* is firm and dry to the touch. Beneath the epidermis, the *dermis* holds glands and hair follicles. Sweat glands produce sweat to keep the body's temperature in a safe range, and oil glands make oil to keep the skin soft and flexible. Hair follicles produce the hairs that cover most of our bodies. Blood vessels in this layer provide nutrients and oxygen to all skin cells. Underneath the skin is a layer of fat that cushions, protects and insulates the body.

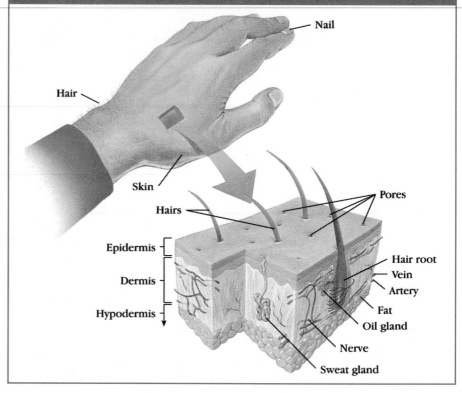

FIGURE B-8 The skin acts as a barrier to bacteria, keeps water inside the body, contains sense organs and regulates body temperature.

How the Integumentary System Ages

As people age, their skin becomes less elastic, the amount of fat under the skin decreases, and their bodies produce less oil. As a result, their skin tends to be dry and looks wrinkled. Older people also develop more skin cancers, usually caused by sun damage that has added up over a lifetime.

The skin is the largest organ in the body; in an adult, it weighs about 6 pounds and, if spread out flat, would cover an area 3 feet wide and 6 feet long. A piece of skin the size of a quarter contains 1 yard of blood vessels, 4 yards of nerves, 25 nerve endings, 100 sweat glands and more than 3 million cells. The skin produces vitamin D when the body is exposed to sunlight. Vitamin D is artificially added to milk and dairy products to ensure that people, especially children, receive an

adequate amount. Human bodies need vitamin D to absorb the calcium that is needed to fill up the spaces created by bone cells.

THE MUSCULAR SYSTEM

Every movement in the human body, from the blink of the eye to the beat of the heart, depends on muscles. The body has hundreds of muscles that come in all sizes, from the delicate muscles in the ear to the thick, powerful muscles in the legs (Figure B-9).

Muscles do their work by getting shorter, or contracting, in response to electrical impulses sent through nerves. To recover from their work, they relax, or get longer. Some muscles, which are under a person's control, are attached to bones by tendons and contract with voluntary actions such as walking. Other muscles, which

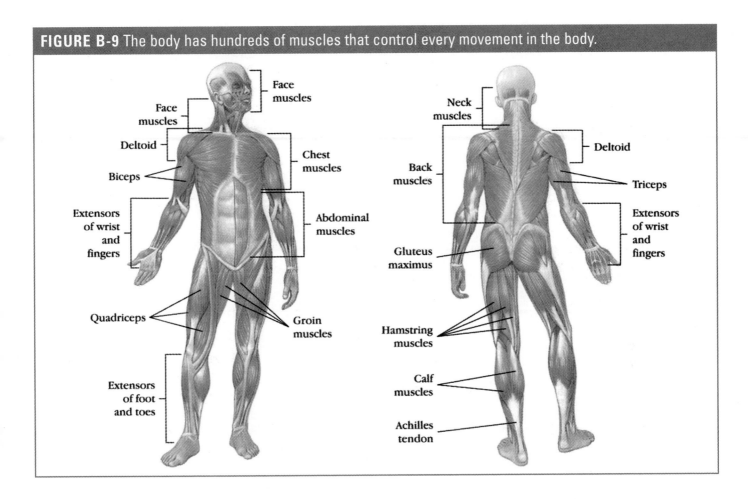

FIGURE B-9 The body has hundreds of muscles that control every movement in the body.

Face muscles

Face muscles

Deltoid

Biceps

Extensors of wrist and fingers

Chest muscles

Abdominal muscles

Quadriceps

Groin muscles

Extensors of foot and toes

Neck muscles

Back muscles

Deltoid

Triceps

Extensors of wrist and fingers

Gluteus maximus

Hamstring muscles

Calf muscles

Achilles tendon

are not under a person's control, surround the blood vessels, digestive tract and other body parts that work involuntarily.

Have you ever noticed your muscles twitching? This normal movement occurs when a single nerve sends its electrical impulse to the muscle. The impulse is not strong enough to make the whole muscle move but is just strong enough to make a couple of muscle fibers contract.

Some muscles, such as those in the arms and legs, work together in contracting and relaxing teams. For example, when a person bends his arm at the elbow, muscles on one side of his arm contract, pulling on the joint and causing it to bend, while muscles on the opposite side relax. To straighten his arm, the opposite happens. These muscle pairs work together to ensure that movement is controlled and smooth. A

person is able to stand straight because teams of muscles around his spine contract and relax in perfect harmony.

How the Muscular System Ages

As people age, their muscles get smaller and less elastic and lose strength. Large muscle loss in the hips and knees affects balance. More fat cells and connective tissue begin to replace muscle fibers. People can help their muscles remain strong with regular exercise and a healthy diet.

THE SKELETAL SYSTEM

The skeletal system supports and protects the body. Without a skeletal system, the human body would collapse like a jellyfish. To support the body, muscles are draped over bones (made mostly of calcium) and carti-

lage, the firm tissue that supports and connects parts of the skeletal system (Figure B-10). To protect vital organs inside the body, the skull surrounds the brain; the twelve ribs and breastbone (sternum) cover the heart and lungs; and the backbone (vertebral column) guards the spinal cord.

Adults have 206 bones in various sizes and shapes. The smallest bones are the ossicles, found inside the ear; they are no larger than the head of a match. The largest bone is the femur, which is the thick, sturdy bone between the hip and the knee. Long bones, such as those in the arms and legs, are not solid structures but have center cavities filled with red marrow (which produces red blood cells) and yellow marrow (which is mostly fat cells).

Joints, the place where neighboring bones are connected by ligaments,

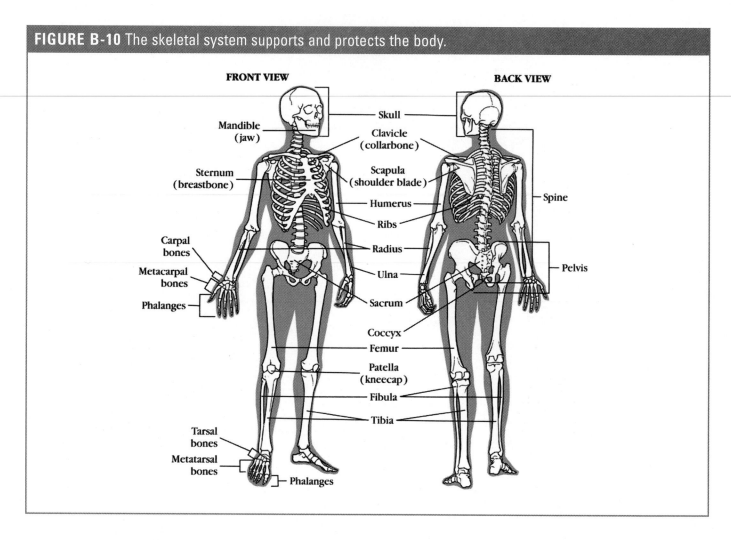

FRONT VIEW   BACK VIEW

Mandible (jaw)
Sternum (breastbone)
Carpal bones
Metacarpal bones
Phalanges
Tarsal bones
Metatarsal bones
Phalanges

Skull
Clavicle (collarbone)
Scapula (shoulder blade)
Humerus
Ribs
Radius
Ulna
Sacrum
Coccyx
Femur
Patella (kneecap)
Fibula
Tibia

Spine
Pelvis

allow the skeleton to move. Some joints work like door hinges, and others are similar to a ball and socket.

How the Skeletal System Ages

As people age, their bones lose calcium, become fragile and break more easily. In addition, without weight-bearing exercise, such as walking, bones tend to lose the calcium that makes them hard. They can take on a sponge-like, porous appearance and become very brittle. Because of this change, the bones of inactive people can break with only small amounts of stress on the bones.

This is especially true for women. Female hormones keep calcium in bones, but after menopause, women's bodies no longer produce these hormones. The vertebrae begin to col-

lapse, and some women actually lose an inch or more in height and may develop a humpback. In addition, their joints become less flexible and begin to wear away, resulting in a form of arthritis. Their walking slows, and their steps may take on a shuffling gait.

THE DIGESTIVE SYSTEM

Every day, we eat, turn food into energy and get rid of wastes our bodies cannot use (Figure B-11). Taking food into our bodies is called *ingestion*. The process of breaking food down is *digestion*. Sending the waste, called *stool* (feces) and *gas* (flatus), out of the body is part of elimination.

We want to eat when the brain sends a message to put food into our mouths. There, our teeth chew the

food and saliva mixes with it to start the digestion process. The tongue pushes food to the back of the mouth.

After we swallow, food travels down the esophagus, a muscular tube, until it reaches the stomach. There, food mixes with chemicals produced by the lining of the stomach, and the "good parts" of the food begin to separate from the "unusable parts," or waste. This process continues as partially digested food passes from the stomach and continues through the small and large intestines. Finally, waste leaves the body through the rectum and anus.

The pancreas contributes to digestion by making digestive juices called *enzymes*. The liver makes enzymes that break down and release sugars, starch, protein and fat and

FIGURE B-11 The digestive system turns food into energy and gets rid of wastes our bodies cannot use.

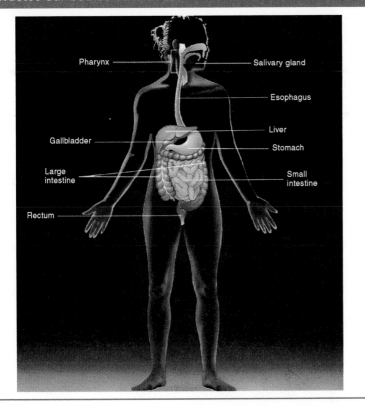

THE URINARY SYSTEM

Every 45 minutes, the body's 5 quarts of blood pass through the kidneys for purification. The kidneys are part of the urinary system, which removes wastes from the bloodstream and eliminates them as urine (Figure B-12).

Two kidneys, bean-shaped organs about 4 inches long, are located at waist level, one on each side of the body. After removing waste materials from the blood, the kidneys mix the wastes with water and turn them into urine. The kidneys produce about $1\frac{1}{2}$ quarts of urine each day.

Urine passes from the kidneys through ureters, delicate tubes connecting the kidneys to the bladder. Urine collects in the bladder until it fills to about $2\frac{1}{2}$ cups. At this point, the person feels the urge to urinate, or pass urine from the body.

Urine passes from the bladder to the outside of the body through the urethra. In women, the urethra is separate from the reproductive system,

also stores starch for later use. The gallbladder makes bile, a green liquid that helps break down fats.

How the Digestive System Ages

The taste buds of the tongue are sensitive to four primary tastes: bitter, sweet, sour and salt. The tongue is not equally sensitive to all tastes in every area. The back of the tongue is more sensitive to bitter, the tip of the tongue to sweet, the sides to sour and the tip and sides to salt.

As we age, these taste buds become less sensitive and saliva production decreases, resulting in a dry mouth and an increase in plaque on the teeth. Intestinal muscle tone decreases, which may lead to constipation and an increase in the time it takes for food to digest. In addition, the digestive juice production decreases, which may result in vitamin and weight loss.

FIGURE B-12 The urinary system removes wastes from the bloodstream and eliminates them as urine.

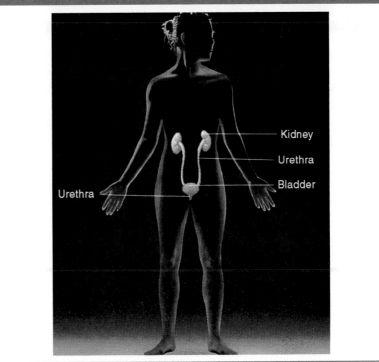

with the opening located anterior (in front) of the vagina. In men, both urine and semen can pass through the urethra, but never at the same time.

How the Urinary System Ages

As people age, they may have trouble with incontinence or dribbling urine. This problem occurs in men when the prostate gland enlarges, squeezing the nearby urethra, creating a need to urinate but an inability to empty the bladder completely. Incontinence can occur in women when muscles near the urethra weaken.

Occasionally, a nurse assistant may work with someone who has had a kidney transplant. Doctors first replaced a failed kidney with a working kidney in the late 1950s. Today doctors replace, or transplant, many kidneys every year. Kidneys used for transplant may be donated by a living person (preferably a family member) or by the family of someone who has died. More than 97 percent of people who receive kidneys from a living-donor and about 94 percent of those who receive kidneys from a deceased donor survive the first year.

INFORMATION REVIEW

Match each body system with its correct description.

nervous
circulatory
digestive
muscular
endocrine
respiratory
urinary
integumentary
skeletal
reproductive

1. The _____ system moves the body in many different directions.
2. The _____ system is made up of the brain and the spinal cord.
3. The pancreas is a part of the _____ system.
4. The _____ system uses food for nourishment.
5. The bones of the _____ system give structure to the body.
6. The _____ system protects the body from cold and germs.
7. The ovum and sperm are a part of the _____ system.
8. The lungs and alveoli are a part of the _____ system.
9. The _____ system pumps blood throughout the body.
10. The _____ system helps rid the body of waste.

Appendix B Answer Key

1. muscular
2. nervous
3. endocrine
4. digestive
5. skeletal
6. integumentary
7. reproductive
8. respiratory
9. circulatory
10. urinary

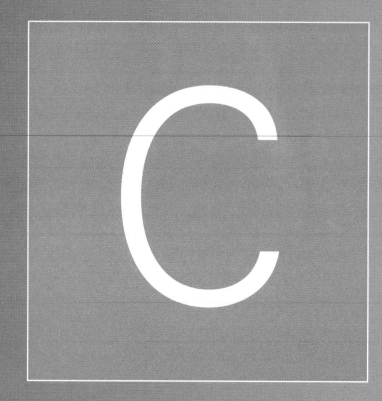

Home Health Care

GOALS

After reading this module, you will have the information needed to:

Follow special procedures for cleaning to prevent the spread of germs, keeping a bed in clean, safe and comfortable condition and doing laundry when providing home health care.

Explain rules for assisting with medications in home health care.

Identify five ways to assist a client with nutrition.

Describe how to read a food label.

Plan a meal for two people in a home.

Write a week's shopping list for two people.

List three ways to store food safely.

Demonstrate the procedure for collecting a urine specimen from an infant.*

Describe how to bathe a child.*

Describe how to comb a child's hair.*

Describe how to dress a child.*

Describe the normal range of respirations for children.*

Describe the normal pulse rate for children.*

After practicing the corresponding skills, you will have the information needed to:

Change crib linens*

Assist with clients' medication needs.

Apply compresses and assist with soaks.

Apply a heating pad.

Apply an aquathermia pad.

Prepare and apply a warm water bottle.

Apply an ice bag.

Collect a urine specimen from an infant or child.*

Note: * *Home Health Care for Infants, Children and Adolescents sections marked with an asterisk throughout Appendix C are optional content that may be skipped, if not required. In some states nurse assistants are not certified to provide home health care of infants, children and adolescents due to the complexity of care necessary. In those states these items may be omitted from the course.*

Mrs. Garcia broke her hip about a month ago. She has been through treatment and rehabilitation and is at last ready to return to her own home. She is looking forward to it, but she is also anxious. Will she be able to take care of her house and herself? How will she cook? It all begins to feel a little overwhelming.

Amber Clark is a single mother who has broken her collarbone in a car accident. She is healing well and is ready to return home, but she knows she cannot yet take care of her 15-month-old daughter Dominique.

Mary Hill and her infant daughter Melissa both are very ill with HIV infection. They are living at home with no one to take care of either of them.

What do these people all have in common? All may be in need of home health care. A home health care agency provides care for people in their homes, usually from a home health aide (a nurse assistant), with the care planned and monitored by a registered nurse. Those individuals who are served by a home health care agency are referred to as *clients*. Most clients need home health care because of a temporary injury, a chronic illness or a terminal illness. Not all of these clients—as you can see from our examples—are elderly.

All of the principles and skills of caregiving you have learned in this book will be valuable should you become a home health aide. For instance, falls and other incidents can happen in the home. Part of your job as a home health aide is identifying

and eliminating safety hazards by observing the precautions that you read in Chapter 8, "Keeping People Safe." However, there are additional things you will need to know.

This optional module will cover specific details about cleaning, laundering and cooking; assisting with medications in the home health setting; and helping with the special needs of children in home health care.

ADMITTING A HOME HEALTH CARE CLIENT

Have you ever had someone come into your home to do repairs? What did it feel like to have a stranger in your home? Were you afraid that he might break something? Were you concerned that he would leave a mess from his work? Did you feel that your home was no longer private? Thinking about your own responses to these questions may help you understand what people experience when they receive home health care and have new people help them in their own homes.

Before Mrs. Garcia is discharged to her home, the discharge planner at the nursing home calls a local home health care agency to arrange for services. After Mrs. Garcia arrives home, the nurse from the agency assesses her needs and, based on her primary care provider's orders and conditions in her home, develops a plan of care. The nurse then discusses the plan with other members of the health-care team, and together they coordinate their activities, including the scheduling of a home health aide. Mrs. Garcia needs a home health aide for personal care, a homemaker for housekeeping, a physical therapist to continue her exercises and a social worker to plan for her health-care needs.

On the first day that you arrive in a new client's home to begin providing care, you must try to help her feel

comfortable and relaxed about your being in her home. Talk with her, ask her about her interests, discuss her preferences and daily rituals, and help her understand what you will be doing in her home.

CLEANING AND LAUNDERING IN A CLIENT'S HOME

When you provide health care to someone at home, your primary responsibility is providing personal care according to the client's plan of treatment (Figure C-1). Light housekeeping chores may play a role in that plan. How much cleaning you do depends on the availability of family members, the amount of time you spend in the home, and the requirements of the client's care plan. You may have to keep the bedroom, bathroom and kitchen clean, since these three areas are important to the client and the care you provide for her. You also may have to do the client's personal laundry and wash her linens.

Maintaining a clean living environment helps promote the client's dignity and discourages the occurrence and spread of diseases such as colds, flu

FIGURE C-1 A client's care plan is often posted in the house so that everybody knows his or her responsibilities. If you are asked to do large jobs that are not listed on the care plan, check with your supervisor first.

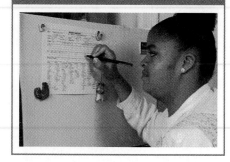

and diarrhea. Also, pests such as roaches, rats, mice, lice and fleas cannot thrive in a clean home. However, your duties as a home health aide differ greatly from those of a housekeeper. You focus your cleaning on eliminating germs, controlling infections and keeping the house free of safety hazards. Under the supervising nurses' discretion you may have to assist in teaching family members proper techniques to clean the household in this manner.

The home health agency that you work for has infection control policies and procedures for client care, housecleaning and laundering. It is important that you understand and practice these policies and procedures. The specific cleaning and laundry duties for which you are responsible are included in the care plan prepared by your nurse supervisor or the home health care team.

Before beginning each day, you must organize your time and thoughts. You have only a limited amount of time to spend with each client. Although your primary responsibility is helping the client with basic personal care, you also have to consider the areas of the client's home you must address after you provide personal care.

When taking care of a client in her home, you must always remember that, just like you, she may feel very strongly about her home and the things in it. Discuss your cleaning duties with your supervising nurse and the client so that you know how much you should do, as well as what the client wants and needs to have done for her. The way that you do things may be different from the way the client does things. If you must do things a certain way to maintain safety or infection control, you may have to explain why. At times, you may have to alter your procedure if the client asks you to handle things differently providing you would not be violating a basic principle of care.

Cleaning to Prevent the Spread of Germs

To prevent the spread of germs and disease always wash your hands before beginning and after completing home maintenance tasks. You may have to carry your own soap, paper towels and disposable hand wipes for handwashing. If there is no running water, use your hand wipes. Always observe the principles of infection control.

Also, observe Standard Precautions and infection control procedures such as wearing gloves if you come into contact with body fluids such as blood, urine or feces. For example, you must put on disposable gloves when handling contaminated laundry or cleaning up vomit. Throw away the disposable gloves in a covered trash can or a plastic trash bag, and wash your hands when you have finished the task. If necessary, put on new gloves for the next job.

In Chapter 7, "Controlling the Spread of Germs," you read about the following three levels of cleaning:

1. Cleaning: To get rid of visible dirt
2. Disinfecting: To remove harmful organisms
3. Sterilizing: To eliminate all organisms

In your job as a home health aide you must use cleaning products safely and store all cleaning products in a safe place (Figure C-2). You also have to know when to use various cleaning agents including the four basic kinds of household cleaning products:

1. All-purpose cleaning agents for general cleaning of many kinds of surfaces
2. Soaps and detergents for bathing, laundering and washing dishes
3. Cleansers for scouring areas that are hard to clean
4. Specialty cleaners for specific tasks and surfaces such as cleaning glass or ovens

Some cleaners also contain disinfectants. If you need to disinfect, but

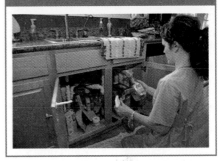

FIGURE C-2 Because some cleaning products are dangerous if swallowed or used improperly, make sure all cleaning products are stored in a safe place. If children or confused people are in the home, use a high shelf or a locked cabinet.

the cleaners you have do not kill germs, use a bleach solution. Household bleach is an inexpensive and effective chemical disinfectant for cleaning.

Because full-strength bleach has a very strong odor and is harsh on the skin, always mix it with water. At the beginning of each visit, prepare the solution by mixing $\frac{1}{4}$ cup of bleach with 1 gallon of water. Put the water in a bucket or other container first and then pour the bleach into it. **Mix bleach *only* with water,** since mixing it with anything else, especially any product containing ammonia, can create a dangerous gas. Make a fresh solution of bleach and water each day, because the disinfecting power of bleach goes away if the solution sits too long.

Before using the bleach solution test a small area to make sure the solution does not affect the color of the surface, and then wash it off. Use the bleach solution to clean the bathroom, floors and counters. Also use it as a disinfectant on a surface that has already been cleaned of visible dirt. To protect your skin wear disposable or household gloves.

Sterilization is a process that kills all germs. A common sterilization process is boiling an item for 20 minutes—this kills most harmful germs. You may have to sterilize baby bottles in the home. Glass bottles may be boiled routinely but check with the client before boiling plastic bottles.

Disposing of Trash

You must dispose of any trash you create while providing care for your client. If time allows, you also may dispose of household trash and possibly teach family members proper techniques for trash disposal. Periodically, you may have to wash trash cans with hot soapy water when they are dirty and rinse them with a bleach solution. Washing reduces germs and odors that grow in trash containers, as well as insects and rodents that may live and breed there. To avoid spreading any germs from handling trash, be sure to wash your hands when you finish disposing of it. In addition, observe the following procedures for different types of trash.

Disposing of Food. To throw away food, first drain off any liquid, wrap the food and put it in a paper- or plastic-lined pail. If your client has a garbage disposal, put only soft foods in it. Never put hard or stringy foods in the garbage disposal because they may damage it.

Disposing of Grease. Pour cooled grease into a disposable container, never into the sink drain or garbage disposal (Figure C-3). Put a lid on the container before disposing of it with the garbage.

Disposing of Cans and Bottles. Rinse cans and bottles to destroy odors that might attract insects, rats or other pests. Put appropriate cans and bottles in containers for recycling and dispose of the others with the trash. Recyclable containers often have the triangular recycle symbol on them.

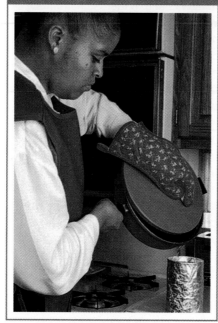

FIGURE C-3 If you must dispose of grease while it is still hot, be sure to use a heat-proof container, such as a metal food can. Allow the container to cool before putting it in the trash.

Disposing of Contaminated and Wet Items. Use plastic bags for contaminated and wet items such as used tissues, sanitary napkins, disposable underpads, adult briefs or dressings. Double-bag and tie these items before throwing them into a plastic trash bag or covered container. Always wear disposable gloves when handling these items, and dispose of gloves properly in a plastic trash bag or covered container.

Doing the Laundry

Part of the care you may have to provide for your client is cleaning and maintaining her linens and clothing. If your client has urinary or bowel incontinence, you may have to do laundry several times a day. To clean contaminated linens:

- Immediately remove contaminated linens from the bed.
- Flush solid waste down the toilet.

- Put the contaminated linens in a plastic bag and take them to the washing machine or to a commercial laundry.

Because you may come in contact with body fluids on contaminated laundry, you must always observe infection control procedures by keeping dirty linens away from your own clothing and wearing a gown and disposable gloves.

When washing a client's linens or clothing, check with her or an appropriate family member about the way she prefers to have her laundry done. You may have to check clothing labels to determine how to wash certain items.

Maintaining a Bed in a Home Setting

In a home setting, in addition to changing the linens on a person's bed, you must maintain the bed so that the mattress remains firm and free from dust that might cause allergies. To maintain the person's bed:

- Brush or vacuum the bed weekly to get rid of dust and dust mites.
- Turn the mattress at least once a month so that the person does not sleep on the same place, which causes uneven wearing of the mattress.
- If she uses an air mattress, make sure the air pump works.

When making a bed in a home setting, remember to use good body mechanics, since the bed may not raise or lower. Protect your back by squatting instead of bending over and by moving around the bed instead of reaching across it.

Some clients in a home setting may sleep on water beds. A soft-sided water bed uses standard bed linens; however, another type of water bed, which consists of a water-filled bladder inside a wooden frame, often requires special linens. You may need to check the water bed thermostat to make sure it is set at the temperature the client prefers. The range of comfort for most people is 75° to 95° F.

When providing care for a client who sleeps on a water bed, you must keep all sharp objects away from the bed, make sure the temperature is comfortable, and check the thermostat daily.

Sometimes you may be required to care for a child who uses a crib. Skill 58 shows you how to change crib linens.

ASSISTING WITH MEDICATIONS IN THE HOME HEALTH SETTING

In addition to home care and the usual types of personal care that all nurse assistants give, a home health aide may have to assist with medications. Only doctors and licensed nurses may actually give medications to people. It is illegal for you, as a home health aide, to give *any* medication to a person in your care—this includes over-the-counter medicines, as well as prescription drugs. The law defining who can give medication protects both you and the person in your care. Giving medication is a big responsibility. If a person is given the wrong medication, he could be injured, and the person who gave him the medication could be held responsible for the injury.

In the home health setting, however, you can *help* the person who must take medication by reminding him to take it. You can bring the medicine container to the person and you can open it, but you *cannot* pour out the medicine or remove it from the container in any way. You also can assist the person by steadying his hand to keep liquid medicine from spilling. Skill 59 talks about assisting with medications in home health care.

If a person asks you to fix some special kind of tea or home remedy, check with your supervising nurse first. Also, notify your supervising nurse if your client:

- Is not taking medication as prescribed.
- Is taking more or less than the prescribed amount.

- Is taking medicine other than what the doctor prescribed, including over-the-counter medicine.
- Is taking medication at times other than those ordered.
- Has side effects after taking medications.
- Says the medication does not seem to be working.
- Has any questions concerning medications.

Also, let your supervising nurse know:

- If a medication container is missing a label or if the label is hard to read.
- When you notice, or your client tells you, that he has just a few pills left from a prescription.
- If a medication has expired, because the strength of the medication cannot be guaranteed after the expiration date. (The expiration date is printed on the container label.)
- If you suspect that anyone in the household is misusing any type of medicine.

ASSISTING A HOME HEALTH CARE CLIENT WITH PHYSICAL COMFORT

As a home health aide you need to help the person to be as comfortable as possible, just as you do in a hospital or nursing facility. In addition to repositioning the person, you must provide personal care. Personal care may include applying comforting measures such as compresses, soaks, aquathermia pad, heating pad, warm water bottle or ice bag. These measures are explained step by step in Skills 60 through 64.

NUTRITION IN HOME HEALTH CARE

On Monday, when you arrive to provide care for Amber Clark and her 15-month-old daughter Dominique,

Amber looks relieved. She says that her sister did the grocery shopping for her on Saturday, but that she has been unable to prepare many dishes because of her broken collarbone.

Together, you and Ms. Clark do an inventory of the food she has in her cupboards and refrigerator and plan menus for her and Dominique. You help her choose a variety of nutritious foods for each meal. You also fix large portions of two meals that she can simply heat at mealtimes.

As a home health aide, you often have the important responsibility to plan, shop for, store, prepare and serve the most nutritious foods possible to help your client regain her health or stay healthy. You also will be responsible for keeping the kitchen area clean.

Planning Meals

To plan nutritious meals, you first must learn the eating habits, likes and dislikes of the person in your care. You also must learn whether she or he has religious or cultural preferences relating to food. Your supervising nurse may be able to give you some of this information, or you may have to ask the client the following questions:

- What do you like to eat?
- How do you like each individual food prepared? (This question should be specific to the foods the client prefers.)
- Do you follow a special diet or have food preferences for health reasons?
- When do you like to eat? How much do you like to eat at each of those times?
- What kinds of snack foods do you like to eat?
- Is there any food you do not like?
- Are there foods you are allergic to? (Allergies should also be documented on the care plan.)
- Do you have any preferences about food storage or handling?

- What foods or brands do you usually buy at the grocery store when you shop? (You should ask this question of the person who usually does the shopping for the household.)

Your responsibility in meal preparation and planning varies, depending on the needs of your client (Figure C-4). At times you may be involved in shopping for groceries. At other times you may plan and prepare meals or you may prepare meals that have been planned by someone else. After your discussion with the client plan the desirable number of meals referring to the five major food groups for guidance in food selection. Finally, plan some meals that are based on leftovers. Using leftovers cuts down on the time spent preparing and enables you to buy larger quantities of items such as meat, rice and pasta which may save money for your client. If your client is on a special diet or is allergic to certain foods or seasoning, this should be documented in their care plan.

Shopping

For some clients, you may have to shop for groceries. Use the information you get from the client and her family to start your shopping list. Check to see what she already has and ask her whether she needs any staple items, such as spices, sugar or flour. Planning meals lets you shop for everything you need at one time.

Shopping wisely saves money. As a shopper, you can follow many practical, money-saving steps for both you and the client. For example:

- Watch newspaper ads for food specials and collect money-saving food coupons.
- Keep an ongoing shopping list. Jot down items to be replaced as you use them, review the list with the client, and complete the list before you go shopping. Follow the list carefully as you shop.
- Use unit pricing. Look at Figure C-5 to compare product prices and sizes and to help you select the most economical product.
- Select less expensive, leaner cuts of meat. These meats may require

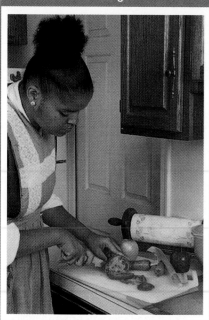

FIGURE C-4 Be sure to consider your client's needs when preparing food in a home health care setting.

FIGURE C-5 If you can efficiently use the 24-ounce can, buy it. However, keep in mind the client's preference for a particular brand and whether she can use the contents of the larger can before they spoil.

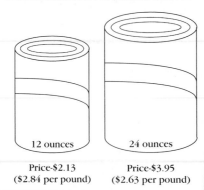

COMPARATIVE SHOPPING

12 ounces	24 ounces
Price-$2.13	Price-$3.95
($2.84 per pound)	($2.63 per pound)

BOX C-1

Product Nutrition Label
Nutrition Information
per Serving

Serving size	9.5 oz
Servings per container	2
Calories	130
Protein	12 g
Carbohydrate	12 g
Fat	3 g
Cholesterol	20 mg
(5 mg/100 g)*	
Sodium	870 mg
Potassium	400 mg

Percentage of U.S. recommended daily allowances (U.S. RDA)

Protein	20
Riboflavin	6
Vitamin A	50
Niacin	30
Vitamin C	†
Calcium	4
Thiamin	4
Iron	15

Ingredients: chicken broth, carrots, chicken, tomatoes, red kidney beans, enriched macaroni product, celery, green beans, green peas, lima beans, food starch-modified, salt, dehydrated onions, hydrolyzed vegetable protein, monosodium glutamate, sugar, autolyzed yeast extract, spice, natural flavor.

* Information on cholesterol content is provided for individuals who, on the advice of a doctor, are modifying their dietary intake of cholesterol.
† Contains less than 2% of the U.S. RDA of this nutrient.

long, slow cooking, such as braising, stewing or overnight marinating to tenderize them.

- Read product labels. Label information lists ingredients, number of servings per container, and the amount of fat, carbohydrates, calories and nutrients in a serving. See Box C-1 for an example of label information.

Storing and Handling Food

Everyone who works in a kitchen and handles food must observe the following basic rules of sanitation and hygiene:

- If you suspect that food has become contaminated or has not been handled or stored properly, wrap it in plastic or aluminum foil and throw it away in a covered trash container. Too many germs in food make it unsafe to eat. Tell your client what foods you are throwing away and why.
- Wash your hands often with soap and water when you are handling food.
- Before and after use, clean and sanitize food preparation surfaces and utensils, especially any surfaces and utensils that come into contact with raw meats, poultry or fish.
- Keep hot foods hot, making sure they stay above 140° F or higher before serving.
- Keep cold foods cold, storing them at temperatures of 40° F or lower. Store appropriate foods in the refrigerator.
- Wash fresh vegetables and fruit carefully before using them.
- Discard any uneaten portion of a client's meal. The food is unsafe to use again and should not be eaten by anyone else.
- Keep all trash covered to prevent attracting insects and rodents.

Preparing Food

Before you start cooking, ask for a tour of the kitchen. If no one can give you a tour, take one yourself (Figure C-6).

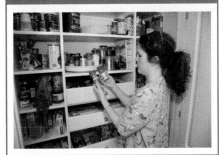

FIGURE C-6 When you work as a home health aide, you may be responsible for cooking. To save time later, get acquainted with the kitchen when first visiting a new client.

Each person organizes her kitchen in her own way. Find out where pots, pans, dishes and utensils are kept so that you are prepared when you must cook or put away clean dishes.

Before beginning to cook, plan and organize all the food and utensils that you must have to do the job. Prepare foods carefully to destroy harmful germs and to retain flavor and nutrients. Use the basic cooking techniques listed in the following paragraphs.

Baking. Baking is a dry-heat cooking process in the oven in which food is not exposed directly to the heat source. Bake foods such as casseroles or breads in oven-proof containers.

Roasting. Roasting is also a dry-heat cooking process, similar to baking, that usually exposes large cuts of meat or poultry to hot air in the oven. Use an oven-proof container without a lid or cover.

Broiling and Grilling. Another dry-heat cooking method is broiling. Place the food (usually meat) on a metal rack in a metal pan. Place the pan on an oven rack, and cook the food directly under the source of heat. For grilling, place the food on a rack directly over the source of heat, as in barbecuing, or place the food in a skillet or on a griddle on a stove burner.

Steaming. Steaming is a moist-heat cooking method that uses a burner on top of the stove. This quick, no-fat way to cook vegetables retains the maximum amount of flavor and nutrients. Place vegetables in a metal steaming basket and set it in a pot over, but not in, water. Cover the pot and bring the water to a boil. Check often to make sure the water has not boiled away.

Boiling. This moist-heat process cooks food directly in boiling water in a pot. Place the pot on the stove burner and bring the water to a full rolling boil. Place the food in the boiling water, cover the pot with a lid (usually), reduce the heat and cook the food until done. Periodically check to make sure the water has not boiled away.

Frying, Stir-Frying and Sautéing. Frying involves cooking foods in preheated fat or oil in a pot or skillet on the stove burner. Because the fat becomes very hot during cooking and can splatter, take extra care when putting food in and removing it from the pan. Stir-frying and sautéing require cooking thin or small pieces of food in a small amount of fat, which may be a combination of butter and oil. Foods brown and cook quickly by these methods.

Microwave Oven. Many of these techniques also may be used in a microwave oven. Follow the manufacturer's directions for proper use of the microwave oven.

Serving Meals

A person usually looks forward to mealtime but food may not seem very appealing to someone who is sick. You can help make mealtime more enjoyable by using some of the following tips:

- Set up a mealtime schedule and stick to it so that your client does not get upset by any changes. However, if your client is not hungry at mealtime and wants to eat at another time, be as flexible as possible.

- Arrange plates and tables attractively so that food looks appealing and appetizing.
- Plan meals that use foods of different colors. If you planned a meal of mashed potatoes, cauliflower and skinned breast of chicken, everything would be white. If you serve carrots instead of, or with, the cauliflower, you add some color. You might also serve brown rice instead of mashed potatoes.
- Always use clean utensils and fresh napkins.
- Make sure that the client is comfortable and that she washes her hands before and after eating.
- Protect her clothing with a napkin or towel.
- Do not hurry the client while she eats.
- Serve hot foods hot and cold foods cold.
- Clear the table or remove the plate as soon as the client has finished eating.

HOME HEALTH CARE FOR INFANTS, CHILDREN AND ADOLESCENTS

Note: In some states nurse assistants are not certified to provide home healthcare for infants, children and adolescents. Find out from your instructor if you need to review this information. If not, you may skip this section and go to Discharging a Home Health Care Client page 535.

NUTRITION FOR CHILDREN

What about children's nutrition needs? You may recall that both Ms. Clark and Ms. Hill have children who will need your care.

Good nutrition often is influenced by food habits acquired in childhood. You can help children in your care establish good eating habits and wholesome attitudes toward food. These attitudes will affect their health throughout their entire lives.

Observing Appetite Characteristics in Young Children

As you provide care for children, you may observe characteristics of appetite in certain age groups. In general, healthy infants have good appetites. Children's appetites decrease toward the end of their first year and continue to decrease in their second year as growth slows down. As toddlers, children may exhibit their need for independence by choosing not to eat. Preschool children frequently eat smaller meals and may want to snack between meals. Children who are 3 or 4 years old may eat slowly but generally show an increase in appetite over the previous year. They generally eat more at one sitting than 2-year-old children. By age 6, most children have developed stable, healthy appetites. Family food preferences and behaviors strongly influence children's likes, dislikes and eating patterns. Children generally learn to enjoy a wide variety of foods if they are exposed to them in pleasant situations.

Feeding Infants

Because infants grow and change at a rapid rate during the first year of life, you must be aware of how their feeding needs change during this time.

0 to 3 Months. Hold the infant during feedings of breast milk or formula. If the family has a history of allergies, breast-feeding the baby is recommended over formula feeding. Cereal is not recommended for a child of this age since it may be too difficult for him to digest.

4 to 5 Months. Continue feeding the infant formula or breast milk and begin baby cereal feedings. The parent should check with the child's doctor before beginning feeding solid foods to the child. Breast milk or formula should be offered before any solid meal. Solid food should be a supplement not replacement for breast milk or formula. Start with 2 tablespoons of rice cereal twice daily and then introduce other single-grain cereals one at a time. Introduce multigrain cereal last. Giving the baby only one new food at a time allows him to get used to the flavor and makes it easier to determine whether he is allergic to any particular type of food. (Signs of food allergy include diarrhea, rash, vomiting and irritability.) During feedings, the baby may push most of the cereal out of his mouth as a result of the tongue's normal sucking action. Use the spoon to gently put the food back into his mouth.

Note: To prevent overfeeding or choking, never put cereal into the baby's bottle.

6 to 8 Months. At this age, the baby may hold his own bottle of breast milk or formula, but he still should be held during bottle feedings to increase his sense of security and to meet his social needs. Introduce apple and noncitrus juices one at a time. Continue feeding the child baby cereal and begin serving him strained fruits, vegetables and meats. Again, introduce new foods one at a time and avoid combination meals. To prepare baby food at home, steam small amounts of food over water and save the resulting cooking liquid. Place the food and vitamin-rich liquid in a blender and puree it. When using commercially prepared baby food, spoon a meal-sized portion into a bowl, and refrigerate the unused food for up to 24 hours. Feeding the infant directly from the jar introduces bacteria into the jar and contaminates the uneaten portion, which must be thrown away.

Note: Do not sweeten foods with honey, because it may cause botulism in infants.

9 to 12 Months. Between feedings, begin offering the child liquids in a cup. Continue feeding the child cereal and slowly advance to chunkier toddler foods. During meals, give the child a separate spoon to encourage self-feeding skills. Introduce small finger foods, such as unsugared adult cereals, cooked vegetables and fruits. Avoid giving the child nuts, raw vegetables, popcorn, grapes and hard candy, which can easily lodge in the throat and cause choking. Make sure the child eats foods such as biscuits, toast and crackers while sitting up (*never* while lying down) to reduce the possibility of choking on crumbs.

Note: *Do not put the child to bed with a bottle of milk or fruit juice. During the night, there is ample time for the sugar in these fluids to attack the teeth and start cavities.*

Feeding Children and Adolescents

When you provide care for children and adolescents, it is important to know what foods they like and how you can make mealtime a pleasant part of the child's daily experience.

Toddlers (1 to 3 years). Begin to wean a toddler from bottle or breast-feeding and offer him whole milk in a cup instead. To encourage the child to eat solid foods limit his milk intake to 16 to 24 ounces daily. Begin serving the child table food that the rest of the family eats keeping a watchful eye on the fat, salt and sugar content. Avoid very spicy foods which can be hard for a young child to digest. To prevent choking do not give toddlers small, round or hard foods, such as hot dogs or hard candy.

Use the child's appetite to gauge how much to serve at mealtime. Typical serving sizes for a 2- to 3-year-old child include 2 to 3 tablespoons of applesauce or cooked vegetables; $\frac{1}{4}$ of a banana or apple; $\frac{1}{3}$ cup of orange juice; 1 to 2 ounces of meat, fish, or poultry; $\frac{1}{2}$ slice of bread; $\frac{1}{3}$ cup of cooked dry peas, beans, or lentils; and 2 to 3 tablespoons of rice or

cereal. Make mealtimes fun and encourage the child to use his own cup and spoon while eating.

Note: *Do not force a child to eat and never use food as a reward or punishment.*

Toddlers are known to be picky eaters. They commonly go on "food jags" and may eat only one type of food for several days. Continue to present the child with a balanced diet by offering nutritious between-meal snacks such as cubed cheese and bread or unsalted crackers spread with peanut butter.

Preschoolers (3 to 5 years). The quality of a preschooler's diet is more important than the quantity. Continue to offer a balanced diet, serving the child approximately 1 tablespoon of each food for each year of his age. You may introduce low-fat or skim milk at this time. A preschool child needs the calcium supplied by two to three 8-ounce servings of milk each day but may not be able to drink an entire serving of milk at one time. To make sure the child gets enough calcium, serve him milk and dairy products as snacks.

Cheese cut into cubes and served with fruit or crackers makes an ideal snack, as do cheese spreads on crackers or bread. (Avoid serving cream cheese, which is full of fat and is more like butter than cheese.) Cottage cheese with fruit or plain low-fat yogurt with fruit added at home is another good snack choice. Make a nutritious frozen dessert by mixing yogurt with crushed fruit in a blender and freezing the mixture in paper cups or other small containers.

To increase the child's iron and protein intake include snacks from the meat group. Cut leftover cooked meat into cubes and serve with fruit or vegetables. Make meat spreads in a food processor and spread on bread or crackers. Another high-protein snack is hard-cooked eggs served with

cheese. Offer sweet, high-fat or salty foods *only* after meeting basic nutrition requirements. Try serving the child yogurt, raisins and graham crackers instead of sweet desserts.

School-Age Children (5 to 12 years). A child grows rapidly during the school-age years, and his appetite often reflects this. When serving meals, increase the portion size of each food served according to how much the child will eat and continue to offer a balanced diet.

During the school-age years, a child's food choices and preferences are often influenced by his peers and by television commercials. Luckily, most children seem to have an avid interest in food and this is a good time to teach them how to make healthy food choices. Encouraging a child to choose nutritious snacks, such as those mentioned previously, is a good way to promote his sense of independence.

Adolescents (13 to 19 years). When serving a meal to an adolescent, plan the meal to allow for the person's need for more protein and iron, which help the body as it continues to grow and mature. Iron is especially important for adolescent girls who begin to menstruate at this time. Adolescents who play sports need to eat more than their non-athletic peers do to keep their energy usage from affecting growth and maturity. Larger meals and between-meal snacks help supply extra calories. Young women who become pregnant also require extra calories and nutrition. To help maintain the mother's and baby's health encourage a pregnant adolescent to have her diet professionally evaluated early in her pregnancy and to receive regular nutrition counseling.

Peers and personal body image influence food selection during adolescence. Even teens who occasionally eat at fast-food restaurants can maintain healthy diets if they make wise menu choices. But adolescents who eat primarily high-fat, high-calorie foods—and those who experiment with dieting—may seriously affect their health. Eating a balanced diet during adolescence is important for promoting good nutrition and maintaining health in the adult years.

Note: *Government food-assistance programs are often available for low-income families. If you provide care for families who are unable to provide their children with a nutritious diet report this concern to your supervising nurse so that she or a social worker can refer the family to the appropriate agency. As a nurse assistant, you may help teach nutrition and meal planning to people receiving assistance from such programs.*

PROVIDING CARE FOR CHILDREN'S ELIMINATION NEEDS

When you work in a hospital or in home health care you often provide care for children. You help infants and toddlers with special elimination needs such as diapering. You may also need to collect urine specimens from infants.

Collecting a Urine Specimen from an Infant

Obtaining a urine specimen from an infant or a child who is not toilet trained requires applying a special self-adhesive collection bag called a pediatric urine collection bag to the infant's perineal area or over the infant's penis. First, provide perineal care cleaning from front to back in girls and from the urethra outward in boys.

To apply the collection bag, position the infant on his or her back and spread the knees apart, exposing the genitals. If the child is very active you may have to ask a co-worker or the child's parent to help hold the child. For a boy, position the penis through the opening at the top of the bag and press the adhesive securely around the base of the penis and the scrotum taking care not to cover the anus. For a girl, position the bag over the urethra and press the adhesive area over the labia to create a seal again taking care not to cover the anus.

Reapply the diaper over the collection bag. If the infant is young enough so that he cannot pull off the bag, cut a slit in the disposable diaper before reapplying the diaper and pull the bag through the slit so that you can see when the infant has voided. Check every 15 minutes to see whether the infant has urinated (Figure C-7).

To remove the bag, loosen the adhesive and gently remove the bag. Seal the top by folding the adhesive area over and placing it in the sterile specimen container. Do not leave the infant unattended to do this. Instead, set the specimen bag down on the crib and put the collection bag in the specimen container later. Some pediatric urine collection bags have a port, or

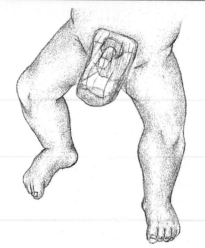

FIGURE C-7 To collect urine from a small child, place a collection bag over the urethral opening for a short period of time. Observe the child frequently until you obtain the specimen.

opening, at the bottom of the bag to empty the urine into the container. Record that you have collected the specimen and report any important observations such as cloudy or foul-smelling urine or blood in the urine.

The specific procedure for collecting urine from an infant or child is explained step by step in Skill 65.

WHO ARE THE CHILDREN WITH HIV INFECTION?

You may recall that Melissa Hill has HIV infection. Providing care for children with HIV infection and AIDS may be challenging for some health-care workers. To be most effective as a nurse assistant you need more information about how HIV infection and AIDS affect children.

Given the length of time between infection and the appearance of symptoms, experts suspect that many of the people diagnosed with AIDS in their 20s actually became infected while they were teenagers. Sharing needles and syringes and having sex with an HIV-infected person are common ways that young people become infected. Teenagers are especially at risk because a number of them experiment with sex, alcohol and drugs. If infected and sexually active they may pass the infection to their children. Not all women who have HIV will give it to their children. Without treatment or breastfeeding about 25% (1 in 4) of pregnant women with HIV will transmit the virus to their babies.

Like their mothers, children born with HIV are also benefiting from early diagnosis and better treatment. Many are living longer and healthier lives due to life-saving drugs and preventive measures.

Babies and children with HIV infection and AIDS most commonly display the following signs and symptoms:

- Various bacterial infections
- Malnutrition and "failure to thrive"

- Pneumonia caused by organisms that may or may not include *Pneumocystis carinii*
- Anemia
- Short time to progress from HIV infection to AIDS
- Short life span
- Heart, liver, kidney or skin problems
- Nervous system damage including developmental disabilities

The reason HIV infection and AIDS progress so quickly in young children is the fact that babies are not born with fully functioning immune systems. Remember that the immune system serves two functions:

1. To develop antibodies against disease agents
2. To surround and attack these disease agents.

Adults tend to lose mainly the second function when they develop AIDS leading to viral, parasitic and fungal infections. However, when babies and children have AIDS, both functions of the immune system tend to fail and they may also display the following signs and symptoms:

- Weight loss
- Persistent diarrhea
- Recurrent fever
- Swollen lymph glands
- Severe thrush (oral fungus infection)
- *Pneumocystis carinii* pneumonia.

How Children Become Infected with HIV

Of the infants and children under 13 who have developed AIDS the vast majority were born to mothers who were at risk of becoming infected or who had HIV infection, including AIDS. Many of these women did not know they were infected until their children were diagnosed; some did not know that they could pass the virus to their babies.

An infected mother can pass HIV to her baby in three ways:

1. During pregnancy the mother's blood nourishes the baby. If this blood is infected with HIV the virus could cross the placenta and infect the baby.
2. During delivery the baby must pass through the mother's vagina. The baby comes in contact with her vaginal fluid, as well as some blood. If these fluids are HIV-infected they could infect the baby.
3. During breast-feeding the baby could receive milk infected with HIV. Other blood-borne viruses have been transmitted from mother to baby through breast-feeding. However, relatively few cases of HIV transmission through breast-feeding have been reported, and experts believe that the relative risk of transmission is small.

All donor blood is now tested and blood that tests positive for HIV is discarded. Also, blood that is used for producing blood products is treated to remove infectious agents, including HIV, which may be present in small amounts from a recent infection and may not have shown up on the test. Thus, it is now unlikely that a child or adult would become infected by receiving either blood products or transfusions.

Providing Care for Children with HIV or AIDS

Infants and children who are infected with HIV or who have AIDS need the same things as those who are well. Infants need to be held and loved and have all the things that they need to grow physically and emotionally. Older children need to play and have friends and, when able, go to school. When you treat the infant or child as you would any other the entire family benefits.

The same infection control principles apply to children as to adults. Remember to practice the principles of care that guide all your caregiving. In addition:

- Pay extra attention to any changes in health or behavior and report these observations to your supervising nurse. For a young child with AIDS these changes could become serious quickly. Watch for breathing problems, fever, exhaustion, diarrhea and changes in appetite.
- Consult the doctor before a child with HIV infection or AIDS receives immunizations or booster shots.
- Wear gloves when changing diapers since blood may be in the child's stool.
- Encourage the child to play with plastic and washable toys because they are easier to clean. Stuffed and furry toys can contain dirt and can be a possible source of other infections to the child with AIDS. If a child plays with stuffed toys, keep them clean and machine washed often.
- Keep the child away from litter boxes and sandboxes to which pets or other animals have access.
- Ask your supervising nurse what precautions you should take if pets live in the home.
- Protect children with HIV infection from getting infectious diseases, especially chicken pox. Report immediately to your supervising nurse if the child has been exposed to chicken pox or shingles. It could be deadly to the child.

Providing care to a chronically ill child can be especially hard for family and other caregivers. Provide support by being trustworthy, dependable and positive and by listening. Remember the anger parents express to you may really be directed at the disease, not at you. Also, try to keep your emotions out of the way while you are providing care. Discuss with your supervising nurse your feelings about caring for an infant or child with AIDS.

PROVIDING PERSONAL CARE FOR CHILDREN

When you go to the home of Amber Clark and her 15-month-old daughter Dominique you provide care for both the mother and her daughter. Ms. Clark broke her collarbone in a car collision and is unable to lift her daughter and provide her personal care. The care that you provide for this child is similar to the personal care that you provide for her mother, but because she is small and at a different stage in her development, you have to do some things differently.

Providing Mouth Care for a Child

Today, when you visit the Clarks, Ms. Clark says that Dominique has been very fussy. She thinks she is cutting more teeth but she cannot hold her to examine her mouth. You hold Dominique on your lap and look into her mouth. Her gums are red and swollen and you can see the white teeth just under the gum. This condition is a clue that you must be very gentle on that area of her mouth when you clean her teeth.

Many children have six to eight teeth by the time they are 1 year old. If a child's gums are not too tender from teething, use a moist cloth or gauze square wrapped around your finger to gently clean the teeth (Figure C-8). If the child is over 1 year of age use a very soft toothbrush dipped in water.

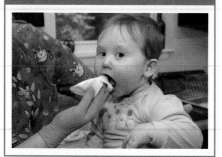

FIGURE C-8 Good mouth care is important for children because it keeps teeth and gums healthy and promotes the development of healthy permanent teeth.

Hold the child on your lap to provide comfort and security.

Babies around 1 year of age frequently go to bed with a bottle, although this is not recommended and should be discouraged. If the baby drinks milk or juice from the bottle, the residue from these liquids can lead to early tooth decay. Because Ms. Clark usually puts Dominique to bed with a bottle of milk, encourage her to give her the bottle before putting her to bed.

Children usually like to try brushing their own teeth and it is important to encourage their independence by letting them do so. However, they usually are not able to clean their teeth effectively until the age of 6 to 10 years. Before then, an adult should brush the child's teeth and the child should be encouraged to brush her own teeth either before or after the parent's brushing. She should brush for 3 minutes. Use an egg timer to let the child know when the 3 minutes have passed and to make brushing a fun time for her. Children should brush their teeth two to three times a day making sure to brush just before bedtime.

You can brush a child's teeth when the child is in bed as you would an adult's teeth. You also can position yourself behind a child who is either seated or standing. Use one hand to cup the child's chin and the other to hold the toothbrush.

Check with your supervising nurse about whether it is advisable to use fluorinated toothpaste and mouth rinses in your geographic area. In many places, dentists recommend the use of fluoride toothpaste and, for children over 6 years, the daily use of a fluoride mouth rinse to reduce the possibility of tooth decay.

When you provide care for a child who is NPO (not eating or drinking by mouth), brush his teeth twice each day with a soft toothbrush dipped in water. Because some medicines are heavily

sweetened to improve their taste children should brush their teeth or rinse their mouths with water after taking these medicines. A child should also brush his teeth after vomiting to remove gastric juices which can wear away tooth enamel. If using the toothbrush causes an ill child to gag, have him rinse his mouth with water and spit it out.

Children with physical impairments may have to use toothbrushes that have been specially adapted with larger or curved handles or self-adhesive fabric fasteners which make them easier to hold. Electric toothbrushes also may be useful.

Bathing and Shampooing a Child

Dominique squeals with delight when you begin to run water into the tub for her bath. She loves bathtime. You gather together the plastic water toys and put them in the tub. After checking the tub water for the correct temperature, you turn off the hot water first, then the cold. You close the bathroom door before undressing Dominique so that she will stay warm. While Dominique plays in the tub, you sit on the toilet lid and watch her as she splashes about. After a few minutes, you kneel next to the tub and start to wash her.

Bathing a Child. When helping children bathe it is important for you to know the age and developmental stage of each child and also his capabilities so that you can safely and appropriately provide care. Generally, older and adolescent children are very concerned about privacy, and younger children enjoy playing at bathtime.

Safety is the most important thing to keep in mind while bathing children. Never leave a child alone in water. Check the water carefully to make sure that it is between 100° and 105°F (or just warm on the inside of your wrist). Fill the tub no more than one-third full and instruct the child, if it is appropriate, not to turn the hot water faucet by himself. To prevent falls, make sure nonskid mats are in the tub. Also helpful are safety rails or specially designed seats to support the child who cannot sit by himself. Do not use bath oils in the tub, because they make the tub and the child slippery and hard to hold on to.

If you have to help a child into a tub be sure to use good body mechanics. If the child is small, bend your knees to squat and lower the child into the tub. Avoid bending over from the waist (Figure C-9). A large tub may be awkward, uncomfortable and unsafe for bathing a small infant. In a home setting, you may use an infant tub on a table top as an alternative (Figure C-10). To hold an infant, place one arm under his neck and back and hold on to the arm on the side farther away from your body. This position gives you a firm grip on the infant and helps to make him feel more secure. Use your other hand to support the buttocks. Gradually lower the infant into the water so that he has a chance to become accustomed to the water temperature and so that he is not startled by the water.

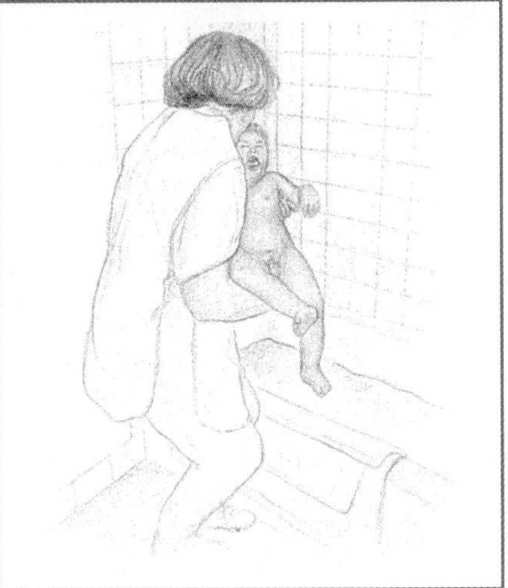

Use one hand to wash an infant or small child who cannot sit without support while holding and supporting him with your other hand. Wash from top to bottom, rinsing each part as you go so that the child does not become too slippery. Also, as with adults, soap is very drying to the skin and may cause vaginal irritation in some little girls. Use soap sparingly and do not let it soak in the bath water. To keep the child warm, wrap him in a towel as soon as you remove him from the tub. Then help him get dressed.

Toddlers generally enjoy playing with unbreakable cups and toys in the bath. Provide time for play if possible but do not leave the child alone. Older children and adolescents, on the other hand, may have strong feelings about privacy, and as you would with adults, you should make every effort to give them privacy as long as you can do so safely.

Use the same basic procedure that you would use to bathe an adult in bed when you give a bed bath to an older child or adolescent or help him with a tub bath or shower.

Shampooing a Child's Hair. If the child is healthy shampoo his hair once or twice a week. Adolescents may wish to shampoo their hair more fre-

quently because the scalp produces more oil at this stage of development. Shampooing can be done during the bath or separately.

Shampoo an infant's hair by applying baby shampoo to the scalp with one hand, while you support him as you did when you lowered him into the tub. Tip him back so that water and shampoo do not run into his eyes. Rinse out the shampoo by using the washcloth or an unbreakable cup to pour water over his head.

If a child is confined to his bed, wash his hair in the bed using the same procedure you use for an adult. Encourage the child to help by holding a washcloth or towel over his eyes. Wrap the child's head in a towel immediately after the last rinse and follow instructions from your supervising nurse about using a blow dryer to dry his hair.

Providing Perineal Care for Infants and Children. For children who wear diapers, it is important to clean the perineal area thoroughly to remove secretions and all traces of urine and feces from the skin. Be sure to observe the condition of the skin as you clean the area and to report all redness or skin irritation. Put on disposable gloves when you provide perineal care.

If a male child has been circumcised, clean the tip of his penis using strokes moving outward from the urethra. Use only a minimal amount of soap, and rinse thoroughly. If the child is uncircumcised, gently retract the foreskin until you feel resistance (the foreskin usually cannot be retracted fully until about the age of 4), and using a clean section of the washcloth or a clean, moist cotton ball, clean around the tip of the penis, moving from the urethra outward. Rinse in the same pattern and dry well. Be sure to return the foreskin to its original position because leaving the foreskin retracted may interfere with circula-

FIGURE C-9 Be sure to hold a child close to your body as you lower him into the bathtub.

FIGURE C-10 Place a specially designed infant tub on a surface that allows you to bathe a child without bending over and straining your back.

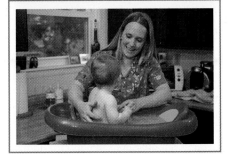

tion in the head of the penis. After washing and rinsing the penis clean the scrotum and then the anal area.

When providing perineal care for a female child, wash any skin folds in the groin first. Then, using a separate section of the washcloth or clean cotton balls for each wipe, separate and clean the labia and then the urethral areas, moving from front to back. Use soap sparingly and rinse thoroughly. After washing and rinsing the labia and urethral areas, clean the anal area. Be sure to remove all secretions, because they can cause skin irritation. Observe the skin for any abrasions or changes in skin color. Report any concerns to your supervising nurse.

Combing a Child's Hair

Dominique hates having her hair combed as much as she loves bathing. Today, you use a new approach to try to get her to sit still so that you can comb her hair. You brought along a blunt-toothed comb with a short handle and an unbreakable hand mirror. You put Dominique on your lap and hand her the new comb and mirror. Dominique begins to "comb" her hair and look at herself in the mirror. While she plays this game, you are able to comb Dominique's hair with your usual comb without having her fuss and squirm.

Periodically comb a child's hair to remove tangles and prevent them from becoming extensive. Some children love to have their hair combed while others do not want to be bothered. As the child gets older, combing is an important part of building good grooming habits and promoting healthy self-esteem.

To remove a stubborn tangle from a child's hair, first wet the hair and then apply conditioner to the tangle, which makes the hair shafts slippery. Applying conditioner often enables you to remove the tangle painlessly with combing. Start combing at the ends of the hair and work your way toward the scalp. When you have removed the

tangle either rinse the conditioner out of that section of hair or give the child a total shampoo.

Dressing a Child

Because Dominique is such an active child, you always sit with her on the floor when you dress her. She has a special floor blanket that you spread out before placing her clothes on top of the blanket. Then you and she sit together on the blanket while you dress her. To help distract Dominique and to keep her busy while you dress her, you also put two or three small toys on the blanket to hand to her, in case she gets bored and tries to wriggle out of your hands.

Dressing a young child on a clean blanket spread on the floor is very safe, because the child cannot fall off or get hurt. With a less active child, you can bring your supplies to the cribside or dressing table and work safely there. Because a child can move very quickly, never leave him unattended and always keep at least one hand on him if he is on a high surface. Infants and children can be very active, and at times you may feel as though you are trying to dress a moving target. Because of their activity, it is essential that you gather all your supplies and have them within your arm's reach yet out of reach of the child's fingers. Older children can be dressed in bed or while seated in a chair.

Stretchy knits or loose-fitting clothes are easier to put on than tight-fitting garments. One-piece garments for infants are convenient and easy to fasten and refasten during diaper changes. Pants for infants and toddlers may have snaps or other closures that make diaper changing easier.

Putting on a Knit Shirt or Undershirt.
Gather up the shirt into a circle at the neck and pull it down over the child's head. Then, starting from the bottom of a sleeve, thread your own fingers through the sleeve until you can gently

grasp the child's hand and guide it through the sleeve. Repeat the process with the other sleeve (Figure C-11).

Putting on a One-Piece Sleeper.
Place the infant on his back. Gather up the leg of the sleeper that has no snaps and put it on his foot and leg. Repeat with the other leg of the sleeper. Bring the sleeper up over the infant's torso. Insert his arms into the sleeves as described in the previous paragraph and fasten the garment. If you dress an older child while he sits in a chair, put the one-piece sleeper on his feet, and then have him stand as you pull the garment up and put his arms through the sleeves.

Putting on Pants.
Place the infant on his back. Put your hand through the garment leg, starting at the bottom, and then grasp the infant's foot and guide his foot and leg through the garment leg. Repeat the process for the other leg. Finish by pulling the waist up over the diaper. If you are dressing an older child, have him sit while you put his feet into the garment legs and then have him stand while you pull the pants up to his waist.

Putting on Socks.
Gather the sock up and place it over the child's toes. Pull it over his heel and leg. Smooth out wrinkles before putting on shoes.

FIGURE C-11 When dressing a child, gently pull his hands through the sleeves rather than pushing them through. This keeps the child's fingers from getting caught in the sleeves.

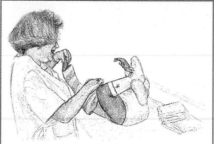

Putting on Shoes. Open the laces and fasteners of the shoe and pull out the tongue. Place the child's foot into the shoe, replace the tongue and fasten snugly but not too tightly. Be aware of how the shoe fits, and report ill-fitting shoes to your supervising nurse.

VITAL SIGNS

What about measuring vital signs? Do the techniques used for children differ from those used for adults?

Taking a Child's Temperature

For children under 5 years of age, take a rectal, axillary or tympanic temperature. The rectal or tympanic methods are preferred, because they provide the most reliable measurement of

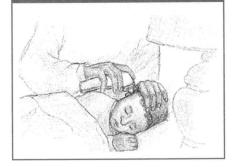

FIGURE C-12 The use of the tympanic thermometer does not require the removal of clothing, which makes it less frightening to children than the rectal or axillary methods.

temperature. The tympanic thermometer is least frightening for children (Figure C-12). However, if a child is very upset or uncooperative and a tympanic thermometer is not available, it is safer to take an axillary temperature rather than a rectal one (Figure C-13). As with adults, do not take a rectal temperature if a child has diarrhea or has had rectal surgery.

To take an infant's rectal temperature, position the baby on her back. Hold her ankles up with one hand and bend her knees to expose the anus. With the other hand, gently insert only the bulb of the lubricated thermometer into the rectum and hold it in place for 3 minutes. Always hold on to the thermometer while it is in the rectum.

To take a child's rectal temperature, have the child lie on his side with his knees flexed, or have him lie on his

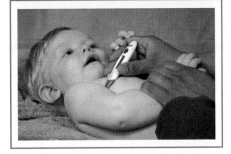

FIGURE C-13 Hold an infant's upper arm close to the body when taking an axillary temperature.

stomach. A child may be more likely to cooperate if he is held across his parent's lap while you take his rectal temperature. Be sure to insert the bulb gently, insert only the bulb, and hold the thermometer in place while the child's temperature is registering.

Whenever possible, use an electronic thermometer for children over the age of 5. Take an oral temperature. If not available, use a flat thermometer, rather than an oral thermometer, because it is easier for a child to hold in his mouth. Always stay with a child who has a thermometer in his mouth to make sure that he remains still, lying down or seated, so that he does not break the thermometer or injure himself.

The normal temperature for a child is the same as it is for an adult, although a child's temperature may change very rapidly. Young children especially may run very high temperatures. If you work in a hospital, be sure to report any temperature changes immediately. In a home setting, refer to the chart in Table C-1 to help you decide when and to whom to report temperature changes.

Taking a Child's Pulse

A small child typically is afraid of an unfamiliar person, especially a nurse assistant approaching with strange-looking equipment, such as a stethoscope. It is difficult to take a child's pulse rate if he is crying or upset. Try to enlist the child's cooperation and

TABLE C-1 WHEN TO REPORT A CHILD'S TEMPERATURE CHANGE IN A HOME SETTING		
Report to Your Supervising Nurse Immediately When the Child Is . . .	**And the Axillary Temperature Is* . . .**	**Or the Rectal Temperature Is . . .**
Under 4 months old	99° F or higher	101° F or higher
Over 4 months old	103° F or higher	105° F or higher

*When the axillary temperature is this high, take a rectal temperature, if possible, to confirm the reading. Report the high temperature immediately to your supervising nurse, or if she is not available, report it to someone else in authority who can take immediate action or direct you to monitor the child's condition.

FIGURE C-14 Being held by a parent may calm a child, allowing you to get a more accurate pulse reading.

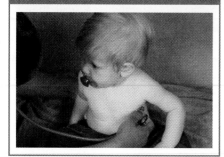

encourage the parent to hold the child (Figure C-14). To help the child relax let him play with another stethoscope or play a listening game. Because activity can affect the reading, report what the child was doing when you took his pulse.

The average pulse rates for children of different age ranges appear in Table C-2.

Counting a Child's Respirations

For an accurate reading, count a child's respirations while she is quiet or asleep. If you also plan to take a temperature or blood pressure reading, count the respirations first in case the child becomes upset and starts to cry. Respiration rates in children are higher than in adults (Table C-3) and may be irregular. Report any abnormal rate or difficulty breathing.

Taking a Child's Blood Pressure

When you take a child's blood pressure, use the right size cuff. A cuff that is too large gives a reading that is too low. A cuff that is too small gives a reading that is too high. Try to get the child to cooperate during the procedure by using words and con-

cepts that he understands. For example, you may tell the child that the cuff is going to give his arm a "big hug" when you squeeze the black ball. Often it helps if the child sits on his parent's lap or is distracted by a toy (Figure C-15).

Table C-4 lists the range of normal or usual blood pressure readings in children. As a group, younger children generally have lower blood pressures than older children do.

As with all vital signs in a child, blood pressure readings can change very rapidly. Report even small changes in blood pressure to your supervising nurse. Also, be sure to note the activity of the child while you

are taking the blood pressure reading so that the significance of any changes can be evaluated.

FIGURE C-15 You can use an object, such as a toy or bottle, to distract a child and gain cooperation while taking blood pressure.

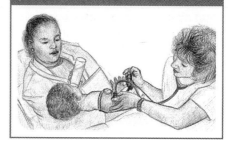

TABLE C-2 PULSE RATES IN CHILDREN

Age	Pulse Rate (beats per minute)
Newborn to 1 year	140 to 170
1 to 2 years	80 to 160
2 to 6 years	80 to 130
6 to 14 years	70 to 110
14 to 18 years	60 to 100

TABLE C-3 RESPIRATION RATES IN CHILDREN

Age	Normal Rate (times per minute)
Newborn to 1 year	35
1 to 2 years	30
2 to 6 years	20 to 25
6 to 10 years	19 to 21
10 to 16 years	17 to 19
16 to 18 years	16 to 18

DISCHARGING A HOME HEALTH CARE CLIENT

After several weeks, Mrs. Garcia no longer needs home health care. The social worker puts her in touch with community resources that can offer ongoing assistance with needs such as transportation.

Although you will not be directly involved with Mrs. Garcia's discharge from home health care be sure to talk with her on your last visit to tell her how much you enjoyed providing care for her. Wish her well and say good-bye to her.

TABLE C-4 BLOOD PRESSURE READINGS IN CHILDREN

Age of Child	Systolic Blood Pressure	Diastolic Blood Pressure
Newborn to 1 year	65 to 91	50 to 56
2 to 5 years	90 to 95	55 to 56
6 to 12 years	96 to 107	57 to 66
13 to 15 years	109 to 114	63 to 67
16 to 18 years	112 to 121	66 to 70

INFORMATION REVIEW

1. If you need to disinfect, but the cleaners you have do not kill germs, you can make your own disinfectant by mixing _____ of bleach with 1 gallon of water.
2. A common sterilization process is to boil an item for _____ minutes.
3. Roasting is a _____ -heat cooking process, and steaming is a _____ -heat process.
4. When collecting a urine specimen from either a male or female infant, be sure not to cover the _____ with the collection bag.*
5. A child should be taught to brush his or her teeth for _____ minutes.*
6. A blood pressure cuff that is too small gives a reading that is too _____.*

QUESTIONS TO ASK YOURSELF

1. Your supervising nurse says you'll need to disinfect a client's bathroom. What is the difference between cleaning, disinfecting and sterilizing?
2. Your client says she wants you to clean the bathroom with a particular cleaner that is not a disinfectant. What can you do to keep her happy and also maintain infection control?
3. Mrs. Garcia asks you to cook her a hamburger for lunch. After serving her the hamburger, you return to the kitchen to clean up. What should you do with the grease left in the frying pan?
4. Your friend Monika, a home health aide, mentions that she "gave" her client his medication on time. Can she really do that? How can a home health aide help with medication?
5. Mrs. Henson does not have much appetite these days. What can you do to make mealtimes as inviting as possible?
6. How can you collect a urine specimen from an infant?*
7. How does an infant's immune system respond differently to AIDS than an adult's?*
8. Describe how you would teach a 6-year-old to brush his teeth.*
9. How old should a child be before you start taking an oral temperature?*

Skill 58*: Changing Crib Linens

PRECAUTIONS

- Always stay with the infant, never leaving him alone.
- Keep clean linens on a clean surface.
- Keep clean and dirty linens from touching the floor.
- Remove and replace linens carefully, without shaking them. Shaking linens causes air currents that may spread dust and germs around the room.
- Wear disposable gloves if linens are wet or soiled. Remove gloves and wash hands before touching clean linens.
- Keep dirty, contaminated linens away from your uniform.
- Use proper body mechanics.
- Be sure the top and bottom rails are in place if you must step away from the crib side.
- Keep one hand on the infant even if you are turning away only for a moment.
- Never use a pillow in an infant crib.

PREPARATION

1. Gather supplies:
   - Bottom sheet
   - Baby blanket
   - Laundry bag (or plastic bag for wet or soiled linens)
   - Disposable gloves, as necessary
2. Follow Preparation Standards (see Chapter 7).

ADDITIONAL INFORMATION
- Always wash your hands before gathering clean linens.
- Talk to the infant as you work.

PROCEDURE

1. Lower the side rail, if used, and raise the upper rail or cover if one is in place. ☐ ☐
2. Place the infant in a safe place, such as in a stroller or playpen, or ask the parent to hold the child. ☐ ☐
3. Remove the dirty sheet from the mattress and put it in the laundry bag. ☐ ☐
4. Place the clean sheet lengthwise on the side of the crib closer to you. ☐ ☐
5. Miter the top and bottom corners of the sheet, or fit the corners of the fitted sheet around the mattress (Figure C-16, A). ☐ ☐

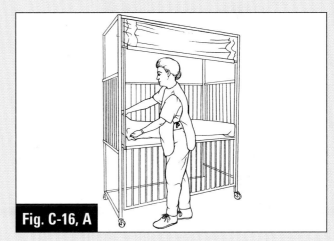

Fig. C-16, A

6. Raise the side rail, if used, and lower the upper rail or cover. Go around to the other side and lower the side rail and raise the upper rail or cover (Figure C-16, B). ☐ ☐
7. Pull the clean sheet across the crib and miter or fit the corners. ☐ ☐

Note: Never use a pillow in an infant's crib because he may suffocate.

8. Place the infant back into the crib. Cover him with the baby blanket if he will be sleeping. ☐ ☐
9. Raise the side rail and pull the upper rail or cover into position. ☐ ☐

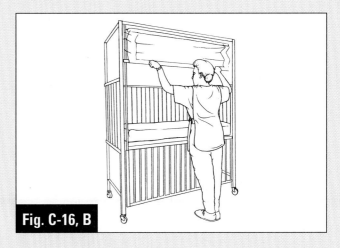

Fig. C-16, B

Skill 58*: Changing Crib Linens—cont'd

 COMPLETION

1. Follow Completion Standards in compliance with your facility. For a complete list of those used in this course, see Chapter 7, "Controlling the Spread of Germs."
2. Before you leave, check:
   - Removal of pillows and other hazards.
   - Top and bottom rails.
3. Report:
   - Drainage on the sheets.
   - Pain.
   - Bleeding.
   - Red or swollen areas.

Skill 59: Assisting with Medications—The Home Health Aide's Role

PRECAUTIONS

- Check the prescription label. Make sure you have the right client, the right medication, the right time, the right amount and the right route.
- Let your supervising nurse know if a medication container is missing a label or if the label is hard to read and if the medication has expired.

PREPARATION

1. Gather supplies:
   - Medication
   - Teaspoon or tablespoon, if needed
   - Glass of water or other cool liquid
   - Straw
   - Tissues or cotton balls, if needed
   - Disposable gloves, as necessary
   - Equipment for handwashing
2. Follow Preparation Standards (see Chapter 7).

ADDITIONAL INFORMATION

1. Check the client's medication list. Identify the correct medication, amount, time and route.
2. Explain that you can help the person as he takes his own medication but that you cannot actually give medicine to the person.

PROCEDURE

1. Provide privacy for the person. Ask visitors to leave the room. ☐ ☐
2. Help the client wash his hands. ☐ ☐

Skill 59: Assisting with Medications—The Home Health Aide's Role—cont'd

3. Place the medications within the client's reach. Make sure the client has his eyeglasses, if they are needed. □ □

4. Loosen container lids, tops or caps. Tell the client the names of each medication. □ □

5. Assist the client with oral medications (tablets, capsules, liquids) as necessary:
   • Support the client's hand, if necessary, as he pours medication into a spoon, cup or other hand.
   • Give the client the glass of water.
   • Make sure the client swallows the medication. □ □

6. Help the client with eye medications as necessary:
   • Position the client so that his head is tilted back.
   • Know which eye will receive the medication.
   • Support the client's hand as he drops the medication into the lower eyelid.
   • Ask the client to close his eyes to help distribute the medication.

7. Assist the client with topical medications (ointments, lotions) as necessary:
   • Help him remove any dressing.
   • Wash the area as instructed by your supervising nurse.
   • Have the client apply the medication.
   • Help him with handwashing. □ □

8. Help the client with a rectal suppository as necessary:
   • Help the client to a side-lying position.
   • Help the client unwrap the suppository.

- Ask the client to put on a disposable glove.
- Guide the client's hand to the rectal area, if necessary.
- Have the client insert the suppository.
- Hold his buttocks together for a few minutes to help the client retain the suppository.
- Help the client assume a comfortable position. ☐ ☐

9. Assist the person to apply a transderm patch.
   - Help the person to remove the patch as directed.
   - Wash the area with soap and water to remove remaining medications. Pat dry.
   - Help the person to apply the new patch, in a different area. Check with the supervising nurse for directions on appropriate areas to replace a transderm patch.

COMPLETION

1. Follow Completion Standards in compliance with your facility. For a complete list of those used in this course, see Chapter 7, "Controlling the Spread of Germs."
2. Report:
   - The medication taken, the amount, the time and the route.
   - Any difficulties the client had in taking the medication (difficulty swallowing, hand tremors).
   - Any observed side effects or client complaints.

a. Notify your supervising nurse if your client:
- Is not taking his medication as prescribed.
- If he refuses to take his medication.
- Is taking more or less than the prescribed amount.
- Is taking drugs other than those prescribed, including over-the-counter drugs.
- Is mixing up prescribed medications.
- Is taking his medication at times other than those ordered.
- Has any questions concerning his medications.

b. Also let your supervising nurse know:
- If you suspect that anyone in the household is misusing drugs.
- When your client has 1 week of pills left from a prescription.
- When a drug is about to expire, because the strength of expired medications cannot be guaranteed.

Skill 60: Applying Compresses and Assisting with Soaks

PRECAUTIONS

- High temperatures can burn skin. Immediately report any signs of burns, pain, redness or blisters to supervising nurse.

> *Note: In most cases, temperature for warm soaks or other heat methods should not exceed 105° F.*

- Babies, young children and elderly people are injured more easily by heat or cold because their skin is more delicate.
- Be especially careful in applying heat to a person who is confused or who has poor sensation in the affected area.
- Prolonged or intense cold can damage skin and cause blisters, pain or redness. Signs of cold damage may include pale, white or bluish color of skin; numbness; or tingling.

PREPARATION

1. Gather supplies:
   - Two towels
   - Washcloth or gauze for compress
   - Disposable bed protector
   - Watch
   - Bath thermometer
   - Laundry bag (or plastic bag for wet or soiled linens)
   - Disposable gloves
   - Plastic trash bag
2. Follow Preparation Standards (see Chapter 7).

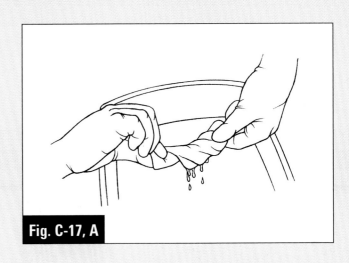

Fig. C-17, A

Skill 60: Applying Compresses and Assisting with Soaks—cont'd

PROCEDURE

Applying a Warm or Cold Compress

1. Place bed protector under body part. ☐ ☐
2. Position a towel halfway under the affected area. ☐ ☐
3. Put on disposable gloves and dip a wash cloth or gauze into a washbasin of warm water (100° F–105° F) or cold water. Wring out any excess moisture (Figure C-17, A). ☐ ☐
4. Place the compress on the affected area of the person's skin (Figure C-17, B). ☐ ☐
5. Place the other half of the towel over the compress and protect it with the disposable bed protector (Figure C-17, C-D). ☐ ☐

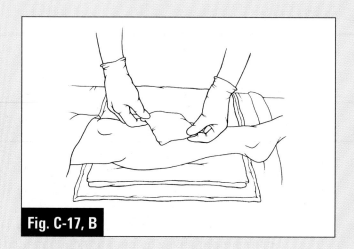

Fig. C-17, B

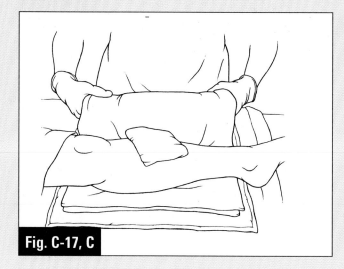

Fig. C-17, C

6. Note the amount of time the compress is to remain on the person's skin.　☐　☐

7. Check on the person every 5 minutes. Report any problem you find to the supervising nurse.　☐　☐

8. Remove the compress after 20 minutes and reapply it as needed.　☐　☐

9. When the time is up, dry the affected area with a clean towel.　☐　☐

Assisting with a Warm Soak

1. Place the disposable bed protector on the bed or a clean surface.　☐　☐

2. Place the washbasin of warm water on the bed protector and place the area to be treated in the basin of water. Provide a blanket to the person for warmth (Figure C-17, E).　☐　☐

3. Check on the person every 5 minutes. Report any problem you find to the supervising nurse.　☐　☐

4. Remove the treatment area from the washbasin after 15 to 20 minutes.　☐　☐

5. When the time is up, gently dry the area with a clean towel.　☐　☐

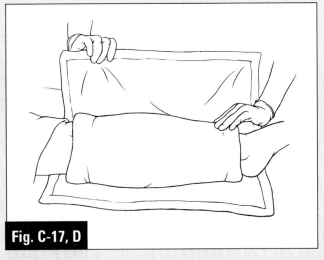

Fig. C-17, D

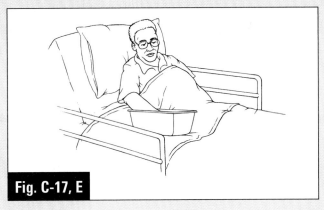

Fig. C-17, E

ADDITIONAL INFORMATION

Check with your supervising nurse for the proper water temperature and the proper lengths of time for applying the compress or for soaking.

 COMPLETION

Follow Completion Standards in compliance with your facility. For a complete list of those used in this course, see Chapter 7, "Controlling the Spread of Germs."

Skill 61: Applying an Aquathermia Pad

PRECAUTIONS

Note: Never use equipment until you have been properly trained to do so.

- Before using electrical equipment make sure equipment works properly and follow the instructions of the manufacturer.
- Secure pad in place with ties, tape or rolled gauze. Never use pins to secure an aquathermia pad.
- Do not place the pad under the person or under a body part. Burns may occur.
- Make sure the temperature setting is correct.
- Immediately report any signs of burns, pain, redness or blisters to supervising nurse.
- Always cover the pad with a towel, pillowcase or flannel cover.
- Follow the rules of electrical safety when using an electrical appliance.

PREPARATION

1. Gather supplies:
   - Aquathermia pad and heating unit
   - Distilled water
   - Towel, pillowcase or flannel cover
   - Tape or roller gauze
2. Follow Preparation Standards (see Chapter 7).

PROCEDURE

1. Fill the heating unit to the fill line with distilled water. ☐ ☐

2. Remove bubbles. Place the pad and tubing below the heating unit. Tilt the heating unit from side to side. ☐ ☐

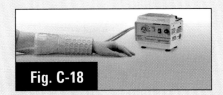

Fig. C-18

3. Set the temperature as directed by supervising nurse (Usually set at 105° F.) Remove the key. ☐ ☐

4. Place the aquathermia pad in the cover. ☐ ☐

5. Plug in the heating unit. Let the water warm to desired temperature. ☐ ☐

6. Keep the aquathermia pad and connecting hoses level with the heating unit. ☐ ☐

7. Apply the pad to the affected area of the person's skin. Secure the pad in place. Do not use pins (Figure C-18). ☐ ☐

8. Place call signal within reach. ☐ ☐

9. Check the person every 5 minutes. ☐ ☐

10. Remove the pad when the treatment time is up. ☐ ☐

ADDITIONAL INFORMATION

Ask your supervising nurse for the proper temperature setting and the proper treatment time.

COMPLETION

Follow Completion Standards in compliance with your facility. For a complete list of those used in this course, see Chapter 7, "Controlling the Spread of Germs."

Skill 62: Applying a Heating Pad

PRECAUTIONS

Note: Never use equipment until you have been properly trained to do so.

- Before using electrical equipment make sure equipment works properly and follow the instructions of the manufacturer.
- Never use pins to secure an electric heating pad.
- Make sure the temperature setting is correct. High temperatures can cause a person's skin to burn. Immediately report any signs of burns, pain, redness or blisters to supervising nurse.
- Keep the heating pad from getting wet.
- Make sure the person's skin is clean and dry before applying the heating pad.
- Do not allow the person to lie on top of a heating pad, because lying on it increases the likelihood of burns.
- If the heating pad does not have a cloth surface or flannel cover, place a towel around it before placing it on the person's skin.
- Follow the rules of electrical safety when using an electrical appliance.

PREPARATION

1. Gather supplies:
   - Heating pad
   - Towel or flannel cover, if needed
   - Watch
2. Follow Preparation Standards (see Chapter 7).

PROCEDURE

1. Apply the heating pad to the affected area of the person's skin. Adjust the position of the heating pad so that its weight is comfortable for the person (Figure C-19). ☐ ☐

2. Make sure the person can contact you using a call signal. ☐ ☐

3. Remove the heating pad when the treatment time is up. ☐ ☐

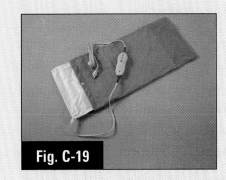
Fig. C-19

ADDITIONAL INFORMATION

Ask your supervising nurse for the proper temperature setting and the proper treatment time. Remind the person not to change the temperature setting.

COMPLETION

Follow Completion Standards in compliance with your facility. For a complete list of those used in this course, see Chapter 7, "Controlling the Spread of Germs."

Skill 63: Applying a Warm Water Bottle

PRECAUTIONS

- High temperatures can burn a person's skin. Immediately report any signs of burns, pain, redness or blisters.
- Be especially careful in applying heat to a person who is confused or who has poor sensation in the affected area.

PREPARATION

1. Gather supplies:
   - Warm water bottle
   - Towel or flannel cover for warm water bottle
   - Bath thermometer
   - Watch
   - Paper towels
2. Follow Preparation Standards (see Chapter 7).

PROCEDURE

1. Fill the bottle one-half to two-thirds full with water of the proper temperature. ☐ ☐
2. Apply the wrapped warm water bottle to the prescribed area of the person's skin. Adjust the position of the warm water bottle so that its weight is not uncomfortable to the person. Make sure that the part of the bottle touching the skin has not become wet. ☐ ☐
3. Make sure there is a call signal within the person's reach. ☐ ☐
4. Remove the warm water bottle when the treatment time is up. ☐ ☐

ADDITIONAL INFORMATION

Ask your supervising nurse for the proper water temperature and treatment time.

 COMPLETION

Follow Completion Standards in compliance with your facility. For a complete list of those used in this course, see Chapter 7, "Controlling the Spread of Germs."

Skill 64: Applying an Ice Bag

PRECAUTIONS

- Do not keep ice bags in place longer than prescribed. Prolonged cold can damage the person's skin.
- Wait 20 minutes before reapplying an ice bag to allow the area to recover from the cold.
- Always cover an ice bag before placing it against the person's skin.
- Make sure the cover is dry because a wet cover can increase the intensity of the cold.
- Check the bag for leaks before using by filling it with water, putting on the cap and turning it upside down.

PREPARATION

1. Gather supplies:
   - Ice bag
   - Crushed ice or chips
   - Towel or cover for ice bag
   - Paper or thin towels
2. Follow Preparation Standards (see Chapter 7).

PROCEDURE

1. Fill the ice bag two-thirds full with crushed ice or ice chips. ☐ ☐
2. Apply the towel-wrapped ice bag to the affected part of the person's body. Note the time. ☐ ☐
3. Make sure that a call signal is within the person's reach. ☐ ☐
4. Remove the ice bag after 20 minutes or after the prescribed time, if different. ☐ ☐
5. Check the skin every 10 minutes. ☐ ☐

ADDITIONAL INFORMATION
Check with your supervising nurse for the proper treatment time.

 COMPLETION
Follow Completion Standards in compliance with your facility. For a complete list of those used in this course, see Chapter 7, "Controlling the Spread of Germs."

Skill 65*: Collecting a Urine Specimen from an Infant or Child

PRECAUTIONS

- Always follow your supervising nurse's instructions for urine specimen collection.
- Remember the principles of infection control when collecting specimens.
- Always wear disposable gloves.
- Always stay with the child, never leaving him alone.
- You may have to ask the parent to hold a very active child.

PREPARATION

1. Gather supplies:
   - Pediatric urine collector
   - Diaper
   - Washcloth
   - Towel
   - Disposable gloves (2 pairs)
   - Scissors, if you plan to pull the collection bag to the outside of the child's diaper
   - Infant's own washbasin
   - Infant's own soap
2. Follow Preparation Standards (see Chapter 7).

PROCEDURE

Obtaining a urine specimen from an infant or a child who is not toilet trained requires applying a special self-adhesive collection bag to a girl's perineal area or over a boy's penis.

1. Fill the washbasin with warm water. ☐ ☐
2. Put on disposable gloves. ☐ ☐
3. Lower the crib rail. ☐ ☐

4. Remove the infant's diaper and place it in the plastic trash bag if it is wet or soiled. ☐ ☐

5. Use the washcloth, soap and water to clean the infant's perineal area. ☐ ☐

Note: *Remember that the same rules for cleaning an adult apply to the infant: clean from front to back for a female, or from the urethra outward for a male.*

6. Use the washcloth to rinse. Dry the area thoroughly with a towel. ☐ ☐

7. Position the infant on his back, and spread his knees apart, exposing the genitals. (If the child is very active, you may need to ask the parent to hold the child.) ☐ ☐

8. Peel the sticky paper off the adhesive area at the top of the collection bag. ☐ ☐
   - *For a male:* Put his penis through the opening at the top of the bag and press the adhesive securely around the base of his penis and his scrotum (Figure C-20, A).
   - *For a female:* Position the bag over her urethra and press the adhesive area over her labia to create a seal (Figure C-20, B). ☐ ☐

Note: *Do not cover the infant's anus with the adhesive area.*

9. Rediaper the infant (Figure C-20, C). ☐ ☐

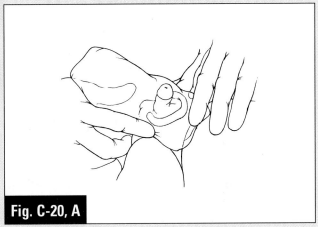

Fig. C-20, A

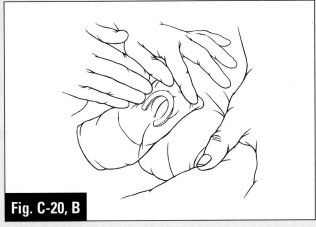

Fig. C-20, B

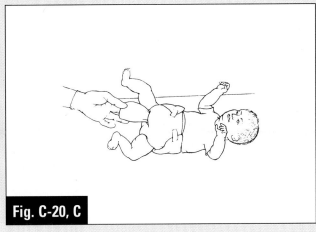

Fig. C-20, C

Skill 65*: Collecting a Urine Specimen from an Infant or Child—cont'd

Note: If the infant is too young to be able to pull the bag off, you may cut a slit in the disposable diaper and pull the bag through the slit to enable you to easily see when the infant has voided.

10. Remove the gloves and put them in the plastic bag. ☐ ☐
11. Raise the crib rail or put the infant in a safe place such as a playpen or infant seat. ☐ ☐
12. Empty and clean the washbasin. ☐ ☐
13. Wash your hands and record when the bag was applied. ☐ ☐
14. Check every 15 minutes to see if the infant has urinated. ☐ ☐
15. Wash your hands. ☐ ☐
16. After the infant has urinated, fill the washbasin with clean, warm water and take it to the cribside. ☐ ☐
17. Put on disposable gloves. ☐ ☐
18. Lower the crib rail. ☐ ☐
19. Loosen the diaper and gently remove the bag (Figure C-20, D).
    - Seal the top by folding the adhesive area over, and place it in the sterile specimen container (Figure C-20, E). ☐ ☐

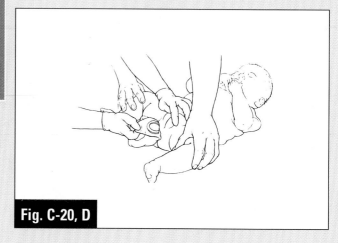
Fig. C-20, D

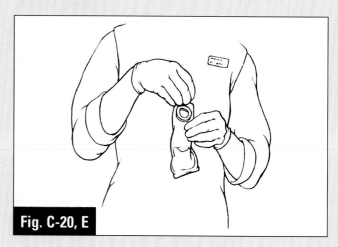
Fig. C-20, E

Note: Do not leave the infant unattended to do this. You may set the collection bag down on the crib and put it in the specimen container later if the infant is very active or if you cannot reach the specimen container without turning your back on the infant.

> **Note:** *Some pediatric collection bags have a port at the bottom of the bag to empty the urine into the container.*

20. Clean and dry the perineal area and put a clean diaper on the infant. □ □
21. Raise the crib rail. □ □

COMPLETION

1. Follow Completion Standards in compliance with your facility. For a complete list of those used in this course, see Chapter 7, "Controlling the Spread of Germs."
2. Before you leave, check top and bottom rails.
3. Report:
   - Any difficulty in urinating.
   - Pain.
   - Bleeding.
   - Red or swollen areas.

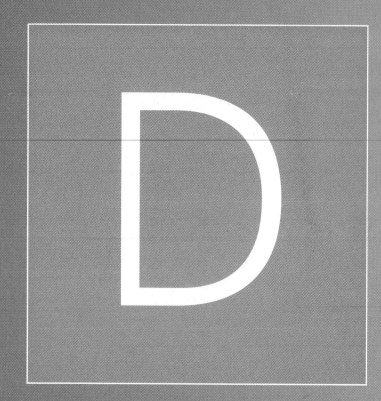

Math Applications

Most nurse assistant students are in the health-care profession because of their love for caring for others, not because of a desire to become doctors or nurses. Even so, they will need some challenging, even complex working skills, such as math. This module is designed to help you sharpen your skills in the calculation of height and weight, food intake measurement, recording time, etc. It also offers help with more general math calculations such as percentage, division, multiplication, fractions, decimals, equivalents, conversions and military time. All these math skills will be used from time to time in your duties as a nurse assistant.

Feel free to challenge yourself in any of the math sections. Your instructor can help you decide which sections are most important for you.

SELECTED MATH VOCABULARY

Vocabulary

Decimal number. A number that contains a decimal point that separates the whole from its fractional part.

3.5

Denominator. The number below the line in a fraction. It tells into how many parts something has been divided.

In the fraction 2/3, 3 is the denominator and tells that the object has been divided into 3 parts.

Difference. The answer in subtraction.

In the math problem 18 minus 8 equals 10, 10 is the difference.

$$\begin{array}{r} 18 \\ -8 \\ \hline 10 \end{array}$$

Digit. One of the figures 0, 1, 2, 3, 4, 5, 6, 7, 8, 9.

For example the number 3 is a digit.

Dividend. The number being divided by another number.

In 9/3, the dividend is 9.

Divisor. The number by which another number is divided.

In 9/3 the divisor is 3.

Fraction. One or more of the equal parts of a whole.

2/3

Minuend. Number from which another number is to be subtracted.

In the example below, 26 is the minuend.

$$\begin{array}{r} 26 \\ -3 \\ \hline 23 \end{array}$$

Multiplicand. Number to be multiplied by another number.

In 8×73, the multiplicand is 73.

Multiplier. Number by which another number is to be multiplied.

In 8×73, the multiplier is 8.

Numerator. Number above the line in a fraction. It tells how many of the parts are in use.

In the fraction 2/3, 2 is the numerator and tells that 2 of the 3 equal parts are being used.

Place value. The position that a digit holds.

In 3.5, 5 is in the tenths position.

Product. The answer in a multiplication problem.

$8 \times 73 = 584$; 584 is the product.

Quotient. The answer in a division problem.

$\dfrac{10}{2} = 5$; 5 is the quotient.

Subtrahend. Number to be subtracted from another number in a subtraction problem.

$26 - 3 = 23$; 3 is the subtrahend.

Sum. The answer in an addition problem.

In $\begin{array}{r} 4 \\ +3 \\ \hline 7 \end{array}$, 7 is the sum.

THE KEYS TO ADDING, SUBTRACTING, MULTIPLYING AND DIVIDING DECIMALS AND WHOLE NUMBERS

Remember to write sums, and differences with the decimal points carefully aligned in a straight line. A digit that is written in the wrong position will produce a wrong answer when working with decimals. A good guide is remembering the "place values." The value of a digit depends on its place, or position, in the number. For example, the place values of 56.89 are as follows: The numbers to the right of the decimal point (.) are a fraction or part of the whole; that is, 89 is 89 parts of 100 (the whole). This number is read "fifty-six and eighty-nine hundredths."

Addition

Decimal tidbits. When adding whole numbers and decimals, place zeros in the decimal positions to the right of the decimal point. (For example to add 6 plus .45 (forty-five hundredths); write 6.00 + .45.)

To add the following two decimals start with the right column of numbers.

```
   ↓
  5.94
+ 2.65
------
     9
```
Think 4 and 5 are 9, then, write the 9 immediately under the first column.

```
  ↓
  5.94
+ 2.65
------
   .59
```
Think 9 and 6 are 15, then, write the 5 immediately under the second column and think "carry" 1 and add it to the third column. (Remember to keep the decimal points in a straight line.)

```
 ↓
 1
  5.94
+ 2.65
------
  8.59
```
Think 1 and 5 are 6 and 2 are 8, then write the 8 immediately under the third column.

To check addition, cover the sums, then add the columns from bottom to top and write the sums in small figures at the top. The sums at the top and bottom should be equal; if not, reverse the addition order and re-add.

```
  8.59
  5.94↓
+ 2.65
------
  8.59
```
8.59 is the sum and is read eight and fifty-nine hundredths.

Note: *Use the same method of carrying when adding whole numbers, regardless of the number of digits.*

Practice Problems Addition

Add and check all problems. See examples, if necessary.

1.	6.83 + 2.98	2.	4.75 + 3.66	3.	3.28 + 2.92	4.	52.94 + 38.66	5.	6.37 + 48.77
6.	78.54 + 14.57	7.	13.96 + 59.57	8.	44.26 + 37.86	9.	67.85 + 28.89	10.	55.47 + 34.73
11.	8.71 + 5.00	12.	75.62 + 14.58	13.	63.48 + 29.61	14.	57.64 + 37.57	15.	38.51 + 46.89
16.	5.27 + .58	17	65.74 + 36.76	18.	83.25 + 57.28	19.	94.16 + 57.28	20.	97.51 + 68.68

Subtraction

Reminder:

Write the differences in straight lines, one digit above with the answer directly below as in the example.

When a digit in the minuend is smaller than the digit in the subtrahend, then it is necessary to "borrow" from the next digit to the left in the minuend. This is the process for subtracting both whole numbers and decimals or mixed numbers.

```
  4,384    minuend
- 2,573    subtrahend
  1,811    difference
```

Example
↓

```
  47.3     Think 5 cannot be subtracted from 3, then "borrow" 1 from the 7, reducing it to 6 and think 1 beside the 3 is 13.
- 21.5     Then, subtract 5 from 13, a difference of 8, which is written immediately under the first column.
    .8
```

↓

```
  47.3     Think the 7 is now 6 because 1 was borrowed, then subtract 1 from 6, a difference of 5, which is written
- 21.5     immediately under the second column.
   5.8
```

↓

```
  47.3     Think 2 subtracted from 4, a difference of 2, which is written immediately under the third column. The
- 21.5     difference is 25.8 and is read "twenty-five and eight tenths."
  25.8
```

Subtracting Tips

The same "borrowing" method is used in problems with four or more digits, and in problems that include whole numbers and decimals.

```
   5.
- 3.28
  1.72
```

↓↓

```
  5.00     When subtracting mixed numbers from whole numbers, place zeros (5.00) to the right of the decimal point (.)
- 3.28     and then borrow as shown to the left.
  1.72
```

Subtracting with Zeros in Three or More Digits

↓

```
  8000     Think 5 cannot be subtracted from 0, then borrow from the next column to the left which is 0 also, thus
- 3725     continue to the next column to the left until a digit other than 0 is available, which in this problem is 8.
  4275     Borrow 1 from 8, reducing it to 7. Think the borrowed 1 beside the 0 in the next column to the right that
           makes it 10 from which borrow 1, reducing it to 9.
```

↓↓↓

```
  7990     Think 10 for the 0 in the right column, now subtract all the columns as usual. Remember to keep columns straight.
- 3725
  4275
```

Practice Problems Subtraction

1.	500	2.	10,500	3.	4,631	4.	4,273	5.	8,126
	− 475		− 6,486		− 1,719		− 3,615		− 5,918

6. 45.78	7. 57.08	8. 24.86	9. 30.78	10. 32.86
− 24.21	− 29.26	− 18.15	− .25	− 26.45

11. Bill helped his father plant 375 boxes of strawberry plants. Bill planted 12.5 boxes. How many did his father plant?
12. Eight thousand people are expected for the convention. By three o'clock, 2975 people were registered. How many more registrants will be needed to achieve the expected attendance?
13. The Marion Anderson auditorium will seat 1578 people. How many chairs will be needed in the aisle to seat a convention of 2000 people?
14. North Central Christian School had 45 boys in the graduating class of 2001 and only 38 girls. How many more boys did they have than girls?
15. The population of a certain city was 20,040 according to the 1990 census and 29,058 according to the 2000 census. How much had the population increased between 1990 and 2000?

Multiplication

Multiplication is a quicker method of addition. For example, if 15 students have 12 pieces of fruit each to share with patients, and it is necessary to know how many pieces of fruit the students have altogether, add 12 + 12 + 12 + 12 + 12 + 12 + 12 + 12 + 12 + 12 + 12 + 12 + 12 + 12 + 12. The quicker solution is to multiply 15 (number of students) times 12 (number of pieces of fruit each student has).

Note: (1) In multiplying decimal numbers by whole numbers, multiply the numbers as if they were all whole numbers.
   (2) In the final product, starting from the right, put your pencil at the decimal position and move the decimal point to the left the number of decimal positions in the multiplicand and multiplier added.

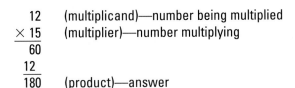

```
    12    (multiplicand)—number being multiplied
  × 15    (multiplier)—number multiplying
    60
    12
   180    (product)—answer
```

Remember to keep digits in a straight line; otherwise the results of each multiplication set can be added incorrectly.

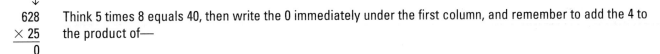

```
      ↓
    628      Think 5 times 8 equals 40, then write the 0 immediately under the first column, and remember to add the 4 to
  × 25       the product of—
      0
```

```
      ↓
    628      Think 5 times 2 equals 10 + 4, or 14, the 4 of which is written immediately under the second column and the
  × 25       1 is to be added to the product of—
     40
```

```
      ↓
    628      Think 5 times 6 equals 30 + 1, or 31, the 1 of which is written immediately under the third column and the
  × 25       3 written immediately under the fourth column.
   3140
```

```
      ↓
    628      Now think 2 times 8 equals 16, and then write the 6 immediately under the second column and below the 4,
  × 25       and remember to add the 1 to the product of—
   3140
      6
```

```
      ↓
    628      Think 2 times 2 equals 4 + 1, or 5, which is written immediately under the third column and below the 1.
  × 25
   3140
     56
```

$$
\begin{array}{r}
\downarrow \\
628 \\
\times\ 25 \\
\hline
3140 \\
\end{array}
$$

Think 2 times 6 equals 12, the 2 of which is written immediately under the fourth column and below the 3, and the 1 written immediately under the fifth column.

$$
\begin{array}{r}
1256 \\
\hline
15700 \\
\end{array}
$$

The answer is the sum of the products.

Decimal Example

First, multiply as if all numbers were whole numbers. Second, count the decimal places in the answer or product. There are 3 decimal places in the multiplier and the multiplicand, so you will put 3 digits behind the decimal point in your answer.

$$
\begin{array}{r}
6.28 \\
\times\ 2.5 \\
\hline
3140 \\
1256 \\
\hline
15.700 \\
\end{array}
$$

Practice Problems Multiplication

1. 276×36	2. 35.84×45.67	3. 48.96×15.94	4. 9.67×5.6	5. 602×3.66
6. 8563×35.79	7. 785.4×14.57	8. $\$50.14 \times 3348$	9. 56.02×9.8	10. 67.85×2.86

11. Sandy spent 4 weeks at summer camp. How many days was she there?
12. Susie counted the tongue depressors that she uses each day. She uses 750 each day. How many are used in March? How many are used in April?
13. Dr. Mendalhouse has 36 boxes of toothbrushes to pass out to his dental patients. Each box contains 24 toothbrushes. How many toothbrushes does he have?
14. The head supervisor, Nurse James, has 50 students in one course. Each course uses 5 notebooks per student. How many notebooks will Ms. James order?

Division

Division problems require both multiplication and subtraction. Like other math computations, it requires you to write the digits in a straight line as in the example below.

$$
\begin{array}{r}
\quad 121 \quad \text{quotient} \\
3\overline{)364} \quad \text{dividend} \\
\underline{3} \\
6 \\
\underline{6} \\
4 \\
\underline{3} \\
1 \quad \text{remainder} \\
\end{array}
$$

divisor $3\overline{)364}$

Example: $3\overline{)7206}$

Divide 3 into the first number in the dividend 7. Write 2 directly over the 7 in the dividend.
Multiply the (quotient) 2 times 3 and write 6 *under* the 7.
Subtract 6 from 7 and write 1 underneath.
Slide the 2 down next to it.

$$
\begin{array}{r}
2 \\
3\overline{)7206} \\
6\downarrow \\
\hline
12 \\
\end{array}
$$

Note: To proceed with the long division repeat the same sequence on each of the digits in the dividend. The sequence is: divide, multiply, subtract and slide.

```
   24
3)7206     Divide 3 into the bottom number 12. Write the 4 immediately over the 2.
   6       Multiply the 4 times the divisor (3) and write that number (12) under the 12.
  12       Subtract 12 from 12 and write 0 under it.
  12↓      Slide the next number in the dividend, 0, down next to it.
  ---
   00
```

```
  240
3)7206     Divide 3 into the bottom number 00. Write 0 immediately over the 0 in the dividend.
   6       Multiply 0 times the divisor (3) and write it in the column directly under the 0.
  12       Subtract 0 from 0 and write the 0 in the column underneath.
  12       Slide the 6 down next to it.
  ---
   00
    0↓
   ---
    06
```

```
 2402
3)7206     Divide 3 into 06. Write the 2 immediately over the 6 in the dividend.
   6       Multiply 3 times 2 and write the product 6 inline under the 6.
  12       Subtract 6 from 6 and the difference of 0, which is the remainder.
  12
  ---
   00
    0↓
   ---
    06
     6
    ---
     0
```

Dividing Decimals

To divide a decimal number by a whole number, follow this example:

```
3)5.1
```

```
    .
3)5.1
```
Put a decimal point directly above the decimal point in the dividend.

```
  1.7
3)5.1      Divide as you would with whole numbers.
  3        Now do the long division as you would with whole numbers. For each digit in the dividend: divide,
  2 1      multiply, subtract and slide.
  2 1
```

Note: *Use zero as a placeholder in the quotient between the decimal point and the first digit of the answer if the decimal point comes first in the dividend.*

For example:
```
  .085
5).425
```

Remainders as Decimals

When you finish with long division and you have a remainder you may continue if you want to express it as a decimal. Put a decimal point and a zero to the right of the last digit in the dividend and a decimal point directly above in the quotient. Continue to divide, multiply, subtract and slide—adding zeroes until there is no remainder.

```
        14.5
    6)87.0
        6
       ‾‾
       27
       24
       ‾‾
        3 0
        3 0
```

Continue to add zeros and divide. A repeating pattern may appear. Either stop dividing at this point or show the quotient with a bar (line) across the top of the repeating part of the quotient. In the example below the full quotient is repeating.

```
       ‾‾‾
       .444
    9)4.000
       3 6
       ‾‾
       40
       36
       ‾‾
        4
```

Dividing by a Decimal Number

```
     ‾‾‾‾
   .2)1.42     Count the decimal digits in the divisor; there is 1 digit in the divisor to the right of the decimal point.
               Place a pointer on the decimal point in the dividend and count 1 place to the right and make a new
    2)14.2     decimal point. Move the decimal point one place to the right, in the divisor too. (This means you will no
               longer have a decimal point in the divisor.)

      7.1
     ‾‾‾
   .2)142      Put a decimal point in the quotient directly above the decimal point in the dividend and divide as whole
     14        numbers.
     ‾‾
      2
      2
     ‾‾
      0
```

Dividing Whole Numbers by a Decimal

```
     ‾‾‾‾
   .5)300

     ‾‾‾‾‾‾
   .5)300.00     Put a decimal point to the right of the last number in the dividend and add at least two zeros, then fol-
                 low the example above.
     ‾‾‾‾‾‾
   .5)3000.0     The new problem will look like this.
```

Note: *Remember to check your work using the original divisor and the quotient. The multiplicand should equal the original dividend. Do not forget to count the decimal places. If the decimals are in the wrong place, the answer will be wrong.*
    Check example from above:

```
      7.1     (quotient)
    × .2      (original divisor)
    ‾‾‾‾
    1.4 2     (multiplicand)
```

Rounding Off Decimals

Decimals are fractions of the whole. They are often used in counting money (cents), and in measuring fluids. To round off decimals, use the following procedure:

1. Find the place you are rounding off to and underline the digit in that place. Then circle the digit to the right.

    Example: 7.3 ② round to the nearest tenth

        8.2 ⑥ 4 round to the nearest tenth

7.3 <u>2</u> ③ round to the nearest hundredth

3.2 <u>5</u> ⑥ round to the nearest hundredth

4.4 4 <u>4</u> ④ round to the nearest thousandth

4.4 4 <u>6</u> ⑧ round to the nearest thousandth

2. If the circled digit is 0, 1, 2, 3, 4, then the underlined digit stays the same. If the circled digit is 5, 6, 7, 8, 9, then add one to the underlined digit. Drop all the digits that follow the underlined digit.

    Example: In 7.32, 7.3 is the nearest round-off to the nearest tenth.

    In 8.264, 8.3 is the round-off to the nearest tenth.

    In 7.323, 7.32 is the round-off to the nearest hundredth.

    In 3.256, 3.26 is the round-off to the nearest hundredth.

    In 4.4444, 4.444 is the round-off to the nearest thousandth.

    In 4.4468, 4.447 is the round-off to the nearest thousandth.

Practice Problems Division and Rounding

1. 9)999   2.   8)692   3. 11)1,134   4. 4)5,144

5. 15)1,286   6. .5)6,329   7. .6)3.87   8.   7).867

9. Betsy bought 6 donuts for $.79. Each donut cost about how much?

10. John bought a box of 8 pens for $3.49. Each pen cost about how much?

11. Undershirts are sold in packages at $6.51 per package with three shirts to a package. How much did each shirt cost?

12. Mrs. Bates needs to buy some dog food for her dog Clementine. She needs to decide which bag is more economical, the large 20 lb. bag for $15.95 or the new small 5 lb. bag for $3.49. Which bag should she buy? Round your answers to the nearest cent.

13. Round to the nearest tenth

     a. 3.82 _____   b. 8.47 _____   c. 13.95 _____   d. 80.333 _____

     Round to the nearest hundredth   Round to the nearest thousandth

     e. 7.893 _____   f. 3.235 _____   g. 6.7356 _____   h. 8.9532 _____

     Round to the nearest whole number

     i. 6.4356 _____   j. 8.9532 _____

Estimates

Rounding off whole numbers can help you make a guess close to the answer to a problem. Making a close guess is called *estimating*. Use the above method to make estimates of whole numbers.

Example:

$$\begin{array}{r} 6.38 \\ + 3.7 \\ \hline \end{array} \quad \text{rounded off to whole numbers becomes} \quad \begin{array}{r} 6 \\ + 4 \\ \hline 10 \end{array}$$

Fractions

A fraction is defined as "one or more of the equal parts of a whole."

 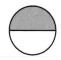 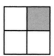

$\dfrac{1}{3}$ One-third $\dfrac{1}{2}$ One-half $\dfrac{1}{4}$ One-fourth

The bottom number of a fraction is the *denominator* and tells into how many parts a certain object has been divided. It names the fraction. The top number is the *numerator* of the fraction and tells the number of parts that are being worked with. The square above has been divided into 4 parts and 1 part is being considered in this explanation.

Remember the denominator *names* the fractions. Fractions with different denominators (names) cannot be added or subtracted until they are given the same name. As items that have different names cannot be added or subtracted collectively, so fractions with different denominators cannot be added or subtracted.

Be sure the denominators are the same before adding and subtracting, as in the examples below.

$$\begin{array}{r} \frac{2}{4} \\ + \frac{1}{4} \\ \hline \frac{3}{4} \end{array} \qquad \begin{array}{r} \frac{5}{9} \\ - \frac{3}{9} \\ \hline \frac{2}{9} \end{array}$$

To add or subtract fractions that do not have a common denominator or name, the first process is to convert the denominators to a common denominator. This process is called finding the least common denominator (LCD). Use the following steps:

Example: Add $\dfrac{3}{4}$

$+ \dfrac{4}{5}$

1. List the first multiples of the larger denominator: 5: 5, 10, 15, ⃝20, 25, etc.
2. List the first multiples of the smaller denominator: 4: 4, 8, 12, 16, ⃝20
3. Circle the first common, or shared, multiples of 5 and 4. The first one that they share, or have in common, is 20. The least common denominator is 20.
4. Then convert each fraction to use that least common denominator (LCD).

Example: $\dfrac{3}{4} \times \dfrac{5}{5} = \dfrac{15}{20}$ $\dfrac{4}{5} \times \dfrac{4}{4} = \dfrac{16}{20}$

Multiplying and Dividing Fractions

Multiplying and dividing fractions does not require that denominators be the same or have a common name.

In multiplying fractions, multiply the numerators and then the denominators.

$$\frac{5}{4} \times \frac{3}{8} = \frac{15}{32}$$

In dividing, rewrite the problem, inverting the second fraction (turning it upside down), and then multiplying.

$\frac{1}{8} \div \frac{5}{6} =$ Rewrite this problem, turning the second fraction upside down and changing the division sign to a multiplication sign.

$\frac{1}{8} \times \frac{6}{5} =$ Now multiply.

$\frac{1}{8} \times \frac{6}{5} = \frac{6}{40}$ Now make the answer as small as possible by finding the largest number that both the numerator and denominator can be divided by. In this case, both 6 and 40 can be divided by 2.

$\frac{6}{40} = \frac{3}{20}$ $\frac{3}{20}$ is the correct answer.

Practice Problems Fractions

Add

1. $\begin{array}{r} \frac{7}{8} \\ +\frac{1}{2} \\ \hline \end{array}$
2. $\begin{array}{r} \frac{5}{8} \\ +\frac{2}{3} \\ \hline \end{array}$
3. $\begin{array}{r} \frac{5}{16} \\ +\frac{3}{4} \\ \hline \end{array}$
4. $\begin{array}{r} \frac{3}{4} \\ +\frac{1}{6} \\ \hline \end{array}$

Subtract

5. $\begin{array}{r} \frac{7}{10} \\ -\frac{1}{5} \\ \hline \end{array}$
6. $\begin{array}{r} \frac{3}{4} \\ -\frac{5}{16} \\ \hline \end{array}$
7. $\begin{array}{r} \frac{2}{3} \\ -\frac{1}{5} \\ \hline \end{array}$
8. $\begin{array}{r} \frac{7}{8} \\ -\frac{2}{4} \\ \hline \end{array}$

Multiply

9. $\frac{15}{16} \times \frac{4}{5} = $ ____

10. $\frac{5}{6} \times \frac{9}{10} = $ ____

11. $\frac{7}{10} \times \frac{1}{4} = $ ____

Divide

12. $\frac{3}{8} \div \frac{3}{5} = $ ____

13. $\frac{5}{16} \div \frac{1}{8}$ ____

14. $\frac{1}{3} \div \frac{1}{6} = $ ____

PERCENTS

Percent is a ratio of a number to 100.

Percent means "per hundred." Sometimes a percent is written using the word "percent," and sometimes it is written using the symbol "%."

You can use graph paper to model percent. For instance, mark off a 10 by 10 square, which will represent 100 squares. Then shade 18 of the squares to represent 18%.

Percents and Fractions

To find the percent for any fraction, you can divide the numerator by the denominator to find the decimal. Then you can write the percent.

Find the percent for $\frac{1}{20} = 20\overline{)1.00}^{0.05} = 0.05 = 5\%$

50% means   50 per hundred
                50 out of every 100

16% means   16 out of every 100 or $\frac{16}{100} = 16\%$

1% means   1 out of every 100 or $\frac{1}{100} = 1\%$

98% means   98 out of every 100 or $\frac{98}{100} = 98\%$

1. 10% of 90 is ____   2. 20% of 90 is ____   3. 30% of 90 is ____   4. 40% of 90 is ____

Practice Problems Metric and English Systems

How many squares will be shaded in for the following percentages?

5. 13% ____   6. 25% ____   7. 75%____   8. 100%____

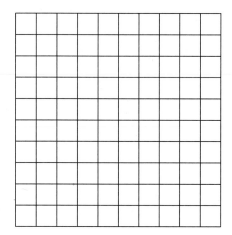

METRIC SYSTEM

The metric system uses the decimal system of weights and measures and is based on the meter as a standard measurement. One meter is 39.37 inches long or about 3 feet, $2\frac{1}{3}$ inches and a kilogram equals 2.2046 pounds.

The metric system is used in this discipline with intake, output and measuring liquids.

BASIC METRIC UNITS OF MEASUREMENT

Quantity	Unit	Symbol
Length	Meter	m
Mass (weight)	Gram	g
Time	Second	S
Temperature	Kelvin	k

Prefix	Multiplier	Symbol
Milli	0.001	m
Centi	0.01	c
Kilo	1,000	k

METRIC SYSTEM CONVERSION CHART

Metric Unit	U.S. Unit*	Metric Unit	U.S. Unit*
1 ml	¼ tsp	1 decimeter	4 inches
1 cc	¼ tsp	1 meter	39 inches
5 cc	1 tsp	180 cc	6 fl oz
5 ml	1 tsp	210 cc	7 fl oz
15 cc	3 tsp	240 cc	8 fl oz
15 cc	1 tbsp	270 cc	9 fl oz
30 cc	2 tbsp	300 cc	10 fl oz
30 cc	1 fl oz	500 cc	1 pint
60 cc	2 fl oz	1000 cc	1 quart
90 cc	3 fl oz	1 liter	1 quart
120 cc	4 fl oz	4000 cc	1 gallon
150 cc	5 fl oz	28 grams	1 oz
1 centimeter	0.4 inches	1 kilogram	2.2 pounds

cc = cubic centimeter   ml = milliliter   fl oz = fluid ounce

*approximate values

Basic Metric Conversion Calculations

Quantity wanted = quantity given × factor unit

Examples:

- Change 40 meters to centimeters.

$$\text{Centimeters (quantity wanted)} = \text{meters (quantity given)} \times \frac{\text{centimeters}}{\text{meters}}$$

Since there are 100 centimeters in 1 meter, write the problem as

$$? \text{ Centimeters} = 40 \text{ meters} \times \frac{100 \text{ centimeters}}{1 \text{ meter}} = 4{,}000 \text{ cm (centimeters)}$$

- Change 430 milligrams to grams. How many milligrams are in 1 gram? The chart shows that *milli* means 0.001, so 1 g equals 1,000 mg. This means there is

$$1{,}000 \text{ mg (which reads 1 g per 1,000 mg)} \qquad \frac{1 \text{ g (gram)}}{1{,}000 \text{ mg}}$$

$$g = mg \times \frac{g \text{ (gram)}}{mg \text{ (milligram)}}$$

$$? \text{ g} = 430 \text{ mg} \times \frac{1g \text{ (gram)}}{1{,}000 \text{ mg}} = 0.430 \text{ g (grams)}$$

- Convert 2.3 kilograms to grams? $g = 2.3 \text{ kg} \times \dfrac{1{,}000 \text{ g}}{1 \text{ kg (kilogram)}} = 2300 \text{ g}$

- Convert 2.3 kilograms to decigrams? $dg = 2{,}300 \text{ g} \times \dfrac{10 \text{ dg}}{1 \text{ g (gram)}} = 23{,}000 \text{ dg}$

- Convert 2.3 kilograms to centigrams? $cg = 23{,}000 \text{ dg} \times \dfrac{10 \text{ mg}}{1 \text{ cg}} = 230{,}000 \text{ cg}$

- Convert 2.3 kilograms to milligrams? $mg = 230{,}000 \text{ cg} \times \dfrac{10 \text{ mg}}{1 \text{ cg}} = 2{,}300{,}000 \text{ mg}$

THE ENGLISH SYSTEM OF MEASUREMENT (AS USED IN THE UNITED STATES)

Length	Weight	Volume
12 inches = 1 foot	16 ounces = 1 pound	16 fluid ounces = 1 pint
3 feet = 1 yard	2,000 pounds = 1 ton	2 pints = 1 quart
5,280 feet = 1 mile		4 quarts = 1 gallon

The English system of measurement used in the United States uses inches, feet, yards and miles to measure length. It uses ounces (oz.), pounds and tons to measure weight. Volume is measured in ounces, pints, quarts and gallons.

Basic English Conversion Calculations

Adding Pounds and Ounces

Steps

1. Add the pounds
2. Add the ounces
3. Subtract number of multiples of ounces (16 oz in 1 pound, 32 oz in 2 pounds etc.) from the original number of ounces

4. Add new number of pounds to the original number of pounds, and keep the remainder of ounces.

    12 pounds 14 ounces
  + 5 pounds   3 ounces
  ‾‾‾‾‾‾‾‾‾‾‾‾‾‾‾‾‾‾‾‾
    17 pounds 17 ounces
              − 16 ounces = 1 pound
  + 1 pound
  ‾‾‾‾‾‾‾‾‾‾‾‾‾‾‾‾‾‾‾‾
    18 pounds   1 ounce   17 lb 17 oz = 18 lb 1 oz

- To convert ounces to pounds and ounces, divide the number of ounces by 16 (16 oz per pound).
  Example: 164 oz

$$\frac{164}{(1\ lb)\ 16} = 10.25 = 10\ lb\ 4\ oz$$

Pints, Quarts, and Gallons

- How many cups are in a quart?
  There are 2 cups in 1 pint and 2 pints in 1 quart; therefore, there are $2 \times 2 = 4$ cups in 1 quart.
- How many cups in 5 quarts? 5 quarts = 5×2 pints = 10 pints, 2 cups per pint $\times$ 10 = 20 cups.
- How many cups are in 1 gallon? 2 pints = 1 quart   4 quarts = 1 gallon

      2 cups in 1 pint   4 cups in 1 quart
    $\times$ 2 pints in 1 quart $\times$ 4 quarts in 1 gallon
    ‾‾‾‾‾‾‾‾‾‾‾‾‾‾‾‾‾‾‾‾‾‾‾‾‾‾‾‾‾‾‾‾‾‾‾‾‾‾‾
      4 cups in 1 quart   16 cups in 1 gallon

- How many pints are in 1 gallon? 2 pints = 1 quart   4 quarts = 1 gallon

      4 quarts in 1 gallon
    $\times$ 2 pints in 1 quart
    ‾‾‾‾‾‾‾‾‾‾‾‾‾‾‾‾‾‾‾‾
      8 pints in 1 gallon

TEMPERATURE SCALES

Fahrenheit Temperature. The freezing point of pure water is at 32 degrees (32° F), and the boiling point of water is at 212 degrees (212° F). There are 180-Fahrenheit degrees between the freezing point and the boiling point of water.

Celsius Temperature. Anders Celsius, a Swedish astronomer, devised the Celsius temperature scale in 1742. On the Celsius scale, the freezing point of water is at zero degrees (0° C), and the boiling point of water is at 100 degrees (100° C). The Celsius scale may be referred to as the centigrade scale.

Converting Celsius and Fahrenheit Degrees

One hundred Celsius degrees cover the same range as 180 Fahrenheit degrees, so that 1 Celsius degree = 1.8 Fahrenheit degrees. 0° C is equivalent to 32° F. Converting temperatures from one scale to the other is based on this fact.

$$°F = (1.8 \times °C) + 32 \text{ and } \frac{°F - 32}{1.8}$$

Example:
- Convert 122° F to degrees Celsius.
  Substitute 122° F into the conversion formula for changing °F to °C

$$°C = \frac{°F - 32.0}{1.8} = \frac{122 - 32.0}{1.8} = \frac{90}{1.8} = 50 \qquad 122° F = 50° C$$

- Convert 100° C to degrees Fahrenheit.
  Substitute 100° C into the conversion formula for changing °C to °F.
  °F = (1.8 × °C) + 32.0; °F = (1.8 × 100) + 32.0 = 180 + 32.0 = 212
  100° C = 212° F

Practice Problems Metric and English Systems

1. Convert 0.25 kg to (a) grams, (b) milligrams.

2. Convert 3.1 m to (a) centimeters, (b) millimeters.

3. Convert 149 mm to (a) centimeters, (b) kilometers.

4. Express 25.0 m in (a) feet, (b) inches.

5. Express 1.2 L in (a) gallons, (b) quarts.

6. Convert 100° F to degrees Celsius.

7. Convert 36° C to degrees Fahrenheit.

8. Change 45 lb to ounces.

9. Change 45 oz to pounds.

10. Add 15 lb 4 oz and 13 lb 7 oz.

11. Add 10 lb 25 oz and 3 lb 15 oz.

12. Subtract 18 lb 3 oz from 42 lb 5 oz.

13. How many cups in 2 pints?

14. How many pints in 16 cups?

15. How many quarts in 14 pints?

16. 20 quarts equal how many gallons?

17. How many feet are in 80 inches?

18. How many feet and inches are in 92 inches?

COMMUNICATIONS IN TIME

The following is a conversion chart from the standard time used in the United States to the 24-hour time used on Activities for Daily Living Flow Charts in some medical facilities and in the military.

The 24-hour clock is read as follows: Hours 1 through 9 are read as "o" 100 to "o" 900 hours ("o" one-hundred hours to "o" nine-hundred); hours from 10 through 24 are read as "10 hundred hours," etc.

US TIME AND MILITARY TIME CONVERSION CHART

US TIME	MILITARY (24-Hour) TIME
7:00 a.m.	0700 Hours
8:00 a.m.	0800 Hours
9:00 a.m.	0900 Hours
10:00 a.m.	1000 Hours
11:00 a.m.	1100 Hours
12:00 NOON	1200 Hours
1:00 p.m.	1300 Hours
2:00 p.m.	1400 Hours
3:00 p.m.	1500 Hours
4:00 p.m.	1600 Hours
5:00 p.m.	1700 Hours
6:00 p.m.	1800 Hours
7:00 p.m.	1900 Hours
8:00 p.m.	2000 Hours
9:00 p.m.	2100 Hours
10:00 p.m.	2200 Hours
11:00 p.m.	2300 Hours
12:00 MIDNIGHT	2400 Hours
1:00 a.m.	0100 Hours
2:00 a.m.	0200 Hours
3:00 a.m.	0300 Hours
4:00 a.m.	0400 Hours
5:00 a.m.	0500 Hours
6:00 a.m.	0600 Hours

Math Module Answer Sheet

Addition:
1. 9.81
2. 8.41
3. 6.20
4. 91.60
5. 55.14
6. 93.11
7. 73.53
8. 82.12
9. 96.74
10. 90.20
11. 13.71
12. 90.20
13. 93.09
14. 95.21
15. 85.40
16. 5.85
17. 102.50
18. 140.53
19. 151.44
20. 166.19

Subtraction:
1. 25
2. 4,014
3. 2,912
4. 658
5. 2,208
6. 21.57
7. 27.82
8. 6.71
9. 30.53
10. 6.41
11. 362.5
12. 5,025
13. 422
14. 7
15. 9,018

Multiplication:
1. 9,936
2. 1,636.8128
3. 780.4224
4. 54.152
5. 2,203.32
6. 306,469.77
7. 11,443.278
8. $167,868.72
9. 548.996
10. 194.0510
11. 28
12. March 23,250; April 22,500
13. 864
14. 250

Division and Rounding:
1. 111
2. 86.5
3. 103.0
4. 1,286
5. 85.7
6. 12,658
7. 6.45
8. .124
9. $.13
10. $.44
11. $2.17
12. 5-lb bag
13. a. 3.8   b. 8.5   c. 14.0   d. 80.3   e. 7.89   f. 3.24   g. 6.736   h. 8.953   i. 6   j. 9

Percentage Problems
1. 9   5. 13
2. 18   6. 25
3. 27   7. 75
4. 36   8. 100

Fractions
1. $1\frac{3}{8}$ 2. $\frac{31}{24}$ 3. $1\frac{1}{16}$
4. $\frac{11}{12}$ 5. $\frac{1}{2}$ 6. $\frac{7}{16}$
7. $\frac{7}{15}$ 8. $\frac{3}{8}$ 9. $\frac{3}{4}$
10. $\frac{3}{4}$ 11. $\frac{7}{40}$ 12. $\frac{5}{8}$
13. $2\frac{1}{2}$ 14. 2

Metric and English Systems
1. a. 250 g   b. 2500 mg
2. a. 310 cm   b. 3100 mm
3. a. 14.9 cm   b. .000149 km
4. a. 82 ft   b. 984 in
5. a. .32 gal   b. 1.3 qt
6. 37.8° C
7. 96.8° F
8. 720 oz
9. 2.81 lb
10. 28 lb 11 oz
11. 15 lb 8 oz
12. 24 lb 2 oz
13. 4 c
14. 8 pt
15. 7 qt
16. 5 gal
17. 6 ft 8 in
18. 7 ft 8 in

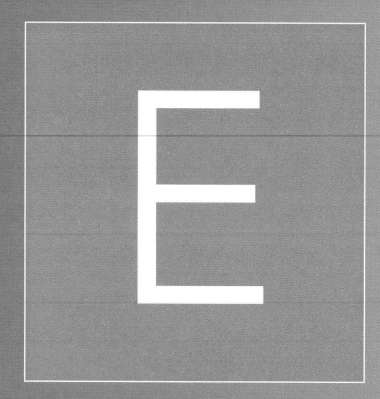

Taking a Temperature with a Glass Thermometer

GOALS

After reading this module and practicing the skills you will have the information needed to:

Read, clean and shake down a glass thermometer.

Take and record a person's oral, rectal and axillary temperature with a glass thermometer.

A glass thermometer is made of clear glass with a hollow shaft in the middle, which contains mercury or another nonmercury substance. In the past, most glass thermometers contained mercury; however, nonmercury thermometers can be purchased in most stores. Nonmercury thermometers may be used in the same way as those containing mercury, but they present less of a hazard to the person, staff and the environment. These thermometers look very similar to the mercury thermometer but use a substance that is nontoxic. This substance travels from a bulb at one end of the thermometer through the shaft toward the other end, called the *stem*. When taking someone's temperature, insert the bulb end of the thermometer into the person's mouth, under her arm or into her rectum. The bulb warms from body heat, and the substance moves further up the shaft toward the stem. Because it takes time for the substance to warm to the same temperature as its surroundings, it is important not to remove the thermometer too soon, or the reading will not be accurate.

Two types of glass thermometers are oral and rectal (Figure E-1). They differ in the shapes of their bulbs. The oral glass thermometer, which you use for taking only oral temperatures, has a long, slender bulb. Rectal thermometers have rounder, stubbier bulbs. Once you use a glass thermometer to take a rectal temperature, you should

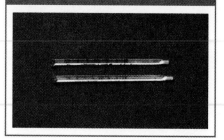

FIGURE E-1 Two types of glass thermometers are top, oral and bottom, rectal.

never use it to take an oral or axillary temperature. To avoid confusion, the thermometer manufacturer often colors the ends of thermometers in red if they are going to be used for taking rectal temperatures. (To remember this clue, think "Red for Rectal.")

Glass thermometers are marked in either degrees Fahrenheit (F) or degrees Celsius (C). The column on a glass thermometer is marked with a series of long and short lines extending from 94 to 108° Fahrenheit or from 34 to 43° Celsius. On a Fahrenheit thermometer, each long line on the thermometer represents 1 degree, and each of the four shorter lines between the long lines represents 0.2 degree. On a Celsius thermometer, each long line represents 1 degree, but each shorter line in between represents 0.1 degree.

Cleaning a Glass Thermometer

Glass thermometers are fragile and can break easily, so they must be stored in holders. In some health-care settings, glass thermometers are all stored together in one container. In most homes, thermometers are stored in individual holders at the bedside or in the bathroom. A holder protects a thermometer from breaking, but it also provides a place for germs to grow. Because of this possibility of infection, you must wash a glass thermometer with soap and water twice: first before you use it—to remove germs that may have grown while it was stored in the holder, and second, after you use it—to remove secretions that may contain germs. Use cold water, because hot water can cause the substance to shoot through the shaft and break the glass. Use soap and water rather than alcohol to clean a thermometer. When cleaning a glass thermometer, follow the specific procedure that is explained step by step in Skill 66. If you should drop and break a glass mercury thermometer, do not touch or let anyone touch the mercury. Report it to your

supervising nurse immediately. The facility will follow special procedures for cleaning up the mercury spill. Nonmercury glass thermometers should be used in place of mercury glass thermometers to prevent this hazard.

Taking a Person's Temperature with a Glass Thermometer

When taking a person's oral temperature, make sure that she has not had recent mouth surgery and does not have a mouth disease. Also make sure that she is not receiving oxygen and is not having trouble breathing, is not confused or unconscious and is not paralyzed on one side of her body or face. Do not take an oral temperature if she is breathing through her mouth or if she has a tube in her nose. Do not take a child's oral temperature if she is under the age of 5. Also delay taking the person's temperature by 15 minutes if she has eaten, smoked or had anything to drink within the past 15 minutes.

To take an accurate oral temperature using a glass thermometer, you must understand how the thermometer works and what conditions can affect the reading. Before using the thermometer, make sure that it is in perfect condition and is not chipped, cracked or broken. Make sure the substance is mostly contained in the bulb, rather than in the column of the thermometer. To move the substance into the bulb, "shake down" the thermometer with a flick of your wrist until the substance column is below 94°.

After placing the bulb of the thermometer in the person's mouth, allow at least 5 minutes for the thermometer to register the person's internal body temperature. If you take the oral temperature of an adult in your care, you usually do not have to hold the thermometer in place. You can make use of the waiting time by measuring and recording other vital signs. (If you take a rectal or axillary temperature you should hold the thermometer in place;

in that case, of course, you will not be able to record other signs at the same time.) When taking a person's oral temperature with a glass thermometer, follow the specific procedure that is explained step by step in Skill 67. Generally, the oral method is the preferred way to measure a person's body temperature, because it is the easiest method and requires little preparation. Taken correctly, it is an accurate reflection of the body's internal temperature.

The rectal method for measuring a person's body temperature also accurately reflects internal body temperature, but it requires more preparation and can be embarrassing for adults and frightening for children. Take a person's rectal temperature when an oral temperature would be inaccurate or might cause injury. When taking a person's rectal temperature with a glass thermometer, always use a rectal thermometer that is in perfect condition. Make sure that the person does not have diarrhea or a blocked rectum. Make sure that she has not recently had a heart attack or rectal surgery or injury or that she does not have hemorrhoids. Allow at least 3 minutes for the temperature to register. Follow the specific procedure that is explained step by step in Skill 68.

The axillary method is the least accurate way to measure a person's body temperature. This method requires you to keep the thermometer in place for 10 minutes. Take an axillary temperature only if the person cannot tolerate either an oral or a rectal thermometer. Make sure the person is sitting or lying down during the procedure and not walking around with the thermometer under her arm. Use only a glass thermometer that is in perfect condition. When taking a person's axillary temperature with a glass thermometer, follow the specific procedure that is explained step by step in Skill 69.

Sometimes certain situations require you to take special precautions when measuring a person's body temperature with a glass thermometer. Read Table E-1 to learn how to respond to these situations.

TABLE E-1 PRECAUTIONS FOR USING A THERMOMETER

Situation	Problem	Solution
Chipped, cracked or broken glass on thermometer	Can cut mouth, lips, rectum, or axilla	Check thermometer before use and discard if chipped, cracked or broken
Broken thermometer	Mercury is a poison that can injure the person who touches or swallows it	Check thermometer before use; follow employer's guidelines for cleaning up broken thermometer
Person just drank hot or cold fluid or smoked a cigarette	Temperature of fluid or cigarette smoke influences temperature of mouth	Wait 15 minutes before taking oral temperature or use another method if permissible
Person has had recent mouth surgery or has a mouth disease	Thermometer may cause injury	Take temperature using rectal, axillary or tympanic method
Confused person	May bite down on thermometer and may injure herself	Take temperature using rectal, axillary or tympanic method
Unconscious person or person paralyzed on one side of body	May not be able to keep mouth closed, resulting in inaccurate temperature reading	Take temperature using rectal, axillary or tympanic method
Person has trouble breathing or breathes through mouth, or person has tube in nose and cannot keep mouth closed	Cannot get accurate temperature reading	Take temperature using rectal, axillary or tympanic method
Person receiving oxygen experiences cooling of the body tissues around the mouth	Cannot get accurate temperature reading	Take temperature using rectal, axillary or tympanic method
Person has a blocked rectum, has hemorrhoids or has had recent rectal surgery	Rectal thermometer can cause injury	Take temperature using oral, axillary or tympanic method
Person has had a heart attack	Rectal thermometer may stimulate the urge to strain and may increase the workload of the heart	Take temperature using oral, axillary or tympanic method
Person is embarrassed about having rectal temperature taken	May be uncooperative	Explain the reason for taking rectal temperature to encourage cooperation
Person perspires under the arms	Moisture can affect the temperature reading	Dry the axilla with a tissue

Skill 66: Reading, Cleaning and Shaking Down a Glass Thermometer

PREPARATION

Gather supplies:

- Thermometer
- Thermometer holder
- Cotton balls
- Plastic trash bag
- Paper towels
- Soap
- Disposable gloves (optional)

PROCEDURE

Reading a Glass Thermometer

1. Follow the steps in Skills 67, 68 and 69 for taking temperatures with a glass thermometer.

2. When you are ready to read a thermometer, remove it from the person's mouth, rectum or axilla. Hold it between your thumb and first finger by the end that was not in contact with the person. Make sure lighting is adequate. ☐ ☐

3. Bring the thermometer to your eye level and slowly turn it until you can see the line made by the substance inside the thermometer (Figure E-2). ☐ ☐

4. Read the temperature where the substance line ends. ☐ ☐

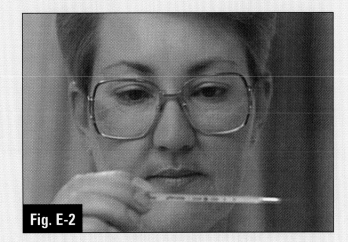

Fig. E-2

Skill 66: Reading, Cleaning and Shaking Down a Glass Thermometer—cont'd

Cleaning a Glass Thermometer

> **Note:** Clean a glass thermometer before and after use. The holder used for storage protects the thermometer from breakage, but allows organisms to grow on it.

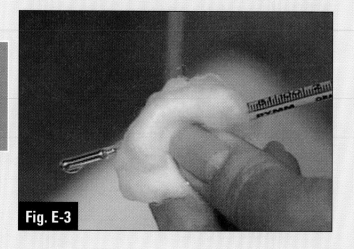

Fig. E-3

1. Wash your hands. Put on disposable gloves (optional). ☐ ☐
2. Place a paper towel in the sink in case you drop the thermometer while you are cleaning it. ☐ ☐
3. Turn on the faucet with a clean paper towel. Adjust the temperature of the water so that it is cool, not hot. ☐ ☐
4. Stand over the sink and hold the thermometer by the stem end (the stem end may be colored). ☐ ☐
5. Wet a cotton ball or tissue with water and apply soap. ☐ ☐
6. To clean the thermometer with soap, wipe down the length of the thermometer, starting at your fingers and working downward over the bulb (toward the tip), with a twisting motion (Figure E-3). ☐ ☐
7. Moisten another cotton ball or tissue with only clean water. ☐ ☐

8. Throw away the cotton balls or tissue in a plastic trash bag. ☐ ☐
9. Rinse the thermometer by using the same twisting motion as before to wipe down the length of the thermometer and the bulb end. ☐ ☐
10. Repeat the entire procedure, both soaping and rinsing, one more time. ☐ ☐
11. Dry the thermometer with a clean cotton ball or tissue, using the same twisting motion. ☐ ☐
12. Remove disposable gloves, if worn, and wash and dry your hands. ☐ ☐

Shaking Down a Glass Thermometer

1. Make sure there is nothing in the way that the thermometer might hit while you are shaking it. Shake down the thermometer after cleaning and before using if it registers above 94° Fahrenheit. ☐ ☐
2. Hold the thermometer by the stem end, not the bulb end. Shake it as if you were shaking water off it. Flex and snap your wrist until the substance is at least below the 94° Fahrenheit mark. ☐ ☐

ADDITIONAL INFORMATION

Dispose of broken mercury thermometers using a mercury spill kit and notify your supervising nurse immediately.

COMPLETION

Follow Completion Standards in compliance with your facility. For a complete list of those used in this course, see Chapter 7, "Controlling the Spread of Germs."

Skill 67: Taking and Recording a Person's Oral Temperature with a Glass Thermometer

PREPARATION

1. Gather supplies:
   - Clean oral thermometer (if the person does not have one at her bedside)
   - Thermometer sheath (optional)
   - Watch with a second hand
   - Disposable gloves (optional)
   - Cotton balls and tissues
   - Plastic trash bag
   - Paper towel
   - Pencil and paper to write down the temperature
2. Follow Preparation Standards (see Chapter 7).

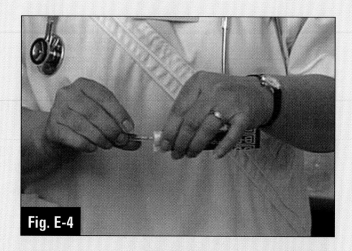

Fig. E-4

PROCEDURE

1. Put the thermometer sheath, if used, on the thermometer (Figure E-4). ☐ ☐
2. Put the bulb end of the thermometer under the person's tongue and slightly to one side. ☐ ☐
   - Ask the person to close her lips and not to bite down on the thermometer with her teeth (Figure E-5).
   - Always stay with the person while you are taking an oral temperature.
3. Note the time on your watch when you put the thermometer in the person's mouth, and keep the thermometer in place for 5 to 8 minutes. ☐ ☐

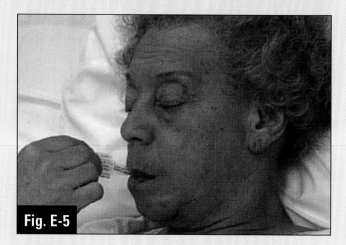

Fig. E-5

4. Remove the thermometer from the person's mouth. Take off the thermometer sheath, if used, and throw it away in the plastic trash bag. If mucus or saliva on the thermometer makes it difficult to read, wipe off the thermometer with a tissue. ☐ ☐

5. Read the thermometer and place it on a clean, dry paper towel or tissue. ☐ ☐ Be sure to write *O* for oral next to the number: Example: 98.6 *O*

Note: *Remember to hold the thermometer at eye level while you read it.*

6. Clean the thermometer, shake it down, and put it back in its holder. ☐ ☐

7. Wash and dry your hands. ☐ ☐

ADDITIONAL INFORMATION

- Use only a glass thermometer that is in perfect condition, not one that is chipped, cracked or broken.
- If you are taking other vital signs in addition to the temperature, do completion steps after you take the last vital sign.

COMPLETION

Follow Completion Standards in compliance with your facility. For a complete list of those used in this course, see Chapter 7, "Controlling the Spread of Germs."

Skill 68: Taking a Person's Rectal Temperature with a Glass Thermometer

PREPARATION

1. Gather supplies:
   - Rectal thermometer (if the person does not have one at his beside)
   - Thermometer sheath (optional)
   - Lubricating jelly
   - Watch with a second hand
   - Plastic trash bag
   - Paper towels
   - Disposable gloves
   - Pencil and paper to write down the temperature
2. Follow Preparation Standards (see Chapter 7).

PROCEDURE

1. Put the thermometer sheath, if used, on the thermometer. Put the thermometer down on a clean paper towel or tissue. Have extra tissues within easy reach. ☐ ☐
2. Lower the side rail, if used, on the side where you will be working. ☐ ☐
3. Help the person lie on one side with his back toward you. Ask him to flex his top knee (Figure E-6). Adjust his clothing and top covers so that he is covered. ☐ ☐
4. Put on disposable gloves. ☐ ☐
5. Put a small amount of lubricating jelly on a tissue. ☐ ☐
6. Turn back the top covers and adjust or remove clothing just enough so that you can see the anal area. ☐ ☐
7. Apply lubricating jelly to the tip of the thermometer from a tissue (Figure E-7). ☐ ☐

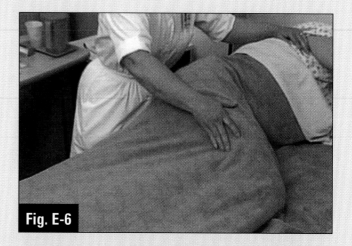

Fig. E-6

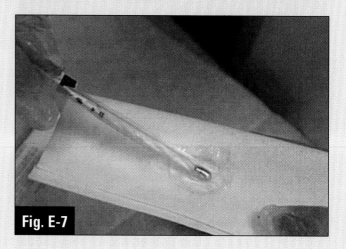

Fig. E-7

8. Lift the person's upper buttock and gently insert the bulb end of the thermometer into the anus, no more than 1 inch (Figure E-8). ☐ ☐
9. Note the time on your watch when you placed the thermometer, and keep the thermometer in place for at least 3 minutes. ☐ ☐

Note: *Always hold on to the thermometer while taking a rectal temperature.*

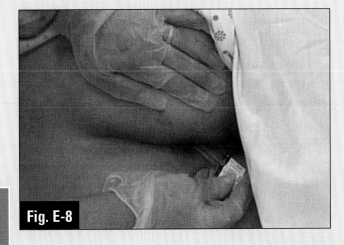
Fig. E-8

10. Gently remove the thermometer and place it on a paper towel.
    • Clean the anal area with a clean tissue.
    • Take off the thermometer sheath, if it was used.
    • Wipe off the thermometer with a tissue, if necessary. ☐ ☐
11. Throw the sheath and all tissues in the plastic trash bag. ☐ ☐
12. Read the thermometer and remember the number. ☐ ☐

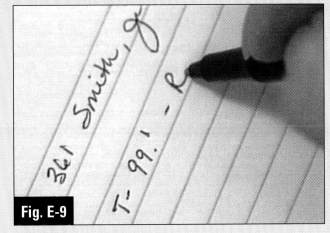
Fig. E-9

13. Place the thermometer on a clean, dry paper towel or tissue. ☐ ☐
14. Remove the gloves and throw them away in the plastic trash bag. ☐ ☐
Follow Completion Standards, including recording the number.
15. Be sure to write *R* for rectal next to the number (Figure E-9). ☐ ☐
    Example: 99.1 *R*
16. Wash and dry your hands. ☐ ☐

Skill 68: Taking a Person's Rectal Temperature with a Glass Thermometer—cont'd

ADDITIONAL INFORMATION

- Use only a glass thermometer that is in perfect condition, not one that is chipped, cracked or broken.
- If you are taking other vital signs in addition to the temperature, do completion steps after you take the last vital sign.

COMPLETION

Follow Completion Standards in compliance with your facility. For a complete list of those used in this course, see Chapter 7, "Controlling the Spread of Germs."

Skill 69: Taking and Recording a Person's Axillary Temperature with a Glass Thermometer

PRECAUTIONS

1. Gather supplies:
   - Clean thermometer (if the person does not have one at his bedside)
   - Thermometer sheath (optional)
   - Watch with a second hand
   - Cotton balls and tissues
   - Plastic trash bag
   - Paper towels
   - Pencil and paper to write down the temperature
   - Disposable gloves
2. Follow Preparation Standards (see Chapter 7).

PROCEDURE

1. Put the thermometer sheath, if used, on the thermometer. ☐ ☐
2. Uncover the person's underarm area and dry it with a tissue, if necessary (Figure E-10). Throw the tissue in the plastic trash bag. ☐ ☐
3. Put on disposable gloves. ☐ ☐
4. Put the bulb end of the thermometer in the middle of the person's underarm (Figure E-11). ☐ ☐
   - Bring person's arm across the chest to hold the thermometer in place.
   - Make sure the person is sitting or lying down during the procedure and not walking around with the thermometer under his arm.

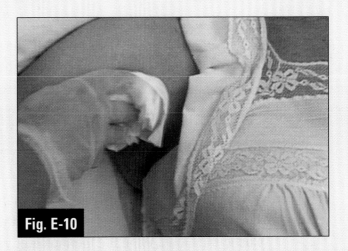

Fig. E-10

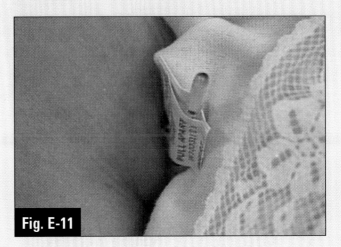

Fig. E-11

5. Note the time on your watch when you placed the thermometer under the person's arm, and keep the thermometer in place for at least 10 minutes. ☐ ☐

> **Note:** *Always stay with the person while the thermometer is in place.*

6. Remove the thermometer. Take off the thermometer sheath, if used, and throw it in the plastic trash bag. Wipe the thermometer with a tissue, if necessary. ☐ ☐

7. Remove gloves and throw them away in the plastic trash bag. ☐ ☐

8. Read the thermometer and place it on a clean, dry paper towel. Write the temperature immediately on the paper that you brought with you. Be sure to write *A* for axillary next to the temperature. Example: 97.6 *A*. ☐ ☐

9. Wash and dry your hands. ☐ ☐

ADDITIONAL INFORMATION

- Use only a glass thermometer that is in perfect condition, not one that is chipped, cracked or broken.
- If you are taking other vital signs in addition to the temperature, do completion steps after you take the last vital sign.

COMPLETION

Follow Completion Standards in compliance with your facility. For a complete list of those used in this course, see Chapter 7, "Controlling the Spread of Germs."

Information Review
Answer Key

Chapter 1

1. hospital, nursing facility, home health
2. patient
3. c
4. b
5. client
6. c
7. c
8. resident

Chapter 2

1. d
2. b
3. supervising nurse
4. OBRA '87
5. cognitive impairment

Chapter 3

1. right
2. c
3. a
4. health-care proxy
5. ombudsman
6. ethical
7. Immediately report what you have seen to your supervising nurse. This is your legal and professional responsibility.
8. neglect
9. confidential

Chapter 4

1. physical, social, emotional, cognitive
2. order, pattern
3. b
4. a
5. b
6. physical, security, social, esteem, self-fulfillment
7. needs
8. sexuality

Chapter 5

1. sender, message, channel, receiver, confirmation
2. b
3. b
4. a
5. d
6. d
7. d

Chapter 6

1. b
2. a
3. care plan, flow sheet, nursing notes
4. a

Chapter 7

1. airborne, droplet, contact
2. clean, disinfect, sterilize
3. b
4. b
5. a
6. d
7. sharps container
8. c
9. a
10. gowns, masks, eyewear, gloves

Chapter 8

1. d
2. back
3. a
4. physical, chemical
5. mind
6. b
7. Any two of the following: bone fracture or dislocation, asphyxiation, tissue damage, nerve damage, chronic constipation, incontinence, pressure sores, pneumonia, decreased appetite

8. emotional
9. 15 minutes
10. c
11. wrist, waist, vest
12. c
13. b
14. c
15. check, call, care
16. physical, chemical

Chapter 9

1. b
2. admitted, change
3. 97.6º F, 99.6º F
4. d
5. rhythm, force
6. brachial
7. a
8. thumb
9. dyspnea
10. c

Chapter 10

1. pressure ulcers, fat, muscle
2. b and d
3. a
4. c
5. d
6. drawsheet
7. explain, help
8. high Fowler's
9. back
10. brakes

Chapter 11

1. b
2. c
3. b
4. c
5. alternating pressure pad

Chapter 12

1. b
2. d
3. c
4. front, back
5. b
6. c

Chapter 13

1. admitting
2. transferring
3. discharging
4. d
5. vital signs
6. a
7. roommate
8. b

Chapter 14

1. c
2. a
3. Fats and oils
4. c
5. 48
6. high-protein
7. pureed
8. d
9. c
10. a

Chapter 15

1. Drinking fluids
2. chart
3. d
4. c
5. toilet, 5
6. tract infection
7. perineal
8. a
9. care plan
10. a

Chapter 16

1. restorative
2. d
3. self-help
4. a
5. d
6. reinforces

Chapter 17

1. d
2. a
3. b
4. b
5. c
6. a
7. independence
8. changes, belongings, inner, medication
9. disease

Chapter 18

1. c
2. a
3. human, virus
4. condoms
5. blood
6. shots/vaccinations
7. a
8. a
9. A
10. d
11. skin

Chapter 19

1. dementia
2. Alzheimer's disease
3. communication
4. social façade
5. c
6. rummaging, hoarding
7. b
8. c
9. d
10. a

Chapter 20

1. d
2. Palliative care
3. a
4. d
5. a
6. hospice
7. lividity
8. postmortem
9. respect

Chapter 21

1. Answers will vary.
2. one, any two of the following: educational history, employment history, type of job desired, individual information, personal history.
3. orientation, probationary
4. proof of work, in-service requirements, continuing education, renewal fee, application and directions on where to send renewal forms and fees.

Chapter 22

1. a
2. schedule
3. a, d
4. prioritize
5. c
6. c
7. a, c
8. schedule, readjust, communicate

Appendix C

1. 1/4 cup
2. 20
3. dry, moist
4. anus
5. three
6. high

Sources

1. Abuse/Neglect
   - CARIE. *Abuse of Nursing Home Residents*—Regulations from State of California. Coalition of Advocates for the Rights of the Infirm Elderly (CARIE) Training Manual, 1991. Philadelphia, PA.
   - *The Identification and Reporting of Abuse: A Training Manual for Nursing Home Aides,* prepared by the Michigan Department for Public Health, 1988.

2. Bed Making
   - *Guidelines for Use of Therapeutic Beds.* http://www.baronhealthcare.com/support.html
   - California Dept. of Health. *A Guide to Bed Safety.* http://www.fda.gov/cdrh/beds/bedbrochure1.html
   - *Therapeutic Beds.* Welfare and Institutions Code. Medi-Cal Policy Division. Department of Health Services, 714 P Street. Sacramento, CA 95814

3. Career Ladders/Retention/Recruitment
   - Fitgerald, Carlson. *Ladders to a Better Life. The American Prospect Online,* Volume 11, Issue 15, June 19, 2000–July 3, 2000. http://www.prospect.org/print-friendly/print/V11/15/fitgerald-j.html
   - Krupa, G. Left Behind—The Forgotten Victims of Poverty. *The Detroit News*; March 25, 2001. http://detnewes.com/specialreports/2001/poverty/lori/lori.html

   - AFT. *Career Ladder Programs.* AFT contract on career ladders. http://www.aft.org/research/models/language/tquality/ladder.htm

4. Diversity and Culture
   - Table 3: Immigrants Admitted by Region and Country of Birth Fiscal Years 1988–98. *Transcultural Nursing.* Published by Homestead Schools, Inc. Torrance, CA.
   - Harry, K. *Communication Skills for Nurses.* Homestead Schools, Inc. Torrance, CA.
   - *Importance of Elders in African Tribes.* http://www.cwrl.utexas.edu/~bill/316/students/elders/tribe.html

5. Emergency and Disaster
   - Emergency and Disaster Preparedness Plan, February 2000. St. John Health System Senior Community.
   - American National Red Cross. Disaster Health Services. ARC 30-3042, 1998.

6. End of Life
   - California Coalition for Compassionate Care. *Recommendations for Improving End-of-Life Care for Persons Residing in California Skilled and Intermediate Care Facilities.* January 2000.
   - Steinhauser, K.E., Christakis, N.A., Clipp, E.C., McNeilly, M., McIntyre, L., and Tulsky, J.A. Factors considered important at the end of life by patients, family, physicians, and other care providers. *JAMA* 2000; 284:2476–2482.

7. Elderly and Aging
   - Fletcher, K., RN, CS, MSN, GNP. The elderly are coming: are nurse practitioners ready? Medscape, 2001. http://www.medscape.com/medscape/CNO/2000/NCNP/NCNP-04.html

8. Facilities
   - *Quality in Nursing Home Care.* http://www.nih.gov.ninr/vol3/NurseHome.html

9. Mental Illness
   - NAMI. *About Mental Illness.* Revised August 18, 2001. http://amimd.nami.org/aboutmi.htm
   - Friends Hospital. *Facts About Mental Illness* July 9, 2001. http://www.fbhs.org/facts.htm
   - Friends Behavioral Health System. *Facts on Mental health of the Elderly.* Friends Behavioral Health System. July 9, 2001. http://www.fbhs.org/elderlyfacts.htm

10. Nursing Assistants
    - 1997 House of Delegates. Unlicensed Assistive Personnel Legislation—1997.

11. Nutrition
    - U.S. Department of Agriculture. *What We Do* Dietary Guideline: Adapted from: Dietary Guideline and Your Diet. Home and Garden Bulletins, NO253-2, July 1993. http://www.miseniors.net/whatwedo/health/DietGuide.asp?CatID=3&SubCatID=2
    - *Building Your Food Pyramid from the Bottom Up.* http://www.miseniors.net/whatwedo/health/eatwell/asp?CatID=3&SubCatID=2

- *Malnutrition Experts Offer Solutions to Malnutrition in Nursing Homes.* Press Release, July 23, 1998.
- Lifland, J. Nursing homes let patients go hungry. Courier/Medill News Service. October 23, 1997.
- *Code of Federal Regulations.* Title 42, Volume 3, Parts 430 to End. Revised as of October 1, 1999. [CITE: 42CFR483.35]
- *Nutrition Care Alerts Warning Signs and Action Steps for Caregivers in Nursing Facilities.* Nutrition Screening Initiative. American Academy of Family Physicians, The American Dietetic Association, National Council On The Aging, Inc.
- Duyff, R.L. *American Dietetic Association Complete Food and Nutrition Guide,* 2006, Wiley & Sons.
- MyPyramid. http://mypyramid.gov/index.html
- USDA National Nutritional Database for Standard Reference. http://www.nal.usda.gov/fnic/foodcomp/search/

12. Pain Management
- State and Consumer Services Agency. Pain management policy. Board of Registered Nursing. State of California, 1994, reprinted from *BRN Report,* Spring, 1997.
- American Society of Pain Management Nurses, Pensacola, FL.

13. Specific Diseases

Cancer
- Lica, L. Radiation therapy. *Gale Encyclopedia of Medicine.* Gale Research, 1999. http://www.findarticles.com/cf dls/g2601/0011/2601001157/print.html

Diabetes
- Bloomgarden, Z.T. Treating diabetes in elderly patients (03/06/01). http://www.medscape.com/medscape/endocrinology?Ask Experts/2001/03/ENDO-ae27.html
- Diabetes Fact Sheets-TIPDOM 1-800-847-3665
- Foot Care for People with Diabetes, LIFECAN Inc., a Johnson and Johnson Company.

Dementias
- U.S. National Institute of Health National Institute on Aging. "Alzheimer's Caregiver Guide." March 9, 2007. http://www.nia.nih.gov/Alzheimers/Publications/caregiverguide.htm.
- Centers for Disease Control and Prevention. "Dementia and its Implications for Public Health." Volume 3: No. 2, April 2006. http://www.cdc.gov/pcd/issues/2006/apr/05_0167.htm
- NINDS. *What Is Dementia With Lewy Bodies?* National Institute of Neurological Disorders and Stroke (NINDS). February 2001. http://cbshealthwatch.medscape.com/cx/viewarticle/402519.
- Lewy Body Dementia. Fact Sheet Number 4. http://dementia.ion.ucl.ac.uk/candid/factsheets/facts4.htm
- Dementia & Alzheimer's—What are they and how do they differ? http://www.angelfire.com/ny2/dementia1/whatisde.html
- CBS Health Watch. Dementia vs. Alzheimer's. Medscape, Inc., June 2000. http://cbshealth-watch.medscape.com/cx/viewe artilcle/215443
- Morris, J.C. *Alzheimer's Disease: Unique, Differentiable, and Treatable.* 52nd Annual Meeting of the American Academy of Neurology; Day 1—April 29, 2000. http://www.medscape.com/medscape/cno/2000/AAN/Story.cfm?story id=1198.
- Spencer, B. and Robinson, A. *Developing Meaningful Connections with People with Dementia: A Training Manual.* Ypsilanti, Michigan, 1998. Alzheimer's Education Program, Eastern Michigan University.
- National Institute on Aging. *Progress Report on Alzheimer's Disease, 1999.* National Institutes of Health. NIH Publication No. 99-4664.
- Creutzfeldt-Jakob Disease in the United States, 1979–1994: Using National Mortality Data to Assess the Possible Occurrence of Variant Cases. http://www.cdc.gov/ncidod/EID/vol2no4/holman2.htm
- Parkinson's Disease Caregivers' Community. Don't face it alone. http://www.webofcare.com/parkinsons.html
- CBS Health Watch. *Special Units for Alzheimer's Patients.* Medscape, Inc., August 2000. http://cbshealthwatch.medscape.com/cx/viewarticle/223411.
- Alzheimer's Disease Fact Sheet. http://www.alzheimers.org/pubs/adfact.html
- CBS Health Watch. *Pick's Disease.* Medscape, Inc., November 2000. http://cbshealthwatch.medscape.com/cx/viewarticle/226728.
- Pick's Disease Information Page. The National Institute of Neurological Disorders and Stroke. National Institutes of Health. Bethesda, MD. June 2000. http://cbshealthwatch.medscape.com/cs/viewarticle/402746 SNL>

Flu and Pneumonia

- Centers for Disease Control. Outbreak of Influenza A in a Nursing Home—New York, December 1991–January 1992. CDC. Update: influenza activity—United States, 1991–92 season. *MMWR* 1992:41:63–5
- _____. "Influenza (Flu)." www.cdc.gov/flu
- HFCA. *Fact Sheet on Influenza and Pneumococcal Disease.* http://www.hcfa.gov/medicaid/smd11220.htm
- National Coalition for Adult Immunization (NCAI). *A Call to Action: Improving Influenza and Pneumococcal Immunization Rates Among High-Risk Adults*: A Special Roundtable Discussion. May 1998, Washington, DC. http://www.nfid.org/ncai/publications/roundtable
- The American Geriatrics Society. *AGS Position Statement: Prevention and Treatment of Influenza in the Elderly.* 1996. http://www.americangeriatrics.org/products/positionpapers/influe96.html
- National Institute on Aging. *What to Do About the Flu.* NIH AgePage. Public Health Service National Institutes of Health, 2000. http://www.aoa.dhhs.gov/aoa/pages/agepage/flu.html

Hepatitis

- CDC National Center for Infectious Diseases. *Viral Hepatitis.* http://www.cdc.gov/ncidod/diseases/hepatitis/index.htm
- _____. "Viral Hepatitis B Fact Sheet." December 8, 2006. http://www.cdc.gov/ncidod/diseases/hepatitis/b/fact.htm.
- _____. *Viral Hepatitis Brochures.* http://www.cdc.gov/ncidod/diseases/hepatitis/resource/brochures.htm
- _____. *Viral Hepatitis A.* http://www.cdc.gov/ncidod/diseases/hepatitis/a/index.htm
- _____. *Viral Hepatitis B.* http://www.cdc.gov/ncidod/diseases/hepatitis/b/index.htm
- _____. *Viral Hepatitis C.* http://www.cdc.gov/ncidod/diseases/hepatitis/c/index.htm
- *Hepatitis A,B, and C: More serious than you think.* http://www.mdch.state.mi.us/bh/hepatitis

HIV/AIDS

- Frequently Asked Questions on HIV/AIDS. http://www.cdc.gov/hiv/pubs/faqs.htm. Updated March 2001.
- Centers for Disease Control and Prevention. A Glance At The HIV Epidemic. CDC HIV/AIDS Update, 2000.
- HIV and AIDS—United States, 1981–2000. MMWR Volume 50: No. 21. June 1, 2001.
- Centers for Disease Control and Prevention. United States HIV & AIDS Statistics Summary. U.S. Department of Health and Human Services. Public Health Service. HIV/AIDS Surveillance Report through December 1999.
- Centers for Disease Control and Prevention. Preventing Occupational HIV Transmission to Health Care Workers. CDC HIV Prevention. June 1999.
- Centers for Disease Control and Prevention. "A Glance at the HIV/AIDS Epidemic." January 2007. http://www.cdc.gov/hiv/resources/factsheets/At-A-Glance.htm.
- _____. "For More Information." March 7, 2007. http://www.cdc.gov/hiv/links.htm.
- _____. "Guarding Against Infections." June 2001. http://www.cdc.gov/hiv/pubs/BROCHURE/care6.htm.
- _____. "HIV and its Transmission." July 1999. http://www.cdc.gov/hiv/resources/factsheets/transmission.htm.
- _____. "HIV/AIDS among Men Who Have Sex with Men." July 2006. http://www.cdc.gov/hiv/topics/msm/resources/factsheets/msm.htm.
- _____. "HIV/AIDS Surveillance Report: HIV Infection and AIDS in the United States and Dependent Areas." http://www.cdc.gov/hiv/topics/surveillance/basic.htm#def.
- _____. "Mother-to-Child (Perinatal) HIV Transmission and Prevention." May 2006. http://www.cdc.gov/hiv/resources/factsheets/perinatl.htm.
- _____. "Pregnancy and Childbirth." February 21, 2007. http://www.cdc.gov/hiv/topics/perinatal/overview_partner.htm.
- _____. "Preventing Occupational HIV Transmission to Healthcare Personnel." February, 2002. http://www.cdc.gov/hiv/resources/factsheets/hcwprev.htm.
- _____. "Updated U.S. Public Health Service Guidelines for the Management of Occupational Exposures to HBV, and HIV and Recommendations for Postexposure Prophylaxis." *Morbidity and Mortality Weekly Report* 50 (2001): 1–42.
- _____. "Zidovudine for the Prevention of HIV Transmission from Mother to Infant." *Morbidity and Mortality Weekly Report* 43 (1994): 1–42. http://www.cdc.gov/MMWR/preview/mmwrhtml/00030635.htm.
- "Human Milk, Breastfeeding, and Transmission of Human Immunodeficiency Virus Type 1 in the United States." *Pediatrics* Volume 112: No. 5, November 2003, pp. 1196–1205. http://pediatrics.aappublications.org/cgi/content/abstract/112/5/1196.

- UNICEF. "Prevention of Parent-to-Child Transmission of HIV/AIDS. http://www.unicef.org/aids/in_preventionMTCT.html.
- _____. "Why it is Important to Share and Act on Information about HIV/AIDS." *Facts for Life.* http://www.unicef.org/ffl/11/.

Multiple Sclerosis:

- Leith, K.C., Cellini, L.A., and Lazzaro R. *Current Concepts in Multiple Sclerosis Clinical Features and Patient Management.* Berlex Laboratories, 2000.

Pressure Ulcers

- *Preventing Pressure Ulcers.* http://www.atlantahealth-pages.org/AHP/LIBRARY/HLTH-TOP/MISC/bedsore.htm
- Cervo, F.A. *Pressure Ulcers-Analysis of Guidelines for Treatment and Management.*
- Cervo, Frank A. *Geriatrics,* March 2000. http://www.findarticles.com/cf dls/m2578/3 55/60122155/p1/article.html

Tuberculosis

- Centers for Disease Control and Prevention. *Tuberculosis.* National Center for HIV/STD and TB Prevention. Division of Tuberculosis Elimination. Last reviewed February 6, 2001.

Urinary Tract Infection

- Gomolin, I.H. and McCue, J.D. *Urinary Tract Infection in the Elderly Patient.* University of California, San Francisco, School of Medicine. http://www.medscape.com/SCP/IIU/2000/V13.N05A/U135a.02.GOMO/U135a.02.GOMO-01.HTML

14. Thermometers/mercury
- Precautions for Health Care Workers. http://www.cocbs.msu.edu/AWARE/pamphlets/hazwaste/mercuryfacts.html
- Mercury: A Fact Sheet for Health Professionals. http://www.cocbs.msu.edu/AWARE/pamphlets/hazwaste/mercuryfacts.html
- Fahrenheit and Celsius Temperature Scales. http://www.athena.ivv.nasa.gov/curric/weather/fahrcels.html
- Mercury-Free Thermometers. http://www.1thermometer.com/Geratherm/geratherm.html; http://www.1thermometer.com/Clinical/clinical.html; http://www.1thermometer.com
- Stanford University Mercury Thermometer Replacement Program—Questions and Answers. http://www.stanford.edu.group/water/hgthermQ&A.htm
- Replace Your Mercury Thermometers Before They Break! http://www.stanford.edu/group/water/hg-therm.htm

15. Residents' Rights
- Code of Federal Regulations Title 42, Volume 3, Parts 430 to end. Revised as of October 1, 1999. From the U.S. Government Printing Office via GPO Access [cite:42CFR483.75]
- Long-Term Care Ombudsman Report Fiscal Year, 1996.

Textbooks

- Lueckenote, A.G. *Gerontologic Nursing*, ed. 2, St. Louis, 2000, Mosby. (Chapter 2)
- Hegner, R., and Caldwell, Needham F. *Nursing Assistant—A Nursing Process Approach*, ed. 8. Albany, 1988, Delmar Publishing. (Chapter 2)

Special Contributors

Life Skills Training– Chapter 21
Ginger Fallesen, RN
Curriculum Development, Health Careers
Educator
Los Angeles County Office of Education
Regional Occupational Program
Marcia Easterling
Job Developer
Los Angeles County Office of Education
Regional Occupational Program
Angie Turner RN, BSN
Assistant Chief Executive Officer
American Red Cross
San Gabriel Valley Chapter
Dana Bas, RN D.S.D.
Consultant
Arriba Juntos
Providing End-of-Life Care–Chapter 20
Mary Cadogan
mcadogan@ucla.edu
Fay Flowers, RN, M.Ed.
Director Health and Community Services
Southeastern Michigan Chapter
American Red Cross
Healthful Eating– Chapter 14
Larissa Barclay, BSN, MSN
American Red Cross
Southeastern MI Chapter
Fay Flowers, RN, M.Ed.
Director Health and Community Services
Southeastern Michigan Chapter
American Red Cross
Math Module– Appendix D
Prof. Edward Hector
Mathematics Dept. Chair
Los Angeles Southwest College
Los Angeles, CA

Miscellaneous

CDC National AIDS Hotline
English (800) 342-AIDS
    (2437 24 hrs/day)
Spanish (800) 344-SIDA (7432)
TTY (800) 243-7889
    Deaf and Hard of Hearing
- The Gerontological Society of America. *The Gerontologist* 40:663–672 (2000). http://intl-gerontologist.gerontologyjournals.org/cgi/content/abstract/40/6/663.
- MedLine Plus. "Medical Encyclopedia." April 5, 2007. http://www.nlm.nih.gov/medlineplus/ency/article/003399.htm#Normal%20Values.

- National Heart Lung and Blood Institute Diseases and Conditions Index. "What is High Blood Pressure?" April 2006. http://www.nhlbi.nih.gov/health/dci/Diseases/Hbp/HBP_WhatIs.html.

- National Institutes of Health, National Kidney and Urologic Diseases Information Clearinghouse. "Kidney and Urologic Diseases Statistics for the United States." NIH Publication No. 06-3895, April 2006. http://kidney.niddk.nih.gov/kudiseases/pubs/kustats/index.htm.

Index

MISSION OF THE AMERICAN RED CROSS

The American Red Cross, a humanitarian organization led by volunteers and guided by its Congressional Charter and the Fundamental Principles of the International Red Cross Movement, will provide relief to victims of disaster and help people prevent, prepare for, and respond to emergencies.

ABOUT THE AMERICAN RED CROSS

The American Red Cross helps people prevent, prepare for and respond to emergencies. Last year, almost a million volunteers and 35,000 employees helped victims of almost 75,000 disasters; taught lifesaving skills to millions; and helped U.S. service members separated from their families stay connected. Almost 4 million people gave blood through the Red Cross, the largest supplier of blood and blood products in the United States. The American Red Cross is part of the International Red Cross and Red Crescent Movement. An average of 91 cents of every dollar the Red Cross spends is invested in humanitarian services and programs. The Red Cross is not a government agency; it relies on donations of time, money, and blood to do its work.

FUNDAMENTAL PRINCIPLES OF THE INTERNATIONAL RED CROSS AND RED CRESCENT MOVEMENT

HUMANITY
IMPARTIALITY
NEUTRALITY
INDEPENDENCE
VOLUNTARY SERVICE
UNITY
UNIVERSALITY